Handbook of the
Brief Psychotherapies

APPLIED CLINICAL PSYCHOLOGY

Series Editors:
Alan S. Bellack, *Medical College of Pennsylvania at EPPI, Philadelphia, Pennsylvania,*
and Michel Hersen, *University of Pittsburgh, Pittsburgh, Pennsylvania*

A Continuation Order Plan is available for this series. A continuation order will bring delivery of
each new volume immediately upon publication. Volumes are billed only upon actual shipment.
For further information please contact the publisher.

Handbook of the Brief Psychotherapies

Edited by
RICHARD A. WELLS
University of Pittsburgh
Pittsburgh, Pennsylvania

and
VINCENT J. GIANNETTI
Duquesne University
Pittsburgh, Pennsylvania

PLENUM PRESS • NEW YORK AND LONDON

Library of Congress Cataloging-in-Publication Data

Handbook of the brief psychotherapies / edited by Richard A. Wells and
  Vincent J. Giannetti.
        p.   cm. -- (Applied clinical psychology)
     Includes bibliographical references.
     ISBN 0-306-43270-6
     1. Brief psychotherapy.   I. Wells, Richard A.   II. Giannetti,
  Vincent J.
     [DNLM: 1. Psychotherapy, Brief.   WM 420 H2362]
  RC480.55.H36   1989
  616.89'14--dc20
  DNLM/DLC
  for Library of Congress   89-23209
                                                                CIP

© 1990 Plenum Press, New York
A Division of Plenum Publishing Corporation
233 Spring Street, New York, N.Y. 10013

Printed in the United States of America

To Sarah and Paul
—RW

To Rita, Vincent, and Anthony
—VG

I can no other answer make but thanks,
And thanks, and ever thanks.
Twelfth Night

Contributors

J. GAYLE BECK, Department of Psychology, University of Houston, Houston, Texas 77204-5341

DUANE S. BISHOP, Department of Psychiatry and Human Behavior, Brown University, Providence, Rhode Island 02912

ANDREW L. BRICKMAN, Spanish Family Guidance Center, Department of Psychiatry, University of Miami School of Medicine, Miami, Florida 33136

CLEON CORNES, Western Psychiatric Institute and Clinic, 3811 O'Hara Street, Pittsburgh, Pennsylvania 15213

CAROL D. DE YOUNG, Colorado Department of Health, 4210 East 11th Avenue, Denver, Colorado 80222

NATHAN B. EPSTEIN, Department of Psychiatry and Human Behavior, Brown University, Providence, Rhode Island 02912

CHARLES PATRICK EWING, Faculty of Law and Jurisprudence, State University of New York at Buffalo, Buffalo, New York 14260

KAREN J. EVANCZUK, Western Psychiatric Institute and Clinic, 3811 O'Hara Street, Pittsburgh, Pennsylvania 15213

LISA A. FELDMAN, Psychology Department, University of Waterloo, Waterloo, Ontario N2L 3G1, Canada

KALMAN FLOMENHAFT, Health Science Center at Brooklyn, State University of New York, Brooklyn, New York 11203

FRANKLIN H. FOOTE, Spanish Family Guidance Center, Department of Psychiatry, University of Miami School of Medicine, Miami, Florida 33136

CHARLES D. GARVIN, School of Social Work, University of Michigan, Ann Arbor, Michigan 48109

VINCENT GIANNETTI, School of Pharmacy, Duquesne University, Pittsburgh, Pennsylvania 15282

OLGA E. HERVIS, Spanish Family Guidance Center, Department of Psychiatry, University of Miami School of Medicine, Miami, Florida 33136

MICHAEL F. HOYT, Department of Psychiatry, Kaiser-Permanente Medical Center, Hayward, California 94545-4299, and the Langley Porter Psychiatric Institute of the University of California, San Francisco, San Francisco, California 94143

STANLEY D. IMBER, School of Medicine, University of Pittsburgh, Pittsburgh, Pennsylvania 15213

NEIL S. JACOBSON, Department of Psychology, University of Washington, Seattle, Washington 98195

NICK KANAS, Department of Psychiatry, University of California, San Francisco, San Francisco, California 94143, and San Francisco Veteran's Administration Medical Center, 4150 Clement Street, San Francisco, California 94121

GABOR I. KEITNER, Department of Psychiatry and Human Behavior, Brown University, Providence, Rhode Island 02912

WILLIAM M. KURTINES, Department of Psychology, Florida International University, Miami, Florida 33199

ADAM K. LEHMAN, Department of Psychology, Yale University, New Haven, Connecticut 06520

RONA L. LEVY, School of Social Work, University of Washington, Seattle, Washington 98195

IVAN W. MILLER, Department of Psychiatry and Human Behavior, Brown University, Providence, Rhode Island 02912

MARLENE M. MORETTI, Psychology Department, University of Waterloo, Waterloo, Ontario N2L 3G1, Canada

RAY NAAR, Medical Center East, 211 Whitfield Street, Suite 635, Pittsburgh, Pennsylvania 15206

ANGEL PEREZ-VIDAL, Spanish Family Guidance Center, Department of Psychiatry, University of Miami School of Medicine, Miami, Florida 33136

PHILLIP A. PHELPS, Child Development Unit, Children's Hospital of Pittsburgh, Pittsburgh, Pennsylvania 15213

FRANK S. PITTMAN, III, 960 Johnson Ferry Road, N. E., Suite 543, Atlanta, Georgia 30342

WILLIAM J. REID, School of Social Welfare, Rockefeller College of Public Policy and Affairs and Policy, State University of New York at Albany, Albany, New York 12222

SHELDON D. ROSE, School of Social Work, University of Wisconsin–Madison, Madison, Wisconsin 53707

ROBERT ROSENBAUM, Department of Psychiatry, Kaiser-Permanente Medical Center, Hayward, California 94545-4299

PETER SALOVEY, Department of Psychology, Yale University, New Haven, Connecticut 06520

R. TAYLOR SEGRAVES, Case Western Reserve University and Metrohealth Systems, 3395 Scranton Road, Cleveland, Ohio 44109

BRIAN F. SHAW, Department of Psychology, Toronto General Hospital, 101 College Street, Toronto, Ontario M5G 117, Canada

JOHN L. SHELTON, Private Practice, Renton, Washington 98055

STEPHEN SOLDZ, Harvard Medical School, and the Mental Health Research Program, Harvard Community Health Plan, One Fenway Plaza, Boston, Massachusetts 02215

JOSE SZAPOCZNIK, Spanish Family Guidance Center, Department of Psychiatry, University of Miami School of Medicine, Miami, Florida 33136

MOSHE TALMON, Department of Psychiatry, Kaiser-Permanente Medical Center, Hayward, California 94545-4299

RICHARD A. WELLS, School of Social Work, University of Pittsburgh, Pittsburgh, Pennsylvania 15260

MARK A. WHISMAN, Department of Psychology, University of Washington, Seattle, Washington 98195

JASON WORCHEL, American Institute of Short-Term Dynamic Psychotherapy, 2101 Arlington Blvd., Charlottesville, Virginia 21903

Preface

The last two decades have seen unprecedented increases in health care costs and, at the same time, encouraging progress in psychotherapy research. On the one hand, accountability, cost-effectiveness, and efficiency have now become commonplace terms for providers of mental health services whereas, on the other hand, an increasingly voluminous literature has emerged supporting the effectiveness of a number of types of psychotherapies. There now exists the possibility for the design and delivery of mental health services that—drawing upon this literature—more closely approximate empirically established data concerning the appropriateness and effectiveness of psychotherapy. The *Handbook of the Brief Psychotherapies* is intended to capture one major thrust of this movement: the development of a group of empirically grounded, time-limited therapies all sharing a common interest in the clinical utilization of a structured focus and an emphasis on time and action.

For many years, professional self-interest, competing theoretical paradigms, and the vagaries of practice, wisdom, and clinical myth have influenced the practice of psychotherapy. A critical questioning of the resulting, predominantly nondirective, open-ended, and global therapies has led to a growing emphasis on action-oriented, problem-focused, time-limited therapies. Yet, ironically, this interest in the brief psychotherapies has not so much involved a radical departure from traditional therapeutic modalities as it has emphasized a new pragmatism about how time, action, and structure operate in life as well as in therapy. These are the factors seen as providing the basic scaffolding for growth and a compelling impetus for change. As reflected in the chapters of the *Handbook*, diverse approaches to therapy and differing theoretical orientations can be adapted to a brief-oriented philosophy, thereby restructuring the therapeutic enterprise in new (yet old) ways.

The *Handbook* is organized so as to address a number of major clinical, research, and organizational issues that have emerged as a result of the increasing shift in practice toward a brief psychotherapy focus. One of the most important of these is the need for the practicing professional and the advanced student of clinical practice to have access to state-of-the-art accounts of the techniques and strategies of established and emerging brief therapies written by outstanding practitioners in each area. The intent is not to offer brief psychotherapy as a panacea for all of the problems inherent in the delivery of mental health services but to stimulate more reflection, research, and experimentation with clinical practice and policy at both micro- and macrolevels. In an age of competing demands for limited resources, any psychotherapy will earn its place not only by a persuasive demonstration of its intrinsic value but by its ability to utilize personal, financial, and emotional resources in a parsimonious manner.

Finally, the *Handbook* is comprehensive in that all of the major theoretical orientations are represented and, in addition, a variety of group, marital, and family therapies are given equal exposure alongside the more familiar one-to-one approaches. Along with a number of well-established methodologies, the reader will encounter such innovative approaches as single-session psychotherapy, One Person Family Therapy, and brief crisis groups; in addition, clinical issues such as engagement, resistance, tasks, and the therapeutic significance of time are discussed in depth. As editors, we believe that the *Handbook of the Brief Psychotherapies* will offer the clinical practitioner a wealth of detail concerning contemporary short-term treatment. Additionally, we hope that this volume will assist in the task of encouraging both practitioners and policymakers to rethink the nature of psychotherapeutic practice and to consider the value of structure, time, and action in delivering mental health services.

RICHARD A. WELLS
VINCENT GIANNETTI

Contents

PART IV. FAMILY AND MARITAL BRIEF THERAPIES

PART V. BRIEF GROUP APPROACHES

I

Introduction

Clinical practice takes place at a number of levels—personal, technical, conceptual, organizational, and philosophical, to name some of the most important. This is the case whether the therapist is engaged in short-term or open-ended therapy but, because of its relative unfamiliarity to many practitioners, the demands of brief therapeutic practice in areas such as these are much less known. The overall purpose of the chapters in this introductory section is to attempt to place brief therapy into a more knowable context in relation to many of these parameters and, in doing so, illuminate the unique ways in which brief psychotherapy operates. Each of the chapters approaches this task from a different perspective.

The overview chapter by Wells and Phelps identifies the major commonalities of concept and therapeutic strategy shared by the seemingly varied approaches that form the family of brief psychotherapies. They sketch out highlights from the historical development of the brief psychotherapies and identify the action emphasis that permeates all of these approaches. From this base, the chapter examines the impact of brief therapeutic practice on the practitioner from technical, moral, and economic perspectives, with a particular interest in its personal impact on the clinician.

Soldz's chapter on research in brief psychotherapy eschews the examination of outcome studies conventionally recounted in such chapters—does it work, with whom, and how much?—and instead plunges into an intensive examination of the process research. Once again, the focus is on the persona of the therapist, in interaction with the client, and an exposition of the key elements in this venture include methods for measuring interpersonal difficulties, examination of key elements in the therapeutic alliance, and best/worst analysis of selected cases. His objectives are to review the most significant findings in the area of process research and to suggest how these might be utilized in clinical practice.

One of the pioneers in the development of planned short-term treatment, William Reid, continues his contributions to the field by presenting an integrative model, incorporating principles applicable to a range of client populations, interventive methods, and theoretical orientations. His chapter outlines and discusses in detail the common conceptual framework and the similar technical operations that characterize brief therapeutic practice in all of these areas. From this integrative perspective, Reid regards individual, family, and group interventions as simply alternative modalities, in service to the needs of the client, rather than competing and unrelated hegemonies.

Finally, Giannetti's chapter looks at the policy issues raised by the development of a cadre of empirically supported brief psychotherapies. He argues that a more rational and cost-effective mental health delivery system can be built around these therapies and that policy considerations should seek ways of providing incentives for both clients and practitioners to utilize time-limited methods. Adding a sense of urgency to his plea for reform of the delivery system is the growing possibility that the various third-party organizations, now so prominent in economic support of the field—and largely unaffected by theoretical biases and allegiance—may well act for us, if we cannot act ourselves.

These chapters set the stage for the succeeding sections of the *Handbook*. The brief psychotherapies may or may not be the wave of the future, but there is no doubt that their very existence and their empirically substantiated effectiveness call into question many of the long-held myths and cherished folklore of the clinical field. The introductory section has critically surveyed broad aspects of this challenge, whereas the remaining chapters will delineate the technical and strategic considerations of a range of well-developed brief therapies.

The Brief Psychotherapies
A Selective Overview

Richard A. Wells and Phillip A. Phelps

Introduction

It is customary in overview chapters to dramatically proclaim that the subject matter of the work, in this case the brief, short-term or time-limited psychotherapies, has "come of age." For better or worse, it is far too late to say this about the brief psychotherapies. They have been in active existence for 30 to 40 years and may more aptly be characterized as facing middle age, perhaps even a midlife crisis. The early roots of brief therapy can be traced back even further and, around the turn of the century, a former patient—a symphonic conductor suffering from psychogenic pain in his conducting arm—described the key session in his brief therapeutic treatment in the following words:

> His advice was—to conduct. "But I can't move my arm." "Try it, at any rate." "And what if I should have to stop?" "You won't have to stop." "Can I take upon myself the responsibility of possibly upsetting a performance?" "I'll take the responsibility." And so I did a little conducting with my right arm, then with my left, and occasionally with my head. There were times when I forgot my arm over the music. . . . So, by dint of much effort and confidence, by learning and forgetting, I finally succeeded in finding my way back to my profession. (Walter, 1946, pp. 167–168)

The preceding passage is drawn from Bruno Walter's autobiographical account of his six sessions of brief therapy with none other than Sigmund Freud and is cited, not to place some sort of legitimizing imprimatur on brief psychotherapy but simply to highlight the essential features of short-term intervention that will be the subject matter of this chapter. There is no doubt that Freud, when he wished, knew how to practice brief therapy and knew how to practice it well (Eisenstein, 1986; Sterba, 1951). The critical elements of brief psychotherapy, directly or implicitly conveyed throughout Walter's description, include the following:

Richard A. Wells • School of Social Work, University of Pittsburgh, Pittsburgh, Pennsylvania 15260. Phillip A. Phelps • Child Development Unit, Children's Hospital of Pittsburgh, Pittsburgh, Pennsylvania 15213.

1. Therapist and client concentrate on a key area of personal or interpersonal concern, providing a clear and impelling focus for the therapeutic efforts.
2. The therapist takes a direct and active role in promoting client function and, at the same time, displays a positive belief in the client's capacity to change.
3. Tasks are given to the client to carry out, outside the therapeutic session, making a clear demand for activity rather than passivity.
4. The therapist works within a time-limited context, usually explicitly conveyed, further emphasizing the immediacy and urgency of the change process.
5. Thus, the brief psychotherapy patient or client is expected to act rather than suffer and to become an involved participant in the therapeutic process.

In the following sections of this overview we will develop on aspects of each of these elements, in some cases relating them to the chapters that follow in this volume, in other instances drawing on our own experiences as brief therapists, or referring to the clinical literature of the brief psychotherapies. Our intent is not to do a systematic overview so much as to offer a provocative discussion of certain factors—past, present, and prospective—that we believe influence the current practice of brief psychotherapy. We are especially interested in the professional and personal impact the practice of brief therapy has upon the therapist, whether that individual is an experienced or neophyte user of brief methods, or practices in public or private settings.

The reader who desires a more systematic exposition of the theoretical and empirical status of the brief psychotherapies is referred to the excellent reviews contained in Budman and Gurman (1983), Koss and Butcher (1986), Kovacs (1982), Marmor (1979), Rogawski (1982), and Sifneos (1981). Cogent criticisms of the brief psychotherapies may be found in articles by such authors as Good (1987), Kanter (1983), and O'Connor and Reid (1986).

A Brief History of Brief Therapy

The brief psychotherapies did not even begin to emerge as legitimate therapeutic method until the decade of the 1950s and only did so when several related changes in therapeutic practice were also taking place. The most important of these other developments were (1) the emergence of two major innovations in therapeutic intervention: behavior therapy and family therapy, and (2) the accumulation of a substantial body of empirical research on the process and outcome of psychotherapy.

Therapeutic approaches do not develop or exist in an ideological or moral vacuum, nor are they devoid of values of many kinds. Every type of psychotherapy contains rules for living, definitions of the good life, ideals concerning how people should act in important relationships and, of course, beliefs about the proper goals of therapy and the correct manner in which therapists should talk and act in assisting their clients in achieving these goals. These constitute the metaphilosophy of psychotherapy and are frequently obscured by the more visible theories and techniques that tend to be the subject matter of most of the clinical literature. Our discussion in this section will survey the historical evolution of those aspects of therapeutic metaphilosophy that define the goals of the therapeutic process and the norms of therapist activity, as it is in these areas that brief therapy most differs from traditional therapeutic approaches.

A compendium of psychotherapies published a few years ago (Herinck, 1980) contains 255 apparently different approaches, ranging from "Active Analytic Psychotherapy," through "Mandala Therapy" (modestly described as "universally applicable"), to "Zaraleya Psychoenergetic Technique." Despite this amazing—and continuing—proliferation of methods, London (1986) has contended that there are still only two major ways of doing therapy: an insight mode and an action mode. The insight approaches emphasize patients or clients developing greater awareness or understanding of themselves, with the therapist, for the most part, playing only a guiding role in this process. The action methods, on the other hand, are problem oriented, concentrate on changes in the here and now of the patient's life, and call on the therapist to take an active, even directive role in the intervention. The brief psychotherapies are preeminently action approaches, even those whose psychodynamic origins might suggest an interest in insight.

These contrasting characterizations of psychotherapeutic mode should not be viewed as simply capsule descriptions of schools of psychotherapies. They stipulate the legitimate and respected goals of the therapeutic process, conceal within themselves a number of highly influential normative or value statements concerning the role of the therapist and, consequently, have major impact on what therapists qua therapists believe and how they think they must act.

For the first half of this century the insight mode of therapy dominated the mental health professions and, if one accepted its metaphilosophy, it was not respectable or allowable for therapists to take a problem-oriented, active stance. Espousing a method counter to the prevailing norms of the time was not easy, and we find Haley, writing in 1962, characterizing the development of family therapy, particularly in its action dimensions, as a covert, secretive affair:

> As a result, since the late 1940's one could attend psychiatric meetings and hear nothing about Family Therapy unless, in a quiet hotel room, one happened to confess he treated whole families. Then another therapist would put down his drink and reveal that he too had attempted this kind of therapy. These furtive conversations ultimately led to an underground movement of therapists devoted to this most challenging of all types of psychotherapy and this movement is now appearing on the surface. (Haley, 1962, p. 69)

Early examples of brief psychotherapy can be found in Freud's own work as we noted at the beginning of this chapter, as well as in the writings of a few other psychoanalytic theorists such as Ferenzi (1920) or Alexander and French (1946). Yet these efforts were largely disregarded or viewed as aberrations and heresies; a book reviewer of the time condemned Alexander and French's ideas for shortening therapy as "not only unsound psychologically but troublesome, if not dangerous" (Oberndorf, 1947, p. 101).

It is, we believe, significant to note that the most fruitful period in the development of the brief therapies has coincided, in large part, with the development of behavior therapy. Although not all of the brief therapies described in this book are avowedly behavioral in orientation or technique, many incorporate the very principles that Bergin and Garfield (1986), for example, identify as behavior therapy's major contribution to the field:

> Its main emphases and contribution have been a clear focus on the patient's complaints, devising specific treatment for specific problems, relatively brief periods of treatment, and systematic appraisals of outcome. (p. 6)

Bergin and Garfield's description of behavior therapy could as easily serve as a summary of the major characteristics of brief therapy, but our point is not to argue that the two are identical. The emergence of behavior therapy, as a recognized contender in the therapeutic field, made it possible for practitioners to begin to subscribe to a different set of values than had been emphasized within what, until then, had been the mainstream of therapeutic metaphilosophy. These included behavior therapy's emphasis on working directly on the client's immediate problems and using a variety of specific change strategies, with the therapist taking a direct and active role in this process.

The simultaneous emergence of family therapy, on the other hand, although calling for practitioners to adopt a radically different theoretical viewpoint concerning the etiology of client problems, most importantly redefined the role of the therapist in a new way. Behavior therapy, with its emphasis on scientific inquiry and technology, has been notoriously unsuccessful in articulating the role of the therapist, except in the most bloodless terms. Much of the behavioral literature simply ignores the persona of the practitioner or, as in Krasner's (1962) characterization of the therapist as a "social reinforcement machine," offers a less than inviting image of the clinician in action. In contrast, family therapy has been able to offer a much more human and compelling vision of what it is like to be an action therapist.

Jay Haley, in such works as *Strategies of Psychotherapy* (1963) and *Problem-Solving Therapy* (1976), is widely regarded as one of the major contributors to the development of brief psychotherapy. Much of his work can be seen as an inspired (sometimes polemical) spelling out of what is entailed in being active and directive as a therapist. Haley, of course, was heavily influenced by the brilliant but often enigmatic work of Milton Erickson and, in one of his (Haley's) lesser known works edited a collection of Erickson's articles on hypnosis and brief therapy (Haley, 1969). In a concluding commentary to this volume, Haley suggests that brief therapy is not so much a set of specific techniques as it is an interrelated series of personal attitudes and values on the part of the therapist, that collectively make brief therapy—of whatever sort—possible. Several of these concern the role the therapist assumes in relation to the client:

1. The therapist must be willing to take charge and direct the client.

2. The therapist approaches the symptom directly and does not discuss what is "behind" it.
3. The therapist must be capable of a wide range of behavior with clients.

Others of the factors identified by Haley characterize the viewpoint the brief therapist takes of clients and the nature of their problems:

1. Within the individual, positive forces are striving to take over.
2. There is a wide range of alternative ways of behaving that are possible for every client.
3. For each client, change is not only possible but inevitable.

Finally, the brief therapist, according to Haley, takes a very specific viewpoint concerning the essential character of the therapeutic relationship:

1. Change occurs in the context of an intense relationship with the therapist.
2. The therapist accepts what clients offer while at the same time diverting them in new directions.
3. The therapeutic relationship is temporary to achieve particular ends.

Along with this growing articulation and acceptance of the action methods, we believe that the accumulation over the past 30 to 40 years of a considerable body of empirical studies of psychotherapy outcome has had an indirect but powerful effect on clinical practice. The beginning of this influence can be traced to 1952 when H. J. Eysenck, the iconoclastic British psychologist, published an article vigorously attacking the effectiveness of psychotherapy that, at that time, was heavily influenced by psychoanalytic theory and avowedly long-term in duration. Eysenck's article was important, not so much for the merit of its argument as for its stimulation of an impressive surge of research into psychotherapy process and outcome. The results of this flowering of studies are initially chronicled in a bibliography published by the National Institute of Mental Health (Strupp & Bergin, 1969) and later in the succeeding editions of the *Handbook of Psychotherapy and Behavior Change* (Bergin & Garfield, 1971; Garfield & Bergin, 1978, 1986).

Any number of guidelines for practice can be drawn from the massive research literature reviewed in these volumes, but the most significant progress has taken place in relation to findings concerning the overall effectiveness of psychotherapy—the question originally raised by Eysenck. As late as 1969, the issue was still clouded, as in Mechanic's bleak, but not unfair social policy analysis of the time:

> We should note, however, the vast disagreement concerning psychotherapeutic effectiveness; no strong evidence justifies public support for this form of service. (Mechanic, 1969, p. 49)

By 1986 the accumulation of studies, and the advent of powerful analytic methods such as meta-analysis, justified a different and quite unequivocal stance:

> Many psychotherapies that have been subjected to empirical study have been shown to
> have demonstrable effects on a variety of clients. These effects are not only statistically
> significant but clinically meaningful. Psychotherapy facilitates the remission of symp-
> toms. It not only speeds up the natural healing process but often provides additional
> coping strategies for dealing with future problems. (Lambert, Shapiro, & Bergin, 1986,
> p. 201)

A series of related findings, specific to short-term interventions, can be drawn from the same research literature:

1. The duration of most therapeutic contact, whatever the intentions or orientation of the practitioner, is relatively brief, averaging 6 to 8 sessions (Garfield, 1986).
2. When clients benefit from psychotherapy, of whatever kind, these positive changes occur relatively early, with 75% of clients being improved within 6 months (Lambert *et al.*, 1986).
3. Finally, comparative studies have consistently found that explicitly time-limited treatments deliver results that are equivalent to those of open-ended or long-term therapies (Gurman *et al.*, 1986; Koss & Butcher, 1986).

As we suggested earlier, the impact of these findings on clinical practice has been indirect. We are no means convinced that the practice of the *average* therapist in any of the helping professions is directly influenced by empirical research but, as in the areas of development discussed earlier in this section, the overall findings from the research literature have played a significant role in shaping the metaphilosophy of therapy. At this value level, they enable psychotherapy to be viewed as a legitimate participant in the scientific tradition of Western civilization while at the same time continuing its many normative and secular functions (London, 1986). In the political arena, psychotherapy no longer has to rely solely on the testimony of its advocates, however fervent they may be, but can point to a substantial body of scientific evidence in its support. A number of the brief psychotherapies have specific bodies of empirical data attesting to their effectiveness and, indeed, have evolved out of a dual concern with empiricism and clinical pragmatism. Moreover, the short-term psychodynamic approaches; (Malan, 1976; Sloane, Staples, Cristol, Yorkston, & Whipple, 1975) are the only area of psychoanalytic practice that can be said to have even a modest base of outcome research attesting to their efficacy and, in this respect at the least, have significantly outgrown their own roots.

Brief Therapy as Action

It is one thing to believe in the legitimacy of an active, problem-oriented approach, but another to have the technical means to implement it. Despite the apparent diversity of the various approaches that can be identified as members of the family of brief psychotherapies, a commonality of technique or strategy pervades all of them. This commonality has three dimensions along which it operates: (1) time is restricted or rationed; (2) a focus of therapeutic effort is selected and maintained; and (3) tasks are employed, both within and outside of the session, to stimulate client change.

It is easy enough to say that brief psychotherapy is time limited but a much more confusing matter to determine what these time constraints are and exactly how they operate. Mental health professionals will almost unanimously register recognition when the term *brief psychotherapy* is mentioned, but further questioning or examination produces quite divergent opinions regarding what it is. Quite obviously, the name implies that brief therapy is short term in duration of contact. The further question arises, however—short compared to what? As numerous studies have affirmed (Garfield, 1986; Koss, 1979; Langsley, 1978), in reality most therapy is time limited, lasting six to eight sessions, on average. This means that most clients, regardless of the setting or the orientation of the therapist, do not stay in therapy for an extended period of time. Furthermore, as Budman and Gurman (1988) point out, the six to eight session average duration of therapy coincides with the number of sessions that other studies have found to be the common *patient* expectation of length of therapy. This might suggest that not only is therapeutic contact brief but that its brevity is being determined, not by the therapist, but by the client.

So what is it that differentiates the use of time in brief therapy from its utilization in other forms of therapies? It would seem the differentiating factor is the *planned* nature of the limited number of sessions that govern the duration of the intervention. Budman and Gurman (1983) emphasize both the time limitation and the underlying therapist attitude:

> What is, in fact, being examined in any discussion of brief treatment is therapy in which the time allotted to treatment is rationed. The therapist hopes to help the patient achieve maximum benefit with the lowest investment of therapist time and patient cost, both financial and psychological. (p. 277)

In other forms of therapies, clients are expected to remain active in therapy for an extended or indefinite period of time. If they terminate before this point, they are considered treatment dropouts, or even failures. In brief therapy, on the other hand, the client's termination is predicted and planned from virtually the entry into therapy and mutually agreed upon by client and therapist. Indeed, in a number of forms of brief therapies the duration is deliberately and explicitly rationed by therapist decree, so to speak, and the client plays no part in determining length.

This differentiation is especially important to keep in mind when exposed to the wide and varied time parameters that can be utilized in various forms of brief therapy: (1) The number of sessions considered brief therapy varies widely from 1 session (Bloom, 1981) to more than 30 (Malan, 1976; Sifneos, 1972). Indeed, an intriguing paper by Frances and Clarkin (1981) describes a number of situations in which, as they put it, *no treatment* is the prescription of choice. (2) It is not always entirely clear whether "brief" is descriptive of the number of sessions or of the amount of calendar time spent in therapy. In other words, is 10 sessions over a 10-week period the same as 10 sessions over the course of 6 months? (3) A number of brief therapists employ a follow-up interview (Wells, 1982), often scheduled months after the termination of the regular therapy sessions, thereby significantly extending the overall duration of contact. (4) Finally, other brief therapists (Budman & Gurman, 1988) work from a primary care perspective in which the client is encouraged to return, on an as-needed basis, for a series of short-term contacts. It is possible for these intermittent contacts to continue over a period of years.

These points are debatable and sometimes controversial. Confusion can be avoided if it is understood that the essential feature of all the brief therapies is their explicit manipulation of time: When therapy will end, and how both the client and therapist will know it is time for it to end, are agreed upon early in the therapy. This is qualitatively different from therapies that determine termination criterion near the end of therapy.

A second major characteristic of brief therapy is its focus. This term can take on several different meanings in its employment in short-term therapy. In one sense, focus is the choosing of an area of importance, selected by the therapist, or jointly agreed upon by therapist and client, that will serve as the target of therapeutic intervention. For instance, in an intriguing account of a single-session intervention, Hoyt (Chapter 6 this volume) describes a 37-year-old married woman, trained as an attorney but working as a teacher's aide, who complained of pervasive feelings of insecurity, anxiety, and low self-esteem. When the client connected some of her feelings to her experience with a very disturbed, irrationally critical mother, the therapist choose to concentrate on this area and quickly moved the client into an emotionally intense exploration of this relationship for the remainder of the session.

In another sense, focus is the application by the therapist of a particular theory of human behavior or personality development in order to make sense out of the client's difficulties. The brief psychotherapies tend to utilize theories that simplify rather than complicate the viewpoint that the therapist takes of the client or patient's difficulties. This process can be seen in a case described by Cornes in Chapter 12 of this volume:

> The patient, a 28-year-old married woman, described increasing symptoms of depression over the past 6 months, which she related primarily to the many difficulties she had working as the assistant manager in a restaurant. . . . Her current symptoms included dysphoric feelings, loneliness, constant worry, feelings of guilt, religious preoccupations, poor self-esteem, pessimistic feelings about the future, and suicidal thoughts (but no plan or intent). She also complained of hypersomnia, increased appetite, weight gain, anhedonia, and anergia and irritability that were both worse in the morning. She related in a defensive, histrionic style, and was often vague and diffuse. (Cornes, Chapter 12, p. 269)

Despite this plethora of symptomatology—which might have led another therapist into considerations of the most negative psychopathology and the lengthiest of treatments—Cornes is quite comfortable in contracting for a 16-week course of interpersonal psychotherapy. Utilizing one of the four problem areas conceptualized by the interpersonal approach as related to depression, he and the client agree that her numerous relationship conflicts might have contributed to her depression and "developed a plan to try to understand more about those disputes and attempt to resolve them."

Finally, focus (more properly *focusing*) may refer to an activity, carried out by the clinician, that involves maintaining therapeutic concentration on the selected and/or agreed upon area of difficulty. As a key therapist activity in brief therapy, focusing may occur repeatedly throughout the therapeutic process, but it is most clearly evident in early stages of contact. Brief therapists, even the most psychodynamically oriented, tend to stay as close as possible to the presenting concerns of the client. Typically, they begin by eliciting this from the patient, as in the following excerpt from the opening moments of an interview conducted by James Mann:

Dr: I would like to ask you this: What is there about the way that you are that you are feeling that you would most want to be helped with? (*An immediate focusing effort.*)

Pt: The anxiety that I have.

Dr: Can you tell me something more about it? (Mann, 1973, p. 90, italicized commentary in original)

The process of focusing is often underlined by an explicit verbal contract with the client, as in the following passage from another of Mann's initial interviews:

Doctor: As I understand it, you have had a very difficult struggle and here you are . . . you're fifty-four years old and feeling very lonely and very hurt.

Mrs. R.: I guess that's it.

Doctor: Would you like to work on that problem to see if you can't find some way to handle it so that you'll feel better about yourself?

Mrs. R.: I sure would. (Mann & Goldman, 1982, p. 134)

The activity of focusing appears most dramatically—and is most obviously necessary—in that briefest of the brief psychotherapies, Bernard Bloom's single-session therapy (Bloom, 1981). He states the issue succinctly in his guidelines for therapists:

> I have had to learn to avoid attractive detours and to remain single-minded about what I am trying to accomplish. There are numerous occasions in every intervention when I find myself wishing I could explore some little phrase for just a few minutes, but such diversions have nearly always turned out to be technical errors. (p. 189)

Finally, brief therapists commonly employ tasks, both inside and outside of the immediate session, as a means of stimulating the change process. Within the therapeutic session these may take the form of enactments or behavior rehearsals—directives from the therapist that require the client to move beyond the confines of descriptive language and literally demonstrate the behavioral, interpersonal, or emotional components of a particular incident or area of concern. Outside of the session clients are frequently assigned tasks or homework, in many instances to further client progress toward therapeutic goals but also as a means of conveying the underlying action message of brief psychotherapy.

In relation to the use of tasks, we believe that a good deal of brief therapeutic practice falls under the rubric of what Kanfer (1979) has called *instigation* therapy:

> This strategy presumes that behavior change occurs *between* therapy sessions and that the "talk sessions" serve mainly to explore objectives, train the client in methods, and motivate him to modify his extra therapeutic environment and to apply learning techniques to his own behavior. . . . During sessions, assigned tasks are practiced, tactics are discussed, and a favorable orientation toward change is created. (p. 189, italics in original)

The emphasis in an instigative therapy is on accurately identifying what is actually taking place in the client's most troublesome life situations in order to devise different ways for the client to deal with these. Doing so requires that the therapist must depend upon some form of enactment—in order to bring representations of life situations into the therapy session in a more accurate and experiential way than can be accomplished through ordinary descriptive talk. Enactments, or behavioral rehearsals, have long been a key component in developing social skills and, in a later chapter of this book, Rose (Chapter 22 this volume) discusses the modeling, rehearsal, and corrective feedback phases of this process within short-term skill-training groups. The family and marital therapies, on the other hand, by their very nature are enactments, as the actual participants in a conflicted situation are assembled, and interact together, in the immediate therapeutic session. Yet another chapter of this volume on one person family therapy (Szapocznik *et al.*, Chapter 20 this volume) describes a number of ingenious enactment devices that are employed to allow for the fact that, in this variant of family therapy, only one member of the family is literally being seen in the therapy session.

On the other hand, the brief therapist characteristically employs tasks as the medium for moving from the therapy session back out into the client's real-life situation. An underlying premise of the action methods is that one cannot count upon the troubled individual to put insights into action—some more compelling device is required. Tasks may be quite direct and specific. For example, in Sigmund Freud's work with Bruno Walter (Walter, 1946), cited at the beginning of this chapter, two key tasks were given over the course of the treatment:

1. At the initial session, Walter was immediately instructed by Freud to leave Vienna and tour Italy for a time, effectively distracting him from his preoccupation with his affected arm.
2. As the sessions continued, Walter was directed to resume conducting, despite his fears, as the therapist, in typical action style, focused attention on the patient's strengths, rather than his difficulties.

As these examples illustrate, many tasks are quite straightforward in their emphasis on restoring client functioning—in a succeeding chapter of this volume Levy and Shelton (Chapter 7) offer a series of clinical guidelines for dealing with the problems of morale and motivation that can hinder client compliance with tasks. In this regard, brief therapists must sometimes exercise considerable ingenuity in tailoring tasks to both the client and the context of the situation.

Rosenbaum (Chapter 16 this volume) describes two cases where the presenting complaint was essentially the same—temper outbursts in a husband that were objected to by his wife. Very different assignments were designed, however, in response to marked differences in the way in which each identified patient viewed his problem. The husband who saw his anger as unconscious and involuntary was asked to practice "projecting his voice and his breathing while doing dramatic soliloquies in their living room at home." The other spouse, who viewed his outbursts as a controlled coping mechanism, was assigned to keep a log so that he could "analyze his behavior and have even more control over it."

As strategies of psychotherapies in Haley's phrase, these three ingredients—time, focus, and tasks—shape the activities of the action practitioner and, of course, place explicit demands and responsibilities upon the client. They interact with each other, especially in the sense that once a time limit is selected, then a clear focus and a demand for action almost necessarily follow—and the latter two elements further commit both therapist and client to the time limit.

TIME FOR SALE

In the preceding section we discussed a number of ways in which time, as a technical device, shaped the practice of brief psychotherapy. Yet time, in a pervasive sense, affects the practice of all of the modes of psychotherapies. That is to say, therapists of any theoretical or technical persuasion, whether they are conducting short-term or long-term therapies, are essentially selling portions of their time to their clients. The typical practitioner in private practice has an established hourly rate, whereas almost all agencies have similar fee schedules for billing either the client or a third-party payer. Economically speaking, it is advantageous to the therapist to sell as much time as possible to each client, especially in private practice contexts where the practitioner is responsible for a variety of overhead costs and, in addition, a steady flow of new clients cannot be assumed. Similar pressures can affect the many clinics and agencies that have responded to the funding cutbacks of the past decade by turning to client fees as an important portion of their financing. Yet brief therapists, if they are to remain true to their beliefs, must deliberately ration or restrict the amount of time available to the client, setting in motion a value conflict between financial renumeration and clinical ideology.

This clash of values has many facets. Although one may argue that most clients, in fact, are seen for relatively brief periods of time (Garfield, 1986), these are *average* figures. With a given client, at a specific moment in time, the practitioner cannot predict, from the empirical data, how many sessions this particular client will remain. The therapist may know that, on average, clients are seen for 6 to 8 sessions, but the particular client being seen might well be one who will remain for 100 sessions. Compounding this dilemma is the fact that it is not at all difficult to identify factors in a given client's initial state of psychological, emotional, or social turmoil that would justify a lengthy period of intervention. Quite aside from the various psychodynamic theories (which have been noteworthy, of course, for their emphasis on long-term treatment), the major alternative conceptual frameworks, whether behavioral or humanistic, have been silent on the question of time or, at the least, allow the practitioner to comfortably predict lengthy interventions (Kopta, Newman, McGovern, & Sandrock, 1986).

As Haley (1976) has suggested, practicing time-limed therapy promotes a rapid client turnover that necessitates the need for more clients and a wider referral base. This may not have an immediate impact on the clinician in the publicly supported organization but can be a serious concern to the private practitioner where referrals are frequently at an uneven and unpredictable pace. When the practitioner has a secure core of longer term clients, this is manageable, but a more "transient" case load could threaten income security. As Budman and Gurman (1983) point out, regardless of the flow of referrals, rent, overhead costs, and salaries must be paid.

The dilemma raised here is by no means confined to the private practitioner of psychotherapy. Many social agencies and outpatient clinics are experiencing financial pressures and expect their staff to maintain a substantial level of direct client contact. The senior author of this chapter has frequently encountered ambivalent reactions to short-term approaches from agency-based clinicians as well:

> While conducting a workshop on brief therapy methods at a community mental health center, discussion arose about the most suitable clientele for these approaches. Most of the participants, who were Master's level social workers and psychologists, had been trained in long-term approaches but were quite interested in acquiring skills in brief intervention. During this discussion, one of the staff suggested that clients could be screened at intake and brief therapy given to those without insurance, whereas long-term treatment could be reserved for those where third-party payments were available. This idea was enthusiastically and uncritically accepted by the participants with no one raising either diagnostic or ethical questions.

Budman and Gurman (1983) identify a number of contrasting values between long-term and short-term therapists and suggest that the long-term practitioner "unconsciously recognizes the fiscal convenience of maintaining long-term patients (p. 279)," whereas, for the brief therapist, "fiscal issues are often muted by either the nature of the therapist's practice or by the organizational structure for reimbursement" (p. 279). They doubt that very many practitioners consciously extend treatment for financial gain but emphasize that clinicians are "in the business of selling time, and business and clinical issues certainly interact, even for therapists who have been psychoanalyzed" (p. 280).

Although we are not aware of empirical data on the subject, it is not difficult to find anecdotal evidence for the value clash we are describing. A recent series of articles in the *Family Therapy Networker* included some frank statements from private practitioners concerning the difficulties of utilizing brief approaches. For example:

> The problem is that while it's exciting to do short-term family therapy, it's difficult to make a living that way. I'm discovering I can afford to see families in no more than a third of my cases. (Brewster & Montie, 1987, p. 33)

We do not mean to suggest, however, that the overriding ambition of thera-pists, especially those in private practice, is to undertake the lengthiest therapy possible with all of their clients. Nowadays the fiscal dilemma can cut both ways. With the growth of a variety of third-party payers who curtail the amount of therapy they will pay for, the practitioner can experience pressure to limit treatment length in order to conform to the strictures of these outside organiza-tions. Unfortunately, we believe, this does not necessarily result in planned short-term intervention but, in many cases, a watered-down version of long-term methodology.

Both Goleman (1981) and Good (1987), in their critiques of brief therapy, have ascribed its development to a desire on the part of third-party payers, whether health insurance companies, health maintenance organizations, or in-dustrial concerns sponsoring mental health benefits for their employees, to save money by limiting therapy length. This places the blame on the demands made by external organizations. We do not believe, however, that therapists have always been the unwilling victims, so to speak, of such outside pressures. Gain-ing access to third-party reimbursement, in one form or another, resolves an uncomfortable fiscal dilemma by assuring a larger and more continuous flow of clients, and practitioners, from time to time, have shown considerable ingenuity in this pursuit (Kutchins & Kirk, 1987; Miller, Bergstrom, Cross, & Grube, 1981; Sharfstein, Towery, & Milowe, 1980).

During the 1970s there was a good deal of political ferment concerning the establishment of a nationwide, federally sponsored health insurance program but reservations on the part of legislators as to whether it was economically possible for this to include any form of psychotherapy. Mechanic (1969), in his analysis of mental health policy, summarized the conventional view of the time:

> Even if we recognize psychotherapy as a solution to psychiatric problems, it is not a feasible approach for most of the patients who require help. Most approaches to psy-chotherapy require a relatively intensive and long-term relationship between a patient and a therapist. (p. 48)

In response, we find Langsley (1978) conducting a study of psychiatric practice with the goal of demonstrating that the duration of psychiatric treat-ment was relatively brief. This, of course, supported the argument that mental health services, at least as offered by psychiatrists, can and should be included in any national health insurance scheme—certainly the most lucrative of any source of third-party payment.

Despite these pressures, there are some creative ways in which even private practitioners can utilize time. The junior author of this chapter, for example, is associated with a private practice group that has attempted to combine the effects of time and task utilization in a manner designed to enhance efficiency, effectiveness, and client compliance. This takes the following form:

> At the close of the diagnostic phase of treatment, each client receives a detailed goal plan that includes the predicted number of sessions, session type (individual, family, marital, etc.), and the estimated cost of the service. For certain diagnostic categories, particularly those involving parental concerns with their child's behavior and/or aca-

demic achievement, the client (or family) is presented with a contract guaranteeing treatment success.

The contract states that specified goals will be achieved by the end of the estimated length of treatment. If not, the client is entitled to continue in therapy, free of charge, up to the original estimated number of sessions or until goals are attained (whichever comes first). For example, if the initial treatment plan called for 15 sessions, and goals are unattained at this point, the client continues free sessions until goals are met or for up to 15 more sessions.

The guarantee contract stipulates certain conditions that must be accepted by the client. The client agrees to adhere to an individualized payment schedule for the contracted sessions, to complete assigned tasks, and to attend scheduled sessions within established guidelines. The underlying message of the plan is to communicate to clients that if they do their work then the therapists will do theirs.

The program has shown promising results. Clients seem to value the expression of confidence the guarantee represents and, in addition, they know from the start of treatment what its total cost will be. The contract affirms the commitment both the client and the therapist have to the process of change. Clients must do their part to bring about change, or they will not achieve their goals and also lose the guarantee. Therapists, on the other hand, must work actively and directly with the client or risk the penalty of donating a significant period of professional time.

SURVIVAL OF THE SHORTEST?

The current economic pressures and their impact on the mental health professions have been widely discussed in the literature (Good, 1987; Kanter, 1983; Kaplan, 1986; Kovacs, 1982) and need not be described in detail here. Suffice it to say, that psychotherapeutic services have benefited from both the community mental health movement of the 1960s and from the overall growth in health care beginning in that same era. Responding to these promising social and political initiatives, however, has not been without its consequences. Governmental support of community mental health centers, particularly for outpatient therapy services, has dwindled significantly in recent years. At the same time, health insurance providers have reduced coverage of psychotherapy as part of an overall attempt to offset the ever-growing cost of health care.

In fact, the concerns about the cost of delivering health care services have resulted in an explosive transformation of the entire health care system. A series of major alternatives to traditional health insurance such as health maintenance organizations (HMOs) and preferred provider organizations (PPOs) have proliferated and grown in popularity and acceptance. Such organizations have produced radical changes in where people go for health care and how the care is paid for. They have also had effects on the character of professional practice and on the relationship between practitioner and client. This has led such commentators as Nicholas Cummings, a former president of the American Psychological Association, to predict that "by 1995 only half of the private practices in the United States will still be around," whereas other writers have suggested that as few as 5% will endure (cited in Adams, 1987, p. 20).

The cost of care has also raised payers' consciousness regarding both the efficiency and efficacy of the services they are supporting. Such devices as diagnostic related groups (DRGs) and utilization review committees were born with the mission to eliminate "waste" in the service provision system by monitoring whether patients are treated in the most cost-effective manner as possible. These developments have placed pressure on mental health professionals to justify the need for extended treatment for clients by establishing treatment plans with specific goals and more accurate predictions of the anticipated length of treatment. Third-party payers also increasingly demand scientific evidence of the effectiveness of psychotherapy (Rogawski, 1982). In short, the old familiar system of clients going to whom they want, when they want, for as long as they want (or of therapists selecting their clients and applying whatever method they may wish, for any length of time), with few questions asked about what services were being provided (or were needed), is rapidly becoming a thing of the past.

On the other hand, the shrinking coverage and growing restrictions have not lessened the demand for services. Employers have become increasingly aware of the losses in production and work efficiency and the increases in absenteeism that are incurred when their employees are experiencing personal or substance abuse problems. The stigma attached to seeking therapy has steadily waned, and "talk shows featuring the quasi-therapeutic musing of psychologists in response to the *angst* of callers have become endemic around the country" (Kovacs, 1982, p. 142).

As a result of these two forces, there has been a sharper focus on the question of efficiency, and many mental health professionals have been expected to provide more units of service at a lesser cost per unit. By increasing client turnover, government-supported agencies can provide service to more people with fewer staff members. Similarly, third-party payers can cover larger groups of participants and, at the same time, save money when their plan participants terminate service sooner. Alternative programs such as HMOs and PPOs by the nature of their structure have the leverage to guide their participants to brief therapy providers or can offer such services through their own professional staff. In the future we may anticipate the following:

1. For clear economic reasons, third-party payers will heavily weigh treatment efficiency when selecting preferred providers, and, as some are already doing, adjust reimbursement schedules so as to favor brevity.
2. Such control efforts as increasing consumer co-payments for treatment as well as decreasing overall benefit coverage will likely continue. These changes have the potential to alter consumers' "shopping patterns" when selecting therapists, as the consumer's personal liability for treatment costs increases.
3. The continued proliferation of HMOs, PPOs, and the like will alter referral patterns as these organizations place greater control and restriction on those mental health professionals eligible for direct reimbursement. Practitioners, used to developing community referral sources, may instead need to place greater emphasis on convincing providers how their proffered services benefit the sponsoring organization, as well as the client.

In summary, the practice of brief therapy would seem to mesh nicely with the current economic trends in health care provision, especially the heightened emphasis on both efficiency and effectiveness. It is not surprising and no coincidence, that during this period of change and turmoil brief therapy has drawn considerable attention from funding organizations—it would seem to be the perfect partner for both public agencies and third-party payers.

FALLING IN LOVE WITH BRIEF THERAPY

The preceding section might suggest that practice is moving toward brief psychotherapy in a major way and that, consequently, there is cause for the aspiring brief therapist to celebrate and perhaps, start looking for a bigger house or a more expensive car. Celebration, however, may be premature. Some of the professional value and economic dilemmas implicit in the practice of brief psychotherapy have already been pointed out but, in addition, we must also note the emotional and psychological hazards involved. These can be especially acute for the less experienced practitioner who is just beginning to practice brief psychotherapy and a common scenario is as follows:

> You are a few years into independent practice and, although your original training emphasized the mainstream long-term approaches, you have recently taken a workshop or two in brief psychotherapy and done a good deal of excited reading in its literature. Imagine yourself shaking hands with your client as a gesture of congratulation for his expedient progress in therapy. He is ready for termination within the predicted time limit, in one of your first brief therapy cases.
>
> You leave the office with a twinge of sadness from the ending of this relationship, but you are more conscious of your sense of accomplishment and your growing enthusiasm for the practice of brief therapy. You experience a sense of defiance in relation to conservative colleagues who claim that lasting and significant growth takes time, and you scoff at the joke, "How many mental health professionals does it take to change a lightbulb? One; but the lightbulb has to want to change, and it takes a long, long time." What you are experiencing is a phenomenon we shall call falling in love with brief therapy.
>
> With your newfound love, you reevaluate your caseload looking for ways to expedite the therapeutic process (especially those clients you don't particularly care for). New cases are viewed from a perspective of where to end as well as where to begin. You find yourself wondering what took you so long to see the light.
>
> But alas, your love is fickle. You soon encounter a case that fits neatly into the model, you clearly specify and contract the treatment goals and use your best clinical judgment to prescribe a length of treatment. During the course of the intervention, however, unforeseen events occur that necessitate time-consuming (even fascinating) detours. You like your client(s) and vice versa; they seem happy with the rate of progress and are in no apparent hurry. Both subtly and overtly they encourage (or even demand) that you forget the time limit and stay with them for as long as it takes.
>
> The treatment "deadline" begins staring you in the face. Suddenly you become less enamored with the word *brief*. Now what do you do? Do you remain steadfast to your commitment and continue to strive toward the deadline or do you forsake the model and go open-ended? Is there a middle road you can take that might allow you to forget the time limit but still stay focused?

Conducting brief therapy on a consistent basis requires the therapist to continually resolve dilemmas similar to the one described here. Moreover, dilemmas of this kind are seldom resolved once and for all as, in succeeding cases, individual differences conjure up the same issue in new and different guises.

The practice of any form of therapy is demanding, of course. Guy (1987) has reviewed, in detail, the effect such factors as physical and psychic isolation, fatigue, one-way intimacy, and the need for emotional control have upon therapists. He also examines the impact these and other factors can have on the therapist's social and family relationships. Along with all of these hazards, we believe that brief therapy places unique demands upon its practitioners, both experienced and neophyte. This is often related to an ambivalence about the fact that time is of the essence. With this recognition comes an underlying anxiety or pressure that can become as imposing as it is motivating. Brief therapy requires an acute awareness of factors in the change process—where they stand, where they are going, how you are to get there, and *when*—which frequently have a tendency to get dulled or ignored in more open-ended work. All therapists have experienced the painful feelings accompanying the recognition that they have fallen short or failed with a particular case. In short-term treatment, the recognition happens more quickly.

Another consideration for the brief therapist is the emotional toll exacted by the inherent frequency of terminating relationships with clients. As Budman and Gurman (1983) point out, the initial interview in brief therapy requires energy and involvement, with a consequent feeling of loss if that client does not return. Moreover, they note, certain aspects of the ongoing process of brief therapy can place compelling demands on the practitioner:

> Additionally, the effective brief therapist cannot remain detached and uninvolved, since activity and planning are two of the central characteristics of brief treatment. The often told joke goes that when the young analyst and the old analyst met on their way out of their respective offices, the young analyst was amazed at how fresh and alert the old analyst appeared (compared to his own exhaustion). He said to him: "Dr. Van Klopfer, how is it that you always appear so chipper after hearing people's problems all day?" Dr. Van Klopfer replied, "Who listens?" Not listening is not a response available to the effective brief therapist. (p. 288)

Finally, brief therapists are also prone to a fair amount of conjoint family and marital work. This work is often fraught with heated sessions and frequent crises that are multiplied by the number of people in the room. This, too, takes its emotional toll on the therapist. Along with these demands, seeing couples and families creates scheduling conflicts, making it difficult to establish a regular and orderly calendar and necessitating primarily evening appointment hours. Such an adjustment requires time away from one's own family on a regular basis, with consequent pressures for therapists in managing their own lives and important relationships.

BRIEF THERAPY AND THE MEDIA

Consider the following statements, appearing in 1986:

The efficacy of any therapy, of course, is highly subjective and has seldom been the topic of serious research—until recently.

Family therapy sees the patient as part of a closed family system in which he or she compulsively reenacts childhood relationships.

Behavior therapy operates on the theory that problematic behaviors are learned and can be unlearned through rigorous mental exercises.

Many psychiatrists view brief therapy as little more than a cosmetic remedy that trims weeds without pulling up the roots, leading to the inevitable reappearance of symptoms.

One might guess that these statements were drawn from a badly prepared term paper by a glib but not very competent undergraduate psychology student. They are not but instead are all direct quotations from a recent *Newsweek* article on the brief psychotherapies (Gelman, 1986). Mental health practitioners receive their most reliable information from the professional literature—books, journals, and so on—or from workshops, conferences, and courses designed for (and restricted to) the active professional. Practitioners may entertain a measure of disdain for the "lay press," yet we must remember that this is the major—if not exclusive—source of information about psychotherapy for the many individuals who comprise the actual or potential recipients of our professional services.

The media has begun to pay increasing attention to brief therapeutic methods. A number of prominent, mass-circulation newspapers and magazines have featured articles about short-term treatment, and it is worth reviewing the picture these widely read sources have presented to the public concerning the methods, effectiveness, and, in essence, the legitimacy of brief psychotherapy.

Perhaps one of the earliest publicly accessible descriptions of brief psychotherapy was in a 1981 article in *Psychology Today*, a publication occupying an ambiguous middle ground between the public media and the professional literature. The article on short-term therapy was written by Daniel Goleman, one of the magazine's senior editors, and presented a relatively accurate description of the major areas of brief therapeutic practice. There are extended illustrations of the brief psychodynamic therapies developed by James Mann and Peter Sifneos, but also descriptions of Budman's employment of time-limited group psychotherapy, based on a life-development model, as well as the Milton Erickson-influenced brief strategic therapy practiced at the Mental Research Institute in Palo Alto. A sidebar recounts Bernard Bloom's experimentation with a single-session psychotherapy. Yet a deep skepticism about even the possibility of brief psychotherapy pervades the article. Its subtitle is "Therapy in the Age of Reaganomics," with the writer ascribing the appeal of brief therapy to the "ascendancy of cost-efficiency as the criterion of value" (Goleman, 1981, p. 60).

An article in *Glamour* magazine (Crump, 1984) offers a much less skeptical account. The essential features of brief psychotherapy—"a focus on a central issue, a time limit, and a high level of therapist activity" (p. 112) are accurately identified. Several illustrations portray short-term therapy with such common problems as depression or reactions to traumatic events. The writer clearly defines the limitations of brief treatment, pointing out that "this type of therapy is [not] helpful to drug addicts, alcoholics, suicidal patients or other people troubled by psychiatric illnesses" (p. 110). The strengths of short-term therapy, the article points out, are in dealing with specific problems in living and such common emotional dilemmas as "bouts of depression, anxiety or low self-esteem, sexual problems, or difficulties in relationships" (p. 110).

In a lengthy article in the *New York Times Sunday Magazine*, Sobel (1982) provides a detailed and admiring account of Habib Davanloo's short-term dynamic psychotherapy. The writer is perhaps overly fascinated with the confrontational elements in the approach. For example:

> In practice, the therapist relentlessly badgers patients to demolish the defense they have built around their feelings. Every time they smile, pause or use an expression that conveys doubt ("I guess," "I suppose") the doctor seizes the opportunity to challenge them, often evoking a storm of emotion. (p. 60)

The overall tone of the presentation, however, is positive, describing the essential thrust of this form of short-term therapy as one of making psychotherapy both more efficient and more accessible to a significant portion of the population.

On the other hand, the most recent article, entitled "Quick-Fix Therapy" (Gelman, 1986) is a curious mixture of accurate information and journalistic excess. It appeared at the time when the initial findings of the NIMH Collaborative Depression Project were being reported to the American Psychiatric Association's annual meeting and gives an accurate and informative account of the effectiveness of the two short-term interventions—cognitive/behavioral therapy and interpersonal psychotherapy—included in that exemplary study of the treatment of depression. Along with this, however, there are some wildly inaccurate statements, a few of which we noted at the beginning of this section. Despite the uneven quality of these samples of the media exposure of brief psychotherapy that we have reviewed, a number of generalizations are possible:

1. After little or no exposure during their formative years in the 1960s and 1970s, the brief psychotherapies are receiving increasing public scrutiny, both positive and negative. Although, as Budman and Gurman (1983) note, short-term therapy has yet to be featured in a movie, potential clients are now much more aware of its existence.

2. Although the brief therapist can expect more clients to be aware of the existence of time-limited methods, one cannot count on any really accurate knowledge. Client education continues to be necessary part of the therapeutic process.

3. The long-term therapies, particularly psychoanalysis, still tend to be the public benchmark for evaluating therapeutic effectiveness. The *Newsweek* article, for example, utilizes the common journalistic ploy of interviewing a couple of classical psychoanalysts who, as one might well expect, caustically denounce all brief therapies as sham and hoax.

4. The media accounts recognize that the emergence of brief methods is signaling a democratization of the clientele of psychotherapy—it is much less

the exclusive prerogative of the small minority of the population who have been economically able to pay for lengthy treatments with a small but prestigious cadre of private practitioners.

5. Another aspect of the democraticization process is also highlighted in two of the articles. This is that legitimate psychotherapy is now offered by a number of professional disciplines, including social workers, nurses, and family and marital therapists, and is no longer the exclusive domain of a particular group of practitioners.

THE FUTURE OF THE BRIEF PSYCHOTHERAPIES

The brief psychotherapies comprise a significant but not major portion of present-day therapeutic practice. As most surveys (Beck & Jones, 1973; Goldemeier, 1986; Langsley, 1978) do not distinguish between planned and unplanned brief therapy, it is difficult to estimate what proportion of therapist/client time is devoted to *explicitly* time-limited treatment—somewhere between 20% to 30% is our best guess. It would be naive and overly optimistic to predict, as some have done, that the brief psychotherapies will become the wave of the future. A number of potential trends can be envisaged, based on our reading of the current factors influencing therapeutic practice, as these interact with historical trends in the development of the mental health field:

1. Although the costs of psychotherapy represent only a relatively small portion of overall health care costs, the continuing crisis in this general area will have fallout effects on therapeutic practice. In large part, this will stem from the proliferation of HMOs, PPOs, and similar organizations and, in general, efforts by third-party payers, both private and governmental, to restrict and control coverage and benefits. As more and more consumers come under the auspices of such organizations, the relationship between therapist and client will be greatly altered.

2. Practicing clinicians will be increasingly pressured to either adopt brief therapeutic methods—under the aegis of a third-party payer—or to restrict their practice to the relatively affluent portion of the population able to finance therapy on their own. This will result in an increase in the amount of brief psychotherapy but conducted, in many instances, by unwilling "brief" therapists.

3. Those therapists who choose to restrict their practice to the economically affluent will be continuing a form of practice not unlike that which existed prior to the advent of the community mental health movement in the 1960s. In addition to limiting long-term therapy to an elite clientele, it also requires a much smaller population of therapists. Along with the co-option of therapists into relationships with HMOs, and PPOs, this possibility has led some analysts, such as Nicholas Cummings, to predict a radical decline in the prevalence of private practice—at least in the sense of an truly "private" relationship between professional and patient.

4. Many clinicians will literally become employees of one or other type of service-providing organization, whereas even those who maintain a semblance

of independence will find significant aspects of their practice governed by their relationship to an external source of remuneration. For example, growing numbers of practitioners may find that competition will force them to think more actively and directly in business terms. The successful therapist will need to define his or her market and, once this is done, develop explicit strategies for capturing a fair share of it. Adams (1987) puts this bluntly:

> Clearly therapists trying to figure out the changing mental health marketplace need to educate themselves about the new health care organizations and become more familiar with who is actually dispensing dollars for mental health care in their community. (p. 25)

5. Psychotherapy will continue to be a legitimate approach to emotional disorders, despite the emergence of biochemical theories and interventions in a number of areas. This is a major implication of the preliminary findings of NIMH's Collaborative Depression Project that found that two purely psychotherapeutic methods (cognitive/behavioral therapy and interpersonal psychotherapy) were as effective as a well-established medication in the treatment of depression. It should be noted that both of these therapies are time limited and are more fully described in later chapters of this volume.

6. From a cost perspective, however, biochemical theories and practice have a decided competitive edge because the treatment mode requires less face-to-face contact with the treating professional. Thus, short-term treatment methods that are "just as good" as medication regimens may not be good enough unless they are equally cost-effective. As mentioned before, the client's insurance company or health care organization have increased leverage to guide participants to providers and, thus, to treatment modalities.

7. At the same time, we anticipate a continued proliferation of psychotherapeutic methods, both within the brief psychotherapies, as well as in the therapeutic field generally. Some of these new interventions will be specific to a particular disorder, but some will be presented as "universal" treatments. In effect, this is simply saying that the future will be much like the past, but it is also a recognition that a driving force in the field is the vision of a unifying theory/treatment that is completely explanatory and universally applicable. Psychoanalysis dominated the helping professions for many years with just such a vision and this, perhaps, was its greatest appeal. Despite its greatly diminished direct influence, its legacy persists in this form.

8. We can also expect that efforts will be made to make the brief therapies more complex and lengthier. This has already taken place in family therapy where the so-called constructivists (Dell, 1982; Keeney & Sprenkle, 1982) are generating theoretical formulations of unparalleled density and obscurity, whereas the advocates of Bowen theory (Bowen, 1975) call for treatment durations rivaling those of classical psychoanalysis.

9. Overall, we expect the brief psychotherapies to continue to flourish as a significant minority position but certainly not as anything even approaching a dominant trend in practice. Their influence will be exerted in such ways as greater eclecticism in theoretical allegiances, a heightened consumer orientation,

and a more conscious awareness of the usefulness of such action methods as tasks and therapist/client activity in inducing change. Despite our own convictions about the great clinical relevance of the time dimension, we believe that the field, as a whole, will continue to be reluctant to adopt brief psychotherapy's emphasis on time limitation.

REFERENCES

Adams J. (1987). A brave new world for private practice. *The Family Therapy Networker, 11,* 19–25.

Alexander, F., & French, T. M. (1946). *Psychoanalytic therapy: Principles and applications.* New York: Ronald Press.

Beck, D. F., & Jones, M. A. (1973). *Progress on family problems.* New York: Family Service Association of America.

Bergin, A. E., & Garfield, S. L. (Eds.). (1971). *Handbook of psychotherapy and behavior change: An empirical analysis.* New York: Wiley.

Bergin, A. E., & Garfield, S. L. (1986). Introduction and historical overview. In S. L. Garfield & A. E. Bergin (Eds.), *Handbook of psychotherapy and behavior change: An empirical analysis* (3rd ed., pp. 3–22). New York: Wiley.

Bloom, B. L. (1981). Focused single-session therapy: Initial development and evaluation. In S. H. Budman (Ed.), *Forms of brief therapy* (pp. 167–218). New York: Guilford.

Bowen, M. (1975). *Family therapy in clinical practice.* New York: Aronson.

Brewster, F., & Montie, K. (1987). A double life: What do family therapists really do in private practice? *The Family Therapy Networker, 11,* 33–37.

Budman, S. H., & Gurman, A. S. (1983). The practice of brief therapy. *Professional Psychology, 14,* 277–290.

Budman, S. H., and Gurman, A. S. (1988). *Theory and practice of brief therapy.* New York: Guilford.

Crump, K. (1984). Short-term therapy. *Glamour* (May), 108–112.

Davanloo, H. (Ed.). (1980). *Short-term dynamic psychotherapy.* New York: Aronson.

Dell, P. (1982). Beyond homeostasis: Toward a concept of coherence. *Family Process, 21,* 21–42.

Eisenstein, S. (1986). Franz Alexander and short-term dynamic psychotherapy. *International Journal of Short-Term Dynamic Psychotherapy, 1,* 179–191.

Eysenck, H. J. (1952). The effects of psychotherapy: An evaluation. *Journal of Consulting Psychology, 16,* 319–324.

Ferenzi, S. (1960). The further development of an active therapy in psychoanalysis. In J. Richman (Ed.), *Further contributions to the theory and techniques of psychoanalysis* (pp. 198–216). London: Hogarth. (Originally published 1920)

Frances, A. J., & Clarkin, J. F. (1981). No treatment as the prescription of choice. *Archives of General Psychiatry, 142.* 922–926.

Garfield, S. L. (1986). Research on client variables in psychotherapy. In S. L. Garfield & A. E. Bergin (Eds.), *Handbook of psychotherapy and behavior change: An empirical analysis* (3rd ed., pp. 213–256). New York: Wiley.

Garfield, S. L., & Bergin, A. E. (Eds.). (1978). *Handbook of psychotherapy and behavior change: An empirical analysis* (2nd ed.). New York: Wiley.

Garfield, S. L., & Bergin, A. E. (Eds.). (1986). *Handbook of psychotherapy and behavior change: An empirical analysis* (3rd ed.). New York: Wiley.

Gelman, D. (1986). Quick-fix therapy. *Newsweek* (May 26), pp. 74–76.

Goldemeier, J. (1987). Private practice and the purchase of services: Who are the practitioners? *American Journal of Orthopsychiatry, 56,* 89–102.

Goleman, D. (1981). Deadlines for change: Therapy in the age of Reagonomics. *Psychology Today, 15,* 60–69.

Good, P. R. (1987). Brief therapy in the age of Reagapeutics. *American Journal of Orthopsychiatry, 57,* 6–11.

Gurman, A. S., Kniskern, D. P., & Pinsoff, W. M. (1986). Research on the process and outcome of marital and family therapy. In S. L. Garfield & A. E. Bergin (Eds.), *Handbook of psychotherapy and behavior change: An empirical analysis* (3rd ed., pp. 565–624). New York: Wiley.

Guy, J. D. (1987). *The personal life of the psychotherapist*.New York: Wiley.

Haley, J. (1962). Whither family therapy. *Family Process, 1,* 69–100.

Haley, J. (1963). *Strategies of psychotherapy*. New York: Grune & Stratton.

Haley, J. (Ed.). (1969). *Advanced techniques of hypnosis and therapy: Selected papers of Milton F. Erickson, M.D.*, New York: Grune & Stratton.

Haley, J. (1976). *Problem-solving therapy*. San Francisco: Jossey-Bass.

Herink, R. (Ed.). (1980). *The psychotherapy handbook*. New York: New American Library.

Kanfer, F. H. (1979). Self-management: Strategies and tactics. In A. P. Goldstein & F. H. Kanfer (Eds.), *Maximizing treatment gains: Transfer enhancement in psychotherapy* (pp. 185–224). New York: Academic Press.

Kanter, J. (1983). Re-evaluation of task-centered social work practice. *Clinical Social Work Journal, 11,* 228–244.

Kaplan, S. J. (1986). *The private practice of behavior therapy*. New York: Plenum Press.

Keeney, B. F., & Sprenkle, D. H. (1982). Ecosystematic epistemology: Critical implications for the aesthetics and pragmatics of family therapy. *Family Process, 21,* 1–20.

Kopta, S. M., Newman, F. L., McGovern, M. P., & Sandrock, D. (1986). Psychotherapeutic orientations: A comparison of conceptualizations, interventions and treatment plan costs. *Journal of Consulting and Clinical Psychology, 54,* 369–374.

Koss, M. P. (1979). The length of psychotherapy for clients seen in private practice. *Journal of Consulting and Clinical Psychology, 47,* 210–212.

Koss, M. P., & Butcher, J. N. (1986). Research on brief psychotherapy. In S. L. Garfield, & A. E. Bergin (Eds.), *Handbook of psychotherapy and behavior change: An empirical analysis* (3rd ed., pp. 627–670). New York: Wiley.

Kovacs, A. L. (1982). Survival in the 80's. On the theory and practice of brief psychotherapy. *Psychotherapy: Theory, Research and Practice, 19,* 142–159.

Krasner, L. (1962). The therapist as a social reinforcement machine. In H. H. Strupp & L. Luborsky (Eds.), *Research in psychotherapy* (Vol. II, pp. 61–94). Washington, DC: American Psychological Association.

Kutchins, H., & Kirk, S. A. (1987). DSM III and social work malpractice. *Social Work, 32,* 205–211.

Lambert, M. J., Shapiro, D. A., & Bergin, A. E. (1986). The effectiveness of psychotherapy. In S. L. Garfield, & A. E. Bergin (Eds.), *Handbook of psychotherapy and behavior change: An empirical analysis* (3rd ed., pp. 157–211). New York: Wiley.

Langsley, D. (1978). Comparing clinic and private practice of psychiatry. *American Journal of Psychiatry, 135,* 702–706.

London, P. (1986). *The modes and morals of psychotherapy* (2nd ed.). Washington: Hemisphere Publishing.

Malan, D. H. (1976). *The frontier of brief psychotherapy*. New York: Plenum Press.

Mann, J. (1973). *Time-limited psychotherapy*. Cambridge: Harvard University Press.

Mann, J., & Goldman, R. (1982). *A casebook in time-limited psychotherapy*. New York: McGraw-Hill.

Marmor, J. (1979). Short-term dynamic psychotherapy. *American Journal of Psychiatry, 136,* 149–155.

Mechanic, D. (1969). *Mental health and social policy*. Englewood Cliffs, NJ: Prentice-Hall.

Miller, L. S., Bergstrom, D. A., Cross, H. J., & Grube, J. W. (1981). Opinions and use of the DSM system by practicing psychologists. *Professional Psychology, 12,* 385–390.

Oberndorf, C. P. (1947). [Review of *Psychoanalytic therapy: Principles and applications*]. *Psychoanalytic Quarterly, 16,* 99–102.

O'Connor, R., & Reid, W. J. (1986). Dissatisfaction with brief treatment. *Social Service Review, 60,* 526–536.

Rogawski, A. (1982). Current status of the brief psychotherapies. *Bulletin of the Menninger Clinic, 46,* 331–351.

Sharfstein, S., Towery, O., & Milowe, I. (1980). Accuracy of diagnostic information submitted to an insurance company. *American Journal of Psychiatry, 137,* 70–73.

Sloane, B., Staples, F. R., Cristol, A. H., Yorkston, N. J., & Whipple, K. (1975). *Psychotherapy versus behavior therapy*. Cambridge: Harvard University Press.

Sifneos, P. E. (1972). *Short-term therapy and emotional crisis*. Cambridge: Harvard University Press.

Sifneos, P. E. (1981). Short-term dynamic psychotherapy: Its history, its impact, its future. *Psychotherapy & Psychosomatics, 35*, 224–229.

Sobel, D. (1982). A new and controversial short-term therapy. *New York Times Sunday Magazine* (Nov. 21), pp. 58, 60–62, 102–110.

Sterba, R. (1951). A case of brief psychotherapy by Sigmund Freud. *Psychoanalytic Review, 38*, 75–80.

Strupp, H. H., & Bergin, A. E. (1969). *Research in individual psychotherapy: A bibliography*. Chevy Chase, MD: National Institute of Mental Health.

Walter, B. (1946). *Theme and variations: An autobiography*. New York: Knopf.

Wells, R. A. (1982). *Planned short-term treatment*. New York: Free Press.

2

The Therapeutic Interaction
Research Perspectives

STEPHEN SOLDZ

Psychotherapy as a profession is nearly a century old. During that time thousands of clinical books and papers have been published. Hundreds of different theories of therapy have been developed. Yet the clinician trying to choose a therapeutic approach has no clear criterion for choosing among the varied alternatives. As matters stand now, such choices are usually made on the basis of where one receives one's training and who one's supervisors were. General trends in therapeutic styles, partly influenced by cultural and economic factors, also influence therapist's choices. Since the 1950s, behavioral and related treatments have challenged the former (brief) predominance of psychoanalytic treatments. In the 1960s the "humanistic-experiential" therapies were popular, at least partly because they were consistent with certain emphases of the popular culture of that time. At present, a biological bias appears to be exerting an increasing influence, as can be seen by the replacement of psychoanalysts by psychopharmacologists in medical school departments of psychiatry.

One common characteristic of humanistic, behavioral, and biological treatments is that, by and large, they are shorter and less intensive than traditional therapies based on psychoanalytic principles. This fact is part of a general trend toward shorter treatments, which is affecting psychotherapy in general. The trend toward explicitly shorter treatments has infiltrated the world of psychodynamic treatment as well. In recent years, numerous theories of short-term dynamic therapy have been proposed (Budman, 1981; Budman & Stone, 1983; Donovan, 1987; Malan, 1979; Strupp & Binder, 1984). In fact, Budman and Stone (1983) claim that short-term psychotherapy has long been the norm, despite the expressed theories of clinicians, because of the simple fact that most patients drop out after a relatively few sessions.

Another change in therapeutic debate in recent years is a rise in claims to scientific support for particular therapeutic practices. Given the importance of science as a justifying ideology in modern society, this is, perhaps, inevitable.

STEPHEN SOLDZ • Harvard Medical School, and the Mental Health Research Program, Harvard Community Health Plan, One Fenway Plaza, Boston, Massachusetts 02215.

Some claimed that there was no evidence that psychotherapy was effective (Eysenck, 1952; Prioleau, Murdock, & Brody, 1983). There have been claims that some psychotherapies have been shown to be more effective than others. Yet, in the 1970s a consensus supported two conclusions: (1) there is substantial evidence that psychotherapy is more effective in helping disturbed people than is no treatment (Lambert, Shapiro, & Bergin, 1986; Smith, Glass, & Miller, 1980); and (2) there does not exist much convincing evidence that one psychotherapy is better than another (Luborsky, Singer, & Luborsky, 1975; Smith, Glass, & Miller, 1980; Stiles, Shapiro, & Elliott, 1986).

These two conclusions left the clinician who desired to use research to help guide clinical choices in a quandary. Offering psychotherapy to patients seemed justified by the evidence, but research provided no guide as to what kind of therapy to offer. Furthermore, these conclusions appeared to suggest that it made no difference what kind of treatment was offered, a conclusion that was radically at variance with the beliefs of most therapists that therapeutic techniques are indeed important to the outcome of treatment. These conclusions may have reinforced the feeling of many therapists that psychotherapy research had nothing to offer them, that research was simply incapable of elucidating complicated and elusive clinical processes. Although not endorsing these feelings about the potential value of their work, several prominent psychotherapy researchers agreed that the research had not yet shown its value (Bergin & Strupp, 1972; Luborsky, 1972). Fifteen years after those pessimistic conclusions regarding the value of research for therapeutic practice, the atmosphere among researchers appears much more upbeat. There seems to be a general feeling among researchers that their work does have something to contribute to clinicians. Furthermore, there is a sense that the field is headed in the right direction(s) and that the next several years will see even greater payoff for their years of effort.

Several factors have contributed to this change in atmosphere. One is the reassurance provided by results supporting the value of psychotherapy. For some, the worst result of research would be evidence that psychotherapy was indeed ineffective, leading to loss of social and economic support for the mental health professions. After the overall effectiveness of psychological treatments was shown, there was a desire to follow the path of medicine and determine exactly which treatments, applied to which patients, were effective. Social pressures from third-party payment sources for therapy made this question an important one for the profession. However, the negative results on differences in effectiveness among treatments raised doubts about the value of this line of investigation. It appeared that, either there were no differences among treatments, or the available research methodologies were not capable of finding them. The search was then on for new research techniques and strategies.

One direction that these efforts have taken is the creation of detailed treatment manuals for particular therapies. Manuals now exist for many therapies, including cognitive therapy (Beck, Rush, Shaw, & Emery, 1979), interpersonal therapy (Klerman, Weissman, Rounsaville, & Chevron, 1984), time-limited group interactional group therapy (Budman, 1987), and psychoanalytically oriented therapy (Luborsky, 1984; Strupp & Binder, 1984). These manuals are often remarkably detailed works, suitable for use as texts for the training of clinicians in clinical training programs, as well as for the research purposes for which they were originally designed. They deal very competently with the technical aspects of therapy. So far, however, none of the manuals has undertaken to describe the process of using the therapist's own feelings during therapy, which has played such a large role in the clinical literature of humanistic and psychodynamic therapies over the last two decades (Epstein & Feiner, 1983). Furthermore, despite rigorous efforts to get therapists in research studies to follow these manuals, there is a limit to which such a complex undertaking as psychotherapy can be precisely specified. Thus, there are, at least at present, natural limits to the degree to which therapy techniques can be standardized. Therefore, it should not be surprising that, after standardization by manual, there is still considerable variability between particular therapy experiences.

Considerable research effort in the last 10 years has gone into exploring the nature of the variability between psychotherapies and between particular stages or sessions of a given psychotherapy, leading to increased research on psychotherapy process as the object of research efforts. Process research has taken many forms, from the investigation, using linguistic techniques, of the first few minutes of a single therapy session (Labov & Fanshel, 1977), to efforts to delineate general dimensions of therapeutic behaviors (Suh, Strupp, & O'Malley, 1986). In this chapter, I will attempt to convey to clinicians some of the nature of the process research of recent years. As several good comrehensive literature reviews already exist (Hartley, 1985; Orlinsky & Howard, 1986), I have chosen not to undertake another. Instead, I have selected a few process studies that illustrate the range of the process research undertaken in recent years. I hope to give clinicians a sense of the variety of techniques currently being used to understand a number of elusive clinical processes. I have concentrated more on the process of the research than on the results, in order to convey to the nonresearcher a sense of both the difficulties and the promise of such research.

In selecting material to be discussed, I have chosen to concentrate on research emanating from a psychodynamic perspective. This decision was taken both for reasons of personal competence and because, in my view, it is in this area, broadly defined, that some of the most exciting work of the last few years has been concentrated. In addition, I have chosen to primarily emphasize the work done by researchers who have been engaged in psychotherapy process research for a number of years. As Kiesler (1973) pointed out years ago, there have been many process researchers who have developed a process measure, carried out one or two studies and moved on to other areas. As a result of this tendency, these research efforts have led to only minimal accumulation of knowledge. In contrast, those researchers who have struggled with this area for years, or even decades, have tended to carry out systematic research programs, involving successive refinements of their instruments, methods, and conclusions. It now appears that it is only out of such perseverance that real knowledge about therapy process will develop.

The research discussed in this chapter, like most psychotherapy research, primarily consists of studies of short-term therapies. However, a few studies of longer therapies, including psychoanalysis, have been included, either because of the paradigmatic nature of the research or its relevance to the general argument of the paper.

MEASURING INTERPERSONAL DIFFICULTIES

There exists little agreement among clinicians about the nature of improvement in psychotherapy. Does it consist of a resolution of symptoms, an improvement in adaptive social functioning, an increase in cognitive complexity, a decrease in subjective distress, an improvement in interpersonal relationships, an increase in self-esteem, or the development of insight into one's wishes, fears, and defenses? Each of these positions has been adopted by some school of therapy. Many, if not most, therapists probably adopt a number of these perspectives in evaluating outcome.

Given this multiplicity of possible dimensions of change, it should not be surprising that measurement of outcome is a difficult matter. Add to this the research finding that different types of improvement are often only moderately correlated, if at all (Lambert *et al.*, 1986), and it might seem impossible. The solution to this problem that has been adopted by researchers with adequate resources is to measure a number of different types of outcome from several different perspectives. For example, a typical outcome battery for a psychotherapy study might include a number of paper-and-pencil tests taken by patients pre- and posttherapy, global ratings of patient benefit by both the therapist and patient, and judgments of patient improvement by an independent clinician rater who interviews the patient before and after therapy (Lambert, Christensen, & DeJulio, 1983; Waskow & Parloff, 1975).

In addition to the problems of multiplicity of types of possible improvement and of perspectives, an additional problem is that it is very hard to measure some of the less overt aspects of patient functioning, such as psychodynamic functioning. For example, many studies investigate the impact of psychotherapy on depression, whereas far fewer look at improvement in patient's subjective difficulties with closeness to others. At least one reason for this disparity is because depression is far easier to measure than is difficulty with closeness. Especially difficult to measure are the type of intrapsychic constructs that are the implicit target of many verbally oriented psychotherapists, especially those of a psychodynamic orientation. Thus, a number of research efforts in the last few years have attempted to operationally define and quantify some of these psychodynamic constructs. In order to illustrate these efforts, this section will discuss two of these techniques, one based on the analysis of psychotherapy transcripts and one using a novel paper-and-pencil test.

Luborsky (1976, 1977, 1984; Luborsky, Crits-Cristoph, & Mellon, 1986) has developed a technique, the Core Conflictual Relationship Theme method (CCRT) for systematically identifying repetitive patterns in intrapsychic representations of personal relationships. In order to use this method, trained clinical judges carefully examine transcripts of portions of psychotherapy sessions in which relationships with others are discussed (relationship episodes, or REs). For each RE, the judge identifies three aspects of the relationship: (1) the wish, need, or intention expressed in the episode; (2) the reaction of the other; and (3) the reaction of the self. After a number of REs have been examined, the judge tries to formulate a brief but comprehensive CCRT formulation for the patient, encompassing the repetitive elements in the REs. Each RE is then reexamined in order to determine the extent to which the CCRT identifies its salient elements, leading to a revision of the CCRT.

Luborsky *et al.* (1986) present examples of two judges' scoring of REs and of their final CCRT formulations. Judge 1's final formulation was "Wish: To be free of being obligated and imposed on. Response from other: Does not respond. Response from self: Feels hassled; compliance." Judge 2's CCRT was: "Wish: To feel free from obligation and the control of others. Response from other: Does not respond. Response from self: Feel hassled; feel compelled to submit" (p. 42). As can be seen, in this example, there is substantial agreement between the two judges as to the central theme in this patient's relationship with others. In Levine and Luborsky (1981), fair to good agreement among independent judges was demonstrated. This is in contrast to previous studies in which unstructured formulations between separate judges showed little similarity (Kaltreider, De-Witt, Weiss, & Horowitz, 1981; Seitz, 1966).

These studies suggest that clinicians, as well as researchers, need a structured format if they are to come up with formulations that are consistent with those of others. This conclusion makes clinical sense. Anyone who has sat in on a case conference has seen the multiplicity of interpretations that can be applied to clinical material. Often the different formulations refer to different aspects or levels of the patient's material, making them, not so much incompatible, as impossible to compare. If, however, a systematic format is specified, different formulations should be comparable, leading, one hopes, to greater agreement. It should be noted though, that CCRT judges have an additional advantage over case conference participants in that their formulations are examined from intensive examination of relevant portions of therapy transcripts, allowing a more leisurely concentration on those portions of the patient's material that is about interpersonal relationships.

It has probably not escaped the psychodynamically astute reader that the CCRT, identified from therapy material, is closely connected to the psychoanalytic concept of transference. The concept of transference implies that a person has one, or a few, patterns of construing and interacting with others, which will tend to become manifest in important relationships and in the relationship with the therapist. In his early work on the CCRT, Luborsky (1977) was extremely hesitant about identifying it with the analytic concept of transference. However, a more recent work (Luborsky *et al.*, 1985) identifies nine different aspects of the concept of transference and presents evidence suggesting that the CCRT is, indeed, a measure of transference. For example, the idea that there should be a similarity between the patient–therapist relationships and the patient's relationship with important others was tested for eight patients. This was done by developing, for each patient, a CCRT from REs involving relationships with others and a distinct CCRT based on the relationship with the therapist. Judges then rated the similarity between each of the therapist-based CCRTs and each of the other people-based CCRTs, without knowing which pairs of CCRTs involved a correct match. The correctly matched therapist–other CCRTs were rated as highly similar, whereas the incorrectly matched pairs received substantially lower similarity ratings.

In contrast to the CCRT, which requires the scoring of psychotherapy transcripts by independent raters, Ryle has developed a simple paper-and-pencil instrument that can be used to determine a patient's repetitive relationship patterns. Arising out of a long-term interest in integrating psychodynamic and cognitive approaches to psychotherapy, Ryle (1975, 1979, 1980, 1981) has explored uses of Kelly's (1955) Repertory Grid (Rep Grid) to identify psychodynamic constructs. Briefly put, the Rep Grid is designed as a way to explore the personal dimensions or constructs that a person uses in construing self and others (Beail, 1985; Landfield & Epting, 1987; Soldz, 1988b). In its classical form, the Rep Grid involves the selection of a representative sample of people (called elements) personally important to the subject (possibilities include self, self as I would like to be, self as I was at age 5, mother, father, best friend of opposite sex, etc.) and the rating of these people on a set of dimensions, or constructs, that are usually elicited from the subject. Statistical analyses can then be performed on these ratings in order to determine the similarities and differences among these people and constructs from the individual subject's point of view (Chambers & Grice, 1986; Fransella & Bannister, 1977). It is an assumption behind this methodology that the underlying dimensions revealed by these analyses represent the fundamental core constructs used by the subject in construing self and others.

One of Ryle's (1975) contributions to the use of the Rep Grid in assessing psychodynamic constructs is his employment of the grid to assess an individual's dilemmas in personal relationships. In order to do this, Ryle has modified the Rep Grid so that the elements to be rated are not people but relationships between people (e.g., "self [in relation] to mother," or "mother to father"). Each relationship is rated on a set of scales, such as "blames" or "is dependent upon." Thus, the rating of the "self-to-mother" relationship on the "is-dependent-upon" dimension measures the extent to which the patient experiences herself/himself as dependent upon her or his mother. A complete grid is generated, consisting of the patient's ratings of each relationship on each scale. Correlations are then generated between each of the scales.

Ryle has described two types of dilemmas in relationships that can be assessed from this Rep Grid. One type of dilemma, called an if-then dilemma, involves a large correlation between certain scales, indicating that one characteristic of a relationship usually involves the other. For example, a high correlation between "looks after" and "is cross with" indicates a dilemma in which looking after others leads to getting cross with them. The other type of dilemma consists of the "either-or dilemma." This type of problem is indicated by an unusually low correlation between two scales. For example, a very low correlation between "looks after" and "is dependent on" indicates a dilemma of the form "either I look after someone or I am dependent upon that person".

Ryle (1981), using the Rep Grid technique, showed that neurotic patients and normal controls demonstrate the same number of dilemmas. However, the patient's dilemmas were more extreme, as measured by the magnitude of the correlations. This conclusion is consistent with the psychodynamic position that all people have repetitive patterns in relationships but that they become problematic most often when they are associated with a lack of flexibility in relationships, so that the dilemmas predominate, to a great degree, in a person's relations with others.

In other studies, Ryle (1979) has used dilemmas identified by the Rep Grid as the focus for brief psychotherapy and has developed pilot data suggesting that patient improvement is indeed related to modification of the extremity of the patient's dilemmas. Given that the Rep Grid is practically unique as an instrument that is capable of generating a map of a patient's conceptual space, the value of Ryle's operationalization of interpersonal dilemmas, and of other Rep Grid techniques in psychotherapy research (Winter, 1985) deserves further exploration.

Both the CCRT and Ryle's Rep Grid technique have so far only been applied to small numbers of therapy cases. Therefore, they need broader application before their true value as operational measures of repetitive relationship patterns can be determined. However, they are both extremely promising techniques for capturing clinically meaningful constructs in a systematic manner. They both deserve future development by researchers. This research is of such potential interest to clinicians in helping them become aware of and refine the processes whereby they make clinical assessments that it deserves to be closely watched by them.

THERAPEUTIC ALLIANCE AND PATIENT ACTIVITY

One of the central areas of process research in the last decade has concerned the nature of the relationship between the patient and therapist. Based on theoretical work of Rogers (1957), a large body of earlier research had focused on the therapist's contributions to this relationship. Rogers had postulated that the necessary and sufficient conditions for successful psychotherapy were certain facilitative conditions provided by the therapist, including empathy, genuineness, and nonpossessive warmth. Research testing these ideas initially looked promising, as it supported Rogers's position on the importance of these factors for therapeutic outcome. However, later research on this topic, by and large, did not support the Rogerian position (Gurman, 1977). When conflicting results occur in a domain of research, as happens not infrequently, researchers generally have two choices: They can either become very concerned with subtle methodological questions regarding the details of the instruments used to measure the constructs and the design of the studies, or they can lose interest in the research topic and move on to an area that appears more promising.

In the study of the therapeutic relationship, the focus of the research gradually changed focus. In addition to the frequently negative findings of studies of the Rogerian facilitative conditions, another reason for the change of focus seems to be a revival of interest in concepts derived from psychoanalytic and psychodynamic theory after a hiatus in which such work was largely out of the mainstream (Bergin & Strupp, 1972). A central theme of the recent work has been the importance of the therapeutic alliance in psychotherapy. Several psychoanalytic theorists have emphasized that an adequate alliance was a necessary prerequisite for successful dynamic psychotherapy (Greenson, 1967). Exact definitions of the alliance have differed (Bordin, 1979; Frieswyk et al., 1986; Hartley, 1985). Luborsky (1976), for example, identified two broad dimensions or types of alliances. A Type I alliance consists of the sense by the patient that the therapist and the therapy are being helpful. A Type II alliance consists of the actual cooperative working of the patient and therapist. Hartley and Strupp (1983) have identified five aspects of the therapeutic alliance: the real relationship between patient and therapist, the working alliance, the patient's contribution to the alliance, the therapist's contribution to the alliance, and the contribution of the therapeutic situation.

In order to study the therapeutic alliance, techniques are needed for precisely specifying the state of the alliance in a given psychotherapy session. One way to accomplish this task is to ask the opinion of either the patient or the therapist, via questionnaire. This technique has been used by several researchers (e.g., Alexander & Luborsky, 1986; Horvath & Greenberg, 1986; Marmar et al., 1986). Another way of measuring alliance is to develop a rating scale that can be applied to a sample of therapeutic material by independent raters, usually either graduate students or experienced clinicians. The rating scale method has also been used by Alexander and Luborsky (1986) and Marmar et al. (1986) and by Hartley and Strupp (1983). The Vanderbilt University group led by Hans Strupp has also constructed another scale, the Vanderbilt Psychotherapy Process Scale (Gomes-Schwartz, 1978; Gomes-Schwartz & Schwartz, 1978; O'Malley, Suh, & Strupp, 1983; Suh, Strupp, & O'Malley, 1986), which bears a certain resemblance to therapeutic alliance scales and which appears to be developing popularity among researchers. In order to illustrate the nature of these scales, I will discuss Luborsky's Penn Helping Alliance Scale (HA) and the Vanderbilt Scale (VPPS).

The HA scale comes in three forms, a questionnaire, a "counting signs" scale, and a rating scale, all of which are intended to measure the same construct. The rating scale is the form that will be presented here. It consists of 10 separate scales (or items), each of which is to be applied, by an independent, clinically sophisticated rater to either transcripts or tape recordings of portions (usually 20 minutes) of psychotherapy sessions. The items consist of 5 purporting to measure Type I and 4 measuring Type II alliance. Among the Type I items are "the patient feels changed by the treatment" and "the patient conveys a belief in the value of the treatment process in helping him or her to overcome problems" (Alexander & Luborsky, 1986, p. 358). Type II items include "the patient experiences him or herself as working together with the therapist in a joint effort, as part of the same team" and "the patient actually demonstrates abilities similar to those of the therapist, especially with regard to tools for understanding" (pp. 358–359). The items for each type of alliance are summed separately, producing total scores for Type I and Type II alliance (HAI and HAII). The VPPS is a scale that is also intended to be applied by trained clinician raters to taped therapy segments. However, it consists of 80 items, designed to measure several different aspects of the therapeutic relationship. These items were then subjected to principal components analysis (PCA), a statistical technique that helps determine which items covary together, or receive similar ratings, across all the rated therapy segments. The results of the PCA led to the construction of seven subscales, representing different dimensions, or factors, of the therapeutic relationship. These dimensions were "Patient Participation," "Patient Hostility," "Patient Exploration," "Patient Psychic Distress," "Therapist Exploration," "Therapist Warmth and Friendliness," and "Negative Therapist Attitude." A couple of the items from the VPPS are "Spontaneous" from the Patient Participation factor and "Tried to help the patient understand the reasons behind his or her reactions" on the Therapist Exploration factor.

When a clinical rating scale like the HA or VPPS is constructed, the first question to be answered about it concerns its reliability. That is, can two different raters be trained to use it and achieve comparable results (Tinsley & Weiss, 1975)? Reliability is essential because, if two raters cannot agree on its use, then the scale will be unduly influenced by idiosyncrasies of the raters. Both these scales were found to be reliable by the original developers.

After the reliability of a therapy process scale is established, its relationship to therapeutic outcome is usually investigated. Both the HA and the VPPS scales have been shown to be related to therapeutic outcome. In a study by Morgan, Luborsky, Crits-Cristoph, Curtis, and Solomon (1982) of psychodynamic therapy with psychiatric outpatients, the HA scale was the only one of several process instruments that was found to be related to patient outcome. Scales purporting to measure therapist facilitative behaviors, patient resistance, and patient insight did not exhibit any relationship with outcome. The relationship of the alliance to pretreatment psychological severity was also investigated. The HA predicted outcome as well as the best predictors among the pretreatment measures of severity. Furthermore, statistical manipulation (partial correlation) was used to demonstrate that the contribution of HA to outcome was relatively independent of pretreatment severity. Thus this study provides evidence that the therapeutic alliance is, indeed, related to the outcome of psychotherapy.

The VPPS has also been shown to be related to outcome. O'Malley, Suh, and Strupp (1983), in a study of short-term psychodynamic therapy with mildly disturbed student volunteers (Strupp & Hadley, 1979), combined the seven VPPS subscales into three broader dimensions, Patient Involvement, Therapist-Offered Relationship and Exploratory Processes. They use outcome measures from three perspectives, that of the patient, therapist, and independent clinical interviewer. They found that, only the Patient Involvement dimension was related to outcome from all three perspectives, whereas Therapist-Offered Relationship and Exploratory Processes predicted outcome only from the therapist's perspective.

Thus these studies provide evidence suggesting that the quality of the patient's involvement in psychotherapy is an important predictor of therapeutic outcome and that patient involvement may be more important than therapist contributions, at least in terms of the dimensions measured by the HA or VPPS scales. Marmar *et al.* (1986) achieved similar results, using a different measure of therapeutic alliance; in that study as well, the patient's contribution to the formation of an alliance was a much better predictor of outcome than was the therapist's contributions.

However, the study of a research domain is seldom neat and clear. For example, a study of brief dynamic therapy for bereavement reactions (Horowitz, Marmar, Weiss, DeWitt, & Rosenbaum, 1984) found that the relation of patient contributions to alliance and outcome varied depending on the level of patient motivation for therapy. Patient positive contributions to the alliance were positively correlated with outcome for lower levels of motivation and negatively correlated to outcome for patients with higher motivation. The results for patient negative contributions to outcome were the reverse. The authors propose that patients with high motivation need to deal with negative reactions to the therapist when they come up but that patients with low motivation cannot deal therapeutically with this material and need a more positive relationship with the therapist in order to sustain them. Therapist contributions to the alliance were not related to outcome in this study, as in the studies discussed before. Another study by Rounsaville *et al.* (1987), which used the VPPS to examine the relation of process to outcome in a study comparing two styles of therapies with depressed outpatients, the patient VPPS factors were, at best, marginally related to outcome, whereas Therapist Exploration and Therapist Warmth were found to predict patient improvement.

It seems likely that differences in therapies and/or patients may explain some of these discrepancies in results. For example, both the Horowitz *et al.* (1984) and Rounsaville *et al.* (1987) studies involved psychotherapies that are largely structured around particular topics and were delivered to relatively homogeneous patient populations. In contrast, the Morgan *et al.* (1982) and O'Malley *et al.* (1983) studies delivered less structured therapies to more homogeneous patient populations. It is thus possible that there is a simple linear relationship of patient involvement and outcome only for less structured verbal therapies, whereas, in the case of more focal therapies, other process factors may be more prominent. Whether or not these speculations are correct, it is clear that differences in patient populations, therapies, and the exact dimensions of therapeutic process measured by each instrument need to be carefully examined in looking at the relation of process variables to outcome.

THERAPIST INTERVENTIONS: WHAT WORKS?

Previous sections have examined the operational definition of repetitive interpersonal patterns and studies of the general dimensions of the therapy session, including the therapeutic alliance. It was pointed out before that most studies of the general dimensions of the therapy session indicated that patient contributions were more important than therapist contributions in predicting therapeutic outcome. The study by Rousaville *et al.* (1987) contrasted with the general pattern by finding that it was therapist, and not patient factors, that primarily predicted outcome. This study differed from the others cited in that the therapy delivered by the therapists were guided by a detailed treatment manual for short-term Interpersonal Psychotherapy for Depression (Klerman *et al.*, 1984). As Rounsaville *et al.* point out, standardizing the treatment may have allowed the effects of general therapist factors to become apparent.

Other studies have attempted to examine the relation of particular types of therapist interventions to outcome. For example, several studies have tested the psychoanalytic proposition that transference interpretations are particularly effective. An early study by Malan (1976) reported a significant relationship between outcome and the proportion of interpretations that linked the patient's feelings about the therapist to feelings about the parents. Marziali (1984) has replicated this study, but Piper, Debbane, Bienvenu, de Carufel, and Garant (1986) cogently criticized the Malan and Marziali studies on methodological grounds and attempted a replication of their own, finding little evidence of the value of transference interpretations. From a clinical perspective, it should not prove surprising that these studies of therapist interventions provide conflicting results. After all, there is much more to therapeutic technique than the content of the interventions. The context in which interventions are delivered, the "accuracy" of the intervention, and the style in which they are delivered are all relevant considerations. It behooves the researcher to find ways of measuring some of these variables. Several recent studies have developed sophisticated techniques to examine these issues. A couple of them will now be examined.

One of the most interesting programs of research on therapy process in the last several years has been a decade-long effort at Mount Zion Hospital in San Francisco to test a modification of the classical theory of psychoanalytic treatment (Weiss, Sampson, and the Mount Zion Psychotherapy Research Group, 1986; cf. Eagle, 1984; Soldz, 1987b). This theory, called the Higher Mental Functioning hypothesis (HMF), postulates that psychopathology is the result of unconscious pathogenic beliefs on the part of the patient that interfere with patient functioning. In the view of these authors, a patient enters therapy or analysis with an unconscious plan to test out his/her pathogenic beliefs with the hope of disconfirming them. The outcome of the therapy, then, will depend on the degree to which the therapist's interventions are consistent with the patient's plan (Curtis & Silberschatz, 1986; Silberschatz & Curtis, 1986). For example, a male patient may have the unconscious belief that any initiative on his part will be intolerable to his father because it would result in harm or death to the father. The Weiss *et al.* theory postulates that this patient would test the therapist by engaging in independent acts, perhaps by disagreeing with the therapist or by doing things that he believed the therapist might disapprove of, in order to see if assertion produced deleterious effects on the therapist. If the therapist does not appear to be ruffled or disturbed by the patient taking the initiative, the patient's pathogenic belief will be gradually disconfirmed, leading to improved functioning.

It should be noted that this theory differs from other cognitive-dynamic theories (Kelly, 1955; Ryle, 1982; Soldz, 1983, 1986, 1987a,b) in postulating a desire on the part of the patient to get better by disconfirming pathogenic beliefs. Weiss *et al.* are analytically orthodox to the extent that they seem to believe that only interpretive interventions (or therapist silence) will be helpful to the patient in this process. They do agree, however, that the appropriate type of interpretation will vary from patient to patient. Also, there is nothing in their theory that requires that only interpretations be used (Donovan, 1987; Soldz, 1987b). Thus attempts to empirically test this theory require that each patient's plan for testing her/his pathogenic beliefs during treatment be determined and that a technique be found to determine if the therapist's interventions are congruent or incongruent with this plan. Furthermore, a measure (or measures) of therapeutic improvement would be needed.

Unlike many other new theories of psychodynamic treatment, the Weiss *et al.* theory has been subjected to an extensive program of empirical research. These research efforts have so far taken two forms. One is the examination, over a period longer than a decade, of one patient's psychoanalysis (Weiss *et al.*, 1986). The other is a program of research into brief psychodynamic therapy, the results of which are only beginning to be reported (Silberschatz, Fretter, & Curtis, 1986).

The Weiss *et al.* (1986) work consists of a number of studies of a psychoanalytic case that was conducted by an analyst who had never heard of their theory and thus could not have been influenced by it. Weiss *et al.* do not have a systematic process for formulating their understanding of the patient's plan for the treatment. Thus their formulation of this case was generated through examination of the case by experienced clinicians familiar with their theory. Their prediction was that the patient, Mrs. C., "would work to change her pathogenic beliefs about her exaggerated sense of responsibility for others and about her fear of hurting them. . . . She would struggle (especially in relation to the analyst) to change the pathogenic beliefs underlying her separation guilt, survivor guilt, and Oedipal guilt" (p. 162). A contrasting formulation, based on classical psychoanalytic theory—called here the Automatic Functioning hypothesis (AF)—was generated by a group of classically oriented analysts in another city. Much of the Weiss *et al.* book consists of various studies examining the relevance of the HMF theory to the first 100 hours of the case, as represented in transcripts of the sessions, and in detailed process notes.

An illustrative study compared predictions based on the HMF formulation of the case regarding the effect of different analyst responses to the patient's transference demands, with the predictions based on the AF formulation. The HMF hypothesis led to the expectation that the patient's in-session behavior would improve to the degree that the analyst's interventions passed the patient's tests. The AF, in contrast, predicted that process would improve, depending on the degree to which the analyst frustrated the transference demands in a neutral manner. The first step in the study consisted of graduate students identifying, from session transcripts, incidents that involved the patient making demands on the analyst, such as attempts to obtain reassurance, support, advice, or more active participation. Analysts who operate from the AF perspective picked those incidents that appeared to them to be attempts to obtain gratification of central unconscious wishes, whereas HMF analysts picked those that were seen as central tests of the patient's pathogenic belief. The overlapping incidents were rated, by other groups of AF and HMF analysts, on the degree to which the treating analyst behaved in accordance with the rival theories.

In order to determine the effect of the analyst's interventions, the patient's behavior was rated on a variety of research scales before and after the interventions. These scales measured such variables as the quality of the patient's here-and-now experiencing, her boldness (vs. inhibition), her freedom and relaxation in the session, and her level of fear, anxiety, love and satisfaction. The difference between her postintervention and preintervention scores on each of the variables was then correlated with the measures of the analyst's behavior. As the AF and HMF theories made different predictions regarding the direction (+ or −) of each of these correlations, the study provided a direct test of the rival hypotheses. The results were that all of the correlations were in the direction of the HMF hypothesis, and four of these eight correlations were statistically significant. The study thus provided strong evidence in support of the HMF theory, as applied to this patient.

In addition to the psychoanalytic studies of Weiss et al. (1986), the HMF theory has also been tested in a study of brief dynamic psychotherapy. Silberschatz et al. (1986) studied three patients in 16-session dynamic psychotherapy. They were interested in comparing the HMF hypothesis regarding the importance of the plan compatibility of therapist interpretations with the rival hypothesis, based on the work of Malan (1976) and Marziali (1984), emphasizing the importance of transference-focused interpretations. As a measure of the quality of the therapy session at a given moment, they used the Experiencing Scale, which taps such aspects of the process as the patient's insight, productive free association, and lack of resistance. They found no evidence that transference interpretations were connected to improved (pre- to postintervention) therapy process. In fact, for one of the patients improved process was associated with nontransference interpretations to a statistically significant degree. In contrast, the study found a strong relationship between the plan compatibility of the therapist interventions and improvement in therapeutic process for each of the patients.

Though the studies performed to date involve only a small number of patients and therapists, they provide intriguing support for the Weiss et al. theory. Should this theory receive additional empirical support, it could play a profound role in reorienting the thinking of many psychodynamically oriented clinicians (Donovan, 1987; Eagle, 1984; Soldz, 1988a). In addition, the methodologies developed by this research group could be adapted to test other theories of the therapeutic process (Sampson & Weiss, 1986). Indeed, a few other researchers have used methods bearing similarities to those of Weiss, et al. For example, in an intriguing study, Meadow (1974) compared the effectiveness of two types of psychoanalytic interventions, interpretations, and joining/mirroring interventions reflective of the patient's resistant attitudes (Spotnitz, 1985; Spotnitz & Meadow, 1976). When Meadow decided to make an intervention, she picked a ball at random from a bowl by her side; the color of the ball determined which type of intervention she made. The patient's speech after the intervention was recorded and rated by experienced analysts on three scales that measured depth and range of affect, quality of insight, and amount of historical material presented. Her analyses showed that joining/mirroring interventions had a much more powerful effect on patient process on all three dimensions. As Meadow was both researcher and treating analyst, the generalizability of this study to other therapists' work is unclear. However, like that of the Mount Zion group, her methodology deserves emulation by other researchers.

Crits-Cristoph (1987) has conducted a study that parallels that of Silberschatz *et al.* (1986) in examining the effect of accuracy of therapist interpretation on patient outcome. The measure of accuracy used was whether the interpretation focused on the CCRT of the patient. They found that the patient Wish and Reaction of the Other were highly related to outcome, whereas the Reaction of the Self was not related. Thus, this study suggests that simply focusing on the patient's feeling states is not sufficient for successful outcome. Instead, the relationship pattern of Wish and Reaction from Others requires attention if patient improvement is to result. Taken together, the studies discussed in this section provide support for the position that the nature of the therapist's interventions are indeed important for the success of therapy. These studies also illustrate the value of developing measures of the elusive clinical processes occurring during psychotherapy. Earlier studies claiming that what the therapist did made no difference were based on very crude measures of therapist behavior. It makes good clinical sense that it is the appropriateness of the therapists' intervention to the process occurring at a particular moment in the therapy that is of decisive importance for therapeutic change to take place. The studies discussed in this section provide evidence that therapeutic appropriateness can be measured. It is to be hoped that other researchers will build on these methods in order to explore what interventions, with what patients, at what point during treatment, are optimally effective.

BEST–WORST ANALYSIS

Previous sections have examined the nature of the therapeutic interaction from various perspectives. Each of the studies discussed there involved the quantification of some (presumed) clinically relevant aspects of the therapeutic relationship. Although the sympathetic clinician may grant the potential importance of the issues examined in these studies, the methodologies they exhibit will most likely appear somewhat alien to clinical modes of working. Strupp (1980a,b,d), in a set of papers, has attempted to close the gap between the clinician and the formal therapy researcher. In these papers, Strupp has created a new genre, the research-informed case study. Among the 18 patients in the Vanderbilt Psychotherapy Project who had been treated by professional therapists (others were treated by lay counselors), 6 were placed in a high-success and 6 in a low-success group on the basis of outcome measures. Three therapists were selected, and a high- and a low-success patient was chosen for each of these therapists. Strupp undertook intensive analyses of these three pairs. The Strupp analyses combine presentation of quantitative data on the process and outcome of the therapy with clinically informed systematic examination of tape recordings and transcripts of these patients' therapies. Thus, these papers differ from traditional case studies in at least two respects. One is that they incorporate the quantitative data, which provide "objective" support for the clinical interpretations rendered therein. Furthermore, unlike most case studies, these papers do not just present successfully treated cases, with the presumption that the treatment was causally responsible for the improvement. Instead, by contrasting successful with unsuccessful cases, they provide evidence regarding the range of applicability of the techniques utilized by the therapists in the Vanderbilt project.

There are a number of striking differences between the successful and unsuccessful cases presented in the Strupp (1980a,b,d) papers. In each pair, the successfully treated patient continued the treatment until the maximum of 25 sessions (one patient received a few more sessions, due to a crisis), whereas the unsuccessful cases terminated after 12 sessions at the most. Thus the unsuccessful cases received substantially less therapy. The differences in length of therapy was reflective of differences that were apparent almost from the commencement of treatment. Each of the successful cases entered into an easy, cooperative relationship with the therapist from the beginning:

> Almost from the beginning, the patient and therapist appeared to establish a good working relationship, and . . . [the patient] appeared animated and capable of relating comfortably to the therapist as a potential helper. (Strupp, 1980b, p. 710)

> From the beginning, Ernest took an active role and seemed to have little difficulty in relating to the therapist. He was articulate in describing experiences and expressing his feelings. (Strupp, 1980d, p. 949)

> Almost from the beginning, there was evidence of a comfortable, mutually respectful relationship—a good therapeutic or working alliance—which gradually deepened, became more animated and relaxed, and eventually led to genuine affection on the part of both participants. (Strupp, 1980a, p. 597)

The ability of these patients to quickly engage in a positive, cooperative relationship with the therapist appeared to be a continuation of a history of basically positive relationships with others. For example, whereas one of these patients was very upset about the recent breakup with his girlfriend, he expressed warm feelings for the young woman and described their relationship as being basically loving.

In contrast, the unsuccessful patients had difficulties in therapy, almost from the very beginning. Each of the three appeared to be uncomfortable in the therapeutic situation. Each of them manifested what appeared to be characterological behaviors that interfered with their ability to comfortably relate to anyone. For example, one of the patients usually acted like a clown, manifesting a persistent tendency to giggle and joke about all aspects of his life. Another patient exhibited a profound demoralization, describing himself as never being successful with the opposite sex because

girls do not have a good time when they are with him. . . . He seemed to say: 'I have
been hurt and rejected; I deserve to be rejected because I am physically repulsive and
no good; yet I am enraged and will seek revenge by provoking anyone who tries to get
near me.'" (Strupp, 1980b, p. 712)

The therapists in this study were all basically psychodynamic in orientation.
They appeared to use clarification, confrontation, and interpretation as their
primary therapeutic techniques. They applied these techniques to each patient
of the pair they treated. In each pair, the successful case was able to comfortably
use the therapist's interventions to further self-understanding and self-exploration. The unsuccessful cases were not able to use the therapist interventions in a
productive manner. Each of these cases responded to therapeutic interventions
with his habitual style of interacting with others. Thus, in one of these therapies,
interpretations were frequently followed by long pauses and a change of topic to
a peripheral issue. The demoralized patient responded to interventions by asserting his worthlessness, whereas the clown giggled and joked in response to
his therapist's interventions.

The therapists appeared to have difficulty dealing with the unsuccessful
patients' resistant behaviors. They seemed to feel that the patient should respond positively to the therapists' interventions. In some instances the therapists got into arguments with the patients, trying to convince them to change
their attitudes.

A further study by Henry, Schacht, and Strupp (1986) of these same six
patients (plus two others treated by a lay counselor [Strupp, 1980c]) sheds further light on differences in the therapeutic process with successful and unsuccessful cases. In this study, Henry, Schacht, and Strupp used a system for
coding the interpersonal interaction implicit in individual verbal utterances, the
Structural Analysis of Social Behavior (SASB; Benjamin, 1974, 1979). The SASB
involves coding each statement on three dimensions: *focus*, that is, whether the
person is concentrating on Self or Other[1]; *affiliation*, or the degree of friendliness
or hostility; and *interdependence* (vs. independence). For each of the Self or Other
foci, the affiliation and interdependence ratings allow the utterance to be assigned to one of eight clusters. Sample clusters on the Other surface are "ignoring and neglecting," "affirming and understanding," and "helping and protecting." Clusters on the Self surface include "disclosing and expressing," "trusting
and relying," and "walling off and avoiding." As can be seen, in traditional
psychotherapy, the patient is more likely to make utterances with a Self focus,
whereas the therapist is more likely to make Other-focused statements.

In the Henry *et al.* (1986) study, the authors had judges rate the first 150
statements (approximately 15 to 20 minutes) from the third session of each of the
eight therapies under examination. They then looked for differences between
SASB clusters used by therapists and patients in successful and unsuccessful
therapies. They found that therapists made more affirming and understanding
and helping and protecting statements in good outcome cases and more belittling and blaming statements in poor outcome cases. The successful patients

---

[1]In fact, a third focus, Introject, is possible, but little research has used this category.

made many more disclosing and expressing statements, whereas the unsuccessful cases made more trusting and relying and walling off and avoiding utterances. These results generally parallel the differences between successful and unsuccessful cases found by clinical examination of the recorded sessions. An additional aspect highlighted by this SASB analysis is the greater dependency of the poor outcome cases, as manifested by their greater frequency of trusting and relying statements.

The SASB analysis revealed another difference between the two sets of cases. SASB analysis allows for an utterance to be coded into more than one category, representing a complex communication. For example a patient asked the therapist "[in a petulant tone of voice] 'Well, what good is it going to do to say something to her'" (Henry et al., 1986, p. 30). This statement is a question (coded trusting and relying), which is also a protest against a previous therapist statement (coded sulking and appeasing). In this study, virtually all of the complex communications occurred in the poor outcome therapies. In fact, for the unsuccessful patients, 22% of therapist responses and 17% of patient responses were complex communications, whereas the comparable figures for successful patients were 0% and 2%. These results suggest that one characteristic of poor outcome cases is that the patients and therapists talk in a complex, indirect manner, communicating more than one message at a time. Perhaps the indirectness of these communications is an element in the inability of the patients to achieve help in these therapies.

The greater use of complex communications among unsuccessfully treated cases probably also is connected to a difficulty that these patients have with hostility. Although frequently acting in subtly hostile ways, these patients have difficulty being overtly aggressive. In fact, hostility seems to be a major component of these patients' relation with the world, though the hostility often takes the form of "passive–aggressive" behaviors that can be especially problematic for the targets, including, evidently, psychotherapists.

In summary, it appears from this series of studies that the unsuccessful patients differed from the successful ones by having major difficulties in sustaining stable, positive relationships, by being unable to respond positively to therapist interventions, and by being more hostile and indirect in their communications. The therapists were not able to deal successfully with these patient behaviors. They appeared to respond with counterhostility of their own, contributing to an atmosphere of conflict and failure. It is sobering to note Strupp's (1980d) statement that "in our study we failed to encounter a single instance in which a difficult patient's hostility and negativism were successfully confronted or resolved" (p. 954).

CLINICAL REFLECTIONS

Research, like other human activities, is not necessarily transparent. What one makes of it depends on the theories, attitudes, and experiences one brings to its interpretation. Previous sections have reviewed some of the recent research on psychotherapy process. I want now to reflect, as a researcher–clinician, on possible meanings of this body of work. The ideas proposed will go beyond the evidence available and will reflect my personal interests and biases, as well as my interpretations of the meaning of the research.

The case studies of Strupp (1980a,b,d) and the related study of Henry *et al.* (1986) raise important issues regarding which patients can benefit from short-term dynamic psychotherapy as currently practiced. In particular, they raise problematic issues about treatment for patients, who have not had a history of dependable, positive relations with others and who prominently display hostility, passivity, and negativity in the therapeutic relationship. Strupp's statement that "in our study we failed to encounter a single instance in which a difficult patient's hostility and negativism were successfully confronted or resolved" (1980d, p. 954) is particularly disturbing. To my mind, it indicates that the development of successful treatments for these patients is perhaps the major clinical and research challenge facing our field today. I want to explore some suggestive aspects of the research literature that may be relevant to the question of treatment of these especially difficult patients.

Much of the research presented supports the position that general dimensions of the therapeutic relationship, including the therapeutic alliance and the degree and quality of the patient's involvement in the therapeutic relationship, are connected to the outcome of the therapy. In particular, greater patient participation, and lesser hostility, are frequently connected with greater improvement during treatment. As noted, this conclusion was replicated in a number, but not in all, studies.

The results on the relation of therapist factors to outcome are less clear. Several studies found little or no relationship, whereas the Rounsaville *et al.* study (1987) found a fairly strong relationship. One explanation of this discrepancy is that the importance of the therapist's activities depends on exactly what the therapist does and the relevance of these activities to the particular patient and to the interpersonal context occurring at the time of the intervention. In fact, a number of studies demonstrated the importance of therapist interventions. For example, Weiss *et al.* (1986) and Silberschatz *et al.* (1986) showed that the compatibility of the interventions with the patient's unconscious plan for treatment was an important determinant of whether the intervention led to improved patient process. Similarly, Crits-Cristoph (1987) showed that interpretations directly related to the patient's CCRT were more effective than other interpretations. Thus possibly it is the particular aspects of therapist involvement—the right intervention at the right time—rather than more general aspects, such as warmth or empathy—that are especially important. It also seems likely that a major effect of therapist interventions is an improvement in the quality of the patient's participation in the therapy, as demonstrated by Weiss *et al.* (1986), Silberschatz *et al.* (1987), and Meadow (1974).

The work of the Mount Zion Hospital group (Curtis & Silberschatz, 1986; Silberschatz & Curtis, 1986; Silberschatz *et al.*, 1987; Weiss *et al.*, 1986; cf. Soldz,

1987b), even though based on the study of only a few patients, raises issues that may be especially important in thinking about the treatment of difficult patients. Weiss, the theoretician of this group, hypothesized that patients enter therapy with an unconscious plan to disconfirm unconscious pathogenic beliefs developed through relationships in childhood. The patient poses tests for the therapist, in order to determine if the therapist will behave differently than the patient's childhood objects. If the therapist passes these tests, the patient's in-therapy process will improve, leading to improved outcome.

The Weiss theory supports speculation that Strupp's therapists failed to pass tests posed by the difficult patients. Assuming that these therapists were at least reasonably competent, one is led to wonder whether many therapists routinely fail tests posed by their more difficult patients. In other words, therapists, in dealing with hostile patients who have difficulty forming positive cooperative relationships, tend to get inducted into the patient's world in such a way as to reinforce, rather than disconfirm, these patients' pathogenic beliefs. A piece of evidence supporting this position is that the therapists exhibited more hostility and use of complex communications in interacting with these patients than they did with easier cases.

Assuming that these speculations are correct, two contributing factors are suggested by studies discussed in this chapter. As previously mentioned, one factor suggested by the results of the Henry *et al.* (1986) study is that the less successful cases used many more complex communications than did the more successful cases. Perhaps these complex communications make it more difficult for the therapists to understand these patients. Use of these communication patterns may also mean that the more difficult patients have more complex unconscious beliefs; consequently, disconfirming one part of the belief could in fact lead to confirmation of another part. For example, "passive–aggressiveness," as seen in Strupp's unsuccessful cases, may involve a belief that independent initiative by the patient will not be tolerated by others, along with the belief that resistance to the demands of others is essential for maintaining one's identity. Interventions responsive to one part of this complex belief may provide confirmation for the other part.

Another possible contribution to therapists' lack of success with difficult patients may be the therapists' inflexibility. The therapists in Strupp's study attempted to apply very similar techniques to their successful and unsuccessful cases. The successful patients responded positively to this; the others did not. It is possible that the very style of the therapist may lead to the therapist's failing certain patient's tests, regardless of the "correctness" of the therapist's interventions. The unsuccessful patients in the Strupp study did not appear to be able to put their therapists' interpretations to constructive use. In fact, unlike the successful cases, self-understanding did not appear to be helpful in producing change in these patients. The therapists of these patients persisted in trying to foster insight and self-understanding, despite evidence of its lack of utility for these patients. Strupp described the attitude of one highly experienced therapist as follows:

> He said, albeit implicitly, to both patients: I am the kind of person and therapist that I am; I use certain techniques [aimed at fostering insight], which I have practiced for a quarter of a century; I am convinced they work; I interact with patients in a particular professional manner and I do not go out of my way to behave differently, I am ready and willing to listen, question, clarify, and interpret; if you can use this approach for your purposes, fine, but I am not prepared to make compromises. (1980a, p. 602)

If, as suggested, dynamic psychotherapists frequently fail their more impaired patients by insisting on using an approach overly oriented toward producing self-understanding, the question arises as to what alternatives exist for treatment of these patients. One possibility is that these patients cannot be treated in short-term therapy and need long-term, intensive treatment where all of the complexities of their complex pathogenic beliefs can be worked out. This position may ultimately be correct. But the fact that all of Strupp's unsuccessful cases prematurely terminated suggests that, for many such patients, long-term treatment of the traditional variety is out of the question. Thus it seems imperative to search for alternative approaches, whether they be applied in short- or long-term treatments.

The same difficulties in forming positive, cooperative relationships that these difficult patients demonstrate in short-term dynamic treatments would likely interfere with their successful participation in some alternative treatments, such as cognitive or behavior therapy, which require the patient to carry out homework assignments in order to fully function. Group therapy is an alternative that is worth exploring. There are suggestions in the clinical literature that group treatment may be successful for some patients who cannot be successfully treated in traditional individual therapy (Budman & Gurman, 1988).

However, there are alternative approaches arising out of the psychodynamic and psychoanalytic traditions that are designed explicitly for the treatment of these patients (Kohut, 1977; Soldz, 1986, 1987a; Spotnitz, 1985; Wolberg, 1973). Although these approaches differ in their details, they all share the presupposition that therapeutic interventions are, among other things, emotional communications to the patient. Thus it is the emotional impact in making the patient feel accepted and understood that is primary, rather than its function in providing correct self-understanding. Another aspect of these therapeutic approaches is that they carefully avoid interventions that lead to premature invalidation of the patient's way of perceiving and making sense out of the world (Soldz, 1983). The assumption is made that these patient's need to cling to their pathogenic ways of seeing the world because they have little alternative psychic structure available to fall back on. Therapy needs to build up an alternative structure before gradually disconfirming the pathogenic beliefs.

There has so far been little research on these alternative therapeutic approaches, though the results of Meadow (1974) are supportive of the position that alternative interventions may be more effective than classical interpretations in furthering the therapeutic process. Given the importance of developing effective treatments for the more difficult patients, it would seem important that research efforts be made to evaluate the possible utility of these techniques and to understand their modes of therapeutic action.

INTEGRATION OF RESEARCH PERSPECTIVE INTO CLINICAL PRACTICE

In addition to using the results of research studies to guide clinical decisions and to suggest areas needing greater attention from clinicians, another aspect of the integration of clinical practice and psychotherapy process research consists of the integration of research instruments and perspectives by the therapist. This is an area that has received little attention from psychodynamically oriented clinicians. From Freud on, therapists have continually claimed that the therapeutic situation is also a research situation. Dynamic therapists have, however, done little to elaborate this perspective.

The behaviorists, in contrast, have systematically integrated research methodologies for investigating the change processes in their patients (Barlow & Hersen, 1984; Barlow, Hayes, & Nelson, 1984). They have developed a number of techniques for studying change in single cases. Although most of these methodologies cannot be directly adapted to the usual dynamic therapies, where treatment cannot usually be conceptualized as consisting of a few discrete interventions, the general idea of integrating research into clinical work can certainly be adapted. Many of the studies discussed in this chapter contain instruments and ideas that can be adapted for this purpose.

Perhaps the easiest way to integrate research materials into the clinical situation would be for the therapist to use some of the new instruments developed for assessing difficulties in relationship patterns. Both the Rep Grid and the CCRT are attempts to systemize the usual forms of clinical inference that presumably occur in the clinical situation. The advantage of using these measures to supplement clinical intuition is that they are more systematic, perhaps helping the therapist to overcome blind spots. Furthermore, these instruments can be used to assess change over the course of psychotherapy. The Rep Grid, in particular, has a long tradition of being used by clinicians to measure change in their patients (Beail, 1985; Neimeyer & Neimeyer, 1987; Ryle, 1975). It has the advantage of being easily adaptable to address a wide variety of clinical questions. Interpretation of the Rep Grid can be done on a qualitative basis, but a computer analysis is very helpful.[2]

The CCRT could also be useful for clinicians to use in determining their patients' repetitive relationship patterns. One could analyze either detailed process notes or tape recordings of therapy sessions in which patients discussed their relations with others. This process could be especially useful for use in supervision to train new therapists to recognize repetitive patterns. Luborsky (1984) has incorporated an informal evaluation of the CCRT into his manual for

---

[2]Fortunately, software for conducting most of the common analyses can be obtained free from Chambers and Grice (1986).

supportive–expressive psychotherapy. There is no reason why this incorporation could not be more formal. The techniques developed for using the CCRT as
a measure of change in therapy could then be adapted by therapists for incorporation into their practice.

The measures of the therapeutic alliance could also be used by therapists to
investigate their own treatment. Several of these instruments have been adapted
to assess the therapist's (and patient's) perspectives on treatment. Therapists
could complete these instruments after each session. Patients could fill out the
analogous set of forms. Therapists could then examine, with colleagues, process
notes of those sessions in which the alliance showed an increase or decrease in
strength. Sessions in which the patients and therapists had differing opinions
could also usefully be examined in order to determine what factors influence the
judgments of each of the participants.

A third way that research perspectives could be integrated into the clinical
situation would be for a therapist to adapt some of the techniques developed by
researchers for the investigation of one, or a small number of cases. For example,
Weiss *et al.*'s (1986) techniques for the study of a single case by examining
change in patient process following therapist interventions of a particular type
could easily be adapted by any therapist who has detailed process notes or tape
recordings available of his/her therapy sessions with a patient. One could either
use the scales that were developed by Weiss *et al.* (their book contains a number
of these as appendixes) or could develop new scales to assess the dimensions
believed to be of clinical interest in the particular case under investigation. The
Meadow (1974) method of studying the influence on patients of two different
types of therapist interventions could also easily be adapted by clinicians.

A study of Hill, Carter, and O'Farrell (1983a; cf. Hill, Carter, & O'Farrell,
1983b; Howard, 1983; Lambert, 1983) provides an interesting example for clinician–researchers to follow. A student volunteer patient was treated by the senior author. The patient completed several outcome instruments before and
after therapy, and at 2 and 7 months after termination. Therapy Session Reports
(Orlinksy & Howard, 1986) were completed by patient and therapist after each
session. Each session was also tape-recorded; the recordings were transcribed
and rated on several content dimensions, measuring anxiety and activity levels
of both participants, the type of verbal response used by patient and therapist
(Hill, 1986), and the therapist's intentions. The relation of therapist interventions to patient process could be examined. One particularly interesting finding
was that the patient's style of using objective description of events appeared to
interfere with the deepening of the therapeutic process. Furthermore, a comparison of the best and worst sessions (as rated by patient and therapist) indicated that the patient engaged in more objective description, whereas the therapist exhibited less variability in behavior during the worst sessions. Perhaps
objective description should be added to hostility as a resistance that requires
flexibility on the part of the therapist. In any event, this case study provides yet
another model of what can be accomplished by systematic research on individual cases.

Finally, the Strupp strategy of systematically examining differences between successful and unsuccessful cases could also be adapted by clinicians. As long as detailed data are available, research groups could be formed in which each member selects a patient from each category. The group could then systematically examine the cases, looking for similarities and differences. The Rep Grid could be adapted by such groups to help systemize their perceptions of the nature of the differences and to compare whether different therapists perceive patient similarities and differences in related ways (Walton & McPherson, 1968).

The different strategies mentioned here for integrating a research approach with clinical work constitute just a few of those possible. Dies and MacKenzie (1983) discuss several such ideas for group psychotherapists that can easily be adapted for application to other forms of therapies. One aspect that all such strategies have in common is that they are probably best engaged in with a group of similarly interested colleagues. An additional advantage of this approach is that it can serve to counteract some of the loneliness that often afflicts therapists. Furthermore, the attempt to precisely codify clinical intuitions that the research process requires can help clinicians become more aware of the implicit assumptions that underlie their work. It can also reinforce a sense of humility about the complexity of human beings and their interactions, counteracting some of the grandiose fantasies of omniscience that therapeutic work can induce in therapists.

ACKNOWLEDGMENT. I would like to thank Simon Budman and Michael Davis for their comments on this chapter. Writing of this paper was aided by the Research Training Program in Social and Behavioral Sciences, National Institute of Mental Health grant MH14246, and by the Mental Health Research Program, Harvard Community Health Plan.

REFERENCES

Alexander, L. B., & Luborsky, L. (1986). The Penn Helping Alliance Scales. In L. S. Greenberg & W. M. Pinsof (Eds.), *The psychotherapeutic process* (pp. 325–366). New York: Guilford.

Barlow, D. H., Hayes, S. C., & Nelson, R. O. (1984). *The scientist practitioner.* New York: Pergamon.

Barlow, D. H., & Hersen, M. (1984). *Single case experimental designs* (2nd ed.). New York: Pergamon.

Beail, N. (Ed.). (1985). *Repertory grid technique and personal constructs.* Cambridge, MA: Brookline Books.

Beck, A., Rush, A. J., Shaw, B. F., & Emery, G. (1979). *Cognitive therapy of depression.* New York: Guilford.

Benjamin, L. S. (1974). The Structural Analysis of Social Behavior. *Psychological Review, 81,* 506–520.

Benjamin, L. S. (1979). Use of Structural Analysis of Social Behavior (SASB) and Markov chains to study dyadic interactions. *Journal of Abnormal Psychology, 88,* 303–319.

Bergin, A. E., & Strupp, H. H. (Eds.). (1972). *Changing frontiers in the science of psychotherapy.* Chicago: Aldine.

Bordin, E. (1979).The generalizability of the psychoanalytic concept of the working alliance. *Psychotherapy: Theory, Research and Practice, 16,* 252–260.

Budman, S. H. (Ed.). (1981). *Forms of brief therapy.* New York: Guilford.

Budman, S. H. (1987). *Time-limited group therapy for personality disorders: A preliminary treatment manual.* Unpublished manuscript. Harvard Community Health Plan, Boston, MA.

Budman, S. H., & Gurman, A. S. (1988). *The theory and practice of brief therapy.* New York: Guilford.

Budman, S. H., & Stone, J. (1983). Advances in brief psychotherapy: A review of recent literature. *Hospital and Community Psychiatry, 34*, 939–946.

Chambers, W. V., & Grice, J. W. (1986). Circumgrids: A repertory grid package for personal computers. *Behavioral Research Methods, 18*, 468.

Crits-Cristoph, P. (1987, June). *How well does "accuracy of interpretation" predict the patient's benefits in psychotherapy?* Paper presented at the Society for Psychotherapy Research, Ulm, F. R. G.

Curtis, J. T., & Silberschatz, G. (1986). Clinical implications of research on brief dynamic psychotherapy I: Formulating the patient's problems and goals. *Psychoanalytic Psychology, 3*, 13–25.

Dies, R. R., & MacKenzie, K. R. (Eds.). (1983). *Advances in group psychotherapy*. New York: International Universities Press.

Donovan, J. M. (1987). Brief dynamic psychotherapy: Toward a more comprehensive model. *Psychiatry, 50*, 167–183.

Eagle, M. N. (1984). *Recent developments in psychoanalysis*. New York: McGraw-Hill.

Epstein, L., & Feiner, A. H. (1983). *Countertransference*. New York: Jason Aronson.

Eysenck, H. J. (1952). The effects of psychotherapy: An evaluation. *Journal of Consulting Psychology, 16*, 319–324.

Fransella, F., & Bannister, D. (1977). *A manual for repertory grid technique*. London: Academic.

Frieswyk, S. H., Allen, J. G., Colson, D. B., Coyne, L., Gabbard, G. O., Horowitz, L., & Newsom, G. (1976). Therapeutic alliance: Its place as a process and outcome variable in dynamic psychotherapy research. *Journal of Consulting and Clinical Psychology, 54*, 32–38.

Gomes-Schwartz, B. (1978). Effective ingredients in psychotherapy: Prediction of outcome from process variables. *Journal of Consulting and Clinical Psychology, 46*, 1023–1035.

Gomes-Schwartz, B., & Schwartz, J. M. (1978). *Journal of Consulting and Clinical Psychology, 46*, 196–197.

Greenson, R. R. (1967). *The technique and practice of psychoanalysis*. New York: International Universities Press.

Gurman, A. S. (1977). The patient's perception of the therapeutic relationship. In A. S. Gurman, & A. M. Razin (Eds.), *Effective psychotherapy* (pp. 503–543). New York: Pergamon.

Hartley, D. E. (1985). Research on the therapeutic alliance in psychotherapy. In R. Hales, & A. Frances (Eds.), *Psychiatry update. American Psychiatric Association Annual Review*. Vol. 4 (pp. 532–549). Washington: American Psychiatric Association.

Hartley, D. E., & Strupp, H. H. (1983). The therapeutic alliance: Its relationship to outcome in brief psychotherapy. In J. Masling (Ed.), *Empirical studies of psychoanalytic theories*, Vol. 1 (pp. 1–37). Hillsdale, NJ: Analytic Press.

Henry, W. P., Schacht, T. E., & Strupp, H. H. (1986). Structural Analysis of Social Behavior: Application to a study of interpersonal process in differential psychotherapeutic outcome. *Journal of Consulting and Clinical Psychology, 54*, 27–31.

Hill, C. E. (1986). An overview of the Hill Counselor and Client Verbal Response Modes Category Systems. In L. S. Greenberg & W. M. Pinsof (Eds.), *The psychotherapeutic process* (pp. 131–159). New York: Guilford.

Hill, C. E., Carter, J. A., & O'Farrell, M. K. (1983a). A case study of the process and outcome of time-limited counseling. *Journal of Counseling Psychology, 30*, 3–18.

Hill, C. E., Carter, J. A., & O'Farrell, M. K. (1983b). Reply to Howard and Lambert: Case Study Methodology. *Journal of Counseling Psychology, 30*, 26–30.

Horvath, A. O., & Greenberg, L. (1986). The development of the working alliance inventory. In L. S. Greenberg & W. M. Pinsof (Eds.), *The psychotherapeutic process* (pp. 529–556). New York: Guilford.

Horowitz, M. J., Marmar, C., Weiss, D., DeWitt, K. N., & Rosenbaum, R. (1984). Brief psychotherapy of bereavement reactions: The relationship of process to outcome. *Archives of General Psychiatry, 41*, 438–448.

Howard, G. S. (1983). Toward methodological pluralism. *Journal of Counseling Psychology, 30*, 19–21.

Kaltreider, N. B., DeWitt, K. N., Weiss, D. S., & Horowitz, M. J. (1981). Patterns of individual change scales. *Archives of General Psychiatry, 38*, 1263–1269.

Kelly, G. (1955). *Psychology of personal constructs*. New York: Norton.

Kiesler, D. J. (1973). *The process of therapy*. Chicago: Aldine.

Klerman, G. L., Weissman, M. M., Rounsaville, B. J., & Chevron, E. S. (1984). *Interpersonal psychotherapy of depression.* New York: Basic.

Kohut, H. (1977). *The restoration of the self.* New York: International Universities Press.

Labov, W., & Fanshel, D. (1977). *Therapeutic discourse.* New York: Academic Press.

Lambert, M. J. (1983). Comments on "A case study of the process and outcome of time-limited counseling." *Journal of Counseling Psychology, 30,* 22–25.

Lambert, M. J., Christensen, E. R., & DeJulio, S. S. (1983). *The assessment of psychotherapy outcome.* New York: Wiley.

Lambert, M. J., Shapiro, D. A., & Bergin, A. E. (1986). The effectiveness of psychotherapy. In A. E. Bergin & S. L. Garfield (Eds.), *Handbook of psychotherapy and behavior change* (3rd ed., pp. 157–211). New York: Wiley.

Levine, F., & Luborsky, L. (1981). The core conflictual relationship theme method—A demonstration of reliable clinical inferences by the method of mismatched cases. In S. Tuttman, C. Kaye, & M. Zimmerman (Eds.), *Object and self: A developmental approach* (pp. 501–526). New York: International Universities Press.

Landfield, A. W., & Epting, F. R. (1987). *Personal construct psychology.* New York: Human Sciences Press.

Luborsky, L. (1972). Research cannot yet influence clinical practice. In A. E. Bergin & H. H. Strupp (Eds.), *Changing frontiers in the science of psychotherapy* (pp. 120–127). Chicago: Aldine.

Luborsky, L. (1976). Helping alliances in psychotherapy: The groundwork for a study of their relationship to outcome. In J. L. Claghorn (Ed.), *Successful psychotherapy* (pp. 92–116). New York: Bruner/Mazel.

Luborsky, L. (1977). Measuring a pervasive psychic structure in psychotherapy: The core conflictual relationship theme. in N. Freedman & S. Grand (Eds.), *Communicative structures and psychic structures* (pp. 367–395). New York: Plenum Press.

Luborsky, L. (1984). *Principles of psychoanalytic psychotherapy.* New York: Basic.

Luborsky, L., Singer, B., & Luborsky, L. (1975). Comparative studies of psychotherapies: Is it true that "Everyone has won and all must have prizes?" *Archives of General Psychiatry, 32,* 995–1008.

Luborsky, L., Mellon, J., Cohen, K. D., van Ravenswaay, P., Hole, A. V., Childress, A. R., Ming, S., Crits-Cristoph, P., Levine, F. J., & Alexander, K. (1985). A verification of Freud's grandest clinical hypothesis: The transference. *Clinical Psychology Review, 5,* 231–246.

Luborsky, L., Crits-Cristoph, P., & Mellon, J. (1986). Advent of objective measures of the transference concept. *Journal of Consulting and Clinical Psychology, 54,* 39–47.

Malan, D. H. (1976). *Toward the validation of dynamic psychotherapy.* New York: Plenum Press.

Malan, D. H. (1979). *Individual psychotherapy and the science of psychodynamics.* London: Butterworths.

Marmar, C. R., Horowitz, M. J., Weiss, D. S., & Marziali, E. (1986). In L. S. Greenberg & W. M. Pinsof (Eds.), *The psychotherapeutic process* (pp. 367–390). New York: Guilford.

Marziali, E. A. (1984). Prediction of outcome of brief psychotherapy from therapist interpretive interventions. *Archives of General Psychiatry, 41,* 301–304.

Meadow, P. W. (1974). A research methodology for investigating the effectiveness of psychoanalytic techniques. *Psychoanalytic Review, 61,* 79–94.

Morgan, R., Luborsky, L., Crits-Critstoph, P., Curtis, H., & Solomon, J. (1982). Predicting the outcomes of psychotherapy by the Penn Helping Alliance Rating Method. *Archives of General Psychiatry, 39,* 397–402.

Neimeyer, G., & Neimeyer, R. (Eds.). (1987). *Personal construct therapy casebook.* New York: Springer.

O'Malley, S. S., Suh, C. S., & Strupp, H. H. (1983). The Vanderbilt Psychotherapy Process Scale: A report on the scale development and a process-outcome study. *Journal of Consulting and Clinical Psychology, 51,* 581–586.

Orlinsky, D. E., & Howard, K. I. (1986a). Process and outcome in psychotherapy. In A. E. Bergin & S. L. Garfield (Eds.), *Handbook of psychotherapy and behavior change* (3rd ed., pp. 311–381). New York: Wiley.

Orlinsky, D. E., & Howard, K. I. (1986b). The psychosocial interior of psychotherapy: Exploration with the therapy session reports. In L. S. Greenberg & W. M. Pinsoff (Eds.), *The psychotherapeutic process: A research handbook* (pp. 477–501). New York: Guilford Press.

Piper, W. E., Debbane, E. G., Bienvenu, J.-P., de Carufel, F., & Garant, J. (1986). Relationships between the object focus of therapist interpretations and outcome in short-term individual psychotherapy. *British Journal of Medical Psychology, 59,* 1–11.

Prioleau, L., Murdock, M., & Brody, N. (1983). An analysis of psychotherapy versus placebo studies. *Behavioral and Brain Sciences, 6,* 275–310.

Rogers, C. R. (1957). The necessary and sufficient conditions of therapeutic personality change. *Journal of Counseling Psychology, 21,* 95–103.

Rounsaville, B. J., Chevron, E. S., Prusoff, B. A., Elkin, I., Imber, S., Sotsky, S., & Watkins, J. (1987). The relation between specific and general dimensions of the psychotherapy process in interpersonal psychotherapy of depression. *Journal of Consulting and Clinical Psychology, 55,* 379–384.

Ryle, A. (1975). *Frames and cages.* New York: International Universities Press.

Ryle, A. (1979). Defining goals and assessing change in brief psychotherapy: A pilot study using target ratings and the dyad grid. *British Journal of Medical Psychology, 52,* 223–233.

Ryle, A. (1980). Some measures of goal attainment in focused integrated active psychotherapy: A study of fifteen cases. *British Journal of Psychiatry, 137,* 475–486.

Ryle, A. (1981). Dyad grid dilemmas in patients and control subjects. *British Journal of Medical Psychology, 54,* 353–358.

Ryle, A. (1982). *Psychotherapy: A cognitive integration of theory and practice.* New York: Grune & Stratton.

Sampson, H., & Weiss, J. (1986). Testing hypotheses: The approach of the Mount Zion Psychotherapy Research Group. In L. S. Greenberg & W. M. Pinsof (Eds.), *The psychotherapeutic process* (pp. 591–613). New York: Guilford.

Seitz, P. (1966). The consensus problem in psychoanalytic research. In L. A. Gottschalk & A. H. Auerbach (Eds.), *Methods of research in psychotherapy* (pp. 209–225). New York: Appleton-Century-Crofts.

Silberschatz, G., & Curtis, J. T. (1986). Clinical implications of research on brief dynamic psychotherapy II: How the therapist helps or hinders therapeutic progress. *Psychoanalytic Psychology, 3,* 27–37.

Silberschatz, G., Fretter, P. B., & Curtis, J. T. (1986). How do interpretations influence the process of psychotherapy? *Journal of Consulting and Clinical Psychology, 54,* 646–652.

Smith, M. L., Glass, G. V., & Miller, T. I. (1980). *The benefits of psychotherapy.* Baltimore: Johns Hopkins University Press.

Soldz, S. (1983, June). *Hostility and the severely disturbed personality: Clinical considerations.* Paper presented at the Fifth International Congress on Personal Construct Psychology, Boston, MA.

Soldz, S. (1986). Construing of others in psychotherapy: Personal construct perspectives. *Journal of Contemporary Psychotherapy, 16,* 52–61.

Soldz, S. (1987a). The flight from relationship: Personal construct reflections on psychoanalytic therapy. In G. Neimeyer & R. Neimeyer (Eds.), *Personal construct therapy casebook* (pp. 76–89). New York: Springer.

Soldz, S. (1987b). Review of J. Weiss, H. Sampson, and the Mount Zion Hospital Psychotherapy Research Group. *The psychoanalytic process. Modern Psychoanalysis, 12,* 108–113.

Soldz, S. (1988a). Constructs and construers. *International Journal of Personal Construct Psychology, 1,* 119–121.

Soldz, S. (1988b). Constructivist trends in recent psychoanalysis. *International Journal of Personal Construct Psychology, 1,* 329–347.

Spotnitz, H. (1985). *Modern psychoanalysis of the schizophrenic patient* (2nd ed.). New York: Human Sciences Press.

Spotnitz, H., & Meadow, P. W. (1976). *Treatment of the narcissistic neuroses.* New York: Manhattan Center for Advanced Psychoanalytic Studies.

Stiles, W. B., Shapiro, D. A., & Elliott, R. (1986). "Are all psychotherapies equivalent?" *American Psychologist, 41,* 165–180.

Strupp, H. H. (1980a). Success and failure in time-limited psychotherapy: A systematic comparison of two cases (Comparison 1). *Archives of General Psychiatry, 37,* 595–603.

Strupp, H. H. (1980b). Success and failure in time-limited psychotherapy: A systematic comparison of two cases (Comparison 2). *Archives of General Psychiatry, 37,* 708–716.

Strupp, H. H. (1980c). Success and failure in time-limited psychotherapy: A systematic comparison of two cases (Comparison 3). *Archives of General Psychiatry, 37,* 831–841.

Strupp, H. H. (1980d). Success and failure in time-limited psychotherapy: A systematic comparison of two cases (Comparison 4). *Archives of General Psychiatry, 37,* 947–954.

Strupp, H. H., & Binder, J. L. (1984). *Psychotherapy in a new key.* New York: Basic.

Strupp, H. H., & Hadley, S. (1979). Specific versus nonspecific factors in psychotherapy: A controlled study of outcome. *Archives of General Psychiatry, 36,* 1125–1136.

Suh, C. S., Strupp, H. H., & O'Malley, S. S. (1986). The Vanderbilt process measures: The Psychotherapy Process Scale (VPPS) and the Negative Indicators Scale (VNIS). In L. S. Greenberg & W. M. Pinsof (Eds.), *The psychotherapeutic process* (pp. 285–323). New York: Guilford.

Tinsley, H. E. A., & Weiss, D. J. (1975). Interrater reliability and the agreement of subjective judgments. *Journal of Counseling Psychology, 22,* 358–376.

Walton, H. J., & McPherson, F. W. (1968). Phenomena in a closed psychotherapeutic group. *British Journal of Medical Psychology, 41,* 61–72.

Waskow, I. E., & Parloff, M. B. (Eds.). (1975). *Psychotherapy change measures.* Rockville, MD: Department of Health, Education and Welfare.

Weiss, J., & Sampson, H., and the Mount Zion Psychotherapy Research Group. (1986). *The psychoanalytic process.* New York: Guilford.

Winter, D. A. (1985). Repertory grid technique in the evaluation of therapeutic outcome. In N. Beail (Ed.), *Repertory grid technique and personal constructs.* Cambridge, MA: Brookline Books.

Wolberg, A. R. (1973). *The borderline patient.* New York: International Medical Book Corporation.

3

An Integrative Model for Short-Term Treatment

William J. Reid

Approaches to interpersonal helping continue to proliferate with literally hundreds of overlapping and competing models currently on the clinical scene. Although therapists, researchers, and clinicians have striven diligently to identify which models may be best suited for which clients, problems, and so forth, these efforts have as yet produced little that is definitive, at least little that is backed by persuasive evidence. These developments have sparked a continuing movement toward eclecticism in practice as well as the rise of "integrative" practice models. The essential function of integrative models is to provide ways of synthesizing this diversity for purposes of practice, training, and research. Although the syntheses they offer are inevitably partial and selective, they can present theoretical horizons and technical combinations not found in single models.

A number of short-term integrative approaches have been developed (Gurman, 1981; Reid & Epstein, 1972; Reid, 1978, 1985; Segraves, 1982, Chapter 18 this volume; Wells, 1982; White, Burke, & Havens, 1981; Szapocznik *et al.*, Chapter 5 this volume). These models reflect a variety of integrative strategies including frameworks for matching types of clients to specific models (White *et al.*, 1983), combining different theoretical perspectives and interventions methods within a single approach (Reid, 1978; Segraves, 1982, Chapter 18 this volume; Szapocznik *et al.*, Chapter 5 this volume; Wells, 1982) and the construction of therapeutic systems encompassing individual, family, and group approaches (Reid, 1978). A major emphasis in this body of work has been the synthesis of different theoretical approaches, especially psychodynamic, behavioral, and cognitive schools.

In this chapter, I will present an integrative model that utilizes a variety of perspectives—problem solving, psychodynamic, behavioral, cognitive, and structural—and presents a single framework for guiding work with individuals,

William J. Reid • School of Social Welfare, Rockefeller College of Public Policy and Affairs and Policy, State University of New York at Albany, Albany, New York 12222.

families, and groups. In presenting the model, I shall give attention to integrative strategies and features that may have value in the development of pluralistic practice.

HISTORICAL DEVELOPMENT AND EVOLUTION

The task-centered approach grew out of a psychodynamic short-term model of clinical social work developed in the early 1960s. This model, which provided eight weekly sessions, was compared in a randomized experiment with long-term, open-ended treatment within the same theoretical orientation, with results that actually favored the shorter service even when the findings of a 6-month follow-up were taken into account (Reid & Shyne, 1969).

In implementing the short-term service, practitioners had made use of a strategy in which they focused on key problems early in the case, developed shared, specific goals with clients and actively helped clients achieve them—a strategy common to many brief treatment approaches. This promising service model was used as a base for developing the task-centered approach. The experiment had suggested that the brief treatment, although comparing favorably to longer term service, still left considerable room for improvement, especially in the degree of change achieved in the client's problems. Moreover, what appeared to be strengths of the model (e.g., focus on specific goals) had been more the result of an imposition of durational limits than the product of a well-articulated design.

Using this psychodynamic model as a base, the author, in collaboration with Laura Epstein, attempted to develop a more systematic, effective brief treatment design, one with its own theoretical framework but still open to concepts and methods from other approaches (Reid & Epstein, 1972).

In constructing this model, emphasis was placed on specific, client-perceived problems and actions or tasks clients could carry out to alleviate these problems (Reid & Epstein, 1972). The model was appropriately called "task-centered" in as much as helping clients plan and achieve these tasks became the main focus of treatment. Whatever appeared to be needed and to be effective in facilitating the client's task work was brought to bear. Straightforward problem-solving, cognitive restructuring, crisis intervention, behavioral techniques, and intervention in the ecosystem eventually supplanted reliance on psychodynamic methods, which increasingly were relegated to a supplementary role. As the model evolved, much of the variation in practice related to the orientation of the practitioner. In a conference held in the mid-1970s, reports of task-centered projects from various parts of the country and abroad spanned a range of intervention methodologies from the psychodynamic to the behavioral (Reid & Epstein, 1977). Both the conference and the model itself provided a way for clinicians with differing points of view to clarify their differences and more importantly to discover common ground in their values and methods.

Additional sources of variation have involved practice setting and modality. Modalities for work with individuals, families, and formed groups have been developed for a wide range of settings including child welfare (Rzepnicki, 1985;

Rooney, 1981; Salmon, 1977), public social services (Rooney & Wanless, 1985; Rooney, 1988), school social work (Epstein, 1977; Reid *et al.*, 1980), corrections (Bass, 1977; Goldberg & Stanley, 1978; Hofstad, 1977; Larsen & Mitchell, 1980), industrial (Taylor, 1977; Weissman, 1977), geriatric (Cormican, 1977; Dierking, Brown, & Fortune, 1980; Rathbone-McCuan, 1985), medical (Wexler, 1977), family service (Hari, 1977; Reid, 1977; Wise, 1977), and mental health (Brown, 1977; Ewalt, 1977; Newcome, 1985).

Basic Concepts and Principles

These variations in orientation, setting, and modality have been bound together by a number of central ideas, which have evolved over time. A current summary follows.

Problem Focus

The main thrust of the model is to help people resolve a limited number of specific, explicit problems that practitioners and clients agree will be the focus of work. Although the definition of these problems may change as the case proceeds, care is taken to keep focus on explicit client-acknowledged problems rather than on what the practitioner may see as the "real" problem underlying them. Avoided is drift into problem areas that may reflect the client's momentary or tangential concerns. Although emergencies are dealt with as they arise, there is no expectation that treatment can accommodate all the client's concerns.

Context

Problems occur in a context of individual, family, and environmental systems that may block or facilitate their resolution. Change in the problem may bring about, or require, contextual change that may have benefits for clients beyond resolution of the target problems. Further, context is viewed in terms of a hierarchy of multiple systems (Tomm, 1982) that enables practitioners to shift focus of attention from one system to another—for example, from individuals to families—thereby avoiding unproductive lock-ins to particular systems.

Problem-Solving and Action

The human being is viewed optimistically as possessing inherent capacities for resolving problems of living or at least reducing them to a tolerable level. Although these capacities are often blocked or utilized in nonconstructive directions, they can be nurtured and channeled. If so, they may be more potent in effecting meaningful problem change than solutions generated by professional helpers. Change is then brought about primarily through problem-solving activities within and outside the session. Engagement of clients in problem solving is a central strategy of the model. Although its main purpose is to help clients resolve specified problems, it also aims to strengthen the client's problem-solving capacities and skills. Tasks are structured forms of problem-solving action that give focus and direction to the client's problem-solving work.

Problem solving is viewed broadly as goal-directed responses to resolve a difficulty. This process needs to be understood at both the individual and social system levels: in terms of the person's wants (motives), cognitions, emotions, and actions, and in terms of the interactional properties of the social systems in which the problems are embedded. Moreover, these processes need to be understood as they generally play themselves out in peoples' efforts to deal with their difficulties rather than in terms of the reconstructed logic of formal problem-solving schemes.

Collaborative Relationship

Client problem solving is facilitated by a collaborative and caring relationship. The practitioner is open and aboveboard about the purposes and nature of service, eschewing hidden agendas and deceptive maneuvers. To the extent possible, she or he shares her/his thinking about assessment and about intervention strategy with the client. Although she/he provides expert knowledge, she/he does so in a way to inform and educate clients rather than direct them. Considerable value is placed on the client's own problem-solving initiatives that are assiduously cultivated. Intervention in the client's life is sanctioned by an explicit agreement with the client on target problems to be dealt with and on the nature of service. Although this position rules out the imposition of unwanted help, it by no means rules out work with "nonvoluntary clients" or "mandated" problems. Even if help was not initially requested, practitioners and clients can often agree on a basis for working together (Rooney, 1981; Rzepnicki, 1985; Epstein, 1988).

Structure

From the initial phase through termination, the model proceeds in a series of well-defined steps. This structure enables practitioners to move ahead systematically and to retrace steps as a means of pinpointing shortfalls and wrong turns. For example, if clients are unable to complete tasks, obstacles are taken up, and an effort is made to resolve them; if this fails, then the practitioner and client consider whether or not the problem definition itself makes sense.

An important element of the model's structure is its planned brevity—6 to 12 weekly or biweekly sessions. The short-term feature of the model is supported by a large amount of research evidence that suggests the following: (1) recipients of brief, time-limited treatment show at least as much durable improvement as recipients of long-term, open-ended treatment (Johnson & Gelso, 1983; Koss & Butcher, 1986; Luborsky, Reid, & Shyne, 1969; Luborsky, Singer, & Luborsky, 1975; Wells, 1982); (2) most of the improvement associated with treatment tends to occur quickly—within the first few months (Howard,

Kopta, Kraus, & Orlinsky, 1986; Meltzoff & Kornreich, 1970); and (3) regardless of their intended length, most courses of voluntary treatment turn out to be relatively brief—the great majority probably last no longer than a dozen sessions—a generalization that suggests that most people exhaust the benefits of treatment rather quickly (Garfield, 1986).

This research evidence is consistent with the hypothesis that problems clients seek help for generally reflect breakdowns in problem coping that set in motion forces for change. These forces, which include the client's own motivation to alleviate his or her distress and resources in the client's environment, operate rapidly in most cases to reduce the problems to a tolerance level, at which point the possibility of further change lessens. If so, then clients might be expected to benefit as much from short-term treatment as from more extended periods of service. Placing time limits on the brief service might be expected to enhance effectiveness by mobilizing the efforts of both practitioner and client.

Empirical Orientation

A strong empirical stance has been one of the essential characteristics of the task-centered approach. In general, this has meant use of scientific knowledge, methods, and perspectives both in the construction of the model and in its use in everyday practice. In respect to practice, clinicians make use of case data derived from standardized instruments, observation, interviews, and systematic recording in assessment and treatment planning. These data are used to evaluate hypotheses about case events. The practitioner is open to alternative theoretical explanations; speculative theorizing is avoided.

These foundation ideas of the model together with its technical procedures provide a framework into which knowledge and methods from various sources can be absorbed. How this is done will be made clear in subsequent sections of the chapter. I shall discuss the basic phases and methods of the model as it is applied to individuals; then I shall take up applications to conjoint family treatment and work with formed groups.

ASSESSMENT

As with most short-term models, assessment in the task-centered approach is problem centered. The first step in assessment is explication of what is troubling the client and what he or she wants to do about it. In the present model, assessment is more than objective study and diagnosis; it is the beginning of a collaborative process of problem and goal clarification.

Principles and Techniques

By focusing on the client's own construction of his or her problems, the practitioner avoids imposing her or his definitions of the difficulty. At the same time, the practitioner does not assume that the client's initial complaints are automatically the problems that are troubling him or her. In the process of problem exploration and specification, the practitioner needs to be sensitive to unspoken agendas and unexpressed feelings. The client's perceptions of the difficulty may then emerge in response to the practitioner's clarifying efforts. In this process, the practitioner may point out possible difficulties the client has not acknowledged.

Coming to terms with the client on what problems will constitute the focus of work is the first and most essential step of assessment. Even though these problems may be redefined as service proceeds, the initial formulation provides direction for further assessment activity.

A good deal will be learned about the client and his or her problems once the initial problem formulation is completed. This information is incorporated into a more systematic explanation of identified problems and their contexts. We are interested in learning the client's view of when, how, and why these problems appeared and developed, especially in events that caused the client to seek help for them. How has the client coped with the problems up until now? What has worked and what has not?

Exploration then proceeds from the problems outward into context. These domains are not examined comprehensively but in relation to the target problems. Additional data may be obtained through standardized instruments, which may be problem specific, such as the Beck Depression Inventory (Beck, 1967) or more general in scope, for example, the Family Assessment Device (Epstein, Baldwin, & Bishop, 1983).

Once the initial "problem survey" has been completed, the practitioner then formulates problems from the raw material of the discussion up to that point. In so doing, the practitioner would try to pull together the client's expressed concerns in succinct statements using concrete language the client can understand. Without doing violence to the client's perception, the practitioner tries to put the problems in the most "solvable" form possible.

The client is then asked to rank the problems in terms of the order he or she should like to see them solved. Up to three problems are then solicited, explored, specified in detail, and become the focus of the short-term intervention.

In short-term approaches, there is usually some form of explicit agreement with the client concerning duration of service and problems or goals to be worked on. The structure of planned brief service almost requires this kind of initial understanding, which in recent years has been referred to as a contract. In the task-centered model, formal contracting usually begins after the problems have been ranked and explored. Emphasis is on contracting as a process—that is, on preceding in terms of a series of explicit agreements subject to modification rather than *the* contract.

Integrative Aspects

During the assessment phase and beyond, the practitioner is encouraged to draw upon whatever theories may help elucidate and define the client's difficulty. In agreement with Wells (1982), we assume that there is no "correct theory" and that no single theory will suffice for the range of problems that practitioners deal with. What practitioners need are "theory menus" that they can select from to find the theory or combination of theories that provides the best fit for the situation at hand. For example, a problem involving a tantruming child and an unskilled mother might call for use of social learning theory; on the other hand, formulations from cognitive and psychodynamic theories may provide the best way of understanding a problem of low self-esteem in an adult.

In the present model, one does not seek a full-blown theoretical explanation of the problem but rather an identification of possible explanatory factors that may be amenable to change. Thus an hypothesis that the child's tantruming behavior may be unwittingly reinforced by the mother's attention may lead to steps to alter her response pattern. The problem of low self-esteem may be seen as growing out of the client's entrenched beliefs that he or she is a loser like his or her father. The latter formulation may lay the basis for cognitive restructuring and insight development.

The practitioner processes such varied perspectives in line with the principles and methods of the task-centered approach. For example, following these principles, theoretical insights would be shared with the client initially as a means of achieving mutual understanding of the problem and later in order to involve the client in collaborative problem-solving and to develop a task plan. Additional perspectives might be applied to other problems in the case. In other words the "borrowed" theoretical understanding would not activate the full practice model connected to the theory but would rather color and shape the application of the task-centered approach. In many cases, a formal theoretical perspective may not emerge. A "commonsense" understanding, perhaps guided by the client's own ideas of what is wrong and why, may provide the basis for problem definition and initial tasks.

INTERVENTIVE METHODS

The treatment process begins with the selection of the problem, usually the one regarded as most important in the client's ranking. The practitioner and clients work collaboratively toward developing a solution.

Task Development and Implementation

The initial role of the practitioner is to help the client generate and evaluate alternative courses of action. Her or his immediate objective is to help the client develop a plan of action or task that can be implemented prior to the next session. Although the practitioner may suggest task possibilities or may even assign tasks if the client is not productive, emphasis is placed on stimulating client problem solving. Often the best tasks are those produced through close client–practitioner collaboration.

The task is spelled out with whatever degree of detail is appropriate to the problem, situation, and the client's problem-solving style. In some cases, a very explicit detailed plan is called for (who does what, when, how, etc.); in others, the task plan is best left open and flexible. Regardless of degree of structure, it is important that the client understands the nature of the plan and its rationale and that he or she expresses a commitment to carry it out. We try to avoid unilateral directives to which the client has made little input or is skeptical about attempting. When tasks involve unfamiliar or anxiety-provoking behaviors, guided practice or rehearsals (through role plays or other means) may be employed. Anticipating and planning for likely obstacles is also a useful device. For example, clients may be asked to think of ways that a task might fail (Birchler & Spinks, 1981). If substantial obstacles appear, techniques of contextual analysis can be used. Alternatively, the task can be modified or another developed.

The same principles are applied to planning of *practitioner tasks* or actions the practitioner will take outside the session in an attempt to bring about desired changes in the client's social system. Although such actions may not be planned in detail with the client, their consideration as tasks not only enables the client to understand and perhaps help shape the practitioner's environmental interventions but makes her or him accountable, as is the client, for task performance.

Problem and Task Review

The client's progress on problems and tasks is routinely reviewed at the beginning of each session. The review covers developments in the problem and what the client has and has not accomplished in tasks to resolve it. Practitioner tasks are reviewed in a similar manner. What the practitioner does next depends on the results of the review. If the task has been substantially accomplished or completed, the practitioner may formulate another task with the client on the same problem or a different problem. If the task has not been carried out or only partially achieved, the practitioner and client may take up obstacles, devise a different plan for carrying out the task, or apply other task implementation activities. The task may be revised or replaced by another, or the problem itself may be reformulated.

Contextual Analysis

During the course of the review of tasks and problems, obstacles to task achievement and problem change are usually encountered. The essential difference between a target problem and an obstacle is that the former is a difficulty that the client and practitioner have contracted to change, and the latter is a difficulty standing in the way of progress toward resolution of a target problem.

Whereas obstacles block progress, resources facilitate it. Resources are usually found in strengths and competencies of individual clients, in the ties of loyalty and affection that hold families together, and in the intangible and tangible supports provided by external systems. However, a given characteristic may serve as either an obstacle or resource, depending on its function in relation to the problem.

In contextual analysis, the practitioner helps clients identify and resolve obstacles as well as to locate and utilize resources. The discussion is led by the practitioner who relies on focused exploration, explanations, and other methods designed to increase the client's understanding. The process may overlap with the problem and task reviews, when obstacles and resources may emerge and be explored. The practitioner may help clients modify distorted perceptions or unrealistic expectations. Dysfunctional patterns of behavior or interactions may be pointed out. Obstacles involving the external system, such as interactions between a child and school personnel or the workings of a recalcitrant welfare bureaucracy, may be clarified, or resources within these systems may be searched for.

Integrative Aspects

Task development and implementation as well as contextual analysis are informed by other approaches. The behavioral movement has produced a rich variety of task possibilities. Among those used extensively in task-centered work with individuals have been various forms of parent training, token economies, techniques for managing disruptive classroom behavior, home notes, self-monitoring, and reward programs. However, in using these techniques, the practitioner normally does not become a pro-tem behavior therapist but rather works them into a task-centered mode of practice. Because clients are collaboratively involved in the planning process and their input utilized, the task plan may depart considerably from standard protocols in using a behavioral technique. Moreover, elements from a behavioral method may be combined with client-generated ideas for tasks. In other words, both practitioner and client make collaborative use of behavioral methods in a problem-solving process. In fact, certain behavioral tenets may be subordinated to basic formulations of the model. For example, children may be given a rationale rather than a tangible reward for doing behavioral tasks, on grounds that taking constructive action because it is in the child's interest to do so—for example, doing homework to pass a course—is more likely to nurture problem-solving capacities and be self-maintained than action motivated by the tangible reward.

To take a rather different illustration, we use paradoxical tasks (Frankel, 1965), especially those based on assumption of compliance (Rohrbaugh, Tennen, Press, & White, 1981). For example, a task for a client with insomnia may be to try to stay awake. Again, following principles of the model, the practitioner and client would discuss the task in an eyes-open fashion—the pun is irresistible—and its paradoxical rationale would be explained. There is research evidence to suggest that such explanations actually increase the effectiveness of such paradoxical injunctions (Ascher & Turner, 1979). By contrast, paradoxical tasks based on the assumption of "defiance" (Rohrbaugh, Tennen, Press, & White, 1981)—asking a truanting adolescent to stay away from school—would be rarely, if ever, used.

In general, task ideas are drawn from various approaches that use tasks including cognitive (Beck, 1976; Sherman, 1984; Werner, 1982); and strategic (de Shazer, 1982; Fisch, Weakland, & Segal, 1982; Haley, 1976; Madanes, 1981; Werner, 1982) as well from specialized literature on homework and the like, (Shelton & Ackerman, 1974; Shelton & Levy, 1981). The borrowed technology is not simply transferred but rather is converted to fit the principles of the model.

Similarly, techniques from psychodynamic and cognitive approaches are used in contextual analysis. Short-term psychodynamic models (Mann, 1973, 1981; Strupp, 1981) have proven more useful than open-ended versions because the former come equipped with methods for dealing with focal issues within brief periods of time. In the task-centered model, psychodynamic methods are used chiefly to work through psychological obstacles to problem definition and task work. Thus a young man unable to complete a task of making an overture to a female coworker might need to work through earlier feelings of failure and rejection in his relations with women. This kind of intervention would be occasioned by an inability of the client to follow through on a course of action he himself agreed to. Development of insight or other outcomes of this analysis would be directed at helping the client move forward with tasks. In the example given and, in general, methods of cognitive restructuring may be used as an alternative to psychodynamic methods, depending on the needs of the client and orientation of the practitioner. The kind of synthesis of these two methods suggested by Segraves (Chapter 18 this volume) is in line with current developments in the model.

TERMINATION AND DURATIONAL LIMITS

The process of termination, as in most planned short-term models, is actually begun in the initial phase when durational limits are agreed on. The termination interview follows a structured format in which first progress on problems is evaluated and rated by practitioners and clients. The clients' accomplishments in respect to their problems is highlighted with an effort made to underscore the clients' sense of mastery. The practitioner then takes up unresolved issues and helps clients plan next steps in dealing with these difficulties. To end the interview and treatment on a positive note, attention is turned to problem-solving skills, self-understanding, and so on, the clients may have acquired during the course of treatment and how they can use these gains in grappling with future problems.

Although the task-centered approach is basically a short-term form of practice, it does have, as an integrative model, an option for extensions. The extensions are themselves time limited, but in some cases renewals can extend service into long-term ranges. Moreover, certain case situations do not lend themselves to routine setting of durational limits, even initially. Decisions about variations from the short-term structure of the model raise questions about length of service, flexibility in the use of limits, and criteria for extensions.

These questions have, of course, ramifications beyond short-term designs because they involve the issue of practitioner responsibility for termination. Should practitioners determine when the end should occur with advantages of stopping treatment at the "right" time with an appropriately structured terminal session (but with the risk of a wrong judgment)? Or should they allow the case to end when the client has had enough, with attendant risks of excessively prolonged treatment, "no-show" termination, and the like?

For most clients who seek help for personal and family problems, a range from 6 to 12 sessions may suffice, but there is a need for tested criteria to decide where within this range to set the limits. Some practitioners, who prefer to keep their options open as long as possible, may delay fixing a specific number of sessions but at a cost of introducing uncertainties and of sacrificing advantages that may be gained from working against fixed limits. Usually a figure is reached on the basis of some judgment about the client's motivation and about the length of service needed to achieve what might be achievable in the case. But this kind of judgment needs refinement, at least to permit one to distinguish between "short" (6–8 sessions) and "long" (10 to 12) brief treatment cases.

Decision making about length of treatment is usually based on a service model consisting of weekly sessions. Increasing frequency of sessions (e.g., twice a week) within a limited period of time (e.g., 6 weeks) can produce a more intensive model that fits well with the strategy used in the present approach; tasks can be tried out, reviewed, and corrected more quickly. (An illustration is provided in Reid *et al.*, 1980.) Experimentation with different variations in session frequency (and session length) with different types of case situations would help create a richer array of options than the standard 6 to 12 or so 50-minute hours once a week.

Setting durational limits in terms of sessions within a time period works well for problems of voluntary clients that can be satisfactorily treated within such time frames. Other standards need to be developed for cases in the following groups: (1) when service duration may be connected to events over which neither practitioner nor client has control (e.g., discharge from a hospital); (2) when the practitioner has mandated protective or correctional functions; (3) when the practitioner and client are part of a long-term care system (e.g., a residential institution); and (4) when the target problem is expressed in terms of a specific goal that may require more time to accomplish than provided by the short-term design (e.g., securing the return of a child from foster care). Although in some of these cases, it makes sense to move to open-ended or goal-related service designs, in others, a short-term contract can be used to work on immediate problems with the option for additional short-term work if needed down the line. We have not yet developed good criteria for making such differentiations or for deciding on the optimum length of service in these situations.

Regardless of the setting or circumstances in which short-term service is used, a perennial issue concerns extensions of service after the agreed-on limit has been reached. Although the present model favors flexibility on this point, it is often difficult to distinguish judicious flexibility from indiscriminate looseness on one side, and, on the other, from rigid adherence to the original service limits. If extensions or "recontracting" are done routinely as long as clients appear willing to continue, the model becomes short term in name only. On the other hand, if little allowance is made for the client's needs for additional time or sessions, client resentment and frustration may ensue, as has been evidenced in client satisfaction questionnaires (O'Connor & Reid, 1986). The issue becomes more subtle when practitioners follow the advice of brief treatment experts and remind clients of agreed on time limits during the course of service. When the last scheduled interview comes, the client may feel that termination is expected and be reluctant to voice needs for additional services (even if asked by the practitioner). The client may then in a postservice follow-up complain that service ended prematurely. In other situations, clients who might be content to terminate on time will respond positively to the practitioner's expectations that more service is needed.

For task-centered practitioners, the recommendation has been to consider extensions (1) when the client explicitly expresses an interest in continuing, (2) when there are unrealized but reachable goals, and (3) when the client has been making progress toward those goals. As noted, the client's responses to the expectation that service will be brief may mask the client's wishes in respect to the first of these criteria; the remaining two are always difficult to evaluate because some unfinished business can almost always be found as well as some signs of progress.

In our experience, it is often the case showing marginal progress at the scheduled time of termination that receives the extension. Cases that have gone nowhere either do not survive to this point, or everyone is happy to quit when it does arrive. And, of course, cases in which presenting problems have been largely alleviated are also likely to exit at this point. Thus criteria that are hard to specify must be applied to cases that are seldom clear-cut. Although the seriousness of the problem may justify continuing the effort in certain cases, frequently the added service adds little to outcome. In particular, there is need to find ways to identify those "marginal gain" cases that appear to have potential for sustained progress beyond the limits of short-term service.

WORK WITH FAMILIES AND FORMED GROUPS

The strategy that has been outlined for treatment of the individual client is applied, with certain modifications, to work with clients in groups. Specific adaptations have been developed for two types of groups: families (or individuals who live together) and groups assembled expressly for the purpose of helping members work on individual problems. This integration across modalities provides a system by which practitioners can apply common concepts and principles to work with individuals, families, and groups. Applications to families and integration with individual methods will be taken up in detail. Work with formed groups will be briefly summarized.

Family Treatment

From its beginning, the task-centered approach has been used as a method of helping families. Early efforts emphasized work with family dyads, principally marital and parent–child pairs. Recently attention has been given to treatment of larger family units (Fortune, 1985; Reid, 1981, 1985).

Treatment of a family unit, like treatment of the individual client, focuses on resolution of specific client-acknowledged problems and associated contextual change. Problems are seen as occurring in a multisystems context in which the family is a major, though not always the most critical, system. To understand problems and their contexts, use is made of research and theory on family interaction as well as specific contributions from behavioral, structural, strategic, and communications schools of family therapy.

In most cases, family members are seen together, and, to the extent possible, problems are defined in interactional terms. In addition to tasks carried out by individual family members and the practitioner, as in the general model, use is made of tasks undertaken jointly by family members, either in the session or in the home. Recent work on the family treatment variation of the model has focused on combinations of tasks in the session and at home. This effort has led to the development of the Family Problem Solving Sequence (FPSS), an intervention that addresses both immediate problems and contextual factors impinging on these problems (Reid, 1987a,b).

Essentially two or more family members work together face-to-face on a target problem in the session (session task). This task provides the basis for further problem-solving work to be carried out either at home or from a home base (home task). When indicated, these tasks are set up to have a positive impact on contextual factors affecting the problem. Although any contextual aspect may be selected, attention is usually concentrated on the family context, especially communication and problem-solving skills and the structure of family interaction. The therapist develops and facilitates the session task and uses it as a basis for other interventions. He or she helps the family plan the home task and reviews its progress in the session following.

For example, a target problem may concern a son's not doing homework regularly. In the session the parents and son work out a plan by which the child agrees to spend 1 hour each weekday evening on the homework with a reward for compliance. This solution is then implemented at home. At the same time, communication and structural factors are dealt with. The father is coached in the use of "I" statements in his communication with the son (Gordon, 1970). At a structural level, the parental alliance is reinforced by having the parents sit together in the session and by praising their efforts to come to an agreement on a plan for the son. This structural emphasis is extended in the home task; the parents are asked to work out together a plan for taking turns in helping the son with his homework.

Practitioners approach each sequence then with a dual perspective. There is always emphasis on an immediate target problem whose resolution is regarded as important in its own right. This may be the only perspective acted on if the target problems in the case are not the product of communication or structural factors or if there are clinical reasons for leaving these factors alone. Usually, however, the target problem currently being worked on (or some other target problem) will be influenced by communication and structural contexts. Thus change in these contexts may need to occur if the target problem is to be resolved or if the resolution is to be maintained.

The communication context is concerned with exchanges of meaning and their effects. It comprises such elements as communication deficits and skills, communication styles, and capacity for problem-solving communication (Jacobson & Margolin, 1979; Robin, 1979, 1981; Wells & Figurel, 1979). Structure comprises rules of interaction among family members, as expressed in such terms as power, control, involvement, alliance, and flexibility (Aponte & Van Deusen, 1981; Minuchin, 1974; Reid, 1985).

An evolving strategy in using the FPSS is to orchestrate session and home tasks and related interventions to have simultaneous impact on the problem and its context. Not all FPSSs may affect both problem and contextual levels, but one is always alert to the potential of this happening. Also, different levels may not receive the same emphasis. For example, in some cases stress will be on the problem, with communication and structure receiving secondary attention. In other cases, work on the problem may be subordinate to work on structural and communication issues.

The dual perspective applies even if the target problem itself involves communications or structural concerns. To illustrate, the problem may be defined as argumentative communication between a husband and wife, and session tasks may consist of guided practice on communication skills. The communication level then becomes aspects of communication not defined as the problem, for example the husband's reluctance to be emotionally expressive with his spouse, which may increase her frustration in the relationship and aggravate the arguments. The same logic applies when a structural issue is the target problem. In other words, there will always be contextual factors to be considered regardless of how the problem is defined.

Types of Tasks

In using the FPSS, it is helpful to distinguish between types of tasks (Reid & Helmer, 1986; Reid, 1985). Session tasks have been divided into two broad categories. One group consists of tasks explicitly designed for purposes of solving substantive family problems or planning activities outside the session. With these tasks, work in the session is preparatory to some form of action outside the session and leads naturally to home tasks. Tasks in this group usually consist of some form of family problem solving and make use of such procedures as problem identification and definition; generating solutions through brainstorming and more deliberate exploration of alternatives; compromising; decision making; and task planning.

The other group consists of tasks involving expressions of affect, enhancing awareness, and skills training. For example, family members may be asked to share feelings, exchange positives about one another, reveal attitudes and expectations, or practice communication skills. Family sculpting, role plays, and other devices to heighten the experiential quality of the task may be used. With these tasks, work in the session is designed to achieve immediate results—for example, learning skills, gaining understanding. The task has intrinsic value even if not followed by a home task. However, home tasks provide an important means of extending accomplishments in the session to the home where ultimately they need to have an impact if they are to be of value. One simple way of doing this is to have participants practice some variation of the session task at home. (This works for some families, but others do not comply well with home-practice tasks.) Another way is to use key elements of the session task as a basis for home tasks involving natural interaction. For example, a session task involving a positive exchange between a husband and wife can lead to a home task in which they agree to compliment one another for specified behaviors. (To ensure generalization, such home tasks would, in any case, eventually replace simple home practice of session tasks.) Not all session tasks of the "immediate learning" variety will lead directly to home tasks. For example, some may be used to work on obstacles arising in the session.

Home tasks are divided into categories of *shared, reciprocal,* and *individual.* Shared tasks are joint activities involving two or more family members. They provide a means for continuing at-home problem-solving and communication tasks worked on in the session or for joint implementation of action plans designed in session tasks. At the same time, they serve contextual goals of increasing closeness, strengthening boundaries, and fostering realignments, depending on which family members share the task. Reciprocal tasks involve exchanges between family members. The exchanges may consist of marital *quid pro quos,* parental rewards for the compliance of children, and so forth. Whatever their form, reciprocal tasks stress the principle of reciprocity, an ingredient essential to successful family functioning. Individual tasks are actions that do not require collaborative activity or specific reciprocation. They may be addressed to either individual or family problems. In addition to providing a vehicle for work on individual problems, tasks of this type are used when conflict is too intense for shared or reciprocal tasks, to promote autonomy, or to allow family members to volunteer independent activity for the family's benefit.

The FPSS is based on the assumption that some problems can be resolved by straightforward family problem-solving efforts but that others will require work on contextual issues. Contextual obstacles to problem resolution are thus identified and addressed. Therapeutic work is then driven by problems and obstacles to their resolution rather than by overall goals concerning family communication or structure. The practitioner begins with the problems and moves "outward" into context.

The FPSS also assumes that informed participation on the part of family members in problem-solving work not only strengthens family competence but preserves family control over the change process. To facilitate such participation, the practitioner encourages the family to develop its own solution in its own way and shares with the family his or her assessments of communication, structural or other changes that may be relevant to problem resolution. At the same time, efforts to foster the family's own problem solving must be balanced against the need to provide leadership to enable the family to achieve its own goals. What is the proper balance for the practitioner between "taking charge" and giving the initiative to the family is an unresolved issue for this model as well as for family treatment generally. In the present model, we try to resolve the issue by providing the family with the optimal amount of structure and input for its problem-solving work.

Finally, it is assumed that an action-oriented approach works better for many families than an approach centered on helping family members develop understanding of their plight or on dealing with its emotional components. Increasing insight and exploration of feelings are rather viewed as essential concomitants of the actions that provide the way to actual solutions.

Combining problem solving in the session with efforts to apply solutions at home is not new. Such a configuration of activities is often a part of problem-solving training (Jacobson & Margolin, 1979; Robin, 1979) and is used in the problem-centered therapy of Epstein and Bishop (1981; Epstein *et al.*, Chapter 17 this volume). What the FPSS work contributes is an integration of emphasis on solving substantive problems, skill development, and structural change. It also focuses specifically on the interrelation between session and home problem solving.

The family treatment variation is viewed as part of a more comprehensive system of task-centered practice. Although work with the family as a unit is generally seen as the treatment of choice when target problems consist of difficulties in family relationships, this method must be evaluated against other options when the target problem involves the behavior of a member outside the family context, such as a child's difficulty at school. Although family treatment may be indicated if the problem is reactive to family processes or if the family can be used as a resource for solving it, work focused on the individual and the setting in which his or her difficulty occurs may prove to be a more effective alternative.

Often some combination of individual and family methods is advisable. In some cases, there may be need for episodic family involvement, such as in individual work with clients in residential or educational settings; in other cases, it may not be feasible to sustain family involvement, as desirable as that may be; in still others, it may make sense to focus on both individual and family problems during a single course of treatment. A unified framework facilitates work in such situations, enabling the practitioner to shift her or his attention and intervention from the individual to the family. Such a framework avoids sterile boundaries between individual and family treatment (Feldman & Pinsof, 1982). We are attempting to achieve the kind of integration in which the treatment plan consists of whatever combinations of individual, family, and community intervention methods appear to be the most effective mode of resolving target problems.

Work with Formed Groups

The principles of conjoint treatment that have been presented can be applied to any situation in which target problems involve interaction of members of natural groups—that is, groups that have a life apart from the treatment session. Somewhat different principles apply when clients are treated for individual problems within the context of a formed group; that is, a group created to help individuals with their own concerns. The ultimate change target against which success is measured is not interaction of group members outside the session but rather resolution of the separate problems of each. Within the task-centered framework, the term *group treatment* is used to describe this form of intervention. The strategies and methods of task-centered group treatment have been presented elsewhere in detail (Fortune, 1985; Garvin, Reid, & Epstein, 1976).

In task-centered group treatment, the group process is used to further the basic activities of the model. Group members, guided by the leader, help one another to specify problems, plan tasks, rehearse and practice behavior, analyze obstacles to task achievement, review task progress, and so on. The leader's role is to make effective use of this process through orchestrating his or her own interventions with the contributions of group members.

In order that the contribution of members can be used to best advantage, groups are made relatively homogeneous in respect to target problems. Thus, a group may be formed around problems of academic achievement or posthospitalization adjustment. As a result, group members have firsthand knowledge of the kind of problems others are experiencing and are thus in a good position to provide support and guidance. Moreover, members can more readily apply lessons learned from the task work of others to their own situations.

Leadership within the group is an important facet that needs to be attended to and used constructively. Although the practitioner normally assumes the primary leadership role in task-centered groups, he or she may use members as co-leaders for particular purposes—one member may be particularly adept at reducing tension in the group; another at keeping the group focused on the business at hand.

Although procedures for forming and conducting groups vary, the following format is typical. Preliminary individual interviews are held with prospective group members to determine primarily if the applicant has at least one problem that would fall within the prospective focus of the group and to orient him or her to the general structure and purpose of the group treatment model. In the initial group meeting, clients are asked to state the problems they wish to work on and to assist one another in problem exploration and specification. A contractual agreement is reached on the purpose of the group and its duration (which is planned, short-term, as in individual treatment). In subsequent sessions, each member, in turn, formulates, plans, practices, and reviews tasks with the help of the practitioner and other group members. In addition, the practitioner may undertake tasks outside the session on behalf of a single client or the group as a whole, or group members may perform extrasession tasks to help another with their problems. Like the individual and family modalities, the group treatment variations draws on compatible approaches (see, for example, Garvin, Chapter 21 this volume).

RANGE OF APPLICATION

As a broad-spectrum, integrative model, the task-centered approach is applicable, as has been suggested, to a wide variety of problems and populations. As with most such models, it is difficult to specify when it may be treatment of choice and when it might be contraindicated.

Well-motivated, well-functioning clients with circumscribed problems usually respond well to almost any kind of therapeutic approach. For such clients, a short-term, problem-centered model like the present one has at least one advantage over models that are longer term and directed to more ambitious goals: The short-term model provides a better fit to what is needed and does not have to be "geared down." Also the planned brevity keeps the practitioner from trying to do more than is indicated, a helpful control with students and beginners.

On the other hand, most approaches find the going tough with clients who are functioning poorly and have pervasive problems. With many such clients, it may make little difference what treatment is offered because gains will be meager in any case.

As a general rule, treatment goals are more important than diagnosis in determining the applicability of short-term models (Koss & Butcher, 1986). For many low-functioning clients with severe chronic problems, limited goals—for example, establishing independent living—may be all that is realistic. The task-centered model, for example, has been used effectively with mentally ill adults to deal with problems of adjustment to community living (Brown, 1977; Newcome, 1985). Similarly, limited-goal, brief therapy (within a psychodynamic framework) has shown promising results with hospital borderline patients (Nurnberg & Suh, 1982). When goals are more far reaching, for example, personality change or major modifications of chronic psychopathology—short-term models are generally not considered as treatments of choice (Clarkin & Frances, 1982). Even though long-term treatment may not, in fact, achieve such goals, one can try it and hope for the best.

As a particular type of short-term treatment that aims to stimulate, guide, and strengthen the client's problem-solving efforts, the task-centered model requires that target problems be alleviated through the client's own actions. Thus the model is not preferred for clients who view treatment primarily as an opportunity to sort out their goals or explore purely interior issues. By the same logic, the model does not work well if the clients are unwilling to take constructive action, as in some types of protective or correctional cases, or if no effective plan of client action can be found, as in some types of psychosomatic disorders.

Research on Task-Centered Practice

There have been over 30 published reports of research on the task-centered model, to which can be added numerous unpublished investigations, including several doctoral dissertations. The effectiveness of the model as a means of resolving specific problems of living has been demonstrated in a variety of experiments in which control groups or single-case controls have been used to rule out the influence of extraneous variables (Gibbons et al., 1979; Larsen & Mitchell, 1980; Reid, 1975, 1978; Newcome, 1985; Reid et al., 1980; Rzepnicki, 1985; Wodarski, Saffir, & Frazier, 1982; Tolson, 1977). Populations in these studies have included psychiatric patients, families in which a member has attempted suicide, distressed marital couples, schoolchildren with academic and behavioral problems, and delinquents in a residential center. A larger number of studies in which controls were not used have provided additional support for the effectiveness of the model with these and other populations (see, for example, Ewalt, 1977; Goldberg & Robinson, 1977; Goldberg, Gibbons, & Sinclair, 1984; Reid, 1977, 1987a; Rooney, 1981; Segal, 1983). However, outcomes have not been consistently positive for family treatment for adolescents acting out in the home and in the community (Reid, 1987a).

Studies of the processes of the model have suggested that certain factors are positively correlated with problem change: the extent to which practitioners and clients focus attention on target problems (Blizinsky & Reid, 1980), degree of task progress (Reid, 1978), and practitioner directiveness (Fortune, 1979). Found to promote task accomplishment has been the degree of client commitment to attempt the task (Reid & Epstein, 1972; Reid, 1978) and repetitions of the task (although the point of diminishing returns in repeated tasks is soon reached). In family interviews, the use of session tasks (face-to-face problem-solving work by clients in the session) has been shown to be positively related to accomplishment of tasks at home, especially tasks involving reciprocal actions (Reid, 1987a). Comparative studies of the practitioner's use of different techniques have shown less use of explanation and greater use of structuring and directive methods than in traditional open-ended practice (Fortune, 1979; Reid, 1978). The relatively high level of practitioner activity is a well-recognized characteristic of short-term models (Koss & Butcher, 1986). The importance of the practitioner's apparent directiveness in the model noted in different process studies requires a word of explanation in view of our emphasis on the client's problem-solving initiatives. Analysis of process tapes has suggested that much of this direction takes the form of suggestions to move the client's problem-solving along. "Have you thought of so-and-so?"—rather than "directives"—for example, "Do this or that."

This body of outcome and process research has provided evidence that tasks can be an effective means of bringing about change in a wide range of specific problems in brief periods of time. There is need to learn more about the impact of the model on client systems as a whole, about the durability of change, and about the contribution of different client factors—for example, motivation and pathology—to outcome.

Although many of the advantages of a broad-range integrative model have been presented, one of its disadvantages becomes apparent when one attempts to study its process and outcomes. There are simply so many client and treatment variables to contend with that it is difficult to build a cumulative body of research evidence about the model as a whole. As the model continues its process of expansion to new populations and incorporation of new theoretical and technical developments, the research agenda falls even further behind.

Given this, it may be better strategy to study the processes and outcomes of specific components of the model than the model as a whole—a strategy reflected in recent research (Reid & Helmer, 1986; Reid, 1987a,b). One may be justified in claiming that the model as a whole works if outcomes are positive and if it utilized core components (including those borrowed from other approaches) that have been found to be effective.

REFERENCES

Aponte, H. J., & Van Deusen, J. M. (1981). Structural family therapy. In A. S. Gurman & D. P. Kniskern (Eds.), *Handbook of family therapy* (pp. 310–360).New York: Brunner/Mazel.

Ascher, M. L., & Turner, R. M. (1979). Paradoxical intention and insomnia: An experimental investigation. *Behavioral Research and Therapy, 17,* 408–411.

Bass, M. (1977).Toward a model of treatment for runaway girls in detention. In W. J. Reid & L. Epstein (Eds.), *Task-centered practice* (pp. 183–194). New York: Columbia University Press.

Beck, A. T. (1967). *Depression: Clinical, experimental, and theoretical aspects.* New York: Harper & Row.

Beck, A. T. (1976). *Cognitive therapy and the emotional disorders.* New York: International Universities Press.

Birchler, G. R., & Spinks, S. H. (1981). Behavioral-systems marital and family therapy: Integration and clinical application. *The American Journal of Family Therapy, 8,* 6–28.

Blizinsky, M., & Reid, W. J. (1980). Problem focus and outcome in brief treatment. *Social Work, 25,* 89–98.

Brown, L. B. (1977). Treating problems of psychiatric outpatients. In W. J. Reid & L. Epstein (Eds.), *Task-centered practice* (pp. 208–227). New York: Columbia University Press.

Clarkin, J. F., & Frances, A. (1982). Selection criteria for the brief psychotherapies. *American Journal of Psychotherapy, 36,* 8–18.

Cormican, E. J. (1977). Task-centered model for work with the aged. *Social Casework, 58,* 490–494.

de Shazer, S. (1982). *Patterns of brief family therapy.* New York: Guilford Press.

Diekring, B., Brown, M., & Fortune, A. E. (1980). Task-centered treatment in a residential facility for the elderly: A clinical trial. *Journal of Gerontological Social Work, 2,* 225–240.

Epstein, L. (1977). A project in school social work. In W. Reid & L. Epstein (Eds.), *Task-centered practice* (pp. 130–146). New York: Columbia University Press.

Epstein, L. (1988). Helping people: The task-centered approach (2nd ed.). Columbus, OH: Merrill Publishing Co.

Epstein, N. B., & Bishop, D. S. (1981). Problem-centered systems therapy of the family. In A. S. Gurman & D. P. Kniskern (Eds.), *Handbook of family therapy* (pp. 444–482). New York: Brunner/Mazel.

Epstein, N. B., Baldwin, L. M., & Bishop, D. S. (1983). The McMaster family assessment device. *Journal of Marital and Family Therapy, 9,* 171–180.

Ewalt, P. L. (1977). A psychoanalytically oriented child guidance setting. In W. J. Reid & L. Epstein (Eds.), *Task-centered practice* (pp. 27–49). New York: Columbia University Press.

Feldman, L. B., & Pinsof, W. H. (1982). Problem maintenance in family systems: An integrative model. *Journal of Marital and Family Therapy, 7,* 295–308.

Fisch, R., Weakland, J. H., & Segal, L. (1982). *The tactics of change: Doing therapy briefly.* San Francisco: Jossey-Bass.

Fortune, A. E. (1979). Communication in task-centered treatment. *Social Work, 24,* 5–25.

Fortune, A. E. (1985). Treatment groups. In A. E. Fortune (Ed.), *Task-centered practice with families and groups* (pp. 33–44). New York: Springer Publishing Co.

Garfield, S. L. (1986). Research on client variables in psychotherapy. In S. L. Garfield & A. E. Bergin (Eds.), *Handbook of psychotherapy and behavior change* (pp. 213–256). New York: John Wiley and Sons.

Garvin, C. D., Reid, W. J., & Epstein, L. (1976). Task-centered group work. In H. Northen & R. W. Roberts (Eds.), *Theoretical approaches to social work with small groups* (pp. 238–267). New York: Columbia University Press.

Gelso, C. J., & Johnson, D. H. (1983). *Explorations in time-limited counseling and psychotherapy.* New York: Teachers College Press.

Gibbons, J., Butler, J., & Bow, I. (1979). Task-centered casework with marital problems. *British Journal of Social Work, 8,* 393–409.

Goldberg, E. M., & Robinson, J. (1977). An area office of an English social service department. In W. J. Reid & L. Epstein (Eds.), *Task-centered practice* (pp. 242–269). New York: Columbia University Press.

Goldberg, E. M., & Stanley, J. S. (1978). A task-centered approach to probation. In J. King (Ed.), *Pressures and changes in the probation service.* Cambridge: Institute of Criminology.

Goldberg, E. M., Gibbons, J., & Sinclair, I. (1984). *Problems, tasks, and outcomes.* Winchester, MA: Allen & Unwin.

Gordon, T. (1970). *Parent effectiveness training.* New York: Peter H. Wyden.

Gurman, A. S. (1981). Integrative marital therapy: Toward the development of an interpersonal approach. In S. H. Budman (Ed.), *Forms of brief therapy* (pp. 415–457). New York: The Guilford Press.

Haley, J. (1976). *Problem-solving therapy: New strategies for effective family therapy.* San Francisco: Jossey-Bass.

Hari, V. (1977). Instituting short-term casework in a long-term agency. In W. J. Reid & L. Epstein (Eds.), *Task-centered practice* (pp. 89–99). New York: Columbia University Press.

Hofstad, M. O. (1977). Treatment in a juvenile court setting. In W. J. Reid & L. Epstein (Eds.), *Task-centered practice* (pp. 195–201). New York: Columbia University Press.

Howard, K. I., Kopta, S. M., Krause, M. S., & Orlinsky, D. E. (1986). The dose-effect relationship in psychotherapy. *American Psychologist, 41,* 159–164.

Jacobson, N. S., & Margolin, G. (1979). *Marital therapy: Strategies based on social learning and behavior exchange principles.* New York: Brunner/Mazel.

Koss, M. P., & Butcher, J. N. (1986). Research on brief psychotherapy. In S. L. Garfield & A. E. Bergin (Eds.), *Handbook of psychotherapy and behavior change* (pp. 627–670). New York: John Wiley & Sons.

Larsen, J., & Mitchell, C. (1980). Task-centered strength-oriented group work with delinquents. *Social Casework, 61,* 154–163.

Luborsky, L., Singer, B., & Luborsky, L. (1975). Comparative studies of psychotherapy. *Archives of General Psychiatry, 32,* 995–1008.

Madanes, C. (1981). *Strategic family therapy.* San Francisco: Jossey-Bass.

Mann, J. (1973). *Time-limited psychotherapy.* Cambridge: Harvard University Press.

Mann, J. (1981). The core of time-limited psychotherapy: Time and the central issue. In S. H. Budman (Ed.), *Forms of brief therapy* (pp. 25–43). New York: The Guilford Press.

Meltzoff, J., & Kornreich, M. (1970). *Research in psychotherapy.* New York: Atherton Press.

Minuchin, S. (1974). *Families and family therapy.* Cambridge: Howard University Press.

Newcome, K. (1985). Task-centered group work with the chronically mentally ill in day treatment. In A. E. Fortune (Ed.), *Task-centered practice with families and groups* (pp. 78–91). New York: Springer Publishing Co.

Nurnberg, H. G., & Suh, R. (1982). Time-limited psychotherapy of the hospitalized borderline patient. *American Journal of Psychotherapy, 36,* 82–90.

O'Connor, R., & Reid, W. J. (1986). Dissatisfaction with brief treatment. *Social Service Review, 60,* 526–537.

Rathbone-McCuan, E. (1985). Intergenerational family practice with older families. In A. E. Fortune (Ed.), *Task-centered practice with families and groups* (pp. 149–160). New York: Springer Publishing Co.

Reid, W. J. (1975). A test of a task-centered approach. *Social Work, 20,* 3–9.

Reid, W. J. (1977). Process and outcome in the treatment of family problems. In W. J. Reid, & L. Epstein (Eds.), *Task-centered practice* (pp. 58–77). New York: Columbia University Press.

Reid, W. J. (1978). *The task-centered system.* New York: Columbia University Press.

Reid, W. J. (1981). Family treatment within a task-centered framework. In E. R. Tolson & W. J. Reid (Eds.), *Models of family treatment* (pp. 306–331). New York: Columbia University Press.

Reid, W. J. (1985). *Family problem solving.* New York: Columbia University Press.

Reid, W. J. (1987a). Evaluating an intervention in developmental research. *Journal of Social Service Research, 11,* 17–39.

Reid, W. J. (1987b). The family problem-solving sequence. *American Journal of Family Therapy, 14,* 135–146.

Reid, W. J., & Epstein, L. (1972). *Task-centered casework.* New York: Columbia University Press.

Reid, W. J., & Epstein, L. (Eds.). (1977). *Task-centered practice.* New York: Columbia University Press.

Reid, W. J., & Helmer, K. (1986). Session tasks in family treatment. *Family Therapy, 13,* 177–185.

Reid, W. J., & Shyne, A. W. (1969). *Brief and extended casework.* New York: Columbia University Press.

Reid, W. J., Epstein, L., Brown, L. B., Tolson, E. R., & Rooney, R. H. (1980). Task-centered school social work. *Social Work in Education, 2,* 7–24.

Robin, A. L. (1979). Problem-solving communication training: A behavioral approach to the treatment of parent-adolescent conflict. *American Journal of Family Therapy, 7,* 69–82.

Robin, A. L. (1981). A controlled evaluation of problem-solving communication training with parent-adolescent conflict. *Behavior Therapy, 12,* 593–609.

Rohrbaugh, M., Tennen, H., Press, S., & White, L. (1981). Compliance, defiance, and therapeutic paradox: Guidelines for strategic use of paradoxical interventions. *American Journal of Orthopsychiatry, 51,* 454–467.

Rooney, R. H. (1981). A task centered reunification model for foster care. In A. A. Maluccio & P. Sinanoglu (Eds.), *Working with biological parents of children in foster care* (pp. 101–116). New York: Child Welfare League of America.

Rooney, R. H. (1988). Measuring task-centered training effects on practice: Results of an audiotape study in a public agency. *Journal of Continuing Social Work Education, 4,* 2–7.

Rooney, R. H., & Wanless, M. (1985). A model for caseload management based on task-centered casework. In A. E. Fortune (Ed.), *Task-centered practice with families and groups* (pp. 187–199). New York: Springer Publishing Co.

Rzepnicki, T. L. (1985). Task-centered intervention in foster care services: Working with families who have children in placement. In A. E. Fortune (Ed.), *Task-centered practice with families and groups* (pp. 172–184). New York: Springer Publishing Co.

Salmon, W. (1977). Service program in a state public welfare agency. In W. J. Reid & L. Epstein (Eds.), *Task-centered practice* (pp. 113–122). New York: Columbia University Press.

Segraves, R. T. (1982). *Marital therapy: A combined psychodynamic behavioral approach.* New York: Plenum Medical Book Company.

Segal, C. A. (1983). *Parent enrichment project: A community based preventative service to families.* Montreal: Allied Jewish Community Services and Ville Marie Social Service Centre.

Shelton, J. L., & Ackerman, J. M. (1974). *Homework in counseling and psychotherapy.* Springfield, IL: Charles C. Thomas.

Shelton, J. L., & Levy, R. L. (1981). *Behavioral assignments and treatment compliance: A handbook of clinical strategies.* Champaign, IL: Research Press.

Sherman, E. (1984). *Working with older persons: Cognitive and phenomenological methods.* Boston: Kluwer-Nijhoff.

Strupp, H. H. (1981). Toward the refinement of time-limited dynamic psychotherapy. In S. H. Budman (Ed.), *Forms of brief therapy* (pp. 219–242). New York: Guilford Press.

Taylor, C. (1977). Counseling in a service industry. In W. J. Reid & L. Epstein (Eds.), *Task-centered practice* (pp. 228–234). New York: Columbia University Press.

Tolson, E. R. (1977). Alleviating marital communication problems. In W. J. Reid, & L. Epstein (Eds.), *Task-centered practice* (pp. 100–112). New York: Columbia University Press.

Tomm, K. (1982). Towards a cybernetic systems approach to family therapy. In F. W. Kaslow (Ed.), *The international book of family therapy* (pp. 70–90). New York: Brunner/Mazel.

Weissman, A. (1977). In the steel industry. In W. J. Reid & L. Epstein (Eds.), *Task-centered practice* (pp. 235–241). New York: Columbia University Press.

Wells, R. A. (1982). *Planned short-term treatment.* New York: The Free Press.

Wells, R., & Figurel, J. (1979). Techniques of structured communication training. *The Family Coordinator, 28*, 273–281.

Werner, H. D. (1982). *Cognitive therapy: A humanistic approach.* New York: Free Press.

Wexler, P. (1977). A case from a medical setting. In W. J. Reid & L. Epstein (Eds.), *Task-centered practice* (pp. 50–57). New York: Columbia University Press.

White, H. S., Burke, Jr., J. D., & Havens, L. L. (1981). Choosing a method of short-term therapy; A developmental approach. In S. H. Budman (Ed.), *Forms of brief therapy* (pp. 243–267). New York: The Guilford Press.

Wise, F. (1977). Conjoint marital treatment. In W. J. Reid & L. Epstein (Eds.), *Task-centered practice* (pp. 78–88).New York: Columbia University Press.

Wodarski, J. S., Saffir, M., & Frazer, M. (1982). Using research to evaluate the effectiveness of task-centered casework. *Journal of Applied Social Sciences, 7*, 70–82.

4

Brief Treatment and Mental Health Policy

Vincent Giannetti

The purpose of this chapter is to discuss brief psychotherapeutic treatment as a means for initiating a cost-effective and integrated mental health delivery system. It is the assumption of this chapter that mental health services are an integral part of the larger health care delivery system. Brief oriented psychotherapy will be used in this chapter to describe the planned and conscious use of time in problem-focused and structured therapy of not more than 20 sessions. The issues of access to services, cost, and quality of services, as well as integration of mental health services with medical services, will form the framework for proposing a mental health delivery system that features brief treatment as the focal point for delivering mental health services. Although the recommendations in this chapter can apply to a centrally financed mental health system, the issue of national health insurance will not be addressed in this chapter.

DEFINING MENTAL ILLNESS

The question of access to mental health services is a function of demand for services based upon need. The question of demand for mental health services becomes quite complex and varies with basic definitional issues such as the nature of mental health and illness as well as what constitutes psychotherapeutic treatment. For example, on one end of the definitional spectrum of mental illness lies the belief that mental health problems are essentially "problems in living." These problems can include a simple lack of access to resources to fulfill personal needs, irresponsible behavior as a result of inadequate socialization, deficits in skill acquisition resulting in interpersonal difficulties, or the inability to cope with excessive stress and demands. Given this broad definition, an increase demand for psychotherapeutic services would exist with a good proportion with the American population fitting into these categories. The President's

VINCENT GIANNETTI • School of Pharmacy, Duquesne University, Pittsburgh, Pennsylvania 15282.

Commission on Mental Health (1978) maintains that, whereas between 10% to 15% of the population requires mental health services, approximately one out of every four Americans suffers from mild to moderate emotional difficulties. In addition to this 25% of the American population who could utilize psychotherapeutic services, there is an increasing social acceptance of psychotherapy in that mental health services have lost their stigma, and people tend to have increased expectations that mental health services can assist in adapting to many of the social pressures and personal problems of modern life (Veroff, Kulka, & Douvan, 1981). Finally, there seems to be a latent demand for mental health services, and it is estimated that approximately only 20% of persons requiring mental health services actually utilize those services and that 29 million persons have been identified as suffering from mental disorders in 1984 (Taube & Burret, 1985).

Utilizing a narrower definition of mental illness, only those persons who could be diagnosed and fit into the current DSM-III diagnostic nomenclature would be considered the target population for psychotherapeutic intervention. Based upon a 6-month prevalence study of mental disorders in three communities, conducted by Myers et al. (1984), using DSM-III categories, this group would vary between 15% and 23% of the adult population (Myers et al., 1984). A similar conservative estimate of 15% of the American population in need of mental health services was established in earlier studies by Reiger, Goldberg, and Taube (1978). Although certainly individuals who define themselves as in distress and who wish to seek the help of a professional in order to resolve their problems in living can do so at their own expense, the issue becomes much more complex when government and third-party payers subsidize all or any part of the fee for professional services.

How one defines mental illness and, on that basis, proceeds to sanction access to psychotherapeutic services through third-party subsidies, creates a problem not unlike the prevention-versus-sick-care orientation with which the practitioners of physical medicine have struggled. Ideally, persons in the beginning stages of emotional stress due to problems in living should have access to psychotherapeutic services in order to treat the emotional distress in the early stages of its natural history of occurrence. The benefits here are obvious in that intervening much earlier in the premorbid, incipient, and early stages of the emotional distress will lead to less costly treatments and a better prognosis for restoration to normal functioning. However, this preventative approach will undoubtedly increase access to the system, thereby increasing short-term costs. It could be argued that long-term costs would be reduced in that problems would be resolved in a more timely and less costly manner. However, the difficulty with this argument is the fact that the delivery of mental health services is plagued by numerous problems that have resulted in inefficiency and lack of cost-effectiveness. These include the following:

1. There is a shortage of psychiatrists with both psychiatrists and psychologists tending to be unequally distributed along rural and urban lines as well as geographically maldistributed.

2. Approximately 80% of Americans who have mental health problems tend to be treated outside the formal mental health delivery system, causing strain on the medical care system as well as other institutions.
3. Third-party coverage is inadequate for mental health care with various surveys demonstrating that 49% of the population is covered for mental health services on a par with coverage for medical services, with patients paying a significant higher proportion of costs for mental health services out of pocket when compared to medical services.
4. The "deinstitutionalization" and "transinstitutionalization" of mental patients have left many people with mental health problems either homeless or in half-way houses or custodially oriented long-term care institutions that are ill-equipped to treat their problems (Koran & Sharfstein, 1986).

THE MENTAL HEALTH DELIVERY SYSTEM

In addition to these problems affecting the organization of mental health services, it is apparent that the method by which mental health services are delivered is not cost-effective. Approximately 75% of all expenditures for mental health services in the United States are for inpatient mental health care. (Frank & Cantlet, 1985). The exemption of mental disorders from the current diagnostic related groups has inadvertently created financial incentives for inpatient mental health care. According to Mechanic (1980), the current method of insurance reimbursement for mental health services is oriented toward a biomedical model and favors inpatient care, providing disincentives for alternative models of care that are less expensive and, in many cases, much less intrusive. In addition, much of the recent increase in coverage for mental health services by private health insurance as a result of state mandate continues to favor inpatient over outpatient care (McGuire, 1981).

Finally, in addition to problems in how mental health services are structured, reimbursed, and delivered, there has been a tendency to exclude certain professions and therapeutic modalities from reimbursement, thereby decreasing availability of services. For example, although psychiatrists and more recently psychologists have received the bulk of third-party payments, there is no evidence that their services are more effective than social workers who tend to be more readily accessible and distributed in the population but have been excluded from third-party payments. In fact, the evidence is that among these three core mental health professions, there is no relationship between professional affiliation and successful psychotherapeutic outcome (Giannetti & Wells, 1985). Also, there is a tendency to exclude problems in living such as described in the V code section of DSM-III from reimbursement and the reluctance of insurance companies to reimburse for marital and family therapy as well as group psychotherapy.

REORGANIZING MENTAL HEALTH DELIVERY

Given these problems in the organization and delivery of mental health services, how can brief-oriented psychotherapy be utilized as a focal point for the reorganization of mental health services along more efficient and cost-effective lines? In an article on the benefits and limitations of psychotherapy, Karasu (1986) listed the advantages of brief-oriented psychotherapy in an era of limited resources for health care. These advantages included reduced costs, ability to treat a greater number of patients, direct focus upon problems of living, applicability to an extended diagnostic base, and the clinical usefulness of planned, time-limited treatment that is believed to accelerate the therapeutic process. In order to discuss the merits of brief-oriented therapy as a focal point for reorganizing mental health services, a number of critical questions must first be answered. Is psychotherapy, in general, effective in treating mental health problems? Is brief-oriented therapy equivalent in effectiveness when compared to long-term therapy? Can brief therapy be integrated with medical care to reduce overall medical care costs? And finally, can brief therapy be utilized in outpatient settings as an alternative to the more costly inpatient treatment of mental health problems?

The issue of the effectiveness of psychotherapy has been researched and debated from the early 1950s. However, recent evidence has suggested that a wide range of psychotherapeutic modalities is effective with a wide variety of emotional problems (Lambert, Shapiro, & Bergin, 1986). The now much quoted meta-analysis of psychotherapeutic outcome research and various reviews of psychotherapeutic outcome research has demonstrated that there is good evidence for psychotherapy's effectiveness in treating a wide range of emotional disorders (Smith, Glass, & Miller, 1980; Saxe, 1980).

Given the general effectiveness of psychotherapeutic interventions, the question of the equivalency of brief psychotherapeutic interventions when compared to long-term intervention has been researched. There is mounting evidence concerning the equivalency of brief-oriented psychotherapy to long-term therapy for a wide range of patient populations and problems. Koss and Butcher (1986) in their excellent review of the research on brief psychotherapy have concluded that "in summary, comparative studies of brief psychotherapy offer little empirical evidence of differences in overall effectiveness between time-limited and unlimited therapy or between alternate approaches to brief therapy" (p. 660). The studies reviewed by Koss and Butcher were generally well-designed studies using a variety of outcome measures and appropriate follow-up. The question of what proportion of the population would be suitable for brief psychotherapeutic intervention remains currently unanswered in that the various approaches to brief treatment utilize various selection criteria, and there is little uniformity in selecting people for brief treatment.

However, one of the more provocative findings of Koss and Butcher's review is related to the issue of time in psychotherapy. According to Koss and Butcher, "regardless of stated time limitations, however, a major proportion of change attributed to psychotherapy appears to occur early in psychotherapy" (p. 654). This finding is most interesting in that it supports the view that there is something analogous to a therapeutic "loading dose," that is, therapeutic gains are most dramatic with initial doses of psychotherapeutic intervention. This fact is paralleled by the finding that the average number of sessions for patients in psychotherapeutic treatment in outpatient settings tends to be between six and eight (Garfield, 1986). In other words, the natural topography of psychotherapeutic treatment seems to favor brevity.

In addition to Koss and Butcher's extensive review of brief-oriented therapy, there have been other findings that tend to substantiate the acceptability and effectiveness of brief-oriented psychotherapy with a variety of patient populations. In one study, 85% of the patient population needing psychotherapy in a national psychological health maintenance organization responded well to brief-oriented interventions (Cummings, 1987). Also, research from the social work literature based upon meta-analysis of social work interventions of 30 controlled studies of outcome of therapy in outpatient settings conducted by social workers yielded the conclusion that "the findings are clear; even with several control variables in place, short-term intervention is more effective than long-term intervention." In the same article, based upon 23 quasi-experimental studies involving social work intervention with the chronically mentally ill, short-term, time-limited intervention proved to be superior to long-term intervention (Videka-Sherman, 1988).

The issue of the integration of brief therapy with medical services as a way to reduce medical care costs has been addressed in the medical offset literature. There is a relationship between stress-related and physical disorders, and under the effects of emotional stress, people overutilize medical services. According to one study, roughly 50% of patients treated by general practitioners have emotional problems contributing to the visit (Follman, 1970). Other studies have demonstrated that the "worried well" excessively utilize health care services such as physicians' visits and extensive testing as well as tend to stay in medical treatment longer (Hankin & Otkay, 1979). In addition, other research has demonstrated that family stress and conflict increases the utilization of both emergency and primary medical care services independent of the presence of medical illness and that life stresses function as a significant factor in increasing utilization of medical services independent of medical conditions (Mechanic, 1978; Roghmann & Hoggerty, 1972).

Of even more significance is the effect of short-term-oriented psychotherapy for the reduction of overall medical care utilization and costs. In one study, both utilization of medical services and medical costs decreased significantly for patients with physical disease such as diabetes, cardiovascular disease, and respiratory disorders as a result of brief mental health treatment (less than 21 days) (Schlesinger, Mumford, & Glass, 1983). In this particular study, there was a 56% decrease in medical services utilized after 3 years for the brief therapy group as compared to the no-therapy group. In a much earlier and frequently cited study, Follette and Cummings (1967) studied the relationship between psychotherapeutic services and medical utilization at the Kaiser-Permanente Clinic in the San Francisco area over a period of 20 years. Examining medical utilization 1 year before and 5 years after psychotherapeutic intervention, researchers demonstrated a significant decrease in medical utilization for people who received psychotherapy as opposed to the control group. The most significant part of this study is that the interviews ranged from 1 session to 34 sessions with the mean of 6.2 interviews. According to the study, the one-interview-only and brief psychotherapeutic groups required no further psychotherapy in order to sustain their low levels of medical utilization over a 5-year period. Finally, Smith and Glass (1977) as part of their large-scale meta-analysis of psychotherapeutic outcome found in their reviews of studies concerning the impact of psychotherapeutic interventions and recovery from surgery that patients receiving intervention based upon brief therapy such as relaxation training and hypnosis were able to significantly decrease the duration of hospitalization after surgery.

Although brief psychotherapy has demonstrated its effectiveness in offsetting medical costs, the ability of brief therapy to be utilized in outpatient settings as an alternative to more costly inpatient mental health services is less documented. However, there is an extensive literature demonstrating that alternate forms of outpatient care are at least equally effective and, in some cases, superior to inpatient care and, in almost all cases, much less expensive. In an excellent review of the literature involving mental hospitalization versus alternate forms of care, Kiesler (1982) reviewed studies that utilized random assignment to condition and involved a variety of patient populations including schizophrenics, depressive disorders, drug and alcohol abuse, and suicidal patients. Treatments included in the alternate forms of care were brief family crisis therapy, day care programs, social skills training, and combinations of drugs and psychotherapy. In the studies, which were well controlled methodologically, alternate forms of care to inpatient hospitalization were found to be more effective, according to standardized psychiatric evaluations, and less expensive than hospitalization. Also, patients in the alternate form of care were more likely to find subsequent employment, independent living, and stay in school longer. This review of the literature states that "in no case were the outcomes of hospitalization more positive than alternate care". Although this review of the literature did not specifically address exclusively brief-oriented therapy, many of the modalities utilized in the study cited were either brief oriented or could be adapted to a brief-oriented focus.

PSYCHOTHERAPY AND THE SOCIAL GOOD

Although the previous sections chronicled problems in the delivery of mental health services and discussed brief therapy's role in alleviating some of these problems, the issue of the social good accruing from the wider distribution and cost-effective delivery of psychotherapeutic services is important to address.

Given the assumptions that, in general, psychotherapy is effective; that there are little differences between brief-oriented psychotherapy and long-term-oriented psychotherapy in terms of outcome; and that psychotherapeutic services could be delivered on an outpatient basis much more cost-effectively, the possibility for a greater distribution of psychotherapeutic services to a larger population can be considered without a precipitous increase in cost of services. However, before an argument can be made for a wider distribution of psychotherapeutic services, the issues of the social costs of not providing psychotherapeutic services and specific "myths" concerning increased insurance coverage for psychotherapeutic services must be addressed.

According to Masi (1984), alcohol-related problems have cost American industry approximately $20.6 billion in lost productivity, and the cost for drug abuse problems is approximately $16.6 billion. Stress-related physical and mental illness costs U.S. businesses $20 billion a year at the managerial levels alone, and finally alcohol, drug, and mental health problems taken together have resulted in a $55 billion loss to American industry in terms of decreased productivity.

Further, there is evidence in industry that with the initiation of employee assistance programs that have traditionally focused on brief-oriented psychotherapeutic intervention, a number of large corporations have documented significant improvements in attendance, decreases in worker's compensation, health care costs, disability cases, job accidents, and significant savings on disability insurance benefits (Follmann, 1978; Witte & Cannon, 1979).

Although the social costs of not providing psychotherapeutic services can be well documented in industry and the savings to industry in providing employee assistance programs is evident, the issue of increased health care costs as a result of the widespread availability of psychotherapeutic services must be addressed. According to Koran and Sharfstein (1986), there are a number of misconceptions regarding health insurance coverage for mental health services. Two widely held myths regarding mental health insurance coverage are important to review. The first myth is that mental health services are essentially uncontrollable and unpredictable in that people will unnecessarily and excessively utilize mental health services. Koran and Sharfstein's review of the literature on this point indicates that, according to a number of studies, only a small percentage of covered populations tend to overutilize mental health services and that essentially mental health costs are stable over time and tend to constitute only a small percentage of total health care costs. Also, as previously cited, mental health services are cost-effective because of the offset in medical care costs as a result of providing mental health services.

Second, the myth that mental health services cannot be accountable to third-party payers is not substantiated in that peer review of psychotherapeutic services has become an integral part of many insurance company's procedures. The most well known is the Champus program that now utilizes a peer review. The evidence cited by Koran and Sharfstein indicates that there has been a significant cost savings from peer review programs and that peer review has been effective in assuring that appropriate care is received.

Policy Issues and Recommendations

The critical question posed in the beginning of this chapter was how can brief-oriented psychotherapy be utilized in order to more widely distribute psychotherapeutic services to the public in a more cost-effective manner. In order to expand psychotherapeutic services, a number of changes are necessary in the current mental health delivery system. First, the reimbursement of a number of different professionals with different ideas about how mental health problems should be treated is necessary. Although psychiatrists and, more recently, psychologists have received the bulk of third-party reimbursement, there is no evidence that their services are more effective than, for example, social workers who have had third-party payments less available (Giannetti & Wells, 1985). Professional affiliation does not bestow clinical competence, and the current cadre of marriage and family therapists, addiction counselors, mental health counselors, and psychiatric nurses provide a base for the expansion of a pluralistic mental health system. With professional organizations increasingly developing advanced clinical credentials involving both supervised practice and competency testing for their respective members and the increase in state licensing laws for a variety of mental health professionals, expansion of mental health providers with state and professional organization monitoring of both the quality and the ethics of psychotherapeutic services can be accomplished.

As the number of qualified and available mental health practitioners increases, the definition of what is a treatable mental illness must change. There is a relatively high degree of dissatisfaction with the current *Diagnostic and Statistical Manual* (III) for diagnosing mental disorders among mental health professionals and evidence that mental health practitioners use the DSM-III to artificially fit clients' problems into categories that are reimbursable, and in some cases deliberately misdiagnose in order to receive payment (Jampola, Sierles, & Taylor, 1986; Kirk & Kutchins, 1988; Miller *et al.*, 1981). An alternate system for classification and reimbursement will be necessary in order to take into account the "problems of living" that can be precursors to later mental illness but are not currently reimbursable. One simple, alternative approach would be to expand, further specify, and include V codes as reimbursable under the present DSM-III system. This would have the effect of legitimately increasing coverage for a wide range of human problems that would be amenable to brief treatment and prevent further and possibly more serious mental illness. The point here is that for many emotional problems, the natural history of onset is slow and gradual, and treating a particular problem in the incipient or early stages will lead to less costly services and a better prognosis for the patient.

A related issue to expanding professionals and changing definitions of mental illness is the types of modalities that are currently reimbursable. A number of insurance companies have traditionally either not reimbursed for group and family therapy or have reimbursed at a much lower rate. There has been a bias toward individual psychotherapy in reimbursement policy and a general lack of understanding of individual psychological problems from a more systems and interpersonal perspective. Encouragement of family and group modalities in treating a wide variety of human problems can result in greater benefit to a wider range of people with less investment of time than traditional individual-oriented psychotherapy. Also, as cited in this book, many family and group modalities tend to be brief oriented in focus.

In addition to expanding the number of professionals, therapeutic modalities, and categories of problems in living that can be reimbursable, financial incentives in psychotherapy must follow the natural topography of practice. As cited earlier in this chapter, there is now an emerging body of evidence indicating that there is something analogous to a "loading dose" in psychotherapy. That is, the greatest amount of benefit in psychotherapy occurs up front in the initial sessions. Reimbursement policy should recognize what the empirical research literature is beginning to discover. Reimbursement for psychotherapeutic services should not provide financial barriers for preventive treatment of emotional problems in the early stages and should recognize that the most benefit often occurs in the initial sessions. As a result, reimbursement should be on a sliding scale with the initial sessions being 100% reimbursable with subsequent sessions involving co-payment. In other words, a reimbursement policy that reimburses the first five sessions at 100% of fee, the second five sessions at 90% of fee, the third five sessions at 80% of fee, and the fourth five sessions at 70% of the fee would provide incentives for problem-focused and brief-oriented therapy. The lack of a financial barrier up front would encourage people to enter treatment for early-stage emotional problems with declining reimbursement providing incentives for brevity.

A number of researchers have already called for a policy where all psychotherapeutic services delivered should initially be brief oriented (Strupp, 1978; Videka-Sherman, 1988). The recommendation here is that all initial psychotherapeutic services should be brief oriented with declining reimbursement and increasing co-payments up to 20 sessions. Past 20 sessions, a peer review system should be initiated for therapists who feel that longer term psychotherapy is necessary for a particular patient's problem and that brief-oriented psychotherapy has not been effective. The therapist should document the nature of the client's problems, the brief interventions utilized, the reasons for lack of therapeutic response, and a rationale for further psychotherapeutic intervention. It could be at this point that further psychotherapeutic intervention may be essentially supportive in nature.

For some clients, long-term supportive psychotherapy is necessary in order to maintain their current level of functioning, but further therapeutic gains may not be possible. For these clients, the current system of both public and private community agencies utilizing paraprofessional counselors under the supervision of practitioners trained, certified, and licensed in the traditional mental health professions could deliver longer term supportive psychotherapeutic services to a variety of client populations. The effectiveness of paraprofessional counselors with a variety of populations has been well documented (Lambert, Shapiro, & Bergin, 1986). In some cases where brief-oriented psychotherapy is clearly not appropriate for a particular client's problem, then certainly longer term therapy could be instituted with the advice and consent of a peer review system. As psychotherapeutic outcome research becomes more refined and available, a peer review of various brief-oriented, as well as long-term oriented, therapies may be able to provide the answer to the critical question of what particular therapeutic modalities, both brief oriented or long term oriented, work for what specific population with what specific problems. As this data becomes validated and more universally accepted, it can be used as a basis for peer review.

The final component of a reorganization of mental health delivery is oriented toward training. Medical professionals must be trained in order to understand the relationship between stress and somatic illness and to appropriately refer to mental health professionals. Mental health professionals, in turn, must be trained through their curriculum to have a thorough understanding of brief-oriented psychotherapy and its value, place, and function in the delivery of quality and cost-effective mental health services.

This chapter has made a number of recommendations concerning the usefulness of brief-oriented psychotherapy in solving some of the organizational problems in the delivery of psychotherapeutic services. The assumption has been that the expansion of reimbursement for a wide variety of mental health professionals, types of psychotherapeutic modalities, as well as a broader definition of what is a reimbursable emotional problem, will result in a greater access to psychotherapeutic services tailored to individual needs. A reimbursement policy that does not set up financial barriers to seeking services initially will encourage more persons to seek therapy at an earlier stage of the natural history of their problem. With an increasing number of diverse professionals and therapeutic modalities, oriented toward brief therapy, there is an increased probability that services will be both cost-effective, more available, and more closely meet the specific needs of a wide variety of persons of diverse cultural and ethnic backgrounds. Although a greater number of persons will have access to psychotherapeutic services, with the emphasis on brief-oriented psychotherapy, the average number of sessions per patient population should decrease, allowing for greater access without an increase in cost. In addition, the more effective utilization of paraprofessions in community agencies and a reimbursement policy that encourages brief-oriented psychotherapy in outpatient settings, as opposed to inpatient mental health care, will increasingly exert a moderating influence on mental health care costs.

This chapter has essentially taken the position that brief-oriented therapy can be the centerpiece of initiating a more rational and cost-effective mental health delivery system. The ideal mental health delivery system would include the following: eliminate fee as a barrier for utilizing initial mental health services; provide incentives for people seeking therapy in the early stage of the natural history of the progression of mental disorders; provide only those services that are necessary in order to achieve therapeutic gains; provide a wide range of mental health services and mental health professions with different philosophies and ideas on how mental health problems should be approached; provide equitable distribution of mental health services to a wider variety of diverse racial, ethnic, and cultural groups; and, finally, encourage accountability and cost-effectiveness through providing financial incentives for brief-oriented psychotherapy and utilizing peer review.

REFERENCES

Cummings, N. A. (1987). The future of psychotherapy: One psychologist's perspective. American Journal of Psychotherapy, XLI, 349–360.

Follette, W., & Cummings, N. A. (1967). Psychiatric services and medical utilization in a prepaid medical plan setting. Medical Care, 25–35.

Follmann, J. F. (1970). Insurance coverage for mental illness. New York: American Management Association.

Follmann, J. F. (1978). Helping the troubled employee. New York: American Management Association.

Frank, R. G., & Kanlet, M. S. (1985). Direct costs and expenditures for mental health care in the U.S. in 1980. Hospital and Community Psychiatry 36, 165–168.

Garfield, S. L. (1986). Research on client variables in psychotherapy. In S. L. Garfield & A. E. Bergin (Eds.), Handbook of psychotherapy and behavior change: An empirical analysis (3rd ed.; pp. 213–256). New York: Wiley.

Giannetti, V., & Wells, R. (1985). Psychotherapeutic outcome and professional affiliation. Social Service Review, 59, 33–43.

Hankin, J., & Otkay, J. (1979). Medical disorder and primary medical care: An analytic review of the literature. ADMHA GPO (no. 78-661) Washington DC.

Jampala, V. C., Sierles, F. S., & Taylor, M. A. (1986). Consumers view of DSM III: Attitudes and practices of U.S. psychiatrists and 1984 graduating psychiatric residents. American Journal of Psychiatry, 143, 148–153.

Karasu, T. B. (1986). The psychotherapies: Benefits and limitations. American Journal of Psychotherapy, XL, 324–342.

Kiesler, C. A. (1982). Mental hospitals and alternate care: Noninstitutionalization as a potential public policy for mental patients. American Psychologist, 37, 349–360.

Kirk, S. A., & Kutchins, H. (1988). Deliberate misdiagnosis in mental health practice. Social Service Review, 62, 225–237.

Koran, L. M., & Sharfstein, S. S. (1986). Mental health services. In S. Jonas (Ed.), Health care delivery in the United States (3rd ed., pp. 263–302). New York: Springer Press.

Koss, M., & Butcher, J. A. (1986). Research on brief psychotherapy. In S. L. Garfield and A. E. Bergin (Eds.), The handbook of psychotherapy and behavior change: An empirical analysis (3rd ed., pp. 627–663). New York: Wiley.

Lambert, M. J., Shapiro, D. A., & Bergin, A. E. (1986). The effectiveness of psychotherapy. In S. L. Garfield & A. E. Bergin (Eds.), The handbook of psychotherapy and behavioral change: An empirical analysis (3rd ed., pp. 157–211). New York: Wiley.

McGuire, T. G. (1981). Financing psychotherapy: Costs, effects, and public policy. Cambridge, Mass.: Bollinger.

Masi, D. (1984). Designing employee assistance programs. New York: American Management Association.

Mechanic, D. (1978). Effects of psychological stress on perception of physical health and use of medical and psychiatric facilities. Journal of Human Stress, 4, 26–37.

Mechanic, D. (1980). Mental health and social policy. Englewood Cliffs, NJ: Prentice-Hall.

Meyers, J. K. et al. (1984). Six month prevalence of psychiatric disorders in three communities. Archives of General Psychiatry, 41, 959–967.

Miller, L. S. et al. (1981). Opinions and use of the DSM III system by practicing psychologists. Professional Psychologist, 12, 385–389.

President's Commission on Mental Health. (1978). Vol 1. Washington, DC, U.S. Government Printing Office.

Reiger, D. A., Goldberg, I. D., & Taube, C. A. (1978). The de facto U.S. mental health system: A public health perspective. Archives of General Psychiatry, 35, 685–693.

Roughman, K., & Hoggerty, R. J. (1972). Family stress and the use of health services. *International Journal of Epidemiology, 1,* 279–288.

Saxe, L. (1980). *The efficacy and cost effectiveness of psychotherapy.* Washington, DC: Office of Technology Assessment Congress of U.S. G.P.O. (no. 052-003-00783-5).

Schlesinger, T. J., Mumford, E., & Glass, G. V. (1983). Mental health treatment and medical care utilization in a fee for services system: Outpatient mental health treatment following the onset of chronic diseases. *American Journal of Public Health, 73,* 422–429.

Smith, J. L., Glass, G. V., & Miller, T. I. (1960). *The benefits of psychotherapy.* Baltimore: John Hopkins University Press.

Smith, M. L., & Glass, G. V. (1977). Meta analysis of psychotherapy outcome studies. *American Psychologist, 32,* 752–760.

Strupp, H. (1978). Psychotherapy research and practice: An overview. In S. L. Garfield & A. E. Bergin (Eds.), *Handbook of psychotherapy and behavioral change: An empirical analysis* (2nd ed., pp. 3–22). New York: Wiley.

Taube, C. A., & Burret, S. A. (1985). Mental health. Rockville, MD: U.S. P.H.H.S. Publ. ADM 85-1378.

Veroff, J., Kulka, R. A., & Douvan, E. (1981). *Mental health in America.* New York: Basic Books.

Videka-Sherman, L. (1988). Meta analysis of research on social work practice in mental health. *Social Work, 33,* 325–338.

Witte, R., & Cannon, M. (1979). EAP's: Getting top management's support. *Personnel Administrator, 24,* 23–26.

II

Technical Issues

As the chapters in the introductory section—each in its own way—strongly suggested, there are commonalities of focus, time, and activity that are shared by all of the brief psychotherapies, whatever their apparent theoretical orientation and their professed strategies of change. Responding to these conceptual and philosophical parameters inexorably propels the clinician into a series of technical dilemmas that must be resolved, if they cannot be avoided through foreknowledge. This section examines a number of the technical issues raised by the need for the brief therapist to assume an active, even directive role in relation to motivating and guiding clients toward their chosen goals of change.

The section begins with a chapter by Szapocznik (5) and his colleagues who describe their work in engaging families in therapy through identifying and challenging their initial misconceptions and structural resistances to change. Like many brief therapists, they view the process of engagement as beginning with the initial telephone contact and frequently foundering at that point, if not effectively managed by the clinician. Although their chapter is written from a family therapy perspective, the clinician utilizing one-to-one approaches can also benefit from their work, especially their underlying notion that engaging and motivating clients is an interactive process in which the clinician must play an active and planned role.

Hoyt's chapter (6) on time in brief therapy is, we believe, one of the most comprehensive and useful considerations that this vital topic has received. He characterizes time as both a medium and a perspective in brief therapy and develops this viewpoint through a detailed discussion of both theory and practice, with a liberal infusion of case vignette and illustration. Although there is no doubt that the explicit time limit of brief therapy affects the client, perhaps its most signal impact is upon the therapist, as a deliberate and open commitment to the possibility of change.

On the other hand, Levy and Shelton (Chapter 7) approach the utilization of tasks as yet another integral part of the core of brief intervention. Just as the therapist must be active within the session for brief therapy to succeed, so must meaningful client participation be stimulated and encouraged outside the session if change is to take place. Their chapter describes in detail the various devices by which the imaginative and enterprising therapist can identify, develop, and assign a variety of such tasks and homework assignments.

Finally, the intriguing chapter by Rosenbaum, Hoyt, and Talmon (Chapter 8) on single-session psychotherapy could have easily been placed in one of the modality sections later in this volume. It is deliberately included in this section as the practice of single-session intervention, certainly the most parsimonious and perhaps the demanding of the brief therapies, highlights dramatically the issues of focus, time, and action that undergird the entire family of short-term psychotherapies.

Many of these topics will reoccur in later chapters of the *Handbook* as the specific types of tasks or time limits favored by one particular brief therapy or another are spelled out. The specific tasks utilized in brief sexual therapy, for instance, are very different from those of general crisis intervention, and, obviously, different clinical issues may arise in their application and management. However, the discussion in this section of these parameters of engagement, time, and tasks is intended to orient the reader to their overall place across the entire spectrum of the brief psychotherapies and, most importantly, to assist in the task of identifying and clarifying the most critical facets of the action dimension in which the brief psychotherapist must always operate.

5

Innovations in Family Therapy
Strategies for Overcoming Resistance to Treatment

Jose Szapocznik, Angel Perez-Vidal, Olga Hervis, Andrew L. Brickman, and William M. Kurtines

The Problem: Resistance to Family Treatment

Regardless of their theoretical orientation or mode and place of practice, every therapist has had the disappointing and frustrating experience of "resistance to therapy" in the form of missed or canceled first appointments. For the family therapist, this becomes an even more common and complex issue because more than one individual needs to be engaged to come to treatment.

Unfortunately the therapist often handles this problem by accepting the resistance on the part of some family members. In effect, the therapist complies with the family's definition that only one member is sick and needs treatment or that only one member is "motivated" to change. Consequently, the initially well-intentioned family therapist agrees to see only one or two people for treatment. With children and adolescents, this usually results in either the child or the overwrought mother becoming the patient who follows through with therapy visits.

The therapist has been "inducted" into the family's definition of the problem, or the family's expectation as to who should "change." Thus the therapist has accepted the family's definition of who is responsible for the cause and/or the solution of their difficulties. The therapist, far from challenging the maladaptive patterns of interaction within the family, literally allies and reinforces the patterns that have kept the family from resolving their problems on their own. It is this perception of their problem that has kept the family "stuck" and unable to come to an adaptive resolution.

Jose Szapocznik, Angel Perez-Vidal, Olga Hervis, and Andrew L. Brickman • Spanish Family Guidance Center, Department of Psychiatry, University of Miami School of Medicine, Miami, Florida 33136.   William M. Kurtines • Department of Psychology, Florida International University, Miami, Florida 33199.

When the therapist agrees to see part of the family, this in effect surrenders therapeutic authority to orchestrate change. Moreover, the well-intentioned therapist who persists in eventually interviewing the rest of the family will be at a great disadvantage because of having begun by establishing a therapeutic relationship with only part of the family. The practitioner will be perceived as having a coalition with the initial allied family member, and indeed, this will be the case. Unable to step back and observe the system as a whole, unable to be a director/choreographer who knows all of the scripts, the clinician will be a player on the stage, familiar with only one of the scripts. The therapist may have thus lost the opportunity to see everyone who lives in a household, to grasp the problem and the patterns of interaction that maintain it.

Unfortunately, many family therapists have resolved the dilemma of the resistant family by taking the position that there are too many motivated families waiting for help, that the resistant families will call back when they finally feel the need, or that there is no need to get involved in a power struggle! The reality for these families is bleak. If they are expected to come to therapy on their own, they will likely fail. Ironically, the families that most need therapy are families in which their patterns and habits are most resistant to change and consequently are most likely to interfere with effective help-seeking behaviors.

There is another alternative to this dilemma for the therapist, one based on the following premises: (1) each family has an organization, a system, comprised of patterns and interactions among the members of the family; (2) the symptom that the family presents to the therapist helps to maintain the family's patterns of interaction; and (3) the family system's resistance to change results from the system seeking to maintain the symptom that in turn preserves the family patterns of interactions. Thus the key to eliminating the resistance to therapy lies within the family's resistant patterns of interactions; overcome the resistance in these patterns of interaction, and the family will come to therapy.

The very same principles that apply to the role of a symptom in maintaining maladaptive patterns of family interactions also apply to the role of resistance to enter treatment as a symptom or mechanism for protecting this very same maladaptive pattern of interaction. Fortunately, however, the very same principles that apply to the understanding of family functioning and treatment, also apply to the understanding and treatment of the family's resistance to change.

In our work, we call a family's repetitive and habitual patterns of interaction the family's structure; and we call the treatment of the family's resistance to coming into therapy *Structural Systems Engagement*.

A SOLUTION: STRUCTURAL SYSTEMS ENGAGEMENT

Structural Systems Engagement (SSE) has been designed to achieve the full involvement of the family in the therapy process. This involvement comes about in a planned and purposeful way. It utilizes the techniques of structural family therapy but focuses on identifying and removing the family's resistance to engaging in a therapeutic contract.

The strategies presented here for engaging adolescent drug abusers into therapy were developed by first extending the techniques of family therapy forward into the engagement process and then determining what patterns emerged that were unique to the engagement of resistant families.

The terminology used in this chapter is consistent with structural theory and techniques. A discussion of these techniques will be presented in this section. In addition, the reader is referred to our work on Brief Strategic Family Therapy (Szapocznik, Foote, Perez-Vidal, Hervis, & Kurtines, 1985; Szapocznik, Kurtines, Foote, Perez-Vidal, & Hervis, 1983; Szapocznik, Kurtines, Hervis, & Spencer, 1984; Szapocznik, Perez-Vidal, Hervis, & Foote, 1983; Szapocznik, Kurtines, Perez-Vidal, Hervis, & Foote, Chapter 20 this volume; Szapocznik & Kurtines, 1989) as well as the original formulations of the theory and practice of strategic and structural family therapy in the works of Minuchin (1974; Minuchin & Fishman, 1981), Haley (1976), Madanes (1981), Aponte (1974), Stanton and Todd (1981), and their colleagues.

In describing SSE in this chapter, it is assumed that the reader is somewhat familiar with the concepts of structural family therapy. Both SSE and structural family therapy rest upon a common theoretical foundation. The core theoretical concepts include that of system and structure. *System* is the most basic concept and refers to a view of the family as made up of individuals who are mutually interdependent. *Structure* refers to the habitual and repetitive patterns of interaction that develop among members of the family system. A third concept that has often been applied to structural family therapy and that is central to our work is that of strategy. *Strategic* refers to a general approach to formulating treatment that includes being problem focused, making careful intervention plans, and being practical.

The sections that follow present a blueprint, using these concepts, for the family therapist to follow in working with families resistant to therapy. We have already described "the problem," that is, the paradox of a family's seeking help and resisting coming to therapy; and the second paradox of the therapist wishing to help and yet surrendering before the battle begins. The next section describes concepts and techniques already familiar to the structural family therapist applied to the treatment of resistance to coming to therapy. These concepts and techniques are thus presented in a new light, highlighting differences and similarities when these techniques are applied to the treatment of a symptom, such as drug abuse, versus the treatment of resistance to coming to therapy. Subsequent sections present the application of SSE to resistant families. Although no two families are alike, a structural analysis of over 100 drug-abusing Hispanic families in the Miami area revealed four basic patterns of resistance. These resistance patterns and how to overcome them are also discussed and illustrated at the end of this chapter.

EXTENDING STRUCTURAL SYSTEMS TECHNIQUES TO ENGAGEMENT

Unlike conventional therapy, which views the treatment process as beginning once the family is in the therapist's office, SSE is built on the assumption that treatment begins with the first phone call or contact between a family member and the therapist. The initial therapeutic challenge is to overcome resistance to therapy. Once families are engaged in therapy, the therapeutic challenge shifts from "resistance to therapy" to "treatment."

When the therapist only has access to one or a few family members initially, rather than commencing treatment on the presenting symptom (e.g., drug abuse), the therapist may consider that having the entire family in treatment is desirable. In this case, SSE can be used initially to (1) join the family through those members who are accessible and available and, through them (2) diagnose the interactive patterns that are keeping the entire family from treatment. With a better understanding of the interactions that are keeping some family members from treatment, the therapist can (3) intervene to overcome the resistant behaviors and bring the whole family into treatment.

The structural systems techniques used in engaging families are modeled after the structural systems techniques developed for use with families in treatment. However, we have modified these techniques to extend them forward in the treatment process. The major techniques can be separated into three types: joining, diagnosing and restructuring. The way in which these techniques are used during engagement are discussed separately later. As illustrated in the cases at the end of this chapter, in actual practice, joining, diagnosing, and restructuring are often intermixed.

Joining

Joining is a process that begins with the therapist's very first contact with the person (i.e., family member) who calls for help and continues throughout the entire experience with the family. While joining a family, the therapist is constantly eliciting its cooperation as well as seeking to discover how the family actually operates. That is, what are its structures, and which ones are maladaptive? Receiving the family's cooperation and diagnosing its structures are, of course, essential in order to pursue making successful and constructive changes. Not until a family has successfully joined with the therapist will the therapist be in a position to assume a leadership role in guiding the family to make changes. The techniques found most useful in joining are the following:

Establishing a Therapeutic Alliance

Because in SSE the therapist will be working initially with and through only one or a few family members, it is important to form a very firm bond with these individuals. The therapist will need to work with these persons in order to bring about the changes necessary to engage the family in therapy. Creating this kind of relationship requires making use of joining because joining techniques have been designed to promote a strong client/therapist relationship. Through joining with various members of the family, the therapist can elicit the cooperation of the entire family in the engagement effort and confirm his or her role as a leader within the family's structure.

Maintenance

Families and family members in most cases are frightened, defensive and may resent having to come in for treatment. A family's confidence can be won by being supportive and accepting; paradoxically, the therapist initially accepts and thereby maintains a family and their way of interacting, even though not agreeing with their life-style or manner of relating with each other. The family is supported when the therapist says something positive, finds something to praise, shows empathy with the family's pain, and identifies with those aspects of the family with which the therapist can resonate. Although this support maintains the family's maladaptive ways, it gains good will for the therapist that can later be used for therapeutic gain.

Mimesis

This refers to adapting to the family or person's style. For example, if a family or family member is serious, the therapist should also be serious. If there is a certain amount of levity, then enter into the mood with an appropriate anecdote or joke. Mimesis reflects clearly the therapist's efforts at gaining mutual acceptance and blending in by imitating the family or person who calls. The therapist, for example, may imitate speech patterns or the mood of the family. In working with a family or family member, these mimetic operations are helpful in joining because the family or family member feels accepted, and thus safe, in cooperating with someone who works within the family's own style, affect, activity, and mood.

When tasks are given, tasks must fit the people being asked to do them. A therapist's description of therapy must fit the family's style as well as the individuals being asked to participate. If the family is rational and logical, then therapy must be offered and proposed in a logical, orderly plan. If the family style is casual, therapy must be presented as spontaneous and casual. If the family is humorous, find the humor in getting together. If the family has a flair for the dramatic, they can be told that therapy is a major "thing" being asked in the lives. For families who are resistant out of fear, therapy may be minimized by describing it as a small thing being asked of them.

In structural terms, this is called *accommodation*. It is a powerful joining technique that aids in rendering the therapist (and consequently the therapy) more syntonic with the family, thus making him or her more comfortable and acceptable.

Tracking

Tracking refers to following the content and interactive process presented by the person or family. If we want to move the family from their present maladaptive interactions to healthy functioning, we do it most easily by moving the family along those "paths" in either content or interactional style it has already established.

There are two kinds of tracking: content and process tracking. In content tracking, the therapist "follows" the content presented by the family member such as their concerns or presenting symptoms (e.g., I am worried about my child's drug abuse) and uses these content concerns as rationales around which to mobilize the family. A frequent example of content tracking in the case of a resistant adolescent is to encourage an adolescent to tell all the ways his parents are interfering in his life and then to say "Well, if you come into treatment we can work on getting them off your back." In this example, the adolescent's own motivation is used to help overcome resistance to treatment. An example of process tracking is to identify in a particular family who is the most powerful family member (it could be the adolescent drug abuser or mother or father) and to strongly ally with this most powerful family member in order to bring the family into treatment. Hence, the therapist tracks the power in the family to get the family mobilized.

Tracking, then, can be used in reaching the various family members who are resistant to coming to therapy. Tracking involves following the natural pathways of the system or person. In engaging family members, the therapist psychologically tracks their needs, agendas, goals, and style. The therapist also tracks physically by adjusting to the client's time, place, or space, reaching the client when and where it is convenient and natural for the client.

With both tracking and mimesis, there is an important point to keep in mind. The therapist wants to become the family's leader and lead them out of their maladaptive behaviors. However, a leader first becomes a leader by knowing when to follow. First, the therapist follows the family through mimesis and by tracking the family's interactional patterns. Then once the family has joined with the therapist and been inducted into a therapeutic system, the therapist can become the leader of this therapeutic system and lead the family to new interactions.

Diagnosing

In the case of engagement, because it is not possible to directly observe the interactions of the family, the therapist very often must track through the caller and any other members who may conjointly or sequentially involve themselves in the process of bringing the family to therapy. Because this often results in the therapist initially not seeing the whole family at once, the actual interactions may not be self-evident at first glance. However, in this case the therapist tracks in two ways:

1. The clinician "follows" from the first family member, to the next available, and the next, and so forth. This "following" is done without challenging the structure and by permitting the structure to open up its available doors, letting the therapist in.

2. The therapist makes use of the concept of *complementarity*. For a family to work as a unit (even though maladaptively), the behaviors of each family member must "fit in" (i.e., complement or supplement) with the behavior of each and every other family member. Thus, within the family, for each action there is

a complementary reaction. The behaviors of members of a family are like the wheels that make up the inner workings of a clock. For the clock to keep on ticking, all the wheels must turn in a certain way. Similarly, for the family to continue to function or dysfunction in a certain way, everyone must behave in a certain way. When a caller tells the therapist that her husband becomes angry at anything she says, the therapist needs to ascertain what the caller said or how the caller said it to elicit an angry response. The task of the therapist is to get as much information as possible and then fill in the missing information using this understanding of complementarity.

Mapping

Engagement mapping is used to identify structural relations impacting on resistance to therapy in order to provide the basis which to plan the types of changes required to overcome resistance. The engagement maps are used to identify the four types of resistant families described in a later section on families with drug-abusing adolescents.

In accordance with the tenets of structural systems theory, the therapist tracks the family's motivation through the initial caller, using the engagement map. In the process of allying with the caller, the therapist asks clarifying questions, evidences interest in the family, and does not challenge existing patterns of behavior. Via an alliance with the caller, information is obtained about the family, or by moving from the caller to other family members, information is obtained directly regarding family interactions that permit the therapist to develop a map depicting the family's interactions and power structure and how these interactions may collude to keep the family from therapy.

Using the map, the therapist moves through the family system attempting to ally with those individuals in the family with the leverage to bring the family into treatment. By using the engagement map to follow the flow of family power, the alliances and the communication avenues, the therapist blends with the family structure without initially challenging the existing system and thus gains position as a leader of the newly formed therapeutic system.

Engagement mapping offers information on the nature of the obstacles to engagement on the basis of which the therapist can make a variety of restructuring decisions. These include reframing, shifting of alliances that either maintain the symptom or can potentially render the patient amenable to therapy, opening of closed but necessary communication channels that are of interest or influence to the patient, and redistribution of power to unbalance the status quo that permits the family to stay out of treatment and remain symptomatic.

Once the engagement/therapeutic alliance is established and the family's maladaptive pattern of interactions—that are keeping the family from treatment—have been identified, the therapist can choose how to move, either by tracking available interactions or by moving around those interactions, that are blocking engagement. In addition, engagement mapping enables the therapist to offer the caller continued support, in a purposeful and clear manner, while together they struggle to bring the family to therapy.

Restructuring

Restructuring refers to operations aimed at challenging the familial status quo, testing its flexibility for change and creating situations that permit more functional alternatives to emerge. Restructuring during the initial or engagement stages aims at making it possible to effect changes in those family interactions that are keeping the entire family from coming to treatment. There are a variety of ways in which change-producing interventions can be made to overcome resistance. A number of the techniques that can be used to restructure and shift family interactional patterns are as follows.

Reframing

The therapist relabels a process, a person, or an event, offering an alternative organization, label, or even essence for the entity. This new conceptualization implies a new way of behaving toward that entity, or a new attitude is brought forth that in turn results in different reactions and behaviors. For example, the therapist may suggest to a son who complains that his parents want him to come to therapy just to get on his case, that "you are right. Your parents are indeed very anxious about your welfare." Hence, the parents' nagging is reframed in terms of anxiety for the son's welfare.

Reversals

The therapist can change a habitual pattern of interacting by coaching one member of the family to say or do the opposite of her or his usual response. A reversal of the established sequence breaks up previously rigid patterns that are pathological and allows new alternatives to emerge. For example, the therapist may recommend to a wife who was berating her husband for not seeking help for their drug-abusing son that she approach him sweetly and "catch him with honey."

Detriangulation

Triangulation occurs when a third person becomes inappropriately involved in a conflict between two other people. Triangles are viewed as being very maladaptive as they prevent dyadic relationships from processing and growth. The conflict between the two people is said to be *detoured* or *diffused* through the third person. Detriangulation prevents the dyad in conflict (e.g., husband–wife) from transacting "business" directly. For example, in a family where there is a close alliance between mother and son, as well as a strong marital conflict, the father may get at the mother through the son by denigrating and belittling him. Conversely, the son and mother are actually pairing up to keep the father distanced from the family. In this fashion, father and mother do not have to discuss their conflict directly, but rather act it out indirectly.

In the case of engagement, however, the family must first be brought into treatment before actual detriangulation can be attempted. At the engagement stage, the existence of such a triangle alerts the therapist to the fact that the father–mother conflict and the mother's desire to keep father distant would not make it feasible to bring father into treatment via mother. Hence, the therapist will have to access each—mother and father—separately to avoid becoming triangulated as well.

Opening Closed Systems

Closed, dormant systems give the appearance of calm so that the tension can be felt somewhere else in the family. One way to open such a system and thus realistically confront the problem genesis is to activate it by magnifying small emotional issues, thereby, creating crises. This, in turn, activates dormant interactions so they can be dealt with openly and in a new manner. Closed systems are those that are bounded solidly so that interaction within is too intense and interaction without is nonexistent. The idea of "opening" refers to opening its boundaries to the outside world so that tension and intensity within is reduced and so that relationships with others can be established to inject new life, new options, and new resources into those individuals who compose it.

An example of a closed system that affects engagement is the case of the wife who calls for help for her son and when asked to bring her husband, expresses fear of letting her husband know about the son's drug use. The nature of the relationship between mother and father is clearly strained, but the strain is dormant. In this case, the therapist might fuel the mother's feelings of not having father's help when she needs him and thus get her to overcome her feeling of not wanting him to know by enhancing previously dormant feelings that he is also responsible.

A similar strategy is to encourage the family members (especially the angry, resistant kind) to talk about how desperate their situation is. Rather than reassuring them it is not so bad, the therapist can agree with them that it is quite bad. If the situation is made to appear desperate enough, they may be more likely to listen and try what the therapist is offering. That is, the therapist uses their desperation as a motivation by emphasizing it and can even project their situation into the future and have the members talk about how disastrous the future will be if something is not done now. Exaggerating the symptom in this manner must be done not only by saying how dreadful it is but also through setting up a scenario where the dreadfulness becomes intolerant. For example: "It is so bad that I think you should turn your son in to the authorities; maybe the court can be something that you can't. I can help you to contact the law enforcement system." Just talking about the situation is usually not good enough because the family have already done that.

EMPLOYING TASKS IN ENGAGING THE FAMILY

Assigning tasks is an essential ingredient of structural family therapy through which the therapist manipulates and reshapes the family in a concrete, behavioral manner. In SSE, tasks are a vital component of the work of reversing resistant structures and are applied, not to the issues of what to do with the family once they are in treatment, but rather, what to do with a family in order to get them into treatment. The first *task* that we give to a family is that of coming together to therapy.

When assigning any task, the therapist must expect that the task may not be performed as requested. Tasks represent direct and sensible actions that relatively well-functioning people can take to correct the unpleasant situations about which they complain. For example, the therapist may give the mother the task of discussing with her husband his participation in therapy on Tuesday in order to bring their rebellious 15-year-old son who is using drugs and skipping school. The implication in the task is that the mother and father will work cooperatively and effectively to achieve their son's adherence to their decision. If it were that simple, the family would probably not need to come to therapy at all. They would already possess the requisite family and parenting skills necessary to control their child. Therefore, it is important that the therapist be prepared for failure and, further, that failure to accomplish this initial task be defined in much the same way as failure to accomplish other therapeutic tasks.

It is amusing and noteworthy to observe that many seasoned family therapists, experienced in defining other family phenomena from a system perspective, quickly revert to individual-type thinking when confronted with systemic *resistance* to therapeutic engagement. Such therapists will use nonsystemic terms like *uncaring father, overwhelmed* or *weak mother, sociopathic youngster, lacking insight into the problem,* and *selfish.* They will feel angry and frustrated and quickly give up working with the resistant family, moving on to a more motivated, better functioning family system. This is beneficial to the therapist's cure record, yet is of no help to the family who cannot mobilize itself to receive help.

From a systems perspective, failure to accomplish the task of bringing the family to therapy can be viewed as another effort of the system to maintain its homeostatic self-regulatory mechanism of nurturing the identified symptom. Refusals to come to therapy always have their roots in the family's interactional conflicts. The failure to come to therapy must therefore be explored in a way that uncovers the conflict, thereby offering solutions. Several facets of task utilization should be kept in mind as the practitioner stimulates such exploration.

Tasks may be given as good advice, or *as directives to change sequences in the family.* The therapist first gives the task of bringing the whole family to therapy to the member calling for help in the form of good advice. The therapist explains why this is a good idea with the usual promises of support. Occasionally, this is all that is needed. Often people do not request family therapy simply because it is not well-known and thus it does not occur to them to take such action. Sometimes, there is fear of what will happen if "all the skeletons are let out." For example, some family members may fear that some dreaded secret may be disclosed (e.g., an extramarital affair) or that old wounds may be reopened. Some of these fears may be real, others may simply be imagined or suspected. In these latter instances, families may respond to reassuring advice in order to overcome their apprehension and consequently come to therapy.

Very often, however, simply addressing the issue at a rational level is not sufficient to mobilize a family. Directives are needed to change the ways in which family members deal with one another. These directives change patterns that are uncovered (or diagnosed) by the very resistance or failure to perform the task.

To motivate a client to do something means to persuade him or her that there is some gain in it. When a therapist wishes to motivate family members to carry out a task, it is necessary to convince them that the task (i.e., coming to therapy) will achieve the ends they want for themselves individually, for each other, and for the family. How to motivate a family depends on the nature of the task (coming to therapy), the nature of the family (to be explored as the task is resisted), and the nature of the relationship the therapist has with the family (to be developed strategically in response to the previously mentioned ones).

A common and very effective approach is for the therapist to convey to the resistant members the knowledge that they want to solve *their* problems and to also say that the therapist wants the same thing. However, it must be recognized that how the problem is defined may vary from one member to another. For example, the mother may want to get her son to quit drugs, whereas the son may want to get his mother off his back. When the therapist and the family members agree on a goal, therapy is offered in the framework of achieving that goal. Even when family members are in conflict over their aims, it is necessary to find some gain for each of them to be achieved from therapy. For example, the therapist can say to the mother that her son should stop using drugs; to the son that his mother should get off his back and stop her nagging; and to the father, that he should stop being called in constantly to referee or play "bad guy." Therefore, they should all come to therapy.

Last, a task must always be clear and precise; never confusing. The task of getting a family to come together for treatment must be presented with clarity and precision. Certainly the date, time, and place need to be negotiated so that there is no ambivalence or inconvenience. In addition, therapy must be explained in a manner that lets the family know exactly what is expected of them and what they can expect in return. Where there is any doubt that someone understands, the therapist should take the initiative to address that person's quizzical look and attempt to resolve any misconceptions or misgivings.

SYSTEMIC PATTERNS OF RESISTANCE

More often than not, the very patterns that emerge in a family to resist change and therapy are the same patterns that give rise to and maintain the symptom that the family seeks to eliminate. An astute therapist will begin to formulate some concepts about these problem patterns from the moment the call for help is received. The therapist will then have an opportunity to validate and elaborate these observations as resistance to therapy unfolds. The presenting problem, family composition, ages of the members, and individual levels of motivation are all clues to the family organization, power distribution, role assignment, and function. The therapist begins to formulate a map that suggests areas of intervention: who to contact, who to join, how to join, what to offer whom, and how to reframe their perception of therapy. In working with a resistant family, the therapist must gain initial entry and map the family before the family ever becomes receptive to forming a full therapeutic alliance. That is, initially the therapist makes enough changes in the family to gain entry that further allows the therapist the opportunity to join the system with the stated purpose of changing how it operates. As a first objective, the therapist changes how the system operates to keep the family from treatment, and once in treatment, the therapist can work on the presenting problem.

This chapter is the result of work done with Hispanic families where the presenting problem was an adolescent known or believed by the parents to be using drugs and/or exhibiting a series of other behaviors associated with the use of drugs such as truancy, delinquency, aggressiveness, frequent fights in and outside the home, and coming home very late at night. As such, the examples to be used are common to Hispanic families with adolescents and are not intended to represent all possible types of structural configurations that work to resist therapy. Therapists working with other types of problems and families are encouraged to review their case load of "difficult to engage" families and to carefully examine the clues that diagnose the systemic resistances to therapy in much the same fashion as those offered in this chapter.

Four general structural organizations emerge from an analysis of families of drug-abusing adolescents who present engagement resistance to the therapist. These patterns are discussed next in terms of what becomes evident to the therapist as the mechanisms of resistance go into effect.

Powerful Identified Patient

These families have within their structure a powerful Identified Patient (IP) and parents who are hierarchically positioned at a lower level of power relative to the IP. The salient characteristic of the lack of parental power at the initial stages of engagement is the inability of the parents to bring the child to therapy without lying to the child. Very often, the mother of a powerful IP will admit that she is weak or ineffective and will say that her son or daughter flatly refuses to come to therapy. We can assume that the IP resists therapy because:

1. It threatens his or her position of power and moves him or her to a "problem-person" position.
2. It is the parents' agenda to come to therapy and thus if followed will enhance the parents' power.

Restructuring needs to be done to alter the existing hierarchical organization in which the IP is in power, thereby eliminating the resistance to initial engagement. In these cases, the hierarchical organization is altered not by "demoting" the IP (that move would be totally rejected) but rather by allying the therapist to the "ruling structure." The therapist brings respect and concern for the IP but also brings an agenda of change that will then, by virtue of the alliance, be shared by the IP.

In order to bring these families into treatment, the IP's hierarchical position is not directly challenged but tracked and allied to the therapist so that the therapist may interject a formulation and solution to the problem. Therefore, the therapist forms an alliance with the powerful IP in order to reframe the need for therapy in a manner that strengthens the IP in a positive way. The reframing is done so that the symptom is transferred from the IP to the family (further supporting the IP's power, to be later challenged in therapy). The other alternative, that of forming an alliance with the parents, would be premature and ineffective at the early stage of the engagement process as the parental subsystem is not strong enough at this point. The pressure to perform while the therapist has no direct access to the IP would render the parents even weaker, and the family would not return for treatment.

Contact Person Protecting Structure

These families are defined by a structure in which the person making the agency contact (usually the mother) is also the person protecting the resistant behavior. The mother gives a double-message to the therapist, "I want to take my family to therapy, but my son can't come because he forgot and fell asleep and my husband has so much work he can't take any time to come to therapy." The mother is expressing a desire for the therapist's help while at the same time protecting and allying with the family's resistance to be involved in solving the problem. The mother "protects" this resistance by agreeing that the excuses for noninvolvement in change are valid. In other words, she is supporting the arguments used for maintaining the status quo. It is worthwhile to note that ordinarily this is the same double bind in the family that perpetuates the symptomatic structure; someone complains of the problem behavior yet supports the maintenance of the problem. This pattern is typical of the family whose patterns of resistance are closely tied to a problem of enmeshment between the mother and the IP.

In order to bring these families into treatment, the therapist must first form an alliance with the mother by acknowledging her frustration in wanting to get help and not getting any cooperation from other family members. Through this alliance, the therapist is then given access to the other members. The therapist can then deal with these other family members directly and, without the mother's "protection," join each family member to then challenge their position of resistance.

Disengaged Parents

These family structures are characterized by little or no cohesiveness or alliance between the parents as a subsystem. In addition, one of the parents (usually the father) refuses to go to therapy. This is typically a parent who has remained disengaged from the problematic behavior. This additional resistance serves to disengage him from another problematic relationship: the other spouse. Typically, the mother is overinvolved (enmeshed) with the IP and either incompetent in parenting or supporting the IP in a covert fashion. For example, if the father moves in to control the behavior, she complains he is too tough or creates mythical fears about his potential violence. Thus the father is rendered useless and again moves out, reestablishing the disengagement between husband and wife. In such families, the dimension of *resonance* is of foremost importance in planning change to bring them to therapy. Very briefly, resonance is that measure of closeness/distance that qualifies any relationship. The closer the relationship (enmeshed), the higher the degree of sensitivity for one another, and conversely, the greater the distance (disengaged), the lower will be the awareness of the other.

In order to engage these families, the therapist must form an alliance with the caller (usually the mother) and bring her closer to the father in tasks that distance her from the IP. To accomplish this, the therapist begins to direct the mother's interactions with the father, changing their patterns of interaction so as to bring him into therapy. The mother is given tasks to do together with the father pertaining *only* to the issue of taking care of the IP's problems. This is done because it must be assumed that if father and mother have become distanced there must be a conflict between them, and it is best during this very early stage for the therapist to avoid any potential confrontation of the marital conflict. The aim at this stage is to provide a task that will restructure mother and father's interaction in a way that stimulates the father to come to therapy.

Although the pattern is similar to that of the contact person protecting the structure, in this instance the resistance emerges differently. In this case, the mother does not excuse the father's distance but, to the contrary, complains about her spouse's disinterest and is usually more willing to do something, given some direction.

Therapy as an Exposé

Sometimes therapy is threatening to one or more individuals, and they resist coming because they are afraid of being made a scapegoat or that dangerous secrets will be revealed. These individuals' beliefs or "frames" about therapy are usually an extension of the "frame" within which the family is functioning.

The therapist must reframe the idea or goal of therapy in a way that eliminates its negative consequences and replaces them for positive aims. This must be done for the member(s) of the family who are feeling threatened by therapy.

CLINICAL ILLUSTRATIONS

In reviewing these patterns, it is evident that considerably more changes are needed to render a family motivated for therapy in some types of families than in others. For example, families with disengaged parents require more therapeutic work than families in which the contact person is protecting the structure. In turn, the latter type of families need more work than those protecting a family secret, where a simple reframing from a position of close therapeutic alliance is likely to be sufficient. Therefore, the notion of degree of change needed by different types of resistant families becomes a highly relevant issue, though not unlike the already accepted reality that some families in therapy need more thorough and deeper restructuring than others. In this final section, we will illustrate how SSE techniques can be applied to each of these types of families.

Case I

Identified Patient in a Powerful Position

Identifying Information. The IP is a 15-year-old male who is living with his father and stepmother. He had previously lived with his mother, her boyfriend, and a half-brother.

Initial Contact. 1/31/84—Mr. L. called the clinic requesting an appointment for his son to be seen by a psychologist. He explained that his son, Raul, had recently been thrown out of his ex-wife's home and had come to live with him and his second wife. Raul was using cocaine and marijuana on a daily basis and alcohol on weekends. The situation was particularly critical because Raul was very disruptive to the father's household. The therapist scheduled an appointment for the following morning. 2/1/84—Family does not show up for appointment; no call or explanation. 2/2/84—Raul's stepmother called the therapist and reported that Raul refuses to come to therapy. Raul told his father, "I am not crazy and don't bother me anymore." The therapist explained that it will be necessary to speak directly with either Raul or the father. If necessary, the therapist explained, he would go to the home.

Assessment. At initial contact, the family appears to be disrupted, and its structure is chaotic by virtue of two divorces, three "parental" figures, and family's apparent inability to maintain order. Often these situations place the offspring in a rather powerful position at an early age as parenting become inadequate and incompetent. Raul, the IP, is both resented and feared, thus increasing his inner sense of worthlessness that is compensated by acting-out anger. Raul has no allies in the family. He holds a powerful yet lonely position. The parents play a game of ping-pong to see who will exercise less parenting. Meanwhile, Raul continues to be left unsupported, undirected and unstructured.

Engagement Plan. The therapist needs to reach Raul directly either through the stepmother or the father in order to create a therapeutic alliance that initially both respects his independence and power, yet has the potential for altering the power structure by placing another powerful person, the therapist, in an allied position to the IP. This new, and also powerful ally (the expert therapist), will then advocate for the parental agenda for change in Raul's behavior from a position inside the power structure (i.e., allied to the IP). In the case of engagement, the therapist advocates for Raul to come into treatment.

The therapist has to be willing to track the communication pathways to the IP through the stepmother, father, and/or whoever else appears necessary and, as needed, has to be willing to show deference to the IP by going to physically meet him wherever he is available. The therapist must follow the lines of communication in the family as they are laid out and also be willing to meet the IP "on his own turf," so to speak.

Implementation of Plan. 2/6/84—Therapist calls father. Mr. L. says that if the therapist makes a home visit, Raul will refuse to communicate and will walk out of the home. The therapist patiently explains to the father the most effective way of discussing the purpose of the therapist's visit. The therapist suggests to the father that when explaining the visit to Raul he deemphasize Raul's role as IP and instead tell him that the visit would be to help all the members of the family. The father agreed to call back.

2/7/84—Mr. L. called the therapist. He followed the therapist's advice on how to engage Raul. Raul agreed, contingent upon the therapist's coming to the father's home at 7:00P.M. that evening.

2/7/84—Home visit: The family was living in a cramped efficiency apartment on Miami Beach. The first strategy of the therapist was to join Raul. This was done by talking about the issues that interested the boy and agreeing with him whenever possible. These included the hassles of finding a job, putting up with parents trying to meddle, how terrible it is to be made to feel like a bum, and so on. The therapist skillfully moved the conversation to "Let's talk more about this in my office where I can give you more time and attention." Raul agreed to come to the clinic.

2/15/84—Raul arrived at the clinic with his father and stepmother. During their first hour together, the following information was revealed to the therapist, either directly or by observation:

1. Because Raul had just recently moved to the father's home, having lived most of his life with his mother, the father–son relationship was very weak.
2. It was only a matter of time before Raul would be expelled from the father's home due to space limitations and the increased tension he was causing.
3. The home in which Raul was raised consisted of his mother, the mother's common-law husband, and the maternal grandmother.

The therapist explained to Raul that it would be necessary to involve Raul's mother in the therapeutic process. He agreed. 2/16/84—The mother telephoned the therapist and explained how glad she was to hear that Raul was getting help and, of course, she would be glad to participate in therapy. 2/17/84—Raul moves back to mother's home. 2/18/84—Raul, his mother, grandmother, and the mother's boyfriend arrive together for intake.

Case II

Contact Person Protects Resistant Structure

Identifying Information. Family is composed of the 17-year-old male IP, father, mother, and two older sisters, ages 21 and 23.

Initial Contact. 4/9/84—Mother, 48 years old, calls the clinic stating her concern for her 17-year-old son, Manuel, who is using cocaine and marijuana. Therapist gives the mother support by listening to a lengthy explanation of her anguish and fears about "How is my son going to end up?" A prompt appointment for the next day is offered to reinforce the therapist's concern and willingness to help. Mother is told that the whole family needs to come. Mother answers with a cooled-down, "Well, I'll see what I can do, my husband and daughters are so busy all the time." Therapist reiterates that the help and involvement of the whole family is most needed and beneficial in treating the situation.

4/10/84—Mother calls the therapist to apologize, but she must cancel the appointment as no one in the family can come. Won't the therapist reconsider and just see her son and herself? Mother adds that her son, Manuel, prefers to come by himself anyway. When asked by the therapist if he could talk to the son directly, the mother explains, "Well, he's not in now, but whatever you and I negotiate will be okay by him." Asked if her husband was available, she again refuses access by saying, "No, he's rarely home anytime before 10:00 P.M., and I don't think he'll like my giving his work number because he doesn't want to deal with this at work."

Assessment. It is evident by the mother's speaking for her son in ways that indicate "special" knowledge of his wishes and control over his decisions that the mother and IP are in an enmeshed relationship. It is also evident by the mother's strong attempts to keep the father out that he has been kept distant from the son and his upbringing and that she wishes it to stay that way. Often in these cases, the son's acting out is an attempt to both gain independence from the mother and to get the father's attention for his support and guidance. To go along with the mother's plan would be a therapeutic mistake that reinforces the existing pathogenic structure and eliminates the possibility of creating a new structure, one that permits access of the son to the father so that a new alliance may aid in the son's acquisition of healthy independence.

Engagement Plan. The therapist must, through an alliance based on the mother's feelings and love for her son, move from the mother to gain direct access to Manuel and his father. From that position, he must help Manuel move closer to the father so as to convince the father to help him by coming to therapy.

Implementation of Plan. 4/10/84—(Same phone conversation.) Therapist suggests perhaps he could help her, "she, who's so concerned and obviously not getting much cooperation from the rest of the family" by talking to the rest of the members directly. The mother is hesitant. The therapist says, "I hear some fears on your part for me to do this; maybe I can help to reassure you that my only concern is to help your family see how important it is that we all work together in resolving Manuel's drug problem.

Often, as there are one or more "hidden" agendas or family secrets, the therapist needs to reassure the caller that other issues will be protected in these meetings unless the family eventually decides to deal with them.

Slowly but surely, the therapist, with warmth and patience, is able to convince the mother that he will be most tactful and "gentle" with the family, and she agrees to help the therapist talk to the father and Manuel directly.

The father will be contacted at home by phone in the evening, and Manuel will be met by the therapist after school in the schoolyard. The therapist, tracking the structure, asks the mother to be in charge of arranging these contacts with the father for this evening and Manuel for next afternoon.

4/10/84—The therapist calls the home and speaks to the father verbalizing the mother's great fears and concerns for Manuel's drug abuse and general emotional state. Initially the father is angry in tone. "I've had enough of hearing about his problems, he's 17 years old and if he wants to ruin his life, there's nothing I can do about it." The therapist hears the father's sense of hopelessness and ineffectiveness (not his anger) and highlights only this aspect of the man's communication to offer support and help and to correct the man's view of his adequacy and importance. "I beg to differ, sir, but it is precisely you who can best help your son, and you can do it with my help, as I have helped so many other fathers before; it is I who can't do it without you."

Father agrees to come to therapy, and the therapist gives him the task to ask Manuel tonight to be sure he keeps his appointment in the schoolyard with the therapist. This task begins to bring father closer to Manuel in a parenting position and thus insures Manuel's compliance with the meeting.

4/11/84—Therapist meets IP after school. Immediately he discovers that Manuel does want help with his drug problem but is afraid to meet with the family because he is homosexual and does not want the family to discover this in therapy. The therapist reassures the IP that the problem to be focused on in therapy is that of his drug use and that his sexual life is entirely his own business and need not be brought up at all. Feeling reassured, Manuel agrees to come to therapy. The therapist asks Manuel to be in charge of telling his family that their first appointment is for the next day at 6:00 P.M. and that he expects all to be there. This places Manuel in a position of power and control, thus reversing his feelings of inadequacy. 4/12/84—Family comes for intake and first session.

Case III

Disengaged Parents

Identifying Information. Family consists of 15-year-old male IP, mother, father, and 6-year-old brother.

Initial Contact. 9/5/84—A mother calls, referred to the clinic by the hospital where her son was treated for an overdose the night before. Therapist gives an appointment for the next day, immediately following the son's release from the hospital at 11:00 A.M. Therapist explains the father must also come. Younger brother is left out given the nature of the presenting problem and his tender age.

9/6/84—Mother and IP come to the appointment without the father. When questioned, mother states that the father refuses to come and be recorded on the records of a drug program that may hinder his career. With mother's permission, the therapist spends a few minutes reassuring the son of his willingness and ability to help him but explains that he must cancel today's session and contact the father directly as his participation is essential. Mother and son agree to proceed this way.

One hour later, the therapist reaches the father at work who refuses to talk in depth with the therapist except to say, "You must work with my son individually, he's old enough." Puzzled by his refusal to cooperate, the therapist confronts the father on the matter of his concern for a son who recently almost killed himself. The father confesses his love for his boy but explains that the marriage to his wife is in a terrible state and that he believes their participation in therapy would be detrimental rather than helpful to his son. The attitude is one of "We can't even help each other much less him and my wife has hurt him enough; keep him away from her."

Assessment. The alienation between the parents is most relevant because their energies are being spent mostly in rejecting each other rather than helping the son. The father's critical anger toward the mother keeps her distant from the husband and probably dependent on the son for emotional meaningfulness and support. The son is probably so locked in this triangulated position that in a sense he is already experiencing his own psychological death. The mother has apparently accepted being labeled as incompetent by the father. The father, in turn, experiences his own nonidentified incompetence in his inability to help his son. The parental conflict has thus been successful in rending the whole family into a state of helplessness and hopelessness. The son's sacrificial creation of a crisis is a cry for help for both himself and the marriage.

Engagement Plan. Therapist must begin to establish a sense of competence and hope in this family quickly, but he cannot use the son for he is already too overwhelmed by his sense of responsibility and centrality. The therapist must thus move to ally strongly with the mother, giving her support and guidance in reaching her husband purportedly on behalf of their son.

If the mother can move her husband to therapy, the son is relieved of his central position, hope is instilled, and husband and wife are engaged in a task that brings them to mutual cooperation, that is saving their son.

Implementation of Plan. 9/6/84—The therapist calls the mother after talking to the father and asks to meet her individually. She agrees to come to the clinic immediately.

In the office, the therapist spends a long time establishing a therapeutic alliance with the mother, reassuring her of his support in a manner that helps her to sense his expertise, ability, and concern. Also, the therapist begins to hear the history of how this marriage has gone wrong so as to look for clues as to where he can link the mother back to the husband. The main clue comes in discovering that some years ago, the husband began to do some heavy drinking after work and weekends, and his wife began criticizing, belittling and distancing him from his son. Although agreeing with the wife that the husband's problem drinking was totally undesirable, the therapist is able to convince the wife that the way in which she has approached the problem is not effective but rather has probably worsened the problem by making her husband feel rejected, disrespected, and alone. The therapist explains to the wife that despite her feelings of anger toward her husband, she must put her son's well-being ahead of her feelings for her husband and help her husband to become involved in therapy for two reasons: (1) the son needs his father, and (2) maybe this could eventually lead to the father working on his drinking, too. The therapist is successful in "selling" this idea to the mother who confesses that despite her anger, she loves her husband and wants to do whatever is needed for her son.

The therapist then directs the mother to prepare her husband's favorite dinner for that evening and afterwards speak to him privately. In this private conversation, she is to ask her husband to please put aside his anger at her, confessing she has not been supportive of him, and to agree to work with her in helping their son. Most important is that the mother make the father feel needed in a way that only he can fulfill.

9/7/84—Wife calls clinic. She carried out her tasks and despite husband's initial reluctance and aggressiveness, strengthened by the therapist's lengthy and strong support, she persisted and has been able to convince him to come. The therapist congratulates the wife and sets up an appointment for the next day. To reinforce the wife's work, the therapist asks her permission to call her husband directly and echo her statements to him about how important and central the father's help is in treating the son as well as how caring a father he is to put aside his marital issues to come forth for his son.

9/8/84—Family shows up for intake and first session.

Case IV

Therapy as an Exposé

Identifying Information. The family is composed of the 14-year-old female IP, mother, father, and 12-year-old brother.

Initial Contact. 1/12/84—The mother calls, worried about her daughter who has a boyfriend who is using drugs heavily. Daughter and boyfriend are also involved in school truancy together. The mother is afraid because the father has said that "either this ends, or I'll go beat up the boyfriend and put an end to this in my way."

Mother is given an appointment and told that the whole family needs to come.

1/13/84—The mother calls back stating that her husband refuses to come to the clinic. The therapist asks the mother for her husband's number at work so he can speak to him directly. The mother agrees.

The therapist calls the father who is initially angry at being bothered at work. The therapist apologizes, explaining that he, too, hates to do this but has heard from the mother about how the girl's situation is so critical: "We should do something now before things get worse." The father agrees and after a while relaxes his attitude and explains to the therapist that he does not want to come to therapy because he has had a mistress for some time now, and although the family knows about it, "Things have been left alone." He is afraid that in therapy this will come up, and "all sorts of feelings are going to be let loose." The therapist acknowledges his understanding of the sensitivity of the situation and agrees to talk to the wife again to see what can be done about keeping the father's affair out of the therapy session.

Assessment. This is a family that is keeping a secret. The daughter, like everyone else, knows about the secret and is angry that she should be scapegoated when there are others in the family also "misbehaving." Very often families deal with a serious conflict by denying the conflict and detouring it in another direction. To deny a conflict is to pretend it does not exist. To detour it is to place the energies and feelings belonging to that conflict into either another realistic problem that is then exaggerated, or alternatively on an issue that is in reality not conflictual but is made to look conflictual.

The mother wishes to enhance her daughter's identified patienthood as a means of moving toward therapy and resolution of the marital issue. The father, on the other hand, threatens to deal with his daughter's problems in a most destructive fashion as a way of quieting the complaint and thus obviating any other solution that may threaten to touch upon his own infidelity. That is, when father threatens to beat up the boyfriend, he is in effect saying, "Either stop complaining, or I'll deal with this in a way that causes even more trouble." This reassures him of being left out of therapy, which is such a threat to him.

Engagement Plan. As a way of getting the father into treatment, the therapist needs to initially present a view of therapy to the family that permits addressing the daughter's problem while still giving the family the alternative to continue the conspiracy of silence about the infidelity, if they so choose.

As a brief and strategic therapy, our approach is problem focused. Thus it is possible to target the therapy to the problems confronting the daughter and to target the engagement efforts to the family's resistance to enter therapy around this issue.

Because the resistance of the father to come to treatment and his attitude in general about the daughter's problem is so affected by his own fears regarding his extramarital affair, the therapist will reframe the father's notion of therapy as an exposé, assuring the father that the matter of his mistress does not need to be disclosed if the family so chooses.

Implementation of Plan. 1/13/84—The therapist calls the mother back and tells her that she must convince the father and daughter to come, if only one time, before things come to a head. The therapist commissions the mother to reassure the father that the clinic will only be interested in the daughter's behavior problems while reassuring the daughter that the clinic is interested in helping not just her but the whole family to get along better. The mother, of course, is to speak to the father and daughter separately. Because the family is expert in keeping secrets, the mother is told to ask each one to keep their thoughts about coming to themselves until the first visit.

1/14/84—The family comes to see the therapist. The therapist takes a lot of time to join each member individually in order to make them feel supported. The therapist makes sure that he behaves nonjudgmentally toward all and rejects all attempts made to get him to take sides, returning to the view, "There are no good guys and no bad guys in families, just people struggling in life who sometimes have difficulty dealing with each other."

The therapist then presents four alternatives to the family:

1. Father can eventually (very soon) have his threatened fight with the boyfriend and risk potential and probably serious trouble for all. "This sort of trouble has a way of going in uncontrolled directions."
2. The family can come to therapy to deal only with the issue of "how to help daughter to make better decisions on her own behalf—so that she may gain some independence without resorting to rebelliousness." Any other issues can be contracted to be left out of the therapy session, in deference to the daughter's emergency, thus obviating any possible excuses to beginning therapy.
3. The family can come to therapy to deal with all the issues that are affecting it, if they feel so moved and ready. The therapist reassures the family of his expertise and experience in dealing with such situations many times prior, thus increasing their sense of confidence in the therapeutic system.
4. The family can negotiate therapy only for the daughter's problem now and agree to renegotiate in the future, when the daughter is fine, whether to continue therapy and move into the other issues.

The therapist asks the family to discuss these four alternatives fully and plans to ally with the daughter and manipulate her into taking the fourth position so that the family is engaged, the daughter is removed from the sole IP (scapegoat) position, and the family feels the assurance of their option to open up later, or not.

The therapist supports the daughter in advocating for the fourth choice. The family, however, agrees to start therapy by adopting the second option. The therapist accepts this choice, which makes it feasible to begin work on the presenting complaint. After all, the family can always choose to open up at a later time, and even if the family chose not to open up, the daughter's problems can be at least partially addressed.

ACKNOWLEDGMENT. This work was funded in part by a grant to Jose Szapocznik from the National Institute on Drug Abuse, Grant No. DA 03224-06.

REFERENCES

Aponte, H. J. (1974). Psychotherapy for the poor: An ecostructural approach to treatment. *Delaware Medical Journal, 46,* 1–7.

Haley, J. (1976). *Problem-solving therapy.* San Francisco: Jossey-Bass.

Madanes, C. (1981). *Strategic family therapy.* San Francisco: Jossey-Bass.

Minuchin, S. (1974). *Families and family therapy.* Cambridge: Harvard University Press.

Minuchin, S., & Fishman, H. C. (1981). *Family therapy techniques.* Cambridge: Harvard University Press.

Stanton, M. D., & Todd, T. C. (1981). Engaging "resistant" families in treatment: II. Principles and techniques in recruitment. *Family Process, 20,* 261.

Szapocznik, J., & Kurtines, W. (1989). *Beyond family therapy: Breakthroughs in the treatment of drug abusing youths.* New York: Springer Publishing Co.

Szapocznik, J., Kurtines, W., Foote, F., Perez-Vidal, A., & Hervis, O. (1983). Conjoint versus one person family therapy: Some evidence for the effectiveness of conducting family therapy through one person. *Journal of Consulting and Clinical Psychology, 51,* 889–899.

Szapocznik, J., Perez-Vidal, A., Hervis, O., Foote, F., & Spencer, F. (1983). *Brief strategic family therapy: Final report.* (NIDA Grant No. R 18 DA 03224). Miami: University of Miami Spanish Family Guidance Center.

Szapocznik, J. Kurtines, W., Hervis, O., & Spencer, F. (1984). One person family therapy. In B. Lubin and W. S. O'Connor (Eds.), *Ecological approaches to clinical and community psychology.* (pp. 335–355). New York: Wiley.

Szapocznik, J., Foote, F., Perez-Vidal, A., Hervis, O., & Kurtines, W. (1985). *One person family therapy.* Miami: Miami World Health Organization.

Szapocznik, J., Kurtines, W., Foote, F., Perez-Vidal, A., & Hervis, O. (1986). Conjoint versus one person family therapy: Further evidence for the effectiveness of conducting family therapy through one person. *Journal of Consulting and Clinical Psychology, 54,* 395–397.

6

On Time in Brief Therapy

Michael F. Hoyt

> Again and again I have had the impression that we have made too little
> theoretical use of this fact, established beyond any doubt, of the unalterability by
> time of the repressed. This seems to offer an approach to the most profound
> discoveries. Nor, unfortunately, have I myself made any progress here.
> —Sigmund Freud (1933, p. 74)

> My interest has been to convince you that you must assume responsibility for
> being here, in this marvelous world, in this marvelous desert, in this marvelous
> time. I wanted to convince you that you must learn to make every act count,
> since you are going to be here for only a short while; in fact, too short for
> witnessing all the marvels of it.
> —Don Juan (Casteneda, 1972, p. 107)

Time is of the essence in brief psychotherapy. The message, by definition, is *brevity:* Do it now, no time to waste, be efficient and parsimonious, seize the moment, be here now, get on with it. At core, brief therapy is defined more by an attitude than by the specific number of treatment sessions. The brief therapist operates with the belief and expectation that change can occur *in the moment*, that the patient has within himself or herself the power to be different or to remain the same (Goulding & Goulding, 1978, 1979). With skillful assistance, the patient will recognize his or her response-ability and thus move from being a victim to a creator of his or her psychological reality (Hoyt, 1977; Kaiser, 1965; Schafer, 1973).

Aspects of time underlie brief treatment across a variety of specific theoretical and technical approaches. My purpose here is to highlight a few of the connections between time and brief therapy, with the hope that heightened awareness of the temporal dimension can help therapists to construct and conduct more satisfying and parsimonious (brief and effective) treatments. What follows is not presented as an all-encompassing review or definitive statement; it

MICHAEL F. HOYT • Department of Psychiatry, Kaiser-Permanente Medical Center, Hayward, California 94545-4299, and the Langley Porter Psychiatric Institute of the University of California, San Francisco, San Francisco, California 94143.

calls attention to a few lines of inquiry and is intended to stimulate thought and experimentation.[1]

THE BRIEF THERAPIST'S BASIC ATTITUDE TOWARD TIME

Time is both a medium and a perspective, and psychotherapies vary in their orientation toward time (Melges, 1982). Psychoanalysis seeks to produce change primarily by directing the patient's awareness toward the past and its persistence in the present—this is the principle Freud (1914) described in his essay, "Remembering, Repeating, and Working Through." Gestalt therapy (Naranjo, 1970; Perls et al., 1951; Perls, 1969), cognitive therapy; (Beck, 1976; Emery & Campbell, 1986), and much of the family therapy movement (Budman, 1981; Guerin, 1976; Gurman & Kniskern, 1981) seek change by focusing on the patient's present experiencing and modes of conduct. There are also methods of treatment such as the Gouldings' (1978, 1979, 1985) redecision therapy, De Shazer's (1985) "crystal ball technique," and Melges' (1982) future-oriented therapy that seek change by having patients actively imagine successful outcomes and their paths to them.

Effective brief therapy may look to the past or the future for clues about where the patient is "stuck" and what experience might be needed for him or her to get "un-stuck" (Hoyt, 1988b, 1989), but the brief therapist knows that only in the present can the patient make a change. Excessive concern outside of the present is counterproductive. The patient may engage in various security operations to remain the same (Gustafson, 1986), especially if he or she feels, as Melges (1982) describes it, that control over the future has been lost. The patient who wants to undo or turn back time interferes with coping in the present (Mann, 1973). Secrets (Hoyt, 1978), obsessions (Hoyt, 1987a), remorse (Hoyt, 1983) and various reality distortions may be clung to in an attempt to avoid movement into a threatening present and future. The therapist will help the patient by assisting him or her to endure and control the present while approaching the future.

Elsewhere (Hoyt, 1985a; also see Budman & Gurman, 1983, 1988), I have contrasted the temporal attitude of brief versus long-term therapists:

> Long-term therapy is based on a number of theoretical assumptions that presuppose that treatment must take a long time to be effective; the belief that pathogenic early

---

[1]The broad topic of the study of time, which has fascinated me for years, goes far beyond the scope of this chapter. The literature is vast, with poets, philosophers, scientists, and that amalgam of the three—psychologists—all contributing richly. The reader interested in the psychological perspective should not miss the books by Fraser (1966, 1975), Mann (1973), Melges (1982), and Hartocollis (1983). Other useful references that will lead in many directions include the following: Becker (1973), Berne (1972), Bonaparte (1941), Boorstin (1985), Cooper and Erickson (1959), Cottle and Klineberg (1974), Doob (1971), Dunne (1973), Fraisse (1963), Freud (1914, 1916, 1917, 1933, 1937), Gorman and Wesman (1977), Heidegger (1927), May, Angels, and Ellenberger (1958), Minkowski (1933), Nannum (1972), Naranjo (1970), Ornstein (1969), Piaget (1946), Pollack (1971), Priestly (1968), Schilder (1936), Spitz (1972), Tart (1969), Wallace and Rabin (1960), and von Franz (1978).

experiences inevitably must be slowly and fully uncovered; the belief that rapport and therapist–patient alliance must form gradually; the belief that the patient must be allowed to regress and that transference takes a long time to develop and should not be interpreted too early; and the belief that the consolidation of gains requires a lengthy period of working through. . . . These theoretical assumptions—which may become self-fulfilling prophecies—are not necessarily always true, and may at times be held as quasi-intellectual resistances to short-term therapy. An alternative set of assumptions suggests that short-term treatment can be effective: the belief that focused interventions can set into motion a whole system of changes; the belief that selected patients can rapidly form a good working alliance and that early transference interpretations can strengthen the alliance; the belief that generalized regression should be avoided and that regression should be restricted as much as possible to the focal area; and the belief that a time limit increases and intensifies the work accomplished, that gains are consolidated throughout the treatment. . . . The differences in these two sets of working assumptions highlight the technical methods that characterize effective short-term work: an explicit understanding that treatment will not be prolonged or "timeless," greater therapist activity and early transference interpretation, selective attention to a central dynamic focus, maintenance of a strong adult-to-adult therapeutic alliance and avoidance of generalized regression, and early attention to termination as part of the working-through process. (pp. 97–98)

There are a series of beliefs or myths (Hoyt, 1985a, 1987b) that are sources of resistance against short-term therapy, factors that are often permeated with therapists' assumptions and anxieties regarding time:

> (a) the belief that "more is better," often held despite the lack of any evidence justifying the greater expense of long-term or open-ended treatment; (b) the myth of the "pure gold" of analysis, the overvaluation of insight and misassumption that change and growth require "deep" examination of an individual's unconscious and psychohistory; (c) the confusion of patients' interests with therapists' interests, the tendency of therapists to seek and perfectionistically treat putative complexes rather than attend directly to patients' complaints and stated treatment goals; (d) the demand for hard work, the need for the brief therapist to be active, intensely alert, selectively focused, intuitive, and risk taking; (e) financial pressures, the temptation to hold on to that which is profitable and dependable; and (f) countertransference and termination problems, the need to be needed and difficulties of saying goodbye. (Hoyt, 1987b, p. 408)

Therapists accustomed to doing long-term or open-ended work will have to suspend or adjust their assumptions about the perspective and pace of treatment if they are to do effective brief therapy. The pursuit of a perfectionistic "cure" through the persistent probing of pathology will need to shift, if one is to work in a "time-sensitive" manner (Budman & Gurman, 1988), to a pragmatic and parsimonious promotion of the patient's strengths and resources vis-à-vis the presenting problem.

THE STRUCTURE OF BRIEF THERAPY

Brief psychotherapy (as well as other, more prolonged or open-ended treatments) can be conceptualized to have the following structure of sequenced phases. In actual practice, of course, the phases blend into one another rather than being so discretely organized. The structure tends to be epigenetic or pyra-

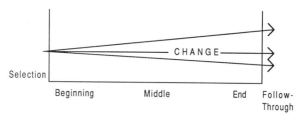

FIGURE 1. The structure of brief therapy.

midal, each phase building on the prior phase, so that successful work in one is a precondition for the next; for example, there is a need for rapport and focusing before working through, and termination will not be meaningful unless a connection and work have preceded. There is often an interesting parallel between the microcosm and the macrocosm (see Figure 1): The structure of each individual session resembles the structure of the overall course of treatment.[2] There is also often a parallel process (Dasberg & Winokur, 1984; Hoyt, 1988a) observable in supervision, wherein brief therapy students/trainees move through the same sequence of phases as do their patients:

1. *Selection.* How well does the patient fit the indications for likely success in brief therapy (high motivation for personal change, circumscribed chief complaint, psychological mindedness, history of beneficial relationships, responsiveness to trial interventions) as described by Sifneos (1979) and Malan (1976)? Is the patient likely to be a spontaneous improver, nonresponder, or negative responder, exclusion criteria that Frances and Clarkin (1981) suggest make no therapy the treatment of choice. Are contraindications or major impediments present (marked inability to tolerate anxiety, guilt, or depression; active psychosis or highly suicidal; active alcohol or drug abuse)? Change often begins with recognition of a problem and the decision to seek therapy, even before the first treatment contact occurs.

2. *Beginning.* Making contact. Forming rapport and a working alliance. Orienting the patient regarding how to use treatment. Confronting resistance and negative transference. Taking history and complaint. Why therapy now? Finding a psychological focus, making a treatment contract. Getting patient's agreement to change. Setting parameters, including time allotted for each session, frequency, and short-term duration. Beginning and ending the session on time, a first encounter with therapeutic time limits. "The battle for structure" and "the battle for initiative" (Whitaker, in Napier & Whitaker, 1978), in which the patient attempts to dictate the parameters of treatment (where, when, who attends, etc.) while trying to get the therapist to set the theme and take responsibility for

---

[2]Gustafson (1986, p. 279) independently has made the same observation: "Just as the entire course of a brief therapy may be seen as having its opening, middle and end game, any particular session may be seen as a microcosm of such thinking. The opening is concerned with where to take hold. The middle is for getting different illuminations of this focus. The end provides a concluding punctuation. Condense, widen, and condense again. Exposition, development and recapitulation."

the work. Giving an initial task or homework assignment to increase patient's active involvement and to promote and accelerate change.

3. *Middle phase.* Working through. Recognition of pattern and choices regarding options. Clarification, confrontation, and interpretation of resistance, discounting, transference. Staying on selected focus, "honoring contract." Homework, behavioral anchors for psychological change. Awareness that time is limited, treatment will end soon.

4. *End phase.* Termination. Continued work on central focus (contract) plus awareness of impending end of therapist–patient contact. Mourning. Arousal of dependency and underlying separation–individuation issues, with possible recrudescence of symptoms. Countertransference pulls to avoid ending, rescue patient, cram "extra" work into last session or two (Hoyt, 1979a, 1985a; Hoyt & Farrell, 1984; Hoyt & Goulding, 1989). Alternatively, last session(s) may be "flat" as participants prematurely detach to avoid genuine ending. Discussion of continuing change, maintaining gains, possible backsliding or "self-sabotage" (Hoyt, 1986). Letting patient know that return to treatment is possible (unless therapist wants for specific reasons to emphasize strongly the separation, as in Mann's [1973] model of Time-Limited Psychotherapy), and sometimes inviting a later follow-up or "check-in" appointment or contact, which may attentuate the emotional impact of termination while implying the therapist's continuing interest in the patient's life and progress.

5. *Follow-through.* Continuation of psychological work and change beyond the formal ending date of therapist–patient contact. Internalization of favorable aspects of treatment: "If I give you a fish you can eat a meal. If I teach you how to fish, you can feed yourself forever." In short-term therapy, much more than in longer-term treatments, change processes may be initiated or set into motion without being completely worked through during the course of actual patient–therapist contact (Horowitz & Hoyt, 1979; Hoyt, 1979a, 1985a; Hoyt, Talmon, & Rosenbaum, 1987; Rosenbaum, Hoyt, & Talmon, 1989; Shectman, 1986; Talmon, Hoyt, & Rosenbaum, 1988). Recognition of differences between treatment goals and life goals (Ticho, 1972), the fact that the consolidation of some benefits of treatment can only occur with lived time. This points to the need for long-term follow-up if therapeutic outcomes are to be thoroughly assessed (Bergin & Lambert, 1978; Butcher & Kolotkin, 1979; Cross, Sheehan, & Khan, 1982). Possible patient return to treatment or "checking in for a booster." The possibility of *serial* short-term therapy—encouraged by quick success for one problem, a patient later seeks treatment for another (Bennett, 1983, 1984; Budman & Gurman, 1983, 1988; Cummings, 1977; Cummings & VandenBos, 1979).

Issues of time may attend each of the five phases. Does the patient have a problem pertaining directly to time (e.g., unresolved mourning, anniversary reactions, procrastination, anxiety about the future, a feeling of hopelessness about the future, impulsiveness, etc.)? Does he or she seek "instant cure" to avoid contact and vulnerability, or does the patient seek "timeless" (open-ended or long-term) treatment to avoid change and maintain dependency? Do sessions begin and end on time? If not, because of whom? Is time "squeezed" or "squandered"? Does change occur? How does the patient respond to the impending termination of treatment? How does the therapist respond? Many of these points are amplified in the following section.

Six Practical Issues Regarding Time and Therapeutic Technique

1. *Duration of contact.* The essence of short-term therapy is an attitude that change is possible and expected now rather than later. There is no magic number of sessions that makes therapy brief—any figure would be arbitrary. Therapy should be as short as possible, and what is possible is determined partially by the expectations and beliefs of therapist and patient. I am reminded of an experience I had several years ago when I visited the Short-Term Therapy Seminar at the renowned Tavistock Clinic in London (Malan, 1976). Cases were presented, and I was asked to comment, which I did with some trepidation. We got into a discussion about length of treatment. I indicated that at the clinic I was then working, we generally saw patients for 12 sessions, a number that followed Mann's (1973) Time-Limited Psychotherapy model and allowed for a good research design (Horowitz et al., 1984). "Here at the Tavistock we allow trainees 35 to 40 sessions. It allows for wasting time and making mistakes," I was told. "Well, in America we're more efficient," I responded, "We find that we can waste time and make mistakes in 12 sessions!"

How many sessions constitute brief therapy? The preceding notwithstanding, there is a range or consensus in the literature. Short-term or brief therapy is often arbitrarily defined as 20 or less sessions. Wolberg (1965, p. 140), for example, refers to "short-term treatment . . . up to 20 treatment sessions." Various insurance plans and health-maintenance organizations (HMOs) also provide for "brief treatment up to 20 sessions." As mentioned before, Mann (1973; Mann & Goldman, 1982) and Horowitz (1976; Horowitz et al., 1984) have reported successful psychodynamic treatments within a 12-session framework. For Wells (1982, p. 99), "short-term treatment comprises three or four sessions up to a maximum of fifteen interviews." There is also a growing literature on *single-session psychotherapy* (Bloom, 1981; Hoyt, Talmon, & Rosenbaum, 1987; Rockwell & Pinkerton, 1982; Rosenbaum, Hoyt, & Talmon, 1989; Talmon, Hoyt, & Rosenbaum, 1988), a maximally brief treatment approach that colleagues and I have been exploring with encouraging results. It should also be noted that for some people no therapy may be the treatment of choice—people who would get better if left untreated, those who do not respond to treatment, and those who get worse with treatment should not be in psychotherapy (Frances & Clarkin, 1981).

There are a variety of ways to establish explicitly the planned brief duration of short-term therapy. One can either speak generally of meeting "for a few times" or "for a month or two," or one can indicate the exact end point at the beginning of treatment either by setting a specific number of sessions ("We'll meet 12 times") or an end date ("We'll meet weekly through November 7"). In any arrangement, there is the question of what to do about missed sessions. I prefer to count them as missed, not to "make them up." If the patient has been making progress, but the desired goal has not yet been reached, I may sometimes negotiate for future sessions, as Wells (1982, p. 100) recommends. Generally, however, one has to be careful not to fall into the trap of simply adding "an extra session" (or two, or three . . .) unless extraordinary circumstances (e.g., a suicidal crisis or unforeseeable emergency) require it because doing so threatens to undermine the integrity of the initial short-term agreement and violates the basic existential truth of time limits:

> For psychotherapy to enable an individual to come to terms with the meaning of his existence, he must come to grips with the reality of non-existence. Psychotherapy is true to this quest insofar as it is a process of termination rather than consolidation of relationship and proliferation of time. (Goldberg, 1975, p. 342)

The therapist can opt not to predetermine the number of sessions but to state "we'll be meeting about half a dozen times" or "we'll only be meeting a few times" and set the termination date as the work draws to completion. Keeping with the idea that "brief" means "no more than necessary," it is interesting to note that two sessions held 6 months apart might be considered more brief than a 12-week treatment consisting of one or more sessions per week.

Scheduling sessions weekly is probably the most common practice, although more frequent meetings can be arranged to intensify treatment, gain momentum, or provide needed support; or less frequently, to attenuate the transference or to allow time for homework and change (see Selvini-Palazzoli *et al.*, 1978). Sessions may be spread out at the end of treatment for a gradual ending, with the probable effect of decreasing the impact of termination. A follow-up session can be arranged for several months later, to help maintain gains, encourage internalization, and assess continued developments. Therapists should be aware that altering the framework of treatment has effects (Langs, 1979) and should consider what purpose (and whose needs) are being served with any temporal arrangement or modification.

When treatment ends, patients can be encouraged to return if needed (and may be helped by exploring what would indicate returning) but often benefit by being counseled to resist returning too quickly so that they can weather some ups and downs and realize their strength. I also prefer to let patients know that they could return for the same problem or a different problem and that they could either contact me or seek a different therapist if desired. In my opinion, someone returning to psychotherapy does not necessarily indicate failure or "unresolved pathological transference" anymore than someone returning to the same restaurant indicates a "failure" the first time they were there.

2. *Duration of treatment sessions.* Most short-term or brief therapists work in conventional "50-minute hours," probably because of convenience and habit. This seems to allow a comfortable amount of time for most therapists and patients to make contact, get (or resume) a focus and contract, engage in exploration and working through, and end the session. (Again, note the parallel between the structure of individual sessions and the overall course of treatment—

see Figure 1.) There is nothing sacrosanct about 50-minute sessions, however, and it is worth considering alternatives. Two well-known and highly effective brief therapists, Robert and Mary Goulding (1978, 1979), like to conduct Redecision Therapy sessions for 20 minutes. Others, often working in understaffed public or private settings, see patients for 5 to 30-minute sessions and need to make therapeutic impact quickly (Barten, 1965; Castelnuovo-Tedesco, 1986; Dreiblatt & Weatherly, 1965; Singh, 1982; Zirkle, 1961). The idea of 50-minute consultations occurring over many meetings is essentially a middle-class notion (Wells, 1982), and persons of different socioeconomic backgrounds may not share this time perspective and may need to see valuable results quickly if subsequent sessions are to occur. Therapists experimenting with single-session therapies (Bloom, 1981; Hoyt et al., 1987; Rockwell & Pinkerton, 1982; Rosenbaum et al., 1989; Talmon et al., 1988) sometimes find it helpful to have 90 minutes or 2 hours for the treatment contact in order to have time to assess, prepare, and complete a substantial intervention. Certain kinds of intense work, such as "re-grief" (Volkan, 1975) or "grief resolution" (Melges, 1982) therapy, can be done in relatively few sessions, but each session may last for a couple of hours. Couples and family brief therapists also find it helpful to have more time per session to deal with the complexities of multiple persons. Would the reader consider a single marathon session, such as the 10-hour treatment reported by Berenbaum (1969), to be a prolonged brief therapy or a brief prolonged therapy?

3. *Conveying the time limit to the patient.* Explicit indication by the therapist that "we will only be meeting X [or "a few"] times" or "until November," or stating that "you have the ability to deal with this pretty quickly if we get right down to work" conveys the message that the patient has the capacity and opportunity to use brief treatment advantageously. It is also honest and ethical in that it lets the patient know the therapist's intentions so that he or she can decide whether or not to engage in treatment. Offering brief therapy apologetically, such as saying, "the clinic will only let me see you five times, but we'll see what we can do," is obviously demoralizing and counterproductive. Clinicians' attitudes toward the value of brief therapy may influence how they communicate with brief therapy patients (Burlingame & Behrman, 1987; Johnson & Gelso, 1980; Sifneos, 1981), and this communication may contribute to a self-fulfilling prophecy. As John D. Rockefeller said: "Whether a man thinks he is going to be a success or a failure, he is probably right!"

A time-limited framework often creates a sense of urgency that helps to foster a rapid and deep involvement. Like the proverbial meeting of strangers on a train, the safety of knowing that the end is clearly defined and in sight sometimes permits short-term therapy patients to become quickly and intensely engaged in treatment (Stierlin, 1968). The operation of "Parkinson's law" in psychotherapy—work expands or contracts to fill the time available for it—was observed by Appelbaum (1975; also see Appelbaum & Holzman, 1967; Hoyt, 1979a; Mann, 1973; Rank, 1945; Wells, 1982), who advocates setting the end point at the beginning of brief therapy to stimulate the patient's will and to counteract passive, timeless waiting for change. This method, of forcing the patient to confront issues of separation by setting a termination date, was first reported by Freud (1918) in his case of the Wolf Man. It is also interesting that Freud, "the father of psychoanalysis," rightfully can be considered the first brief therapist in that many of his early cases (Breuer & Freud, 1893–1895/1955) only lasted from a single session to a couple of months.

In setting a time limit or conveying the idea of "a few sessions" or "a couple of months," the brief therapist does not need to appear arbitrary or ruthless. Indeed, the therapist should believe genuinely that he or she is able to render professional assistance in the time offered and be willing to discuss the recommendation with the patient. Iatrogenic resistance is minimized if therapy is a cooperative, bipersonal venture. Following the principle of informed consent, initial assessment should include asking patients what bothers them, what they want, how long they think it will take to accomplish, and discussing with them their ideas and reasons. Patients' beliefs and goals merit due respect, to be sure, but they may be inaccurate or colored by their pathology; for example, many patients with borderline personality structures hope for a magically quick cure, whereas dependent patients almost always are sure that they will need to be seen "for a long time." When told that, say, 12 sessions of therapy are recommended, most patients will respond, "that many?" (see June & Smith, 1983; Pekarik & Wierzbicki, 1986). Nowadays, most patients (except, perhaps, mental-health professionals!) seek and expect rapid results, a trend consonant with both economic realities and with the "do it now" ethic of our "instant society" of high-speed computers, drive-thru fast food, "one minute managers" (Blanchard & Johnson, 1982), and 30-minute TV dramas. Even the popularization of digital clocks and timing devices may affect the conceptualization of temporal experience, as the cyclical nature of the sweep of the analogue clock is replaced by the dizzying blur of the digital display (Hoyt, 1979a). Oh, how right Bob Dylan was back in 1963 when he told us, "The times they are a-changin'"!

4. *Selecting the time limit.* As Wells (1982, pp. 134–135) has noted, the setting of time limits in brief treatment is far from an exact science. Experienced short-term therapists seem to rely primarily on "clinical judgment" or "intuition" when deciding whether a particular patient will be offered, say, 10 sessions, rather than 8 or 12 sessions. It is generally agreed among brief therapists that a foreseeable limit should be set and that the expectation of success should be conveyed with firm confidence, but how does one decide how many sessions?

Sometimes the number is determined by external factors, such as a research design or agency policy, or by the patient's preference, ability to pay, or expected time to be available. Therapists should not automatically accede to such constraints—sometimes they are put forward as reality resistances that can be modified. If the therapist does not feel that successful treatment is likely in the amount of time being considered, he or she should so advise the patient and refer him or her elsewhere or suggest that the patient delay treatment until a more propitious time.

Inexperienced practitioners often set too *long* a time limit (e.g., 15 to 20 sessions) and thus lose the structuring effect that a shorter time limit (6 to 8 sessions) might provide. It is also important, of course, especially while learning to work briefly, not to err too far in the other direction by setting time limits that are unrealistically too brief, which might result in treatments that are frantically rushed and incomplete rather than pleasantly urgent and efficient. Factors that need to be taken into consideration include what the patient wishes to change in the treatment, his or her motivation and apparent abilities (and weaknesses), the therapist's level of skillfulness and sense that rapid change is possible, and the "friendliness" (supportiveness and malleability) of the circumstances the patient is confronting.

A fixed (usually 12-session) time limit is useful if the therapist wants to engage the patient in a process (Mann, 1973; Mann & Goldman, 1982) that will restimulate, via the transference, unresolved mourning and other separation–dependency issues. The reactivation of latent maladaptive cognitive-affective schemata (Horowitz et al., 1984) permits their reworking, even if, as Westen (1986) has questioned, the 12-session limit may not allow enough time for a fundamental internalization of the therapist as a replacement for previous and less-benign figures. A "dozen sessions" does seem to offer enough time, if skillfully handled, for a meaningful engagement and mourning process to take place:

> In our culture, a "dozen" carries some extra meaning, and there is some greater sense of a gestalt being completed with the culmination of a dozen. This may relate to some other frequent measures of time, such as 12 months in a year and 12 hours in the sweep of a clock. It seems that the choice of exactly 12 sessions may somehow capitalize on and heighten the existential impact of termination within the time-limited model. (Hoyt, 1979a, p. 217)

Perry (1987; also Frances, Clarkin, & Perry, 1984; Budman & Gurman, 1983, 1988) provides a useful discussion of factors that tend to increase versus decrease the duration of psychotherapeutic treatment. He notes that therapy tends to be shorter under the following conditions: when the diagnosis focuses on acute symptoms, when there is a precipitating stress, treatment goals are limited, premorbid functioning was good, the patient expects brief therapy and believes that change should occur quickly, the patient has limited time and money, the therapist takes an actively directive approach and is not easily available for sessions, the goal of treatment is reparation or return to function, techniques are more behavioral/directive than "exploratory," and the identified patient is a minor or senior and a family/marital format is used.

This is not to say that brief therapy should necessarily avoid stirring up affect or uncovering painful material. As I have summarized elsewhere:

> There has been controversy in the short-term therapy literature about patient selection, therapeutic techniques, and expected outcomes. . . . Simply stated, the "conservative" position has been that brief treatment generally is appropriate only for the mildly and recently distressed, that techniques should be supportive rather than uncovering or anxiety-producing, and that expected results are basically superficial and symptom suppressive. The "radical" position, on the other hand, is just what the name literally implies: "going to the root"; the radical view is that the skillful clinician working within an explicitly short-term treatment framework can use a full range of psychodynamic methods with a variety of neurotic patients, often achieving some genuine and lasting personality modifications as well as symptomatic relief. While there is more research to be done, the general thrust of the evidence is clear: Many patients benefit from brief, focused, psychodynamic therapy. (Hoyt, 1985a, p. 95)

During the initial assessment, the therapist has to estimate the patient's capacity for work and integration when selecting the time limit. It is probably better to err slightly on the cautious side because it is easier and more reassuring to declare the job done "ahead of schedule" and to stop earlier than planned rather than have to extend or prolong a treatment. Wolberg's (1965, p. 140) recommendation is wise:

> The best strategy, in my opinion, is to assume that every patient, irrespective of diagnosis, will respond to short-term treatment unless he proves himself refractory to it. If the therapist approaches each patient with the idea of doing as much as he can for him . . . he will give the patient an opportunity to take advantage of short-term treatment to the limit of his potential. If this fails, he can always then resort to prolonged therapy.

What is most important in selecting a length of treatment is attention to the needs of the particular patient at the particular time (de la Torre, 1978, p. 192). "Fixed duration" should not be a Procrustean bed, with some patients fitting nicely, whereas others are needlessly stretched or cut short. Flexibility and a genuine belief that lasting change can occur rapidly are paramount. Therapists should also know their own personal strengths and weaknesses but should not impose their preferences or predilections in the name of "policy" or "style." In this connection, it is worth noting that Brodaty (1983, quoted by Hatcher, Huebner, & Zakin, 1986, p. 514) reviewed the brief therapy literature and concluded that "rigidity of a therapy timetable seems to be based more on the character of the therapist than on any theoretical evidence."

Generally speaking, the exact time limit is of less importance than the increased awareness of patient and therapist that there is a time limit. The element of time can be highlighted from the very first contact with the patient by referring to the treatment being "brief" or "time-limited." This will help convey the basic attitude and expectation of brief therapy, that change can occur within the moment. Some ways that this emphasis can be accomplished during sessions are described in the next section.

5. *The language of time limits.* The brief therapist and patient should both be aware that time is limited, not endless, and that *now* is the time to move forward. (As Shectman [1986, p. 521] has put it, "Necessity is thus becoming not only the mother of invention but of intervention as well.") Setting a time limit or agreeing to meet "just a few times" helps instill this awareness. The language that therapists use during sessions can reinforce (or undo) the therapeutic impact or thrust of time limit setting.

Eric Berne (1961, 1972), the originator of Transactional Analysis, would ask himself before each session, "What can I do to cure this patient today?" Single-session "cure" did not always result, of course, but the question focused therapist and patient on making rapid changes. Goulding and Goulding (1978, 1979) have developed Berne's concept of *contractual therapy* and ask patients, as they begin each treatment session, *"What are you willing to change today?"* In this one brilliant sentence the key elements of brief therapy all occur! Here they are, spelled out:

> *What* [specificity, target, focus]
> *are* [active verb, present tense]
> *you* [self as agent, intrapsychic, personal functioning]
> *willing* [choice, responsibility, initiative]
> *to change* [alter or be different, not just "work on" or "explore"]
> *today* [now, in the moment]
> *?* [inquiry, open field, therapist receptive but not insistent]

The effective brief therapist often includes references to time limits in setting the focus or contract with the patient. Consider, for example, this statement made to a bereaved and betrayed widow at the beginning of a 12-session time-limited therapy:

Th: Let's have an agreement that we might meet say a dozen times, and keep our focus pretty much on what your husband's passing and what this affair meant in your life, and who you are now and how that is affecting it, and who you can be in the next few years, and not spend a lot of time talking about other problems. (Hoyt, 1979a, pp. 211–212)

Time can also be used as a resistance (Appelbaum, 1975). Stalling, to avoid the present and the future, will need to be confronted and given up for therapy to progress. Consider these interchanges:

Pt: Let me ask you a question in a round about fashion.
Th: You want to duck it slowly? (Mann, 1973, p. 37)

Th: You tell me, I mean look, we have spent fifteen minutes, you tell me what we've accomplished?
Pt: My goodness, many people come to psychiatrists for years on end . . .
Th: Uh hmm.
Pt: . . . and ah . . .
Th: So what you say is this, that we have to come for years until we understand.
Pt: No, I, I hope not. (Davanloo, 1986, pp. 119–120)

Some other statements made with similar purpose might include:

Th: You seem to be filling our time together with small talk rather than confronting the problem that brought you here.
Th: With all the serious problems you mentioned before, I'm wondering why you are spending so much time talking about X.
Th: We're already half-way through our 6 sessions. You're going to have to really get going to get this worked out. What do you want to change today?
Th: I'm not willing to keep meeting if you're going to waste time. Do you want to work?

Therapists sometimes convey the message that problems with a long history will necessarily require a long time to resolve, as in these statements by a therapist from transcripts of a 100+ session marital therapy (Fanshel, 1971):

"And I really think [sighingly] we ought to allow ourselves more time for this because it's only going to make trouble" (p. 108) and "if it's a *long* story, it's a *long time* getting out in the open" (p. 287, italics in original). Sometimes long-term treatment is desired and necessary (as certain patients undergo self-exploration and characterological change or to help them weather a difficult life passage or maintain a tenuous psychosocial adjustment), but the therapist should also have the theoretical ability, practical skill, and interest to consolidate a protracted storyline into a treatable central issue. One might begin to do this by asking:

Th: What's most important is not how far back this goes, but how much further you're going to continue to do it. Are you willing to look at your part in it right now?

Once therapy gets underway, it sometimes continues, week after week, simply because the time is reserved and appointments scheduled. As I learned from Carl Whitaker (personal communication), the patient's initiative and involvement can be strengthened by asking occasionally:

Th: Do you want to keep the appointment next week? We could cancel it if you don't want to work.

There are other brief therapists, such as Cummings (1977) and Austin and Inderbitzin (1983), who also advocate letting patients set appointments for when they are willing to work.

The language of brief therapy also gains therapeutic impact by being present centered. Psychotherapy is more likely to be effective if the patient has a here-and-now experience rather than just a there-and-then explanation. Experience results in genuine learning and growth, whereas explanation or information simply leads to recognition. This is why the well-timed psychodynamic transference interpretation can be so powerful: It brings the patient into the present. Malan (1976), for example, found the use of transference interpretations to be positively correlated with successful outcomes in short-term dynamic psychotherapy. Similarly, Hoyt (1980; Hoyt *et al.*, 1983) reports data indicating that short-term dynamic therapy sessions are judged to be particularly "good" when the activities of therapist and patient emphasize the patient's expression of thoughts and feelings and the collaborative exploration of the meaning of this expression in terms of the patient's self-concepts, reactions to the therapist, and links between past and present.

Mental imagery can serve the same purpose: It brings the patient's outside world into the therapist's office and increases the likelihood that a range of meaningful emotions will be experienced (Hoyt, 1986). This is consistent with what Whitaker and Malone (1953, p. 204) contend: "Any technique which succeeds in equating in the patient all time, whether past or future, with the present time, seems to have validity." William James (1890, p. 293) recognized the same thing: "Each world whilst it is attended to is real after its own fashion."[3] Brief therapists who are skillful in using mental imagery (see Singer [1974] for a good overview of methods and Shorr [1972, 1974] and Goulding [1985] for some particularly creative applications) will be able to help patients rapidly generate therapeutic experiences. Gestalt therapists and redecision therapists (Goulding & Goulding, 1978, 1979), for example, know that it is often much more effective for producing change to have people talk *with* their introjects in the present, via double-chair work, rather than having them talk *about* them in the past tense. It is also helpful, both generally and when doing imagery work, to attend to patients' rate of speech. Sometimes patients will slow down or speed up to avoid particular images, feelings, or a "loss of control" that might actually be a step into the warded-off present.

There are a number of quotations and pithy statements about time that I have found to be helpful, when judiciously shared with patients, for heightening the existential impact of brief therapy. The "zingers" include:

> Killing time isn't murder. Killing time is suicide.
> —William James

> If you don't change directions, you'll wind up where you're heading.
> —Old Chinese saying

> If not you, who? If not now, when?
> —Rabbi Hillel

> Teach us to number our days that we may get us a heart of wisdom.
> —Moses (Psalm 90: 12)

> Brevity is the soul of wit.
> —Shakespeare (*Hamlet*, II, ii, 90)

> There is no time like the present.

> You don't have to change, but you know what happened to the dinosaurs.

> Growing old isn't bad, when you consider the alternative.
> —Maurice Chevalier

> Well, no one lives forever. But even if you believe in reincarnation, there is still the question: Is there life *before* death?

Once I consulted with a man, about to turn 40, who complained that he was feeling old, that life was rushing by despite his increasingly "Type A" freneticism. He also complained of difficulty making commitments. I asked him to be specific: What commitment?

Pt: Well, my girlfriend wants to get married, but I'm not sure.

Th: How long have you been together?

[3]Recognition of the present-centered construction of all time may have also inspired T. S. Eliot's (1943) famous lines:

> Time present and time past
> Are both perhaps present in
>   time future
> And time future contained in time past.

Pt: Eight years.

Th: Oh, I see. Well, you certainly don't want to rush into it. Why don't you wait to see how she handles menopause and retirement. You certainly don't want to get stuck with a crotchety old lady, do you?

He laughed, first at my gentle mockery, then harder, at himself. "It is crazy, isn't it?", he said. I tried to keep a straight face but added: "Well, I don't know. You can't tell what's going to happen in the future." Many months later he telephoned to let me know that he had gotten married and was happy. He offered thanks for "bringing me to my senses." I told him I was glad to hear that he was happy but that the credit was his because "you're the one who got the joke."

6. *When does most change occur in psychotherapy?* It is now well documented that change *does* occur in psychotherapy. Perhaps the most impressive study is that of Smith, Glass, and Miller (1980), who performed a "meta-analysis" of almost 400 controlled psychotherapy outcome studies involving more than 25,000 patients and control subjects. Their conclusive finding was that the patients who received psychotherapy did better on various outcome measures than 75% of those persons who remained untreated, demonstrating the benefits of psychotherapy. Of special interest was the fact that the mean length of these effective treatments was approximately 17 sessions. Howard, Kopta, Krause, and Orlinsky (1986) found 75% of patients to show improvement within 26 sessions. Along the same vein, the Vanderbilt Psychotherapy Research Project (Gomes-Schwartz, 1978; Hartley & Strupp, 1983; Strupp, 1980a–d; Strupp & Binder, 1984; see Frieswyk *et al.*, 1986) found overall outcome to be predictable in time-limited dynamic psychotherapy from aspects of the first three interviews, a finding that jibes with the common experience of therapists that one often can tell pretty quickly if a case if going to "go anywhere." Several studies (Bloom, 1981; Hoyt *et al.*, 1987; Malan *et al.*, 1975; Rockwell & Pinkerton, 1982) have found significant changes to occur after one session, and although Howard *et al.* (1986) do find a positive correlation between number of sessions and amount of improvements in their meta-analysis of studies (they suggest 26 sessions as a practical limit), there is no research evidence (Butcher & Koss, 1978; Luborsky, Singer, & Luborsky, 1975; Meltzoff & Korneich, 1970) that long-term therapy produces more changes than short-term therapy. Given these findings, it seems reasonable to speculate that most change in psychotherapy occurs relatively quickly, within the period of time usually considered to be brief treatment. Additional changes sometimes may occur in longer-term treatments, and there may be different criteria for assessing these changes, but there may also be diminishing returns as one approaches a psychotherapeutic asymptote. This was recognized by Appelbaum (1975), a psychoanalyst impressed by his experiences with brief therapy, who noted that even if long-term treatment were to produce some added gains, it would be questionable whether these gains would often be commensurate with the added expenditure of time and money. Appelbaum's (1975) observation of "Parkinson's law" in psychotherapy is worth repeating: Work expands or contracts to fill the time available for it.

Three Models of Brief Therapy That Explicitly Address Issues of Time

Time plays a role in all psychotherapies and particularly in those therapies that are planned to be brief or time limited. Some forms of short-term therapy are even more explicitly time oriented in that they deliberately address aspects of the patient's temporal experience as a central feature of the treatment. In this section, I highlight three of these approaches.

Mann's (1973; Mann & Goldman, 1982) Time-Limited Psychotherapy

This is a psychodynamic-existential model built on the theory that the experience of time has central meaning in our psychological development. Mann (1973, p. 25) believes that "in this kind of time-limited psychotherapy, mastery of separation anxiety becomes the model for the mastery of other neurotic anxieties, albeit in a somewhat derived manner. Failures in mastery of this basic anxiety must influence both the future course in life of the individual as well as the adaptive means he employs, more or less successfully." The reworking of the separation–individuation phase, according to Mann, is manifested in four universal conflict situations: (1) independence versus dependence; (2) activity versus passivity; (3) adequate self-esteem versus diminished or loss of self-esteem; and (4) unresolved or delayed grief.

Mann believes that therapy should focus on the "present and chronically endured pain" of the patient's self. He posits that "all short forms of psychotherapy, whether their practitioners know it or not, revive the horror of time. . . . One way of understanding the failure to give time central significance . . . lies in the will to deny the horror of time by the therapists themselves" (Mann, 1973, pp. 10–11).[4]

He describes his approach clearly:

> My method of time-limited psychotherapy includes more than the use of twelve sessions with the termination date known from the start of the first therapy session and the importance of the termination phase in rekindling the affective state that brought the patient for help. Of equal importance is the selection of a central issue, extracted

---

[4]Mann's concern with the "horror of time" resonates with the depiction of the ancient Greek god of time, Chronos, who would eat his children. In the *Metamorphoses*, Ovid speaks of "time, the devourer of all things." A similar image is provided in Indian mythology, where Kali (the feminine form of the Sanscrit word *Kāla*, meaning "time") is depicted as gruesome with her tongue out ready to lick up the world (Von Franz, 1978, illustration and caption 29).

For many adults, there is a reversal in the sense of directionality of time, usually in middle age (Neugarten & Datan, 1974). As children and youngsters, we measure time as time lived since birth. Sometime in adulthood—a profound moment of truth—we experience time as time left to live. This is our mortality, the recognition of the finiteness of our being, an awareness that is often thrust upon us by a personal existential crisis, such as an illness, death of a friend or parent (Malinak, Hoyt, & Patterson, 1979), the birth of a child, or beginning to work (Sarason, Sarason, & Cowden, 1975). Psychotherapy can help one to make this recognition constructively, the importance of living every moment. In this spirit, Castenada (1987, p. 262) has Don Juan advise: "If you think about life in terms of hours instead of years, our lives are immensely long. Even if you think in terms of days, life is still interminable."

out of the patient's history, which includes the elements of time, affects, and the image of the self; invariably a negative self-image. The goal of treatment in the twelve sessions becomes one of reducing as much as possible the negative self-image. The time restriction and the adherence of the therapist to this kind of central issue result in a telescoping of events and a heightened affective state that makes for an intense in vivo experience. (Mann, 1984, p. 207)

Mann delineates three phases of treatment, each lasting approximately four sessions. In the first trimester, a positive transference emerges as the patient experiences the unconscious fantasy of endless nurturance. This gives way to the more ambivalent affect of the second phase, wherein the therapist frustrates the patient by sticking to a focus and not gratifying the patient's desire for unending contact. Finally, in the last third of treatment, the patient deals constructively with the termination of therapy and reworks previous experiences of loss. Schwartz and Bernard (1981) have reported some empirical evidence to support this three-stage model; Westen (1986) has questioned it on theoretical grounds and Hatcher *et al.* (1986) have reported data suggesting that for many therapists the central focus of time-limited psychotherapy tends to undergo significant revisions across the course of treatment.

In addition to Mann's (1973; Mann & Goldman, 1982) own case reports, an extended example is provided by Hoyt (1979a; also see Leon, 1987) who described the termination work across a 12-session time-limited psychotherapy conducted with a 69-year-old woman 5 months after the death of her husband. The initial setting of the 12-session time limit has already been described. The following quotations, taken from the therapist's remarks across the latter half of the 12 sessions, convey some of the unfolding emphasis on a reworking of the mourning/separation/self-esteem theme that was central to this treatment. There was much more work done than these few comments convey, of course, although they may portray some of the typical activity of a therapist working within this particular short-term model:

Th: Well, it sounds as if you're doing pretty well. You joke about a postgraduate course. I think that you're thinking about the fact that we will be ending pretty soon.

Th: We are going to have five more meetings. From some of the things you've said, I imagine that you are beginning to have some feelings about the fact that we are going to end, and this is going to be another person that you have come to know and trust, and then it's going to end.

Th: You said you don't feel sad now?

Th: You look at your watch a lot.

Th: A minute ago you cried when we talked about separating, and then you kind of quickly talked about going back East.

Th: I think that as things come to an end over time we'll miss this relationship, but also it can remind you of other times when you've been involved with someone or cared about someone.

Th: It sounds like you're saying that you don't want to get too attached.

Th: Just because I'm the Doctor and you're the Patient doesn't mean you have to put up with me. There are times when I'm wrong, and you want to stand up for yourself.

Th: And the fact that you are getting a lot from this relationship may make it difficult for you to let yourself sometimes be annoyed with me or be angry with me.

Th: I imagine your getting involved in that relationship with him has changed your feelings about ending therapy here, having someone else you're talking to.

Th: What are your feelings about ending, terminating?

Th: I understand that you'll take some things away with you, but there is also the reality that we will stop seeing each other, that it will end.

Th: It's good that you see the difference between our relationship and what you had with M. You depended on him so much.

Th: Have you thought much about our finishing?

Th: Talking about his death and that time seems fitting, since we are almost at the end of our relationship.

Th: It has been very good for me, too. I've not only been helpful, but I have also gained personally from spending time with you.

Th: I think you *took* it back, and I helped you.

This case had a very favorable outcome, documented with long-term follow-up. The patient's age raises an interesting point:

> The successful outcome again demonstrates the value of psychotherapy with older persons. Her age also may be relevant in regard to our emphasis on temporal experience. With advanced age and the realistic awareness of the finitude of life, time may be experienced differently and may in some ways take on more value (Scott-Maxwell, 1968). The utility of a time-limited model thus would make sense both theoretically and practically with geriatric patients. (Hoyt, 1979a, p. 217)

Melges's (1972, 1982) Future Oriented Psychotherapy

This approach conceptualizes time distortions as altering consciousness and impairing reality testing. Melges posits that a person's inner sense of the future influences the present, a model that provides "a framework for focusing psychiatric treatment on time and the future. The restoration of control over the personal future can be accomplished through the correction of time distortions and the harmonization of future images, plans of action, and emotions. The restoration of control over the future is the key to interrupting psychopathological spirals" (Melges, 1982, p. xxi).

Melges's cybernetic model is that "psychopathological spirals occur when problems with sequence, rate, and temporal perspective disrupt the normal interplay between future images, plans of action, and emotions" (1982, p. 49). The following table (from Melges, 1982, p. 51) indicates a hierarchy of time problems, with the most severe at the top.

Melges describes a number of methods for assessing patients' time sense, and provides a brilliant exposition of the biopsychosocial treatment of time distortions, including the use of medication and hospitalization, psychodynamic therapy, transactional analysis, cognitive therapy, hypnosis, and family therapy. By focusing on the temporal aspects of the patient's functioning, particularly

TABLE 1. Different Problems with Time and the Personal Future
in Psychiatric Disorders

Time problem	Personal future	Psychiatric disorder
1. Time disorientation	Confused	Organic brain disease
2. Temporal disintegration of sequences	Fragmented	Schizophrenic disorders
3. Rate and rhythm problems:		
Increased rate	Overexpanded	Mania
Decreased rate	Blocked	Depression
4. Temporal perspective problems:		
Overfocus on future	Threatened	Paranoid disorders
Overfocus on past	Dreaded (uncertain)	Anxiety disorders
Overfocus on present	Disregarded	Antisocial personality
5. Desynchronized transactions	Ambivalent	Adjustment disorders

From Melges, 1982, p. 51.

the patient's impaired future sense, Melges often is able to achieve significant improvements with brief treatment.[5,6]

Seeman (1976) illustrates through a case example how much of the disordered reality testing and thought process of a schizophrenic can be understood as manifestations of a defective time sense. Pathognomic experiences regarding permanence versus change, unidirectionality versus bidirectionality, periodicity, simultaneity, duration, continuity versus atomicity, uncontrollable inevitability, sequencing versus causality or intentionality, clairvoyance, "marking time" and "doing time," and confusions of past/present/future are all seen as reflections of disturbances underlying perceptual-cognitive schemata. Seeman describes a therapeutic approach that "can be viewed as a form of cognitive repair focused on the perception, interpretation, and integration of the sense of time" (p. 193), noting that a treatment explicitly directed toward a schizophrenic patient's cognitive-temporal organization helps to structure the patient's experience while defocusing from affect that might otherwise become too intense and stormy. Seeman sees this psychotherapy of time sense as also being consistent with the use of antipsychotic medications that aim to "damp down affects but

[5]A related analysis is provided by Thomson (1983), who illustrates how overabsorption with either the future, the present, or the past can result in a respective excess of fear, anger, or sadness. From a psychoanalytic perspective, Hartocollis (1983) draws similar parallels between future versus past-time orientation and anxiety versus depressive affects.

[6]"Time therapy" is a fourth-dimensional meta-therapy that provides a form of hierarchical control over what occurs in three-dimensional space. Linear, unidirectional time is a Western invention, and time was not so neatly regularized before Galileo invented the mechanical clock (Boorstin, 1985). I think that the Church was so able to organize and dominate Europe partially by the ringing of bells to mark the hours. Uniform time structure was thus institutionalized, the assertion of a common external structure permitting more precisely coordinated social functions and profounding influencing the patterning of consciousness.

remove interferences with perceptual and cognitive functioning" (p. 194). Her case example is not short-term treatment, but her principles may be applicable to brief therapy, as Melges (1982) demonstrates.

Lesse (1971) has also used the term *Future Oriented Psychotherapy* to describe a treatment approach. He uses the term in a more global sense, not basing his therapy (which is essentially psychodynamic) on a theory of time, but rather providing a "prophylactic" function by guiding patients over a relatively brief number of sessions to consider their role in the future in order to prepare for the impending stresses and challenges. Lesse sees such a futurologic perspective as especially valuable because "the ever accelerating rate of change that characterizes our society makes it necessary that the psychotherapy patient have a general idea of what his or her role is likely to be in the world of tomorrow" (p. 192).

Berne's (1961, 1972) Transactional Analysis and Goulding and Goulding's (1978, 1979) Redecision Therapy

The description of Berne's model of human development, intrapsychic organization, and interpersonal dynamics goes far beyond the scope of this exposition (see Woollams & Brown, 1978). There are three elements of Berne's work, however, that pertain directly to time and brief therapy.

Contractual Therapy

Berne favored the explication of specific, obtainable goals in treatment, ones that could be conceptualized in a manner such that they could be accomplished and recognized. He wanted patients to set their own treatment goals and to recognize their ability to make changes rapidly. "What can I do to cure this patient today?" was a question that Berne liked to ask himself before sessions.

Time Structuring

Berne theorized that patients early in life form a life plan or *script* that guides much of their subsequent course. He felt that scripts could be recognized and discarded or changed. To avoid the pain of boredom, people need to structure time. Essentially, there are six possible ways to structure time: withdrawal, ritual, pastime, activity, rackets/games, and intimacy. Because humans apportion their energy among these six alternatives and some are more satisfying and growthful than others, understanding of these concepts will reveal a great deal about a person's psychological way of being in the world. Woollams and Brown (1978, p. 91) explain the psychotherapeutic significance of this:

> Analyzing a client's time structuring provides information about how she exchanges strokes, which in turn tells us how she maintains her script decisions. Helping the client understand and change how she structures her time provides new ways for her to give and get the kinds of strokes which her Free Child wants and needs. Invariably, as clients change their ways of structuring time and exchanging strokes, they need to

work through the feelings connected with giving up their old patterns and relating in new ways.

Script Time

The script concept was central to Berne's later (1972) thinking. He saw that many people organize their life plan in terms of an approach to time:

> Winning or losing, the script is a way to structure the time between the first Hello at mother's breast and the last Good-by at the grave. This life time is emptied and filled by not doing and doing; by never doing, always doing, not doing before, not doing after, doing over and over, and doing until there is nothing left to do. This gives rise to 'Never,' and 'Always,' 'Until' and 'After,' 'Over and Over,' and 'Open-Ended' scripts. (Berne, 1972, p. 205)

Brief therapists who wish to help patients make major changes quickly may find it helpful to recognize and focus directly on modifying basic aspects of temporal perspective such as script time orientations.

A patient in her late 30s complained of procrastination and feeling stagnant. She was bright and articulate but doing a job that lacked excitement for her. She had a number of years earlier left her marriage for another man, but that had not worked out and now she was without a partner or likely prospects. Despite her efforts to be "rational" and "positive," she obsessed, looked sad, and sighed unhappily. The therapist, trying to gain ingress to the patient's deeper feelings, asked if there were any scene she could think of that expressed her situation (see Hoyt, 1986). "Yes," she responded almost immediately. "Did you see the film *Superman?* It's like the scene where he flies backward and stops time! God, I wish I could do that!" With tears in her eyes she described the scene where the hero flies backwards around the earth so quickly that time is somehow reversed, thus allowing him to intervene in something that had already happened.[7] This image opened wide the patient's regret for mistakes past and her attempts to avoid risks and stave off future misfortunes.

Robert and Mary Goulding (1978, 1979) have provided a major contribution by combining the theory of Transactional Analysis (Berne, 1961, 1972) with Gestalt techniques plus their own unique innovations. Their approach is built on the basic theory that as children people often make key life decisions (such as Don't Feel, Don't Think, Don't Be Close, Don't Grow Up, Don't Be Important, Don't Enjoy, or Don't Be) in order to survive or adapt to perceived and often veridical parental pressures. In treatment, the patient reenters and reexperiences the pathogenic scene as a child, via imagery and Gestalt work, and with the encouragement and support of the therapist makes a *re*decision that frees the patient from the pernicious injunction that he or she has earlier accepted. This here-and-now work involves a powerful combination of affect and insight, with support and behavioral anchors maintaining the gains achieved.

---

[7]This is an old motif, done one better: Zeus once held the sun back so as to spend a longer night with a lover.

Oftentimes patients recognize in redecision therapy that they have been trying magically to change the past or control the future. An example would be the man who, after reliving an early scene, was asked to experiment by the redecision therapist with saying to his imagined father, "I'm going to stay angry at you until you treat me differently when I was 6!" Hearing himself tilt absurdly against a long-gone windmill, he laughed, recognized his "craziness," and claimed his freedom. Like the Zen monk who finds himself seeking permission from Another for what only he can control (Hoyt, 1979b, 1985b), the patient suddenly realizes that "it's all in my mind, and I control my mind!" This is the basic truth behind the title of Mary Goulding's (1985) book, *Who's Been Living in Your Head?* Another well-known TA/Gestalt therapist, James (1985), has also suggested the possibility of rapid change through the title of one of her books, *It's Never Too Late to Be Happy*.

Motivated patients sometimes make a forceful redecision within a single session. The following case example occurred recently in my office:

The patient was a 37-year-old married woman. She came for an initial appointment complaining of "insecurity, anxiety, and low self-esteem." She reported that she was married to a man with strong macho tendencies, who sometimes verbally abused her. She also reported being bored and dissatisfied with her job, a teacher's aide in a school. Remarkedly, she revealed that she was a licensed attorney, that she had graduated from a major law school and had passed the bar on her first attempt. She had then married and had children, however, and had only practiced law part-time for a short while before staying home with the kids and then returning to work as a teacher's aide.

She again described herself as insecure and said that she "couldn't do anything right." The therapist asked her to repeat that phrase, which she did, and he then asked where she had heard it as a child. The patient then reported that her mother had been a very disturbed, highly critical woman, one whose irrational beliefs, fears, and occasional behaviors suggested schizophrenia. Indeed, the patient's mother had been hospitalized in mental institutions on and off throughout her childhood. The father had divorced and left the family. What a remarkable accomplishment for this patient, to have done so well given such a rough start: She had married, mothered two children, and had become an attorney. The therapist complimented her success. "I know," she replied, "but I still hear my mother telling me how I can't do anything right." She gave several examples of things her mother would irrationally criticize.

At this juncture the therapist decided that talking *about* the problem would not generate a strong enough experience to produce a genuine change in this bright woman. He announced that he wanted to meet the patient's mother. When she responded that "mother would never agree to come here," the therapist said, "I want to meet the woman you carry around in your head. Do an experiment. Change seats. In that seat, *be* your mother. Hi, Mother, what's your name?" The therapist then proceeded to interview "Mother" for about 15 minutes. At first the patient was hesitant, but she quickly got into the part. She even surprised herself with the richness of characterization of Mom: her gestures, her words, her easy flow of irrational ideas. Mom felt her daughter [the patient] was always wrong, wouldn't go to her house or hold her children because they might have germs on them, felt it was "just wrong" for a girl to go to college or work with men, thought law school was because the patient had not done well in college, and kept insisting that all her children were "exactly the same." The therapist listened respectfully and then added, "I'm not a lawyer, so I'm not defending her, but I've heard that you have to be very smart to even get into that law school, and even smarter to graduate." Mom didn't know that. The therapist also commented that he could see how much Mom wanted to love all her children and that it must be hard to see that in some ways they were different from one another (Mom has even given them all the same middle name). After a bit, the therapist thanked Mom, asked her if she would be willing to come back sometime "if we need to hear from you," and had the patient resume her own chair in the office.

The patient was stirred up by the experience. She stared at the now empty chair where "Mom" had been, shook her head, and said, "I didn't realize how crazy Mom actually is." The therapist then said to her: "Do this. Say 'I *am* an attorney. I got into law school and I graduated,' and see how it feels." She said it once, with hesitation, then repeated it with conviction and added: "I *am* an attorney, I'm smart, I got into law school, I graduated, and I passed the bar on my first try!" She was sitting up straight and alert, confident and strong. The therapist noted the change, saying "Do you feel how different you are? You look stronger, more attractive. I feel that now I'm sitting here with a professional woman, not the scared daughter of your crazy mother."

The patient understood but attempted to discount her change. She remarked: "It's a role that I'm good at playing."

The therapist nodded and said, "I think that you're right except that you've got it 100% reversed. *This* is the real you, and you were playing a role to get along with your mother. You know, like they say, putting a bushel over your light. You were playing dumb so Mother wouldn't get upset or be threatened. Smart people can play dumb. This is the real you, not what you said [gesturing toward the empty seat "Mom" had occupied]."

The patient looked transformed. She was grasping a basic truth and liking its feel. "You're right. I am smart. I am. I *am* an attorney, and I can be a damn good one, too. I'm not going to buy into Mom's crazy ideas anymore."

The therapist complimented her on her insight and awareness. They talked briefly about how she could start using her confidence and intelligence. She was full of good ideas. When asked if she wanted another appointment, she said, "Not now. I can handle what I have to do. I'm an intelligent woman. I'll be making calls to get my career back on track."

Comment

This interaction, which took no more than 1 hour, from start to finish, is an example of effective single-session psychotherapy (see Bloom, 1981; Hoyt *et al.*, 1987; Rockwell & Pinkerton, 1982; Talmon *et al.*, 1988; Rosenbaum *et al.*, 1989). It was useful to have the patient vividly see how unhealthy her mother's messages were and to help the patient make a new decision about her own competency and importance. This was an application of the Redecision model of therapy developed by Goulding and Goulding (1978, 1979), although it was not technically a full redecision because the patient did not make her new decision while actively in the child ego state. Still, reinforcing the patient's strengths and helping her to sort out her true self from an archaic pathological introject allowed her to rapidly make the change in self-image necessary for her to get unstuck and to resume movement in her life.

Concluding Remarks

Time is of the essence, in therapy and in life. To be intimate one must be, literally, "in-time-mate." Brief psychotherapy is true to this quest insofar as it calls for participants to "Be Here Now." This is the message of this chapter, as indicated by its title: "On Time in Brief Therapy."

ACKNOWLEDGMENTS. Grateful acknowledgment is made to Richard Wells for inviting me to write this chapter and for his many helpful suggestions. Additional thanks to Sidney Blatt, who long ago encouraged my study of the psychology of time; and to Bob and Mary Goulding, who have greatly expanded my appreciation of the therapeutic possibilities of the present. Finally, love and kisses to Alexander Lillard Hoyt (born May 18, 1987), who has changed my experience of past, present, and future time forever.

References

Appelbaum, S. A. (1975). Parkinson's law in psychotherapy. *International Journal of Psychoanalytic Psychotherapy, 4*, 426–436.

Appelbaum, S. A., & Holzman, P. S. (1967). "End-setting" as a therapeutic event. *Psychiatry, 30*, 276–282.

Austin, L., & Inderbitzin, L. (1983). Brief psychotherapy in late adolescence: A psychodynamic and developmental approach. *American Journal of Psychotherapy, 37*, 202–209.

Barten, H. (1965). The 15-minute hour: A brief therapy in a military setting. *American Journal of Psychiatry, 122*, 565–567.

Beck, A. T. (1976). *Cognitive therapy and emotional disorders.* New York: International Universities Press.

Becker, E. (1973). *The denial of death.* New York: Free Press.

Bennett, M. J. (1983). Focal psychotherapy—terminable and interminable. *American Journal of Psychotherapy, 37*, 365–375.

Bennett, M. J. (1984). Brief psychotherapy and adult development. *Psychotherapy, 21*, 171–177.

Bergin, A. E., & Lambert, M. J. (1978). The evaluation of therapeutic outcomes. In A. E. Bergin & S. L. Garfield (Eds.), *Handbook of psychotherapy and behavior change* (2nd ed. pp. 139–190). New York: Wiley.

Berenbaum, H. (1969). Massed time-limit psychotherapy. *Psychotherapy: Theory, Research & Practice, 6*, 54–56.

Berne, E. (1961). *Transactional analysis in psychotherapy.* New York: Grove Press.

Berne, E. (1972). *What do you say after you say hello?* New York: Grove Press.

Blanchard, K., & Johnson, S. (1982). *The one minute manager.* New York: William Morrow.

Bloom, B. L. (1981). Focused single-session therapy: Initial development and evaluation. In S. H. Budman (Ed.), *Forms of brief therapy* (pp. 167–216). New York: Guilford.

Bonaparte, M. (1941). Time and unconscious. *International Journal of Psycho-Analysis, 21*, 427–468.

Boorstin, D. J. (1985). *The discoverers.* New York: Random House.

Breuer, J., & Freud, S. (1955). Studies in hysteria. *Standard Edition of the Complete Psychological Works of Sigmund Freud* (Vol. 2. pp. 1–319). London: Hogarth Press. (Originally published 1893–1895)

Brodaty, H. (1983). Techniques in brief psychotherapy. *Australian and New Zealand Journal of Psychiatry, 17*, 109–115.

Budman, S. H. (Ed.). (1981). *Forms of brief therapy.* New York: Guilford.

Budman, S. H., & Gurman, A. S. (1983). The practice of brief therapy. *Professional Psychology, 14*, 277–292.

Budman, S. H., & Gurman, A. S. (1988). *Theory and practice of brief therapy*. New York: Guilford.

Burlingame, G. M., & Behrman, J. A. (1987). Clinician attitudes toward time-limited and time-unlimited therapy. *Professional Psychology: Research and Practice, 18,* 61–65.

Butcher, J. N., & Kolotkin, R. L. (1979). Evaluation of outcome in brief psychotherapy. *Psychiatric Clinics of North America, 2,* 157–169.

Butcher, J. N., & Koss, M. P. (1978). Research on brief and crisis-oriented psychotherapies. In S. L. Garfield & A. E. Bergin (Eds.), *Handbook of psychotherapy and behavior change: An empirical analysis* (2nd ed., pp. 725–768). New York: Wiley.

Castelnuovo-Tedesco, P. (1986). *The twenty-minute hour: A guide to brief psychotherapy*. Washington, DC: American Psychiatric Press.

Casteneda, C. (1972). *Journey to Ixtlan*. New York: Simon & Schuster.

Casteneda, C. (1987). *The Power of Silence*. New York: Simon & Schuster.

Cooper, L. F., & Erickson, M. H. (1959). *Time distortion in hypnosis* (2nd ed.). Baltimore: Williams & Wilkins.

Cottle, T. J., & Klineberg, S. L. (1974). *The present of things future: Explorations of time in human experience*. New York: Macmillan.

Cross, D. G., Sheehan, P. W., & Khan, J. A. (1982). Short- and long-term followup of clients receiving insight-oriented therapy and behavior therapy. *Journal of Consulting and Clinical Psychology, 50,* 103–112.

Cummings, N. A. (1977). Prolonged (ideal) versus short-term (realistic) psychotherapy. *Professional Psychology, 4,* 491–501.

Cummings, N. A., & VandenBos, G. (1979). The general practice of psychology. *Professional Psychology, 10,* 430–440.

Dasberg, H., & Winokur, M. (1984). Teaching and learning short-term dynamic psychotherapy: Parallel processes. *Psychotherapy, 21,* 184–188.

Davanloo, H. (1986). Intensive short-term psychotherapy with highly resistant patients. I. Handling resistance. *International Journal of Short-Term Psychotherapy, 1,* 107–133.

de la Torre, J. (1978). Brief encounters: General and technical psychoanalytic considerations. *Psychiatry, 41,* 184–193.

De Shazer, S. (1985). *Keys to solution in brief therapy*. New York: Norton.

Doob, L. (1971). *Patterning of time*. New Haven, CT: Yale University Press.

Dreiblatt, I. S., & Weatherly, D. (1965). An evaluation of the efficiency of brief contact therapy with hospitalized psychiatric patients. *Journal of Consulting Psychology, 29,* 513–519.

Dunne, J. S. (1973). *Time and myth*. Notre Dame: University of Notre Dame.

Dylan, B. (1963). *The Times They Are A-Changin*. Record album. New York: Columbia.

Eliot, T. S. (1943). *Four quartets*. New York: Harcourt.

Emery, G., & Campbell, J. (1986). *Rapid relief from emotional distress*. New York: Rawson Associates.

Fanshel, D. (1971). *Playback: A marriage in jeopardy examined*. New York: Columbia University Press.

Fraisse, P. (1963). *The psychology of time*. New York: Harper & Row.

Frances, A., & Clarkin, J. F. (1981). No treatment as the prescription of choice. *Archives of General Psychiatry, 38,* 542–545.

Frances, A., Clarkin, J., & Perry, S. (1984). *Differential therapeutics in psychiatry: The art and science of treatment selection*. New York: Brunner/Mazel.

Fraser, J. T. (Ed.). (1966). *The Voices of Time*. New York: George Braziller.

Fraser, J. T. (Ed.). (1975). *Of time, passion, and knowledge*. New York: George Braziller.

Freud, S. (1914). Remembering, repeating and working through. *Standard edition of the complete psychological works of Sigmund Freud* (Vol. 12, pp. 145–156). London: Hogarth press, 1953–1974.

Freud, S. (1916). On transience. *Standard edition* (Vol. 14, pp. 303–308).

Freud, S. (1917). Mourning and melancholia. *Standard edition* (Vol. 14, pp. 237–258).

Freud, S. (1918). From the history of an infantile neurosis. *Standard edition* (Vol. 17. pp. 3–122).

Freud, S. (1933). The unconscious. New introductory lectures. *Standard edition* (Vol. 22, pp. 3–184).

Freud, S. (1937). Analysis terminable and interminable. *Standard edition* (Vol. 23, pp. 209–254).

Frieswyk, S. H., Allen, J. G., Colson, D. B., & Coyne, L. et al. (1986). Therapeutic alliance: Its place as a process and outcome variable in dynamic psychotherapy research. *Journal of Consulting and Clinical Psychology, 54,* 32–38.

Goldberg, C. (1975). Termination—A meaningful pseudodilemma in psychotherapy. *Psychotherapy: Theory, Research & Practice, 12,* 341–343.

Gomes-Schwartz, B. (1978). Effective ingredients in psychotherapy: Prediction of outcome from process variables. *Journal of Consulting and Clinical Psychology, 46,* 1023–1035.

Gorman, B. S., & Wesman, A. E. (1977). *The personal experience of time.* New York: Plenum Press.

Goulding, M. (1985). *Who's been living in your head?* (Rev. ed.). Watsonville, CA: WIGFT Press.

Goulding, R., & Goulding M. (1978). *The power is in the patient.* San Francisco: TA Press.

Goulding, M., & Goulding, R. (1979). *Changing lives through redecision therapy.* New York: Grove Press.

Guerin, P. J., Jr. (Ed.) (1976). *Family therapy: Theory and practice.* New York: Gardner Press.

Gurman, A. S., & Kniskern, D. P. (Eds.). (1981). *Handbook of family therapy.* New York: Brunner/Mazel.

Gustafson, J. P. (1986). *The complex secret of brief psychotherapy.* New York: Norton.

Hartley, D. E., & Strupp, H. H. (1983). The therapeutic alliance: Its relationship to outcome in brief psychotherapy. In M. Masling (Ed.), *Empirical studies of psychoanalytic theories* (pp. 1–37). Hillsdale, NJ: Analytic Press.

Hartocollis, P. (1983). *Time and timelessness.* New York: International Universities Press.

Hatcher, S. L., Huebner, D. A., & Zakin, D. F. (1986). Following the trail of the focus in time-limited psychotherapy. *Psychotherapy, 23,* 513–520.

Heidegger, M. (1927). *Being and time.* New York: Harper & Row, 1962.

Horowitz, M. J. (1976). *Stress response syndromes.* New York: Jason Aronson.

Horowitz, M. J., & Hoyt, M. F. (1979). Book notice of Malan's "The frontier of brief psychotherapy." *Journal of American Psychoanalytic Association, 27,* 279–285.

Horowitz, M. J., Marmar, C., Krupnick, J., Wilner, N., Kaltreider, N., & Wallerstein, R. (1984). *Personality styles and brief psychotherapy.* New York: Basic Books.

Howard, K. I., Kopta, S. M., Krause, M. S., & Orlinsky, D. E. (1986). The dose-effect relationship in psychotherapy. *American Psychologist, 41,* 159–164.

Hoyt, M. F. (1977). Primal scene and self-creation. *Voices, 13,* 24–28.

Hoyt, M. F. (1978). Secrets in psychotherapy: Theoretical and practical considerations. *International Review of Psycho-Analysis, 5,* 231–241.

Hoyt, M. F. (1979a). Aspects of termination in a time-limited brief psychotherapy. *Psychiatry, 42,* 208–219.

Hoyt, M. F. (1979b). 'Patient' or 'client': What's in a name? *Psychotherapy: Theory, Research & Practice, 16,* 46–47.

Hoyt, M. F. (1980). Therapist and patient actions in "good" psychotherapy sessions. *Archives of General Psychiatry, 37,* 159–161.

Hoyt, M. F. (1983). Concerning remorse: With special attention to its defensive function. *Journal of the American Academy of Psychoanalysis, 11,* 435–444.

Hoyt, M. F. (1985a). Therapist resistances to short-term dynamic psychotherapy. *Journal of the American Academy of Psychoanalysis, 13,* 93–112.

Hoyt, M. F. (1985b). 'Shrink' or 'expander': An issue in forming a therapeutic alliance. *Psychotherapy, 22,* 813–814.

Hoyt, M. F. (1986). Mental-imagery methods in short-term dynamic psychotherapy. In M. Wolpin *et al.* (Eds.), *Imagery* 4, pp. 89–97. New York: Plenum.

Hoyt, M. F. (1987a). Notes on psychotherapy with obsessed patients. *The Psychotherapy Patient, 3,* 13–21.

Hoyt, M. F. (1987b). Resistances to brief therapy. *American Psychologist, 42,* 408–409.

Hoyt, M. F. (1988a). Book review of Gustafson's "The Complex Secret of Brief Psychotherapy." *American Journal of Psychiatry, 145,* 374–375.

Hoyt, M. F. (1988a). *Teaching and learning short-term psychotherapy: Resistances and phase-specific parallel processes.* Paper presented at annual convention of the American Psychological Association, Atlanta.

Hoyt, M. F. (1989). Psychodiagnosis of personality disorders: A guide for the perplexed. *Transactional Analysis Journal, 19,* 101–113.

Hoyt, M. F., & Farrell, D. (1984). Countertransference difficulties in a time-limited psychotherapy. *International Journal of Psychoanalytic Psychotherapy, 10,* 191–203.

Hoyt, M. F., & Goulding, R. L. (1989). Rapid resolution of a transference-countertransference impasse using Gestalt techniques in supervision. *Transactional Analysis Journal,* in press.

Hoyt, M. F., Xenakis, S. N., Marmar, C. R., & Horowitz, M. J. (1983). Therapists' actions that influence their perceptions of "good" psychotherapy sessions. *Journal of Nervous and Mental Diseases, 171,* 400–404.

Hoyt, M. F., Talmon, M., & Rosenbaum, R. (1987). *Single-session psychotherapy: Increasing effectiveness and training clinicians.* Workshop presented at annual convention of the American Psychological Association, New York.

James, M. (1985). *It's never too late to be happy.* Reading, MA: Addison-Wesley.

James, W. (1890). *The principles of psychology* (Vol. 2). New York: Holt.

Johnson, H., & Gelso, C. (1980). The effectiveness of time limits in counseling and psychotherapy. *The Counseling Psychologist, 9,* 70–83.

June, L. N., & Smith, E. J. (1983). A comparison of client and counselor expectancies regarding the duration of counseling. *Journal of Counseling Psychology, 30,* 596–599.

Kaiser, H. (1965). The problem of responsibility in psychotherapy. In L. B. Fierman (Ed.), *Effective psychotherapy: The contribution of Hellmuth Kaiser* (pp. 1–13). New York: Free Press.

Langs, R. (1979). *The therapeutic environment.* New York: Jason Aronson.

Leon, I. G. (1987). Short-term psychotherapy for perinatal loss. *Psychotherapy, 24,* 186–195.

Lesse, S. (1971). Future oriented psychotherapy—a prophylactic technique. *American Journal of Psychotherapy, 25,* 180–193.

Luborsky, L., Singer, B., & Luborsky, L. (1975). Comparative studies of psychotherapies: Is it true that "everyone has won and all must have prizes"? *Archives of General Psychiatry, 32,* 995–1008.

Malan, D. H. (1976). *The frontier of brief psychotherapy.* New York: Plenum Press.

Malan, D. H., Heath, E. S., Bacal, H. A., & Balfour, H. G. (1975). Psychodynamic changes in untreated neurotic patients. II. Apparently genuine improvements. *Archives of General Psychiatry, 32,* 110–126.

Malinak, D. P., Hoyt, M. F., & Patterson, V. (1979). Reactions to the death of a parent in adult life: A preliminary study. *American Journal of Psychiatry, 136,* 1152–1156.

Mann, J. (1973). *Time-limited psychotherapy.* Cambridge, MA: Harvard University Press.

Mann, J. (1984). The management of countertransference in time-limited psychotherapy: The role of the central issue. *International Journal of Psychoanalytic Psychotherapy, 10,* 205–214.

Mann, J., & Goldman, R. (1982). *A casebook in time-limited psychotherapy.* New York: McGraw-Hill.

May, R., Angel, E., & Ellenberger, H. F. (Eds.). (1958). *Existence.* New York: Simon & Schuster.

Melges, F. T. (1972). Future oriented psychotherapy. *American Journal of Psychotherapy, 26,* 22–33.

Melges, F. T. (1982). *Time and the inner future: A temporal approach to psychiatric disorders.* New York: Wiley.

Meltzoff, J., & Kornreich, M. (1970). *Research in psychotherapy.* New York: Atherton Press.

Minkowski, E. (1933). *Lived time: Phenomenological and Psychopathological Studies.* Evanston, IL: Northwestern University Press, 1970.

Nannum, A. (1972). Time in psychoanalytic technique. *Journal of the American Psychoanalytic Association, 20,* 736–750.

Napier, A. Y., & Whitaker, C. A. (1978). *The family crucible.* New York: Harper & Row.

Naranjo, C. (1970). Present-centeredness: Technique, prescription, and ideal. In J. Fagen & I. L. Shepherd (Eds.) *Gestalt therapy now.* (pp. 47–69). New York: Science and Behavior Books.

Neugarten, B. L., & Datan, N. (1974). The middle years. In S. Arieti (Ed.), *American handbook of psychiatry* (Vol. 1, 2nd ed, pp. 592–608) New York: Basic Books.

Ornstein, R. E. (1969). *On the experience of time.* New York: Penguin.

Pekarik, G., & Wierzbicki, M. (1986). The relationship between clients' expected and actual treatment duration. *Psychotherapy, 23,* 532–534.

Perls, F. S. (1969). *Gestalt therapy verbatim.* Lafayette, CA: Real People Press.

Perls, F. S., Hefferline, R. F., & Goodman, P. (1951). *Gestalt therapy.* New York: Julian Press.

Perry, S. W. (1987). The choice of duration and frequency for outpatient psychotherapy. *Annual review of psychiatry, 6*, 398–414.

Piaget, J. (1946). *The child's conception of time.* New York: Basic Books, 1969.

Pollack, G. H. (1971). On time and anniversaries. In M. Kanzer (Ed.), *The Unconscious Today* (pp. 233–257). New York: International Universities Press.

Priestly, J. B. (1968). *Man and time.* New York: Dell.

Rank, O. (1945). *Will therapy.* New York: Knopf.

Rockwell, W. J. K., & Pinkerton, R. S. (1982). Single-session psychotherapy. *American Journal of Psychotherapy, 36*, 32–40.

Rosenbaum, R., Hoyt, M. F., & Talmon, M. (1989). *The challenge of single-session therapies: Creating pivotal moments.* In R. Wells & V. Giannetti (Eds.), *Handbook of the brief psychotherapies.* New York: Plenum Press.

Sarason, S. B., Sarason, E. K., & Cowden, P. (1975). Aging and the nature of work. *American Psychologist, 30*, 584–592.

Schafer, R. (1973). The termination of brief psychoanalytic psychotherapy. *International Journal of Psychoanalytic Psychotherapy, 2*, 135–148.

Schilder, P. (1936). Psychopathology of time. *Journal of Nervous and Mental Diseases, 83*, 530–546.

Schwartz, A. J., & Bernard, H. S. (1981). Comparison of patient and therapist evaluations of time-limited psychotherapy. *Psychotherapy: Theory, Research & Practice, 18*, 101–108.

Scott-Maxwell, F. (1968). *The measure of my days.* New York: Knopf.

Seeman, M. V. (1976). Time and schizophrenia. *Psychiatry, 39*, 189–195.

Selvini-Palazzoli, M., Cecchin, G., Prata, G., & Goscolo, L. (1978). *Paradox and counterparadox.* New York: Jason Aronson.

Shectman, F. (1986). Time and the practice of psychotherapy. *Psychotherapy, 23*, 521–525.

Shorr, J. E. (1972). *Psycho-imagination therapy: The integration of phenomenology and imagination.* New York: Intercontinental Medical Book Corporation.

Shorr, J. E. (1974). *Psychotherapy through imagery.* New York: Intercontinental Medical Book Corporation.

Sifneos, P. E. (1979). *Short-term dynamic psychotherapy.* New York: Plenum Press.

Sifneos, P. E. (1981). Short-term anxiety-provoking psychotherapy. In S. H. Budman (Ed.), *Forms of Brief Therapy* (pp. 45–80). New York: Guilford.

Singer, J. L. (1974). *Imagery and daydream methods in psychotherapy and behavior change.* New York: Academic Press.

Singh, R. N. (1982). Brief interviews: Approaches, techniques, and effectiveness. *Social Casework,* December, 599–606.

Smith, M. L., Glass, G. V., & Miller, T. I. (1980). *The benefits of psychotherapy.* Baltimore: Johns Hopkins University Press.

Spitz, R. A. (1972). On anticipation, duration, and meaning. *Journal of the American Psychoanalytic Association, 20*, 721–735.

Stierlin, H. (1968). Short-term versus long-term psychotherapy in the light of a general theory of human relationships. *British Journal of Medical Psychology, 41*, 357–367.

Strupp, H. H. (1980a–d). Success and failure in time-limited psychotherapy. *Archives of General Psychiatry, 37*, 595–603(a), 708–716(b), 831–841(c), 947–954(d).

Strupp, H. H., & Binder, J. L. (1984). *Psychotherapy in a new key.* New York: Basic Books.

Talmon, M., Hoyt, M. F., & Rosenbaum, R. (1988). *When the first session is the last.* Symposium presented conference on Brief Therapy: Myths, Methods, and Metaphors (Fourth International Congress on Ericksonian Approaches to Hypnosis and Psychotherapy), San Francisco.

Tart, C. T. (Ed.) (1969). *Altered states of consciousness.* New York: Wiley.

Thomson, G. (1983). Fear, anger, and sadness. *Transactional Analysis Journal, 13*, 20–24.

Ticho, E. A. (1972). Termination of psychoanalysis: Treatment goals, life goals. *Psychoanalytic Quarterly, 41*, 315–333.

Volkan, V. D. (1975). "Re-grief" therapy. In B. Schoenberg (Ed.), *Bereavement: Its psychosocial aspects* (pp. 334–350). New York: Columbia University Press.

von Franz, M.-L. (1978). *Time: Rhythm and respose.* New York: Thames & Hudson.

Wallace, M., & Rabin, A. I. (1960). Temporal experience. *Psychological Bulletin, 57*, 213–226.

Wells, R. A. (1982). *Planned short-term treatment*. New York: Free Press/Macmillan.

Weston, D. (1986). What changes in short-term dynamic psychotherapy? *Psychotherapy, 23*, 501–512.

Whitaker, C. A., & Malone, T. P. (1953). *The roots of psychotherapy*. New York: Blakiston.

Wolberg, L. R. (1965). The technic of short-term psychotherapy. In L. R. Wolberg (Ed.), *Short-term psychotherapy* (pp. 127–200). New York: Grune & Stratton.

Woollams, S., & Brown, M. (1978). *Transactional analysis*. Ann Arbor, MI: Huron Valley Institute Press.

Zirkle, G. (1961). Five-minute psychotherapy. *American Journal of Psychiatry, 118*, 544–546.

7

Tasks in Brief Therapy

Rona L. Levy and John L. Shelton

Rationale and Theory for the Use of Tasks

Our stance on the importance of tasks is simple: We do not see tasks as an adjunct, even a critical adjunct to brief psychotherapy. Rather, we see them as *the basis for action in brief psychotherapy*. If therapy is to be effective in a short period of time, the therapist *must* encourage the efficient conduct of the client's therapeutic activities—both in and outside of the therapy session. The opportunity that tasks provide for the productive use of time outside regularly scheduled hours is extensive. Therapists and clients may use this time for such activities as the observation of naturally occurring events or the practice of skills learned during the therapeutic session. (A more extensive discussion of different types of tasks follows in the next section.)

Another advantage to the use of tasks is that they actively involve the client in the work of therapy. Thus, rather than the client seeing therapy as something done "to" him or her, clients can see themselves as actors in the therapeutic process. As we also mention later on, this "active patient orientation" has been shown to be positively related to clinical outcome (Schulman, 1979).

Aside from this discussion of practical reasons for using tasks in the brief psychotherapies, Bandura's theory of self-efficacy (Bandura, 1977) offers a theoretical rationale for the use of tasks. He explains how "psychological procedures, whatever their form, serve as means of creating and strengthening expectations of personal efficacy" (p. 193). Furthermore, performance-based treatments (which include tasks) "not only promote behavioral accomplishments but also extinguish fear-arousal, thus authenticating self-efficacy through enactive and arousal sources of information. . . . This source of efficacy information is especially influential because it is based on personal mastery experiences" (Bandura, 1977, p. 195). Bandura's concept of "mastery experiences" is

RONA L. LEVY • School of Social Work, University of Washington, Seattle, Washington 98195. JOHN L. SHELTON • Private Practice, Renton, Washington 98055. Portions of this chapter originally appeared in *Applications in Behavioral Medicine and Health Psychology*, edited by D. C. McKee and J. A. Blumenthal, Professional Resource Exchange, Sarasota, Florida, 1987, and *Behavioral Assignments and Treatment Compliance*, by J. L. Shelton and R. L. Levy, Research Press, Champaign, Illinois, 1981.

similar to Liberman's (1978) use of this concept in his theoretical analysis of tasks in psychotherapy. Simply, assigning tasks that are successfully accomplished can build an individual's sense of self-efficacy.

Types of Tasks

Tasks were originally defined as "assignments given to the clients which are carried on outside the therapy hour" (Shelton & Ackerman, 1974, p. 3). The types of tasks that may be given under this broad aegis are as varied as the directions that each individual therapist may take in the therapeutic process. Wells (1982) has classified tasks into three categories: (1) observational or monitoring tasks; (2) experiential tasks, which are "designed to arouse emotion in the client or to challenge beliefs or attitudes" (Wells, 1982, p. 171); and (3) incremental change tasks, "designed to stimulate change directly toward a desired goal, in a step-by-step manner" (Wells, 1982, p. 171). We include in this incremental category all assignments that are related to practicing any social or interpersonal skill and that are intended to lead to ultimate competence in that skill.

Several other categories may be added to these. A fourth group of "one-shot" tasks can be designed simply to get something done and provide an end in themselves. For example, making an appointment, starting a job, and the like. A fifth category of assignments might be called "mediator assignments." Tharp and Wetzel (1969) defined a mediator as "some person naturally articulated into the client's social environment" (p. 3). Mediators are often given assignments on behalf of someone else. For ethical reasons, of course, we assume the client has agreed to the participation of such individuals. When this has occurred, mediators may be very useful for monitoring, recording, and collecting data, providing assistance (such as transportation), feedback, and other relevant activities. It is important to not forget this category of tasks, as nearly all important issues concerning tasks, such as compliance (discussed in a later section), must also be considered with this category.

Another category of tasks may be called *paradoxical* and are familiar to most readers from the work of Jay Haley (1963, 1973, 1976), among others. This type of task really is a form of compliance enhancer and is discussed in a later section. The intent of the therapist is not to have the assignments carried out as given but actually in some manner contrary to what is given. The idea behind such assignments is that in some situations, such as when the therapist is faced with a resistant client, the resistance is utilized to reach the desired therapeutic goal. By assigning a paradoxical task, the resisting client is expected to act contrary to the task and hence in a manner consistent with therapeutic goals. Paradoxical tasks may also be a useful way of reducing performance anxiety. For example, a client who has trouble falling asleep may be told to "try to stay up as long as possible." Elsewhere (Shelton & Levy, 1981), however, we have cautioned against the use of these tasks unless other alternatives have failed. Results from using them are simply less dependable and have less empirical data to support their use.

Another way to "cut the pie" on types of tasks might be to look at the types of assignments given from different theoretical approaches to therapeutic practice. However, one must be careful not to be too simplistic in making these distinctions. Certainly, cognitive/behavioral therapists give more assignments that involve practice in specific behaviors. For example, a shy man might be asked to do an "incremental change task" such as beginning social contacts with women, with the eventual goal being increased social competence. Yet, a non-behaviorally oriented therapist might also ask a client who has recently gained insight into his anxiety around women to begin social contact with them.

Tasks that involve thoughts or feelings also might cut across differing theoretical frameworks. Cognitive/behavioral, as well as insight-oriented therapists might well ask clients to monitor their own thoughts or feelings at a particular time or under particular circumstances. Differences may arise in the stated reasons for the monitoring, however. One therapist may have as a goal changing the thought, whereas another might claim "insight" as the intended goal.

Another perspective on categorizing different types of tasks is to consider how many individuals are the goal for change. Specifically, is the client an individual, a couple, a family, a group, or some segment of society, as in social policy change. Tasks for individuals are the ones that most commonly come to mind in clinical practice. Clients are asked to record their thoughts, eat a low-calorie diet, speak to someone with assertiveness, study for 2 hours a night, congratulate their spouse for following a task, and so on. All of these assignments, whether given to the client or a mediator, are designed to move an individual toward some goal.

From the perspective of assignment type, group therapy may be considered a special type of individual therapy, in that the target of change is an individual. One task-related difference between individual and group therapy is that assignments for individuals may be given to groups of people. (This is done, of course, only as appropriate for clinical purposes or to test the effectiveness of a standardized research protocol.) Tasks may also be individualized to clients within the group. Another way group therapy and individual therapy differ dramatically from our perspective is in the availability of the groups to promote compliance with the assignments. This aspect will be discussed later in our presentation on compliance enhancement.

Tasks may also be devised that are designed to bring about change in two or more individuals, such as in family or marital therapy. In addition to completing treatment-related questionnaires, couples in family or marital therapy are typically asked to practice certain communication as well as problem-solving skills learned in the therapeutic session (Jacobson, 1981). Couples may often be asked to monitor each other as well, particularly in respect to behaviors critical to the relationship.

Finally, there are types of assignments that are designed to bring about social change. With broad sweeping goals such as influencing social policy, one is, perhaps more than in other areas, forced to think in terms of "incremental change tasks." Final goals such as "social equality for minorities in the community" must be broken down into finer steps until manageable tasks for individuals and groups can be constructed. For example, a first change in achieving this end goal might be "measurement of the ratio of minority children in the different school programs."

The Ethics of Task Giving

Two aspects of the ethics of task giving should be considered. First, we expect therapists to consider the ethical implications of their assignments in the same manner as they consider all aspects of their therapy. One's professional code of ethics provides a good checklist for reviewing this aspect of the appropriateness of an assignment. For example, the social worker must consider a client's perspective in selecting an assignment, as well as in the overall course for therapy. Also, we have already mentioned the importance of being sensitive to issues of confidentiality when giving an assignment. A clear, explicit treatment contract is critical both ethically as well as to enhance effectiveness. Another aspect of ethics to consider is the recognition of the values one is conveying when giving a task. The type of task selected, the manner in which tasks are given, and even the giving of tasks can convey important messages about such things as what clients ought to be doing for themselves, how persons should treat each other, the respect the therapist has for the client, and so on. Sensitivity to gender roles is one key area to be considered in this regard (Jacobson, 1983). Thus careful thought must go into this entire process.

Enhancing Compliance

Compliance has been defined elsewhere as "carrying out an assignment in the way described by the assignment giver(s)" (Shelton & Levy, 1981, p. 37). Although most of this definition seems fairly straightforward, note the phrase *by the assignment giver*. Thus, the reader should note that the assignment giver may be the therapist, the client him- or herself, or the two in combination. Aside from the ethically desirable position of having the client, rather than the therapist, be the assignment giver, there are also practical reasons for this. As we will discuss later, the client as assignment giver may actually enhance compliance.

Why Don't Clients Comply?

One may think of there being as many reasons for not complying as there can be reasons for individuals doing, or not doing anything. Haynes, Taylor, and Sackett (1979) reviewed several studies where patients had given reasons for noncompliance. Although there are many ways for categorizing these reasons, we have found the following system useful.

Group 1: The Client Does Not Know How to Complete the Task

Within this category might fall those situations where someone (1) was not instructed on how to do something; (2) was instructed, but insufficiently to produce knowledge transfer; or (3) was instructed, did learn, and then "lost" the knowledge. For example, within this group would fall those patients given an appointment slip that was then misplaced, clients who forgot a once-learned assignment, or clients who could not understand the therapist because the task-giving language was not sufficiently clear.

Group 2: The Client Does Not Believe Complying Will Help

Several factors may result in this cognition. To name a few: the client does not regard the clinician as credible; the client thinks the clinician does not understand him or her, or the problem. On some occasions, relatives give contradictory advice. On other occasions, the client does not feel similar treatment has helped (or may have even made them worse), or the client is already improving and does not feel he or she needs to do anymore. Finally, in Haynes *et al.*'s (1979) review, several studies reported that clients stated they simply were not interested or "motivated" to change. (We view *motivation* as a generic term that serves to cover explanations for other reasons in this group and the other two.)

Group 3: Factors in the Patient's Life Make Compliance Difficult, or at Least Do Not Support Compliance

Included in this category certainly are many of the areas that practitioners should often be addressing: financial, transportation, or child care problems. Often, the client's job situation makes it difficult to comply. Clients may believe complying will help, but they are afraid of the response from others in their environment. Potential ridicule or hostility are also often major concerns.

All of these potential reasons for noncompliance need to be considered by the clinician. What follow are some of the steps that could be taken to counteract these factors.

Steps to Enhance in Compliance

Several authors have devised systems for enhancing client compliance. In his task-centered approach, Reid (1975) first recommended a five-part sequence using the following steps: (1) enhancing commitment—the client is "to consider the potential benefits of carrying out the task" (p. 3); (2) planning task implementation—"the client is helped to specify the task and develop a plan for carrying it out" (p. 3); (3) analyzing obstacles—the client is asked "to consider problems that may be encountered in carrying out the task" (pp. 3, 4); (4) modeling—rehearsal and guided practice—"the caseworker may model possible task behavior or ask the client to rehearse what he is going to say or do" (p. 4); and (5) summarizing—"the caseworker restates the task and the plan for implementation" (p. 4).

Wells (1982), drawing from the work of Liberman (1978), has also made the following suggestions for the therapists: (1) utilize assignments that are directly related to the clients' goals, (2) adequately explain the relevance of the task, (3) carefully select tasks that are not too easy and not too difficult, (4) take into account the reactions of significant others, and (5) the therapist should attempt to assure self-attribution in task success or failure.

We believe all of these suggestions by Reid and Wells are excellent and should be incorporated into any therapist's task-giving activities. We have developed our own recommendations that expand on some of those discussed or add to them. They are all suggestions for content that should be included in the giving of assignments.

One final, yet critical point before we get to these assignments: All of these recommendations must occur within the context of a good therapeutic relationship. Otherwise, any efforts are highly likely to fail. Others have extensively discussed the therapeutic relationship in relation to task compliance and we refer the interested reader there (Di Matteo & Di Nicola, 1982; Meichenbaum & Turk, 1987).

Recommendation 1: The Therapist Should Be Sure Assignments Contain Specific Details about the Desired Behavior

Assignments should specify how, when, where, and for how long something is to be done. Studies in the medical literature show considerable variation in the interpretation of doctors' instructions (typically medication taking). In one study (Mazzulo, Lasagna, & Griner, 1974), it was found that patients had many different interpretations of apparently simple instructions such as "take four times a day."

When we ask patients to keep an ongoing record of some activity, it is important to ask where they plan to keep their monitoring sheet. This encourages them to plan the specific details of how they will keep the assignment. Many men, for example, prefer to keep a three-by-five card in a shirt pocket. We also encourage patients to do their recording as close as possible in time to when the event of interest occurred. Otherwise, they may forget to record or are more likely to record inaccurately.

Contracts have been very successful in obtaining compliance, as demonstrated in an antihypertensive regimen study by Steckel and Swain (1977). One way that contracts may work is that they provide a way of specifically outlining a patient's responsibilities so that the chances of misinterpretation are reduced. One caution should be noted here: Simplicity should not be sacrificed for specificity. Extreme detail and complexity may actually make a behavior too difficult (Haynes *et al.*, 1979). For example, "at exactly 5 minutes past every hour I want you to sit in that chair in your office we were discussing and take exactly 60 seconds to relax" may be far too detailed to obtain compliance. If this occurred, we would most likely instruct a client that we wished her or him to take a relaxation period approximately 1 minute in length at the rate of once an hour but would usually leave the exact timing to her discretion.

Exactly how the client is asked to carry out the assignment is another aspect of being specific that we also feel is important and may be conceptualized as a "delivery style" issue. We believe there will be a difference in outcome between telling someone "I would like you to . . ." or "call . . . ," and "if you feel like doing X, you may want to . . ." More directiveness exists in the first two statements, which clearly imply the therapist's preference. There is no ambiguity present, and it reduces the room for the client to think, "well, he said if I *want to* . . . and I don't, so I won't!" In most circumstances, it is more likely to produce compliance. However, for those clients where control is an issue, the therapist may find that being *less* directive is more effective.

Recommendation 2: The Therapist Should Give Direct Skill Training When Necessary

This recommendation is essentially an elaboration of Reid's (1975) modeling, rehearsal, and guided practice. A frequent mistake made by therapists who utilize home practice is the assumption that the patient has the skills necessary to complete the desired task. It is therefore wise to practice the behavior in the office before asking the patient to engage in the task in the natural social environment. This practice is particularly recommended in cases where the assigned behavior is so complex that verbal instructions alone are inadequate.

1. The therapist assesses the level of patient skills relevant to the upcoming assignment (skill training is not always necessary).
2. If the decision is made to proceed with skill training, the therapist begins by giving the patient verbal and written instructions.
3. The therapist models the skill.
4. The patient then imitates the skill, with coaching, prompting, and reward for approximations toward the desired goal.

For example, staying with the relaxation example, a patient who is almost constantly in interaction with other people was asked to take "brief relaxes" throughout her day. She was told this could even be done when in a face-to-face interaction. She expressed doubt about how she could do this. Thus it was determined that skill training was appropriate. The patient was then given verbal and written instructions (e.g., "take a slow deep breath, exhale slowly, let your tension be released," etc.). The therapist then modeled this behavior, demonstrating that this relaxation did not need to interrupt their interaction. Finally, the patient was asked to perform the behavior, with appropriate feedback from the therapist.

Recommendation 3: Compliance Should Be Rewarded

The rate of compliance is influenced by the consequences that immediately follow compliant behavior. Missed opportunities to reward compliance may lead to a decrease in the frequency and duration of home practice activities and an overall reduction in effectiveness.

A number of reward opportunities exist for encouraging the patient to adhere to the prescribed task. The sources of reward can be the therapist, the client himself or herself, or significant others.

Therapist Reinforcement

Because the patient may not gain immediate reward from persons in his or her social environment, he or she should always be told in advance that the criterion for success is the execution of the behavior (compliance) and not the outcome of compliance. The therapist, at least initially, is frequently the most important source of reward. The therapist should keep a careful record of all prescribed assignments so that patients should never have to "fish" for reinforcement by reminding the therapist of what they were asked to do. Recording task assignments also spares therapists having to struggle to remember specific tasks or losing credibility with clients if they have to confess they've forgotten. A therapist who has lost credibility is one who has significantly reduced reward potential.

Initially, patients should be reinforced for *all* approximations to desirable compliance efforts. For example, if a patient was assigned to keep a daily journal of food consumed for 1 week but completed only 1 day's record, he or she should be rewarded at first for this approximation to carrying out the assignment (see next recommendation).

Therapists should also make use of the telephone to offer reinforcement, either by calling patients or having them call in. A telephone call can provide the therapist with an opportunity to provide social reward to the client in a natural setting. Phone calls should, however, be used carefully because some patients may use homework failure as an excuse to obtain more contact with the therapist. Whenever possible, phone calls should therefore be made at a scheduled time, preferably after completion of a task rather than when there is difficulty in doing the task. Patients can be instructed to call when they finish a difficult task, not "whenever the homework doesn't go well." Thus, although problems arising from homework should be understood and empathized with, the emphasis remains on the positive aspects of performance of assigned tasks. We have found patients to be generally delighted to receive at-home calls. They have said that this seems to show caring when the therapist is willing to step outside of the scheduled hour-long weekly meeting.

In addition to the therapist's praise, other avenues of therapist-initiated reward exist. A contingency statement in the homework format is one good way of assuring that the homework will be completed, and several contingencies can be designed to increase adherence. Rather than seeing the client at a scheduled time, the therapist may not schedule the client for the next appointment until he or she calls to say that the assignment is done. This contingency is based on the assumption, of course, that the client finds it rewarding to talk to the therapist.

Other rewards can also be considered. For example, the therapist may give a money rebate upon completion of agreed-upon homework. He or she can also make a regular appointment with the client but reduce the length of the session if the client does not attempt the homework. This latter type of reinforcement is useful for agency workers who cannot manipulate the fee and also for situations in which the therapist chooses to make some contact with the patient, although for only a short time.

Reward structures should be clearly outlined. One way to do this is to use a behavioral contract. Although contracts require more time and effort to construct, they can provide the additional structure and contingencies needed to foster the completion of home activities. Contracts generally emphasize the positive rewards for achieving compliance with assigned tasks. In addition, they help clarify the consequences of completing the assignment, and they provide clear-cut criteria for achievement of the stated therapeutic activities.

Contracts can be unilateral or bilateral. A unilateral contract is one in which the client obligates himself or herself to complete the homework and is rewarded for such completion. Bilateral contracts specify the obligations and the mutual rewards for each of the parties involved.

Contracts should be very specific, determined by negotiation and fully understood and accepted by the patient. Contracts should be written down, and both the therapist and the patient should have a copy. Successful contracts should also have short-range goals, as well as ultimate therapeutic goals. The achievement of short-range goals, which are the result of task completion, can give the client a positive expectation of change—and self-efficacy.

Other elements of a successful contract include the following:

1. A very clear and detailed description of the homework should be stated.
2. The contract should specify the reward gained if the homework is completed.
3. Some provisions should be made for some consequence for failure to complete the assignment within a specified time limit or behavior frequency.
4. The contract should specify the means by which the contract response is to be observed, measured, and recorded.
5. An arrangement should be made so that the timing for delivery of rewards follows the response as quickly as possible.

Patient Reward

Another important source of reward is the patient himself or herself. Self-reward is vital to the success of homework and may actually be the key to maintaining therapeutic behaviors after treatment has been terminated.

Conceptually, it is helpful to look at a model first provided by Johnson (1971) in which overt behaviors and covert behaviors (thoughts) can be rewarded overtly or covertly. The reward possibilities and contingency relationships generated by this model are extensive:

1. An assertive response (overt behavior) is followed by self-praise (covert

behavior) such as "I did a beautiful job on that assertive response. Dr. ——— would be proud of me."

2. A thought such as "I will be successful as long as I concentrate on the task" (covert behavior) could be rewarded by a pleasant activity, such as having something desirable to eat (overt behavior).

3. A thought such as "I am very attractive when I smile" (covert behavior) could be followed by an instance of self-praise (covert behavior) such as "keep up the good work of thinking good thoughts."

Reward by Others

Involving others in the client's treatment can be a very effective part of therapy. Family members or friends can help in various ways to support completion of homework assignments (Levy, 1983, 1985). Other persons' participation may even be formalized by being built into a contract.

Brownell and his colleagues (Brownell, Heckerman, Westlake, Hayes, & Monti, 1978; Brownell & Stunkard, 1981; Wilson & Brownell, 1978) have systematically involved partners of overweight spouses in weight reduction programs, with mixed results across studies. Each week, patients were given homework assignments, and partners are also given their own homework assignments, many of which include rewards to the overweight partner for compliance with assignments. Although these procedures seem to logically have value, more research into their most effective components is needed.

Group therapies provide a unique opportunity for reinforcement of task compliance. In many programs, clients are expected to make public statements of their successes or failures. This can provide a powerful reward (or punishment). Group members can also be used as new significant others, much as Brownell used spouses in the preceding example. Group members can call each other for support and encouragement in following a buddy's progress.

Recommendation 4: The Therapist Should Begin with Homework That Is Likely to Be Successfully Accomplished

One technique in this approach is referred to as the "foot-in-the-door" (Freedman & Fraser, 1966) technique. Patients are first asked to comply with a small request. If the request is complied with and rewarded, they are then more likely to comply with a subsequent task.

Another good way to look at this suggestion is to always work for success. The therapist should give assignments that he or she believes have a high likelihood of being successfully completed. This will increase the opportunity for the development of self-efficacy as discussed earlier.

Recommendation 5: The Therapist Should Use a System That Will Remind Patients of the Assignment

The therapist should take steps to insure that the client is reminded, cued, or prompted to carry out an assignment at the appropriate time and place. One cue to assignment compliance that can be carried into the natural environment would be a copy of the written assignments. Therapists may use either a xerox copy of their own record, made in session while assignments are given, or they might utilize NCR (no carbon required) pads when writing down assignments. Thus the therapist and the patient immediately get one copy. Patients may then be asked to post this list in a convenient place. The senior author has a place on her appointment cards where assignments are to be recorded. The following is printed on the cards: "Between now and _____ you have been asked to" (if the list is long and would not fit on the card, simply write "complete assignments on your assignment sheet").

Phone calls by the therapist, in addition to being rewards, may also be useful to remind and prompt the client. Significant others can be helpful by providing needed reminders at appropriate times. Finally, various devices have been used as aids to compliance, including timed buzzers, calendars, and dated pill dispensers (Epstein & Cluss, 1981).

Although the evidence has been mixed, several studies have found increased appointment-keeping compliance when clients receive reminders in the form of postcards or phone calls (Levy & Claravall, 1977). As it likely does not decrease appointment keeping, it certainly appears worthwhile to remind clients of their appointments, if therapists have the facilities to do so.

This is another area where the use of a group is helpful. Group members can be utilized to call each other up to remind them of tasks.

Recommendation 6: The Therapist Should Have the Client Make a Public Commitment to Comply

Public commitments, such as verbalizations of a concrete plan, can serve two purposes. First, they can provide considerable evidence about how someone intends to behave. Such information can provide a basis for further discussion if it appears that the client may not intend to adhere to prescribed assignments. One of the best ways to predict compliance is to simply ask the client whether or not he or she intends to comply with the assigned outside activity. The therapist may also ask for specifics such as frequency and duration.

An overt, publicly given commitment may also serve to enhance the likelihood of compliance. In many situations such a commitment, if given verbally and written down, is sufficient to bring about completion of assignments (Levy, 1977; Levy & Clark, 1980; Levy, Yamashita, & Pow, 1979). However, despite assurances from the patient that he or she intends to comply with the stated assignment, the therapist may doubt the accuracy of the prediction. In some cases, the patient may have repeatedly promised to complete the assignment and failed to follow through. As with reminders, the evidence is mixed on the relationship between overt commitment and improvement in compliance rates (Shelton & Levy, 1981). Yet, it "costs" so little to simply ask a patient, "will you do it?", that it seems useful to use this technique in all situations along with other techniques that may be appropriate.

Recommendation 7: The Patient Should Believe in the Value of the Assignment for Treating His or Her Problem

First the patient needs to have a belief structure that supports the task. He or she must believe that the assigned task is useful, that it is acceptable to others, that it has a high probability of successful completion, and that the entire treatment program is valuable. Therapists should take considerable time to elicit the patients' beliefs, fears, and expectations regarding compliance. Questions should be encouraged, and good rapport, as always, is critical. After being given the assignment, the patient should be questioned regarding his or her reaction to the assignment. This intensive discussion will also provide the opportunity to further enact other compliance-enhancement steps, such as more direct training, if needed. Well-chosen bibliotherapy regarding the benefits of treatment or the consequences of an untreated problem may alter beliefs. In addition, some people benefit from listening to audiocassettes designed especially for patients.

Any relationship-building activities in which the clinician can engage are likely to increase the chances of compliance. Kanfer and Goldstein (1975) provide a good framework for demonstrating how a client's liking, respecting, and trusting a therapist will lead to client change. This point seems obvious and should not be overlooked in a consideration of enhancement strategies.

A final and critical aspect of this recommendation for compliance enhancement is that clients should help select homework assignments. Rather than just hand out assignments, therapists should work with clients to develop assignments, perhaps using phrases such as "now, what do you think would be a good way to keep track of . . . ?", or the therapist may offer a range of assignments from which the client can choose.

This active participation (Schulman, 1979) by the client may have several positive consequences. First, clients should have an increased perception of control. No one is *making* them do this—they have chosen to do the assignment and are thus more likely to follow through. Second, clients will have selected assignments that they can imagine occurring in their own world. This fact reduces the possibility that, after a reflecting on an assignment, a client will think, "The therapist doesn't really know how difficult it would be to do that," and then fail to comply. In this way, the client actually becomes the assignment giver.

Recommendation 8: The Therapist Should Use Cognitive Rehearsal Strategies

This is another elaboration on Reid's recommendation for rehearsal, with an emphasis on cognitive rehearsal. Having a patient take some time in the office to actually imagine carrying out the assignment can lead to several positive results. First, the patient may be able to raise possible difficulties that could arise, and these may be "problem-solved" (see Recommendation No. 9). The patient may also recognize some confusion with aspects of the assignment and may be able to ask clarifying questions. Finally, imagining a difficult activity in the relaxed atmosphere of the therapeutic office, with the support of the therapist readily available, may be an easy first step, consistent with Recommendation No. 4.

In addition to rehearsing cognitively in the office, several techniques for cognitive rehearsal outside of the therapist's office have also been recommended. With Suinn's (1972a,b) approach, the client is asked to carry out a specific cognitive strategy just before engaging in a self-directed assignment. This procedure asks the client to:

> RELAX
> VISUALIZE (the successful completion of the assignment)
> DO (the assignment)

For example, the client who is fearful of failure in some athletic event would be asked to first relax immediately before the event, then to visualize successfully completing the event, and then to do, or to initiate, the athletic response.

Meichenbaum's (1977) Self-Instructional Training is considerably more complex than that just discussed, and it has shown a great deal of merit. In this approach, patients are taught to focus on the assigned task. The strategy consists of the following:

1. *Preparing for a stressor.* In this first step, the client is urged to prepare a "game plan" for anticipated anxiety and inability to focus on the assigned task (e.g., taking an exam). The client might, for example, rehearse the more frequent distractors likely to be faced when the stress mounts. The patient will then remind himself or herself what he or she plans to do when the distractors occur (e.g., "I must remember to read the directions twice and do the easiest questions first").
2. *Confronting the stressor.* In the second phase, the patient actually activates the coping strategy rehearsed earlier. Cues such as written notes can be used as reminders of what self-control interventions to employ during the stressful time. Self-statements such as "don't worry about the clock; just concentrate on the exam" and "don't worry if they are already finishing; that doesn't mean they have done well" may be useful.
3. *Rewarding self-statements.* This third step requires the patient to reward himself or herself for the successful completion of homework.

Recommendation 9: The Therapist Should Try to Anticipate and Reduce the Negative Effects of Compliance

Again, we see this as an example of Reid's recommendation to analyze obstacles. Efforts should be made to anticipate barriers to compliance in the natural environment and facilitate the integration of the assignment into the patient's normal activities. Many potential punishment pitfalls can be avoided by following some of the strategies already discussed. For example, patients who have received thorough training in performing a task are likely to find it less difficult. Patients who have tried techniques such as Meichenbaum's (1977) or Johnson's (1971) self-reward system, discussed in Recommendations 8 and 3, respectively, are less dependent on external rewards as they generate their own reward intrinsically. Thus a client who complies with a very difficult task can be encouraged to say to herself or himself something like "Good for me! That was tough, but I did it!," even if persons around her or him, such as a spouse, are less rewarding.

Sometimes modifications that help avoid punishment for compliance are very easy. One client reported that it was difficult to put the yellow monitoring sheets provided by the therapist out on her desk to monitor her task completion. She said she worked in an office where people were always writing on white sheets of paper, and if she pulled out a yellow sheet, people would know that it was something different. This was handled by simply xeroxing the form and giving her copies of the form on white sheets of paper.

Recommendation 10: Compliance Should Be Closely Monitored by as Many Sources as Possible

Monitoring may include direct observation of the client's compliance behavior or some indirect method of assessing the behavior. It may be carried out by the client (self-monitoring), by someone else in the client's environment who has the opportunity to observe compliance (or noncompliance) behavior, or both.

Monitoring is critical because of the therapist absence feature of many brief therapies. If the therapist cannot directly observe compliance, he or she must rely on some system of monitoring to determine that it has occurred and whether congratulations or further instructions are appropriate. Monitoring can also provide several direct benefits to the patient. He or she can engage in self-reward when monitored data are good and will also be made more aware of the importance of the task being assigned.

One example of monitoring by the patient might occur in a smoking-reduction program, where the assignment might be to reduce smoking by two cigarettes per day. Compliance could be self-monitored by having the patient count the number of cigarettes smoked per day and may be co-monitored by having the client's spouse count the number of cigarettes remaining in the client's cigarette pack (assuming, of course, that the patient was not smoking any cigarettes other than his or her own).

For medication compliance, blood serum or urine assays may be directly observed. Of course, the timing on when such samples are taken will affect their accuracy as a measure of compliance (Epstein & Cluss, 1981). Tracer or marker procedures, typically used with urine-detection methods also may be employed. With this method, the clinician or others may directly observe tracers or have patients do the monitoring of, say, urine color. Therapists could, for example, give pills to patients with tracer colors ordered in a sequence known only to the therapist. If the patient reports the correct sequence, compliance is assumed to have occurred (Epstein & Masek, 1978).

Spouses can easily monitor eating behaviors during mealtimes or other appropriate periods when the spouse is present (such as during evening TV watching or a social gathering). Brownell and Stunkard's (1981) system, mentioned under Recommendation 3, relies heavily on spouse observation. If available to the therapist, trained observers may sometimes be placed in the patient's environment. Finally, other methods discussed in Gordis (1979) and Dunbar (1979), such as collecting data from permanent products (physical results from some behavior—e.g., a candy bar wrapper may be taken as evidence that a candy bar has been consumed) or mechanical devices, may also be used to monitor compliance. Patients should be involved in the planning of any methods such as these to monitor their behavior.

When monitoring for compliance is conducted by the patient, several issues come up. One issue is that self-monitoring may be reactive—it may actually change the behaviors being observed (Barlow, Hayes, & Nelson, 1984). There is also some evidence that monitoring increases a desired behavior and decreases undesired behaviors (Kanfer, 1980, pp. 353–357). Thus, monitoring has some positive effect on task achievement and can offer an initial reward (through the previously noted effects) that will tend to encourage further task compliance.

Another issue to consider in using self-monitoring to improve compliance is accuracy. For example, it would certainly be undesirable if the therapist were rewarding the client for desirable eating habits, as reported on the patient's self-monitoring sheet, if the client were not eating as indicated on the assignment. In this case, the patient would be being rewarded for inaccurate recording and poor eating habits. Thus it is important for the therapist to know how to determine and enhance the accuracy of the data received from the patient.

Monitoring by others raises many of the same issues as self-monitoring. Monitoring by others may also be reactive and could thus be utilized by the therapist to affect compliance in a desirable direction. Observers also need to be trained in accurate recording methods. Finally, the therapist needs to be aware of many of the factors that can affect the accuracy of information.

As a final point, in working with a patient or other persons to set up many of the compliance enhancements such as monitoring (Recommendation 10), reward (Recommendation 3), and reminders (Recommendation 5), the therapist needs to be aware of the importance of viewing these activities as assignments themselves. Thus if the therapist wishes compliance with activities such as monitoring one's compliance, rewarding oneself after completing an assignment, or putting up reminder notes, compliance-enhancement recommendations should be utilized to enhance these activities as well.

One Additional Suggestion: Paradoxical Intention

We have listed this as a suggestion rather than a recommendation because we feel it is not something the therapist should consider in all situations. However, on some occasions, a therapist may resort to strategies for change that are not openly agreed upon. Most of these procedures may be labeled *paradoxical* and spring from the work of Haley (1963, 1973, 1976). They use the client's uncooperative behavior in such a way as to discourage resistance and produce therapeutic results. When the therapist accepts the resistance, the client is caught in a position where resistance becomes cooperative.

These procedures should be used only as a "last resort." To date, little empirical evidence has been found to support their effectiveness, and they are often extremely complex and have the potential to be very harmful to clients. Judgments regarding when and with whom to use these procedures require long-term experience with clients and specific training in paradoxical procedures.

An article by Ascher (1979) provides some evidence for the effectiveness of paradoxical intention in the treatment of urinary retention. In this study, five individuals were selected for paradoxical intention therapy, who had previously tried, and failed, at a traditional behavioral regimen consisting of *in vivo* assignments, control of fluid intake, and systematic desensitization. The paradoxical intention procedure utilized by Ascher (1979) consisted of requesting that each client enter a bathroom in which he felt uncomfortable and engage in a number of activities that were commonly associated with urination. However, he was prohibited from actually urinating. For example, a male client was given the assignment to enter a men's room, walk to the urinal, unzip his fly, perform the appropriate manipulation and, stand there as if to urinate, but under no circumstances was he to allow himself to pass urine. After a reasonable period of time, he was then instructed to readjust his anatomy, return his pants to the proper order, flush the urinal, wash his hands, and leave the bathroom. The assignments given the subjects in the ensuing 2 to 3 weeks consisted of very frequent opportunities to practice the paradoxical intention activity. They were never actually given the permission to urinate. Ascher (1979) assumed that when performance anxiety was sufficiently low and urgency to urinate was great, the clients would then violate the prohibition. They were instructed to inhibit the flow of urine for as long as possible each time they entered a restroom associated with anxiety. These instructions were continued for a period of 2 to 3 weeks, after which the program was discontinued. Ascher (1979) reports that all five subjects improved significantly within a 6-week program.

Wells (personal communication, 1988) has also found some paradoxical tasks to be useful. In one case, he reports on a woman who successfully carried out a task involving being more assertive with a family member. It was helpful to predict a relapse, giving the client the task of watching for the relapse (i.e., a return to former behaviors) and acting assertively again. He has also used monitoring tasks in situations where it is believed the client is skeptical or uncertain about acting or might even resist a direct assignment. Thus a couple were instructed to observe instances of "incomplete messages" between them, that is to say, times when one or the other was not clearly conveying a need. They were instructed that they "didn't have to do anything about the message, other than observe its happening." Not surprisingly, they reported at the next interview few instances of unclear or vague communication and a much more conscious effort to make requests in a straightforward manner.

WHAT TO DO WHEN NONCOMPLIANCE OCCURS

The first point to be made here is to call attention to the placement of this section: It is at the end of this chapter. By this we hope to convey the message that compliance issues need to be considered at the beginning of task assignment in a preventive manner, before noncompliance occurs. By implementing compliance-enhancement activities in this way, the likelihood of noncompliance is greatly reduced.

Nevertheless, noncompliance still will occur even when the clinician feels he or she has utilized a compliance-enhancement protocol. The answer to what to do at this point is both simple and complex: The clinician must first consider possible reasons for noncompliance, often with the client, to determine the source of the problem. The client may simply report, "I forgot. I didn't notice the reminder I had posted." Utilizing the active participation model in Recommendation 7, the therapist could seek the client's assistance to determine other reminders that might be more effective. Then the clinician should review other enhancers to make sure all "bases" were truly covered. The clinician should also be sure that the context in which enhancers occur, the therapeutic relationship, is a good one.

During this review, the clinician must also consider the appropriateness of the task. For example, a client who has been asked to monitor something may report that he or she "has never been good at writing things down." Theoretically, the clinician could try to increase the reinforcement value of task completion. However, if one is working against a long-standing history of not being a recorder, it might be more prudent to put one's resources elsewhere and alter the assignment. Phone call-ins, verbal reports, or using others as data collectors are just some possible options.

Finally, Meichenbaum and Turk (1987) include an interesting discussion on why health care providers do not follow compliance-enhancement strategies. Providers' beliefs, expectations, memory, and inertia are all factors considered in their discussion. When noncompliance occurs, the clinician must examine his or her actions to see if everything that was reasonable and appropriate for that situation had been completed.

REFERENCES

Ascher, L. M. (1979). Paradoxical intention in the treatment of urinary retention. *Behaviour Research and Therapy, 17,* 267–270.

Bandura, A. (1977). Self-efficacy: Toward a unifying theory of behavioral change. *Psychological Review, 2,* 191–215.

Barlow, D. H., Hayes, S. C., & Nelson, R. O. (1984). *The scientist practitioner.* New York: Pergamon.

Brownell, K. D., Heckerman, C. L., Westlake, R. J., Hayes, S. C., & Monti, P. M. (1978). The effects of couples training and partner cooperativeness in the behavioral treatment of obesity. *Behaviour Research and Therapy, 16,* 323–333.

Brownell, K. D., & Stunkard, A. J. (1981). Couples training, psychotherapy, and behavior therapy in the treatment of obesity. *Archives of General Psychiatry, 38,* 1224–1229.

Di Matteo, M. R., & Di Nicola, D. D. (1982). *Achieving patient compliance. The psychology of the medical practitioner's role.* New York: Pergamon.

Dunbar, J. M. (1979). *Issues in assessment.* In S. J. Cohen (Ed.), *New directions in patient compliance* (pp. 41–57). Lexington, MA: Lexington Books.

Epstein, L. H. & Cluss, P. A. (1981). A behavioral medicine perspective on adherence to long-term medical regimens. *Journal of Consultation and Clinical Psychology, 50,* 1–10.

Epstein, L. H., & Masek, B. J. (1978). Behavioral control of medicine compliance. *Journal of Applied Behavior Analysis, 11,* 1–9.

Freedman, J. L., & Fraser, S. C. (1966). Compliance without pressure: The foot-in-the-door technique. *Journal of Personality and Social Psychology, 4,* 195–202.

Gordis, L. (1979). Conceptual and methodologic problems in measuring patient compliance. In R. B. Haynes, D. W. Taylor, & D. L. Sackett (Eds.), *Compliance in health care.* Baltimore: Johns Hopkins University Press.

Haley, J. (1963). *Strategies of psychotherapy.* New York: Grune & Stratton.

Haley, J. (1973). *Uncommon therapy: The psychiatric techniques of Milton H. Erickson, M.D.* New York: Norton.

Haley, J. (1976). *Problem-solving therapy.* New York: Norton.

Haynes, R. B., Taylor, D. W., & Sackett, D. L. (1979). *Compliance in health care.* Baltimore: Johns Hopkins University press.

Jacobson, N. S. (1981). Marital problems. In J. S. Shelton & R. L. Levy, *Behavioral assignments and treatment compliance* (pp. 147–166). Champaign, IL: Research Press.

Jacobson, N. (1983). Beyond empiricism: The politics of marital therapy. *American Journal of Family Therapy, 11,* 11–24.

Johnson, S. M. (1971). Self-observation as an agent of behavioral change. *Behavior Therapy, 2,* 488–497.

Kanfer, F. H. (1980). Self-management methods. In F. H. Kanfer & A. P. Goldstein (Eds.), *Helping people change* (2nd ed., pp. 334–389). New York: Pergamon.

Kanfer, F. H., & Goldstein, A. P. (1975). *Helping people change: Methods and materials.* Elmsford, NY: Pergamon.

Levy, R. L. (1977). Relationship of an overt commitment to task compliance in behavior therapy. *Journal of Behavior Therapy and Experimental Psychiatry, 8,* 25–29.

Levy, R. L. (1983). Social support and compliance: A selective review and critique of treatment integrity and outcome management. *Social Science and Medicine, 17,* 1329–1338.

Levy, R. L. (1985). Social support and compliance: Update. *Journal of Hypertension, 3*(Suppl. 1), 45–49.

Levy, R. L., & Claravall, R. (1977). Differential effects of a phone reminder on patients with long and short between-visit intervals. *Medical Care, 15,* 435–438.

Levy, R. L., & Clark, H. (1980). The use of an overt commitment to enhance compliance: A cautionary note. *Journal of Behavior Therapy and Experimental Psychiatry, 11,* 105–107.

Levy, R. L., Yamashita, D., & Pow, G. (1979). Relationship of an overt commitment to the frequency and speed of compliance with decision making. *Medical Care, 17,* 281–284.

Liberman, B. L. (1978). The role of mastery in psychotherapy: Maintenance of improvement and prescriptive change. In J. D. Frank, R. Hoehn-Saric, S. D. Imbar, B. L. Liberman, & A. R. Stone (Eds.), *Effective ingredients of successful psychotherapy* (pp. 35–72). New York: Brunner/Mazel.

Mazzulo, S. M., Lasagna, L., & Griner, P. F. (1974). Variations in interpretation of prescription assignments. *Journal of the American Medical Association, 227,* 929–931.

Meichenbaum, D. H. (1977). *Cognitive-behavior modification: An integrative approach.* New York: Plenum Press.

Meichenbaum, D., & Turk, D. C. (1987). *Facilitating treatment adherence. A practitioner's guidebook.* New York: Plenum Press.

Reid, W. J. (1975). A test of a task-centered approach. *Social Work, 20,* 3–9.

Schulman, B. (1979). Active patient orientation and outcomes in hypertensive treatment. *Medical Care, 17,* 1205–1207.

Shelton, J. L., & Ackerman, J. M. (1974). *Homework in counseling and psychotherapy.* Springfield, IL: Thomas.

Shelton, S. L., & Levy, R. L. (1981). *Behavioral assignments and treatment compliance.* Champaign, IL: Research Press.

Steckel, S. B., & Swain, M. A. (1977). Contracting with patients to improve compliance. *Hospitals, 51* (23), 81–84.

Suinn, R. M. (1972a). Behavioral rehearsal for ski racers. *Behavior Therapy, 3,* 519–520.

Suinn, R. M. (1972b). Removing emotional obstacles to learning and performance by visuo-motor behavior rehearsal. *Behavior Therapy, 3,* 308–310.

Tharp, R. G., & Wetzel, R. J. (1969). *Behavior modification in the natural environment.* New York: Academic Press.

Wells, R. A. (1982). *Planned short term treatment.* New York: The Free Press.

Wilson, G. T., & Brownell, K. D. (1978). Behavior therapy for obesity including family members in the treatment process. *Behavior Therapy, 9,* 943–945.

8

The Challenge of Single-Session Therapies
Creating Pivotal Moments

ROBERT ROSENBAUM, MICHAEL F. HOYT, AND
MOSHE TALMON

> . . . [H]e felt a faint shiver, a matutinal coolness and sobriety which told him
> that the hour had come, that from now on there could be no more hesitating or
> lingering. This peculiar feeling, which he was wont to call 'awakening,' was
> familiar to him from other decisive moments of his life. It was both vitalizing and
> painful, mingling a sense of farewell and of setting out on new adventures,
> shaking him deep down in his unconscious mind like a spring storm. . . . a line
> of verse suddenly sprang into his mind:
>
> In all beginnings dwells a magic force
> For guarding us and helping us to live . . .
> So be it, heart: bid farewell without end!
> —H. Hesse, *The Glass Bead Game*, 1943/1969, pp. 370–371

INTRODUCTION

The psychotherapeutic facilitation of "decisive moments of life," such as that
described above, is not necessarily a function of treatment duration. Even a
single session of therapy can sometimes provide a pivotal moment, invoking the
"magic force dwelling in beginnings" that guards us and helps us to live.

Accounts of profound changes occurring in one session of therapy have
existed at least since Freud's meeting with Katarina (Breuer & Freud, 1893–
1895/1944) and his cure of Gustav Mahler's sexual problem on a single long walk
(Bloom, 1981). Therapists as diverse as Davanloo (1986), Erickson (Haley, 1973),

ROBERT ROSENBAUM, MICHAEL F. HOYT, AND MOSHE TALMON • Department of Psychiatry, Kaiser-
Permanente Medical Center, Hayward; California 94545-4299. Portions of this chapter have been
presented by Rosenbaum, Hoyt, and Talmon (1987) and Talmon, Hoyt, and Rosenbaum (1988).
Address reprint requests to Robert Rosenbaum, Department of Psychiatry, Kaiser-Permanente Medical Center, 27400 Hesperian Blvd., Hayward, California 94545-4299.

Winnicott (1971), and Sullivan (Gustafson & Dichter, 1983; Gustafson, 1986) have all reported anecdotal single-session therapy successes, and studies (e.g., Kogan, 1957; Spoerl, 1975; Cummings & Follette, 1976; Bloom, 1981) have indicated that in most outpatient settings, single-session encounters—whether planned or not—are extremely common. Within our own psychiatric clinic, part of a large health maintenance organization, approximately 30% of our clients are seen for only a single session, despite having prepaid coverage entitling them to additional sessions if indicated.

There are a number of reasons a therapist and a client may meet only once. Sometimes a referral to another practitioner is made; sometimes a second appointment is scheduled, but the client chooses not to come back despite the therapist's advice. However, there are also many occasions where the therapist and client mutually agree that enough has been accomplished in the single session so there is no immediate need for further sessions. This chapter will focus on the issues involved in planning for and successfully conducting these intentional single-session therapies (SSTs).[1]

Much as recognizing one's mortality can "concentrate the mind" and intensify our appreciation of life, so an awareness that the first therapeutic session with a client may be the last can heighten our involvement and efficacy with the client. Many therapists almost automatically regard clients who come in for but a single session as "dropouts," "premature terminations," or "treatment failures." Often, however, if these clients are seen on follow-up, they show impressive gains. Change may occur more rapidly than many therapists expect. Even without psychotherapy, psychological difficulties have a spontaneous remission rate of around 40% (Lambert, 1986). Research evidence has been accumulating indicating that some patients make significant life changes facilitated by a single therapeutic encounter (Bloom, 1981; Cummings & Follette, 1976; Hoyt, Rosenbaum, & Talmon, 1987; Hoyt et al., 1987; Hoyt et al. (n.d.); Malan, Heath, & Balfour, 1975; Rockwell & Pinkerton, 1982; Talmon et al., 1988), and that this may occur rather more frequently than might be expected. Other than mental-health professionals and selected character pathologies, who comprise the bulk of the people in psychoanalysis and other long-term therapies, the average client wants change "yesterday" and expects just a few sessions of therapy will do the job (Garfield & Wolpin, 1963; Garfield, 1978). "Yesterday" may not be possible (although often clients appear at their first session having already made important changes), but the therapist needs to be ready for changes "today."

Therapy is an ongoing process, which persists after sessions end (see Hoyt, Chapter 6 this volume; also Rosenbaum, 1983) and is independent of treatment duration (Shectman, 1986). Clients often display a vivid sense of the therapeutic encounter long after it has terminated, even when only a single session has

---

[1]Some patients may be better off without *any* treatment. As Frances and Clarkin (1981) point out, patients who are nonresponders, negative responders, and spontaneous improvers do not need therapy and may, in fact, incur needless expense and/or be harmed if treatment is attempted. Other patients may require one session for evaluation and referral for medication or other nonpsychotherapy services (e.g., legal, vocational, financial, or spiritual counseling).

taken place. Consider the following example taken from a follow-up interview 2½ years after a single psychotherapeutic session:

> "My first [and only] interview here was like having to do a very complex algebraic problem, and somebody sits down with you and tells you how to work it out and get the answer. I didn't realize that my feelings were quite so strong and that my father was there behind things. Since that time I have been able to see it. This has helped. . . . The interview . . . made a tremendous impression on me. . . . [it] upset me, not because someone told me something I didn't want to know, but I felt as if I had been *run over*. You know, if you have a small accident, you feel sort of shaky afterwards." (Malan *et al.*, 1975, p. 121, italics in the original)

THERAPIST RESISTANCES TO SINGLE-SESSION THERAPIES (SSTs)

Planning for the possibility of an SST may enhance the efficacy of the initial encounter, whether further sessions are held or not. Many therapists, however, have difficulties accepting the fact that change can occur in a single session Sifneos (1987, p. 88) has stated the problem succinctly:

> We should do all we can to spot these individuals who have a potential to resolve their problems rapidly. One of the difficulties, however, is the incredible speed with which changes can take place in these patients. Psychiatrists who have been trained to believe that psychological reactions take a long time to be modified become suspicious when they see such speedy resolutions and tend to undermine the patient's confidence by implying that they represent a "flight into health" or a "counterphobic reaction," or doubt that the positive results will be maintained. On the contrary, the role of the therapist should be to encourage such patients to do their own problem solving and not to urge them to accept long-term psychotherapy instead.

Although some caution in approaching SST is wise, denying the existence of meaningful SSTs with automatic emotional intensity and rigid closed mindedness may be evidence of a kind of "resistance." Such resistances are often due not to reasoned disagreement with the *content* of the idea but rather to a need to maintain a consistent professional identity or personal self-image (Rosenbaum, 1988a). It is easy to form a syllogism, "Long-term therapy is good therapy; I am a long-term therapist; therefore I am a good therapist." We become attached to certain ways of doing things, and these procedures then become a statement about ourselves. To be willing to entertain the idea that clients can change even in a single session, we must be willing to entertain changes in our images of ourselves as therapists.

Therapist resistances to brief therapy in general have been characterized by Hoyt (1985a, 1987, Chapter 6 this volume) and Winokur and Dasberg (1983). They include the following erroneous beliefs and barriers:

1. For therapy to be effective, "deep" character changes must be accomplished.
2. "More is better."
3. It is important to develop a therapeutic alliance cautiously; working relationships are fragile and hard to come by.
4. Client resistance is inevitable.

5. Countertransference to termination, including therapists' "need to be needed."
6. Brief therapy is hard work and requires special brilliance on the part of the therapist.
7. Confusion of the patient's interests with those of the therapist.
8. Economics and other payoffs.

Parsimony comprises part of the art of therapy; a single pithy sentence has more impact than a 5-minute lecture. Wagner is "more" but not necessarily "better" than Mozart. Should our patients meander, in fear of losing their wits, we may find it helpful to recall, with *Hamlet* (II, ii, 90), that the soul of wit is brevity. Although a consumer society such as ours tends to promulgate the idea that "more is better," it is our responsibility to bear in mind that more is not better; *better* is better.

In therapy, the idea that "more is better" is often expressed as the belief that "deeper is better" and "inner truth" is superior to "mere, superficial" appearance. In fact, however, our inner selves are *less* individualistic than our surface appearances (Arendt, 1978). Inside, we are all more human than otherwise (Sullivan, 1954). Individual distinctiveness and psychological identity is a matter of qualitative "surface" details creating differing styles (Hoyt, 1989; Rosenbaum, 1988a; Shapiro, 1965); it is precisely these specific individual details as they are expressed in the here and now that successful SSTs must address. Freed from the idea that change can only occur through the alteration of "deep" structures, we can identify the small idiosyncratic perturbations that lead to large differences. The following story sometimes instills hope in patients who worry about having "deep-seated" problems:

> Imagine if you had an old car which began to stall out on you. You don't know it, but while driving along a country road, some insects flew into your carburetor and blocked the proper airflow. If you didn't know what was wrong, you might turn your engine over again and again, and in the process burn out your starter. Now it would really have a problem starting up! If you took it to a mechanic who said, "Your car's pretty old, it's at a stage in its life-cycle where we're going to have to do an engine overhaul," you might be inclined to believe that mechanic, and let yourself in for a lot of unnecessary expense. All this could have been avoided by simply removing the fly in the ointment. After repairing the problem, you might prevent future recurrences by redesigning your entire engine, removing its carburetor and using fuel injection. You could get equally effective results, however, by installing a cheap plastic shield on your front hood to catch insects before they get to the engine. (Rosenbaum, Chapter 16 this volume)

Even when short treatments do not result in lasting "character changes," SSTs may help a person resolve an immediate problem. Therapists need not feel they have failed if further brief treatment is needed in the future. This kind of "life-cycle psychotherapy" (Bennett, 1984; Budman & Gurman, 1988; Rosenbaum, 1983; see also Hoyt, Chapter 6 this volume) capitalizes on the fact that different kinds of therapeutic interventions may be appropriate to different life circumstances. It is not just that the content of a person's concerns changes at different stages of the life cycle: The style with which the client approaches problems also changes. Contrast, for example, the urgency of the adolescent with the caution of the middle aged in dealing with an "identity crisis." The former may need to be slowed down supportively in therapy; the latter may need to be urged on through confrontation. One needs reins; the other, spurs.

Rather than keep a person in psychotherapy for many years during which you accompany the client on their journey through life, SSTs and other brief therapies provide what is needed when it is needed (Ticho, 1972). Doing so meets the client at his or her view of the world (Lankton & Lankton, 1983) in an empathic fashion that helps build rapport and a therapeutic alliance rapidly (Mann, 1973; Mann & Goldman, 1982) while reducing resistance. We find we can often get whatever work needs to be done accomplished in SSTs before untoward "resistance" arises, especially if we meet the patient in his or her framework of understanding and establish a mutually agreed-upon treatment contract (Berne, 1972; Goulding & Goulding, 1978, 1979; Polster & Polster, 1976). If strong resistance does arise, we either utilize it strategically (Haley, 1977) or make it the focus of psychodynamic confrontation and interpretation (Davanloo, 1986). We conceptualize resistance as one more part of the change process: All stability is maintained through change, and all change is maintained through stability (Keeney, 1983). To be effective in an SST format, then, the therapist needs "the wit and deftness to 'work the opposing currents'" (Gustafson, 1987, p. 413).

HELPFUL THERAPIST ATTITUDES FOR PROMOTING SINGLE-SESSION THERAPIES

> The therapist must be alert to the possibility [of SST occurring], must assess quickly when s/he has a [potential SST] case in hand, set the process in motion, and determine a satisfactory stopping point. (Rockwell & Pinkerton, 1982, p. 39)

Recognizing when a patient may benefit from SST involves a number of factors:

1. What is the patient's motivation and expectation? Clinical experience and research (Pekarik & Wierzbicki, 1986) have shown the single best predictor of therapy duration is the patient's expectation of the likely number of sessions necessary.
2. What is the focus? What specifically does the patient want to accomplish? Can the therapist and patient formulate the problem in a concise manner? What (if any) is the patient's "hidden agenda?"
3. Is the patient's difficulty best conceived in terms of intrapsychic, characterological, interpersonal, or systemic processes (Gustafson, 1986)? What precisely triggers the patient's pain; what will allow the therapist access to that painful state, and what will provide a route out of the pain (Gustafson, 1987)?
4. What solutions have been attempted in the past: Which have been successful and which ineffectual? Can something that proved helpful in the

past prove helpful once again? (Don't reinvent the wheel!). What technical approach(es) will be most helpful: educational, behavioral, cognitive, psychodynamic, interpersonal, strategic, systemic, and so forth?

5. Are there contraindications for SST, such as psychotic, suicidal, or assaultive risks? Is there an opportunity for other treatment approaches and/or additional sessions to be used if needed?

6. Timing and pacing: Is the desired change possible now, or do other things need to happen first? Are the goals realistic, or do they reflect overly large expectations on the part of the client and/or the therapist?

In summary, the therapist asks: Where does the patient get stuck? What is needed for him or her to get unstuck? How can I, as a therapist, facilitate the patient's change process (Hoyt, 1988a, 1989)?

Before asking these specific technical questions, in order to "be alert to the possibility" of SSTs, therapists must acknowledge the possibility that people can change in the moment and that change may occur through sudden discontinuous shifts of being. This is not to say we should deny that many people change gradually. We have no desire to create a psychotherapeutic schism paralleling those Buddhist disputes over the virtues of sudden, as opposed to gradual, enlightenment (Suzuki, 1956). We must, however, be alert to the possibility of the proverbial "bolt from the blue." Even though we often think of nature as existing continuously and changing in gradual increments, recent geological evidence suggests that the world has changed not only through gradual evolution but also through "punctuated evolution" where sudden discrete events such as meteorite strikes cause long-term changes (Gould, 1980).

> One of the authors (RR) was trained in short-term psychotherapy but still had his doubts about SSTs. He was walking in the mountains one day, indulging his doubts on the subject: "Perhaps some change can occur in a single-session, but surely not *significant* change. Lasting change requires the gradual processes that mold mountains: time, slow erosion, wind and rain sculpting the face of the stone over and over again." At that point, the trail turned around a bend. A huge avalanche chute came into sight. Half of a mountain, seemingly, had slid down into the valley last winter, changing both mountain and valley forever, all in the course of less than 30 seconds.

The human experience is also sometimes marked by such quantum shifts in being. All our lives begin with a discrete event: birth, which provides a model for the emergence of truly new beginnings (Arendt, 1978; Hoyt, 1977; Rank, 1914, 1929/1964, 1973), where something that was previously only imagined becomes tangible and fully present. There is a gestation period prior to birth, but compared to the life that will follow it, the actual birth process is short. Furthermore, in most cases the birth process proceeds more or less naturally, without undue intervention by medical professionals. The therapist who is interested in doing SSTs can take a lesson from this. Clients come to us at different stages in the gestation process of changing; some of them will require a certain amount of waiting and preparation before giving birth, but others will be virtually fully dilated. Wherever the client may be in the birth process, it is seldom our task to "do something" to create change; rather, our role is more similar to that of the midwife, who attends the process, eases the transition, and provides a helping hand in case anything gets temporarily stuck. This was well recognized by Berne (1966, p. 63):

> The patient has a built-in drive to health, mental as well as physical. His mental development and emotional development have been obstructed, and the therapist has only to remove the obstructions for the patient to grow naturally in his own direction. . . .
>
> The therapist does not cure anyone, he only treats him to the best of his ability, being careful not to injure and waiting for nature to take its healing course. . . . Hence in practice "curing the patient" means "getting the patient ready for the cure to happen today" . . . When the patient recovers, the therapist should be able to say, "My treatment helped nature. . . ."

BASIC HEURISTIC AND TECHNICAL PRINCIPLES FOR SST

Keeping these general ideas in mind, we can now discuss some aspects of how the therapist should conduct him- or herself in performing SSTs. Bloom (1981) has made the following helpful concrete recommendations:

1. Identify a focal problem
2. Do not underestimate client's strengths
3. Be prudently active
4. Explore, then present interpretations tentatively
5. Encourage the expression of affect
6. Use the interview to start a problem-solving process
7. Keep track of time
8. Do not be overambitious
9. Keep factual questions to a minimum
10. Do not be overly concerned about the precipitating event
11. Avoid detours
12. Do not overestimate a client's self-awareness [i.e., don't ignore stating the obvious]

In addition to these excellent specific suggestions, we have found certain heuristics particularly helpful in facilitating the SST process. One may or may not express all these attitudes in specific statements to the client, but it is essential that the spirit of the overall SST stance permeate the therapeutic encounter. We discuss each of these later, with illustrative case material.[2]

1. *Expect change.* People are not unvarying beings but rather, like every stable phenomenon, changing all the time. In order to maintain stability, it is necessary to make constant small adjustments and changes: To steer a sailboat in a constant direction, you must constantly trim your sails and move your rudder. In therapy, the client has taken a new, temporary passenger (the therapist) into the boat: This will change the ballast of the boat and require the client to adjust

---

[2]The therapist for each case is indicated by the initials of the author at the end of the case material.

the sails and pull on the rudder, thus increasing the probability of a change of course. The therapist need not explore theories of celestial navigation to help a client who is sailing in circles; if you move the rudder, pull on the sheets, or lean over the side of the boat, it is rather likely a change in direction will occur.

The effective SST therapist's attitude is that not only is change inevitable, but in fact it is *already* happening, though the client may not have noticed yet. In hypnosis, for example, it is common to say to a patient "I don't know if you've noticed *yet* how deeply you've begun to go into trance . . . how your rate of breathing is different *now*. . . ." The hypnotherapist takes an inevitable phenomenon (the fluctuation in the rate of respiration), then punctuates it as a sign of something else (the beginning of trance), which ratifies and creates the phenomenon it purportedly is describing. Use of the word *yet* allows patients the freedom to experience the new phenomenon any way they want but has a strongly implied suggestion that if they haven't noticed up until now, they will in the future.

The client's first visit to the therapist presents a similar situation. As soon as the client considers entering therapy, the change process has already started; an aspect of his or her experience is being thought of as troublesome and changeable. The client's problem is being presented in a novel context: the very act of coming to the therapist makes a change for the client, so the therapist's job becomes helping the client pursue the change profitably. The therapist does not structure the therapy to continue *until* change occurs because change is *already* occurring. Therapy focuses and amplifies the ongoing change process.

In terms of specific techniques to create an expectation of change, it is best to begin at the first therapeutic contact. Early in the meeting, we say something like the following:

> We've found a large number of our clients can benefit from a single visit here. Of course, if you need more therapy, we can provide it. But I want to let you know that I'm willing to work hard with you today to help you resolve your problem quickly, perhaps even in this single visit, as long as you are ready to start doing something different or whatever's necessary.

We find this message contains a number of efficacious elements. In the first sentence, it immediately lets the patient know that change is possible. At the same time, we leave the door open to not change (by temporizing with "perhaps" and by making more therapy potentially available); this seems to minimize resistance and dependent passive aggression and also helps clients feel any changes they make are made autonomously rather than coerced. Telling the client that we are willing to work hard with him or her is evidence of our sincerity and helps build an alliance. Finally, we let the patient know that change is in his or her hands: he or she must be an active participant. We purposely keep the kind of participation vague: "Something different or whatever's necessary" provides an illusion of alternatives (Lankton & Lankton, 1983) in that it allows almost anything the patient does to be helpful, but it does not give the client the option of doing nothing.

Other similar messages include: "What are you willing to change today?" (Goulding & Goulding, 1978, 1979), "What will you be doing differently when you don't come here any more?", and "We've scheduled plenty of time today so we can sit here and keep working until we get this thing dealt with." Sometimes it helps to emphasize growth by speaking with the client about what he or she wants to "accomplish" or "create" in therapy, rather than "change" or "improve."[3] All of these messages highlight client autonomy and responsibility by emphasizing that it is what the *client* does (rather than what is done to him or her by the therapist) that is crucial. Asking "what do you want to change today?" orients the client to the present and future and creates an expectation of change by talking about *when* not *if* change happens.

It is often helpful to have an explicit "contract," an agreed upon operationally defined goal that is attainable. Unspecified or overly vague goals (such as "to be more open" or "to know myself better") may keep therapy unfocused and promote interminable treatment.

A woman sought therapy wanting to "sort out my thoughts" about whether to continue at a certain job or to seek a different position. In one session, a semistructured "motivational balance-sheet procedure" (Hoyt & Janis, 1975) was used to help her weigh the instrumental and emotional implications of her options. Within an hour she came to her decision, which she recognized as what she had thought she wanted to do. Her choice now felt more "solid," however, and she ended by saying that she had gotten what she had come for and that she would call again if she needed help in the future. (Hoyt, 1989)

In many situations, clients have difficulty specifying a clear goal. In those cases, using the session to help clients clarify their goals can be quite helpful. However, there are times when despite both parties' best efforts, therapy goals remain vague. The therapist may then elect to help the client by seeding suggestions for nonspecific change, with the idea that *any* alteration in the patient's system will result in new and potentially useful directions for the client.

A woman in her mid-30s, when asked what she wanted to accomplish, began her therapy session by handing the therapist a 10-page single-spaced typed narrative describing her early life history, her unhappiness at still being single, of being blocked creatively, of feeling unappreciated at her low-paying job, and of feeling embarrassed that she was still financially and emotionally dependent on her parents. She had been seeing another therapist for over a year, but that relationship had become attenuated (without actually terminating) due to the therapist's illness. She presented in an overcontrolled ruminative manner, with very tangential thinking, anxious mood, and depressed affect.

Repeated attempts to establish a focus failed. The patient tended to obsess about whether to stay or leave her current job, but this was tied to so many issues regarding her self-worth and conflicts about being independent that a "balance-sheet approach" such as the one described in the case above seemed unlikely to be effective. The patient felt torn between her "common sense" and her "feelings" and tended to feel alternately

---

[3]Sometimes the SST therapist, faced with a truly insoluble problem, can be helpful by acknowledging the impossibility of change. By aiding the client to cease useless or compulsive attempts to solve the impossible, the client may attain a measure of equanimity and acceptance by letting go of further treatment and attempts at "cure."

grandiose about her "inner, hidden abilities" and deflated at her lack of accomplishments and acknowledgment by others.

The therapist noticed the patient wore a pretty crystal on a necklace, and the patient described how she used crystals for meditation. She pulled out a variety of crystals from her purse. The therapist decided to use hypnosis to indirectly further psychodynamic goals (Wolberg, 1980) and had the patient choose two crystals, "of differing character," and hold one in each hand. A trance was induced by having her focus on the different sensations in each hand, where one crystal "could be thought of as hard, but ordinary, common sense," while the other "feels like it gives brilliance, healing, and comfort." The patient was then asked to combine the two inside herself; she then reported strong sensations of strength and energy with accompanying imagery. She was then given suggestions that she would be able to use this experience in the near future, together with posthypnotic cues for regaining the sensations at need. After arousing from the trance, she was given an assignment: to either submit one of the stories she had already written for publication or to create something new.

By the end of the session, her rumination had given place to curiosity and mild excitement. On follow-up she was markedly less depressed, less conflicted about her job, and had written some new children's stories she was attempting to get illustrated and published. (RR)

It is also important, at the end of the session, to leave the client with the idea that change will occur. Thus when we close the session, we mention we will be contacting the patient to find out *what* has changed and *how* he or she has progressed (rather than *whether* there has been any improvement).

A young woman, employed as a hair stylist, was seen about a year after she had been struck by a drunk driver in an automobile accident. She had retreated from social activities, feeling ashamed about the scarring on her legs. She experienced intrusive thoughts about the accident, nightmares, and struggled to suppress displaced rage by becoming quite passive. She had continued her work but was feeling angry at her boss for not appreciating what she was going through.

The session utilized hypnotic trance for abreaction of her anger and indirect suggestions that reframed the scarring as a "badge of experience." At the end of the session, she mentioned that the anniversary date of the accident was approaching. I gave her the open-ended suggestion that "sometime soon, you'll notice a difference in the way you're feeling or thinking . . . . I'm not sure exactly what the difference will be: Perhaps you'll find yourself having more thoughts about the accident in preparation to letting go of it when the anniversary comes; or perhaps you'll find yourself having less thoughts shortly after the anniversary. You may notice a difference in your dreams, or maybe just a general feeling of the beginnings of relief. You know how you don't notice your hair getting longer, and then one day all at once you say: My hair's grown! This may be sort of like that. Or you can enjoy the changes when you notice a particularly nice job your hands have done on a customer."

On follow-up, the patient reported a number of improvements in her symptoms and a general increase in well-being. Note that the above suggestions were given when the patient was no longer in a formal trance. As should be clear from the wide variety of approaches illustrated by our clinical vignettes, we do not feel hypnosis is a necessary component of SSTs. What is necessary is to help alert patients to change in general while allowing them to pick and choose which changes will occur. (RR)

2. *View each encounter as a whole, complete in itself.* Bion (1967, 1970) suggested the therapist enter each session "without desire, memory, or understanding" so that each interaction would have "no history and no future." This "is a matter of approaching each hour with the openness . . . which will best serve therapist and patient in the pursuit of the unknown" (Langs, 1979). Such an attitude allows the therapist to seize the moment while fostering creativity and new learning.

By definition, effective single-session therapists do not have separate sessions for the gathering of information and history taking, the formulation and communication of a diagnosis, and then the "therapy proper." Rather, the problem must be elicited and its resolution derived in one meeting. Each move by the therapist, together with the client's response, includes both a probe for information (about each other, the problem, etc.) and an intervention requiring a response, providing feedback for succeeding interactions. Treatment begins when the client first telephones in and continues through the final words of the leave taking. The attitude for successful SSTs was succinctly stated by Berne (quoted by Goulding, Goulding, & Silverthorn, 1983, p. 67) who said that, before each session, "I ask myself what I can do this day, so that all patients are cured this day."

A patient complained of people not liking him, but not knowing why. As he sat down in the therapist's office, he commented, "I guess you're a psychologist because you couldn't get into medical school, huh?" and smiled. The therapist stopped him, saying, "What effect do you think it had on me to start our meeting with that comment?" The patient said he didn't understand. The therapist decided to go along with the patient's ploy of innocence [avoiding the discussion of whether or not it was 'unconscious'] by explaining that sometimes a person has an interpersonal style that annoys other people without realizing it, but that once they know about it, then they are responsible for what they do. He repeated the comment and asked the patient if there were other times the patient could think of when his 'jokes' might have been misunderstood. The patient quickly learned about his counterproductive behavior and began to modify it. (MFH)

3. *Do not rush or try to be brilliant.* It may seem paradoxical to advise practitioners of SST not to act too quickly, but sometimes it is helpful to remember the saying, "Don't just do something—sit there!" Too often therapists jump at the first bit of material they feel competent to comment on, rather than surveying the situation and picking carefully where to exercise their expertise. The tendency to find quick solutions to problems can have the effect of perpetuating or even creating problems (Watzlawick, Weakland, & Fisch, 1974). We agree with Sullivan (1954, p. 224) that therapeutic skill sometimes consists of "making a rather precise move which has a high probability of achieving what you're attempting to achieve, with a minimum of time and words," but we also agree with Spoerl (1975) that SSTs often succeed without heroic measures, by providing needed reassurance, catharsis, and problem solving.

If a therapist goes into a session thinking he or she must do something extraordinary or brilliant to make a change, it decreases the chance that change will occur, for it denies the client's autonomy. Trying too hard to be brilliant often is counterproductive; polishing a surface overmuch can scratch and dull its sheen. The therapist need only facilitate the *client's* natural tendency to keep changing. The therapist does not attack a client's problems or sculpt a client to fit an idea; rather, as stated before, the therapist is akin to a midwife attending a birth. Overly eager therapists would do well to remember to let the patients do the work, simply guiding and helping them to keep moving. It is counterproductive for therapists to do for patients what they can do for themselves; better to assist the patient to "stretch" a bit past his or her usual stopping point.[4]

SST may engender a sense of pleasant urgency, but it is important for the therapist and patient not to feel desperately rushed. Each session has its unique qualities, including pace, and enough time needs to be allotted to do the job well. Effective sessions can sometimes be accomplished relatively quickly, although scheduling 90 minutes or 2 hours is usually optimal to allow enough time for a complete, impactful meeting.

A 60-year-old woman was referred by her physician, who had successfully treated her breast cancer 2 years ago. Since that time, however, she had become chronically anxious, fearful of a recurrence, and hypervigilant to all aches and pains. She had never been to a therapist before and was skeptical about the psychotherapeutic enterprise. The therapist, on hearing the presenting complaint, and noting the patient's apparent minimal psychological mindedness and motivation for insight, quickly made a decision to treat the somatic preoccupations with hypnosis, a technique he had found useful in similar cases. The patient "rambled," however, and he was unable for a bit to get a word in edgewise to either establish the treatment focus or to initiate trance.

In her "ramblings," the patient mentioned that her elderly mother was living with her. The therapist asked how that was for the patient, and the patient related how she had been taking care of her mother since she (the patient) was 14 years old when her mother had ejected her alcoholic husband from the home. A simple question from the therapist, inquiring about the patient's father, elicited a tearful response. The patient described how much she had cared for her father, and how hard it had been to see him die on Skid Row shortly after the divorce. She had been her father's favorite. She had been angry at her mother for leaving her father but had never expressed these feelings. Instead, she had gone to great lengths to take care of her mother, at considerable self-sacrifice. The patient would not go out by herself because the mother would demand to be taken along. The patient had many things she wanted to do, especially travel with her husband who was due to retire but feared that, obligated to her mother, she might die or become ill before she had the opportunity.

The patient felt guilty about her resentment of her mother and hid the feelings; she was fearful that admitting to her anger would cause her to take actions that would be overly hurtful to her mother. It became clear she had never had the opportunity to discuss these feelings before with anyone, including her husband. The therapist gave her permission and encouraged her, commenting: "You have the right to figure this out." The remainder of the session involved working through, in affective imagery and detailed planning, how the patient could carve space for herself and deal with her mother in a fashion that was both assertive and caring.

---

[4]Single-session interventions in supervision may help therapists resolve transference–countertransference impasses involving the overassumption of responsibility and caretaking (Hoyt & Goulding, 1989; Hoyt, 1988b).

In all of this, the therapist's interventions were minimal as the patient used the opportunity to think through her situation in a way that had not been available to her previously. At the end of the session, the patient stated, "You mean, I have to look out for myself more." She stated her immediate plan: Instead of going directly from the session to pick up her mother, she would take a little time for herself. On follow-up, the patient had worked out a viable arrangement to allow her the freedom to engage in some of the activities she had wished for, while still taking appropriate care of her mother. The anxiety symptoms had remitted.

If the therapist had jumped in with hypnosis too soon, the patient might have achieved some symptom relief but would have been denied a significant experience of autonomy and growth. By waiting, the therapist provided an opportunity for the patient to "ramble" herself free. (RR)

4. *Emphasize abilities and strengths rather than pathology.* It is important to ask, "How can this client create a solution?" rather than stopping at "How does this patient create this problem?" Faced with a client in pain, overwhelmed by his or her problems, diagnostic labels may seem to leap out at the clinician; it is easy to overlook client efforts at adaptation and coping. All too often, "assessment" means a lengthy description of all the manifestations and sources of illness, with at best a short sentence or two cursorily depicting "ego strengths" or "support networks." On a more profound level, we must realize that the very distinction between healthy and pathological behavior is itself problematical.

Drawing distinctions is the first step in any assessment process, and the kinds of distinctions one makes helps determine the range of intervention options that can be perceived (Bateson, 1979). If you focus on distinguishing between pathological and healthy behavior, you will then devote much of your time to seeing pathology. Therapists should attempt to avoid creating diagnostic labels that create patients (Szasz, 1970). To the extent that we try to find a formulation of the *problem*, we will be looking for problems rather than solutions, and the formulation—whether it be psychodynamic, DSM-III-R, behavioral, or systemic—will tend to foster pathology by highlighting difficulties. In contrast, to the extent that we try to find past successes and present client resources, we will be fostering flexibility and health. The kind of data one collects helps create the "reality" being investigated, which in turn influences the kinds of data one looks for. Even the terms *patient* or *client* may have important implications (Hoyt, 1979b, 1985b), connoting certain assumptions regarding dependency and responsibility in psychotherapy. Potential dangers (suicidal risk, alcohol/drug abuse, psychosis) should not be overlooked, of course, but neither should potential strengths.

The SST therapist looks for the information necessary to help the client make a change, rather than focusing on pathology. The focus is on finding solutions, not problems (DeShazer, 1985). One way of doing this is to find skills the client already has that he or she can use. Strategic therapists have listed a variety of ways of doing this: by looking for past client successes, by finding something the client already is doing that would be useful to do more of, or by looking for "exceptions to the rule" of the problem. Positive connotation and reframing look for the health-seeking intent in problematic behavior (Selvini-

Palazzoli, Boscolo, Cecchin, & Prata, 1978); therapists must recognize that clients make the best choice for themselves at any given moment, given the resources and circumstances they perceive as available to them (Lankton & Lankton, 1983).

All of these techniques presuppose that the therapist has a strong belief that the power is in the client (Goulding & Goulding, 1978, 1979): that ultimately, the client knows himself or herself more than you do, and that your task is to facilitate the client's finding his or her own solution. Whether stated explicitly or not, this therapist attitude encourages client autonomy and refuses to buy into the idea that clients are not in control of their lives. Because clients often come into treatment feeling like victims controlled by other persons, this affirmation of their ability to make a difference in their experience is itself helpful, countering the sense of powerlessness that results in clients feeling "stuck." Helping people feel autonomous rather than victimized is itself salutary and serves as a precondition for many further changes. Sometimes the therapist can facilitate a single-session "ceremony" or ritual that will mark a passage and help the patient to reclaim his or her sense of self-determination. The therapist may use a preliminary consultation to set the stage for the single-session intervention.

A woman in her late 20s mentioned a series of problems and then said, "What's really bothering me is something I've carried as a secret for years. My father molested me for a long time, when I was in my late teens." She described a situation of terrible abuse and exploitation and made the connection between the sexual abuse and her subsequent low self-esteem and various personal problems. She had made repeated attempts as an adult to confront her father and discuss what had happened and her feelings about it, but each time he rebuffed and mocked her. In fact, he continued to make occasional attempts to exploit her, promising to loan her money but then withholding the loan unless she gave him sexual "favors."

"I'm tired of this shit," the patient exclaimed. "I want to put it behind me and be done with it. I want to get him and what he did out of my life, once and for all!"

At this point the therapist, who had listened sympathetically, suggested she needed a way of divorcing her father and breaking the bond. What was needed was something that would make the break total and permanent *for her*. "Some people might want to say certain words, or burn a picture, or do whatever would mean to them they were free and done with him. You need to create a personal ceremony, one that will let you be free all the way through your mind and your soul. Spend some time really thinking about what you want to do and bring it in. We'll meet in a week, OK?"

A week later the patient arrived, with her husband, a portable stereotape player, and an envelope. She looked nervous but indicated she was ready. The therapist gave a brief speech like a clergyman at a wedding but instead expounded on the significance of divorce ("an ending, a separating, one voice becoming two from this day on," etc.). He then, as master of ceremonies, nodded to the patient to proceed, only occasionally directing, pacing, pausing for emphasis and heightened impact.

An extraordinary experience unfolded. The patient read aloud a several page account of her betrayal and outrage, giving witness to what she had never before dared to reveal. While she read, taped music played, song lyrics about love and betrayal poignantly coordinated to her reading. Several times she paused, overcome with emotion, and then she would continue. At the end of her reading, she produced a photograph of her father, along with a lighter. The therapist held the picture with a scissors while she lit it. Eerily, his face was the last portion to burn. The ashes fell into the office trashcan, a glass of water was poured over the ashes, and (for good measure and to the delight of all) the therapist spit into the ashes. The patient and her husband laughed. She said she felt "free," reached into the envelope and pulled out several copies of a printed "Decree of Divorce" she had written and had professionally printed. It declared her "No longer the daughter of XXX except through biology." She signed each copy, as did her husband, and then the therapist. Happy music was played. She explained that one copy was for her, to be displayed at home next to her graduation diplomas, another copy was for her sister, a third was to be sent to her father (the last time she would contact him, she said), and the last copy was for the therapist (who was honored to accept it).

The mood in the room was exceptionally positive, a marked contrast to her state earlier in the hour and at the initial consultation. Before closing the ceremony, however, the therapist asked her to close her eyes and to get a vivid picture of herself when she was a little girl, before "all the bad things happened." When she indicated having a clear image, he then asked her to keep that image and "now also see yourself as you are now, a strong grown-up woman." When she got that image he continued: "Now I want you to do two more things. First, notice that you're now grown up, no longer a little girl, no longer vulnerable. You're strong now, adult and able to take care of yourself. And now, in your mind's picture, see the grown-up you bend over and pick up the little girl and hold her close and lovingly, and in a nice way, the little girl just sort of blends into you and your arms are around yourself. And you know that she is safe inside of you and that you will always protect her."

Tears ran down the patient's cheeks. She opened her eyes. Her face looked beatific. She laughed freely, looked around, and hugged her husband. After a couple of minutes of celebrating and expressing their appreciation, the session ended. No further treatment was sought. (MFH)

5. *Life, not therapy, is the great teacher.* Although SST therapists view each encounter as complete in itself, they do not regard it as completely fulfilling, a cure-all or final solution. Therapists who perform SSTs are not megalomaniacs nor magicians. Rather, SST therapists believe that what happens in the therapy session can provide the *impetus* for the client to begin making significant changes in his or her daily life, outside the session. The purpose of SST is to help clients access healthful experiences in both their inner life and their daily interactions with others that they may have overlooked. We therefore often give assignments to be performed after the SST meeting, which are designed to introduce some new element into a client's usual routine.

A young couple came in who described themselves as happily married. Over the past year, however, the husband had developed severe complex partial seizures. As part of the seizures, he had suffered a transient psychosis from which he was now recovered. However, he had residual obsessional symptoms, most prominently intrusive suicidal thoughts that he had no intention of acting on but that he would mention to his wife. She was anxious and depressed, quite tearful, and feared his seizures (which he was having every other day), as well as being concerned about his obsessional thoughts. She coped with the situation by emotionally smothering her husband, worrying over his seizures, and trying to "take care of him." The more she did this, the more he told her of any symptoms, and the worse the situation became.

The therapist praised how much the couple cared for and took care of each other, while worrying aloud that the wife's hovering might prove draining to her or occasionally irritating to her husband. The therapist also shared his concern that the wife would feel guilty and depressed if, trying to pull back, she felt she was not helping enough.

The therapist then gave them a paradoxical assignment, in which the husband was to pretend to have minor seizures several times a day, while the wife was to guess whether the seizure was genuine or not, helping out if it were genuine and ignoring it if it had been initiated purposefully by the husband. They were told this would help the husband learn more about the signs and symptoms of his seizures, while giving the wife an opportunity to learn when she need and needn't worry.

On follow-up, the couple said they had practiced the assignment faithfully for about a week but then had found it "silly" because the husband's obsessional thoughts had virtually vanished, and his seizures had markedly decreased. The wife was no longer tearful, and she discussed detaching from her husband's condition enough to establish some independent plans for herself (such as attending school). These gains were maintained at follow-up 1 year after the intervention.

Talking about the seizures and the couple's relationship within the session was useful, but it was important to give the clients something different to do to alter their interactions in everyday life. (RR)

6. *Focus on pivot chords.* In music, the pivot chord is an ambiguous chord that contains notes common to more than one key and so can imply several "directions" to the music and facilitate the transition from one key to another. An important task of the SST therapist is to construe the client's difficulty in such a way that it can function as a pivot chord for change. The therapist can be helpful by putting the symptom into a larger pattern in which the problem contains the seeds of new directions for the client.

In the case of the couple with seizures just described, the occurrence of seizures acts as a pivot that allows the couple to achieve greater differentiation, rather than as an occasion for helplessness and smothering. In another case described by Hoyt (Chapter 6 this volume), an insecure attorney who feels she is "dumb" is told that "smart people can play dumb." This transforms the patient's experience of herself as "dumb" into a pivot; "dumbness" becomes evidence of being smart. Sullivan provided a classic example when he was able to highlight a stifled housewife's strength in her presenting complaint:

> Her feeling of helplessness to get going in the morning rather encourages me than otherwise. Has she never heard of a woman who preferred something else to domestic preoccupation? (quoted by Gustafson, 1986, p. 47)

Psychotherapy involves a reframing of clients' experience of themselves and their world (Frank, 1973). The task for any kind of reframing, of course, is to simultaneously meet the client at their view of the world, so they feel understood and validated, while at the same time offering a new perspective. All therapies face the challenge of joining and empathizing with the patient's attitude while trying to change it. The therapist wants to initiate some element of doubt or openness to alternative meanings in the patient's world view without denying the client's experience or confronting it in a way that leads to a battle over which view of the experience is "right." In the behavioral therapies this may go under the rubric of "orientation and the correction of misconceptions"

(Wolpe, 1973); in psychodynamic therapies it is accomplished by means of interpretations. Strategic therapies offer many varieties of reframing, ranging from positive connotation (Selvini-Palazzoli *et al.*, 1978) to "splitting the symptom" (Lankton & Lankton, 1983).

The therapist focuses on that portion of the client's problem that has sufficient ambiguity to be reconstrued as a bridge to new behaviors and experiences. The technique chosen is not so important as the attitude the therapist adopts: The therapist can convey the central experience of reframing—namely joining with the client even while introducing doubt and the possibility of viewing events differently—as simply as by raising the eyebrows while maintaining a sympathetic facial expression.

A couple came in for treatment bitterly divided and distant from each other. They didn't even argue any more, since they couldn't resolve a particular issue: Their 7-year-old son slept in bed with his mother, whereas the husband slept on the couch. This had continued for years, ever since the child had had nightmares as a 3-year-old. The husband wanted the boy out, but while the mother complained of lack of sleep and regretted the growing distance from her husband, she felt she could not be a "bad mother" and, for "selfish" reasons, subject her son to the "rejection" she felt sending him to his own bed would entail. She also worried she would not be able to deal with the "loss" of her last child.

The therapist praised the woman for her motherly concern. He sighed and noted sadly how it was a parent's job to give their children the strength to cope with the inevitable losses and griefs of life. Tolerating the loneliness of his own bed was important practice for this. The therapist suggested it was the mother's painful duty to teach her child how to be on his own. At least, though, when her son slept in his own bed through the night, they could both value their morning snuggles more highly, when her son would come all that distance from his room to be with her. "Absence does make the heart grow fonder."

The woman quickly seized on this reframing as a "cross she would have to bear" to be a good mother. She and her husband were able to devise a 2-week transition period for their son. On follow-up, the adults were in one bed, having both more arguments and more love making, while the boy was enjoying his own room. The wife was delighted, and said, "This is great. I never knew this is what God meant bedtime to be for." (RR)

Pivots are particularly useful when clients are troubled by ego-dystonic affects they regard as shameful, destructive, or otherwise "wrong." Many patients come in with symptoms related to unsuccessful attempts to ban all anger from their lives. For patients phobic about anger, the following story often proves helpful:

You know about Alfred Nobel, the inventor of dynamite? He woke up one morning to read his own obituary. Another man named Nobel had died, and a newspaper editor, thinking it was Alfred Nobel, had penned a piece in which he severely excoriated Nobel, condemning him as a creator of misery and destruction because of the explosive qualities of dynamite. Nobel was so upset by the article he used part of his fortune to establish the Nobel Peace Prize.

The interesting thing about all this is that the European editor had it all wrong.

Americans in the 1800s greeted dynamite as the answer to their prayers. You see, Americans were just then trying to explore and settle the West, but it was very difficult cutting roads through hills with pickaxes, or blowing up tree stumps and boulders in farm fields with gunpowder, the only extant explosive at the time. Dynamite allowed you to control the amount and the direction of the explosive charge quite effectively, and so it enabled Americans to build the railroads and highways which could connect people from distant places and bring people together.

Now, dynamite is a very safe substance generally, except in one instance. If you store it in a shed and never attend to it, over the years the active ingredients slowly leak out and leach into the surrounding soil. When that happens, dropping something on the soil or walking onto it can result in an unplanned, destructive explosion. It's important to use dynamite constructively, setting it off usefully rather than letting it just sit around.

That's just the way it is . . . usually, to make something, you have to tear something else up first. The trick is to use the power creatively. Of course, we've known that ever since taming fire for our uses. (RR)

7. *Big problems do not always require big solutions.* It is often useful to consider the possibility that symptoms may not be part of a person's psychological "essence" but instead may represent a response to some kind of intrusion, much as we get physiological symptoms when our body is invaded by a virus. Such symptoms do not represent pathology but instead a healthy attempt by our body to restore normal functioning.

A psychological symptom may fulfill a purpose in an individual or family negotiating a stage in the family life cycle (Carter & McGoldrick, 1980), of course, but sometimes it may be helpful to think of a symptom as having been introduced by a chance fluctuation that became more fixed as people put excessive unproductive energies into solving it. The meanings people assign to a symptom may be self-fulfilling and contribute to their difficulties, so calling something a "random glitch" is less likely to make a person feel stuck than calling it a "problem whose deeper meaning we will have to gradually uncover and work through."

We know small changes can have large effects: A small addition to a radioactive pile can achieve a critical mass with a self-sustaining chain reaction. In a similar way, any small change in a client's life can lead to exposure to new life circumstances, which will lead to new client reactions, which will lead to new life circumstances, and so forth. The advantage of adopting the attitude that a small change is sufficient is threefold: (1) it takes the pressure off both therapist and client, so that neither one falls over their feet in the process of trying too hard; (2) a client is more likely to be undaunted and thus willing to make a small change rather than a large one; and finally (3) any kind of movement may suffice to ignite hope in the client.

Consider the following follow-up interview with a patient 1 year after a SST, quoted verbatim:

I remember at the time I came in I was feeling overwhelmed, the kids were getting under my skin. I had been a 24-hour-a-day mother for 5 years. I felt I was isolated, the only mother with such problems.

I remember the session well. . . . I took your suggestion [making an appointment with herself, away from home]. Every month I make two appointments with myself of 2 hours each. I get my nails done, meet with a friend in a cafe, and we chat about everything except the kids. If I feel the kids are getting under my skin, I take a walk or switch to some other activity.

I realized nobody can be a 24-hour-a-day mother. We all need time and space.

When I stopped feeling the kids were getting under my skin, I started feeling better as a mother. That freed me to take care of other parts of myself; like, I started paying more attention to taking care of my looks. That led me to start feeling better about myself. And that seems to have made my marriage better.

You see how the little things make a big difference? (MT)

A corollary to the idea that big problems do not always require big solutions is that some patients can only tolerate a small change. In such cases, more would be less. Frequently, SSTs provide such patients with a positive, nonthreatening experience that can also set the stage for additional therapy should it be needed.

A very intense and outspoken woman arrived complaining bitterly of mistreatment by her current boyfriend. Employers and past lovers were also all described as abusive. She rapidly displayed many strong affects and said that she needed answers *now*, that she didn't have the patience to spend weeks talking about her problems. The therapist complimented her on her direct, nonnonsense approach and her obvious emotional honesty and commitment to being treated fairly. They then discussed the patient's situation and her possible courses of action. The therapist also indicated to her that more sessions might be useful, if she wanted. She declined, saying the meeting had been very helpful but "I don't like to get dependent on anyone." The therapist said, "Fine. Not now. But if you sometime want another session, call me." (MFH)

8. *Termination is about the structure of memory and the realization of implications.* In order to make a single session of therapy complete in itself, it must contain a fitting ending. This requires that SST therapists confront their countertransferences to termination: the disappointment of not being able to prolong what is pleasurable, having to leave some things incomplete, and experiencing loss. Too many therapists are not well trained in the art of termination and have particular difficulties in this critical phase of treatment (Hoyt 1979a, 1988b; Hoyt & Farrell, 1984).

Many therapists think of termination almost exclusively in terms of the content of the themes that emerge and therefore focus on issues of loss, longing, and incompleteness. In addition to thematic content, though, termination has processive and structural aspects as well (Rosenbaum, 1988b), and these often come to the fore in the context of SSTs. Our understanding of the meaning of an event includes not only what actually occurred (the realized implications) but also what might have happened but did not. In SST, as in any psychotherapy, patients present problematical patterns; these patterns may have many possible repercussions, outcomes, and pathways, but the client tends to expect certain outcomes and therefore repeats patterns unsuccessfully in a particular way. The therapy process, when successful, consists of the realization of some new subset of the possible pathways implicit in the patient's repertoire. There are always important alternative implications that might have occurred in a relationship but did not appear. As Sampson and Weiss have noted (Sampson, 1976), if a patient expects certain responses from a therapist (e.g., to be criticized for being autonomous) and if the therapist "passes the test" by avoiding enactment of the feared response, patients may experience a sense that it is safe to continue their "unconscious plan" for growth. What did not happen becomes the mutative experience. However, the therapist cannot "pass the test" before completing it; only when the therapy is ended can the patient review what occurred and what did not, and then realize none of the expected, dreaded consequences have transpired. As long as the therapy is ongoing, even when the therapist passes test after test, until termination is completed successfully, the patient may wait for the other shoe to fall. The therapy must end in order for what did not happen to have meaning; this is the processive aspect of termination.

The structural aspect of termination refers to the architectonic sequence in which therapeutic events are organized in time: what happened when. Because therapy, like most human experiences, is quintessentially temporal, it involves endings and thus invokes memory. Memory is a key to our experience of time, and the structure of sequences of events influences how they will be remembered. The effects of context, of primacy and recency, distinctiveness, interference, priming, and depth of encoding all play critical roles (Cermak & Craik, 1979). Saying something at the beginning and then again at the end of a session is very different from saying the same thing several times in the middle of the session; the former will be much more likely to be remembered than the latter. Termination, by creating an ending point, punctuates experience and so structures how we remember and interpret what has occurred, both within the therapy session and in the passage of our lives.

Beginnings cannot be understood without endings; it is only after you have completed a journey that you can look back on the route you have traveled and put it in proper perspective. Termination allows both client and therapist to achieve a retrospective understanding of the therapy process. Understanding what did happen and what did not can give new implications to what can happen in the future, as well as to what problems need not be repeated any more.

There is a paradox in remembrance: Memory is an *immediate*, present-time experience that recalls the past and in so doing can affect our actions in the future. The SST therapist, by highlighting certain events and deemphasizing others, attempts to help the client focus on what will be useful while letting go of whatever needs to be left behind. In terminating the session, the SST therapist may help a client remember to remember, forget to remember, remember to forget, or forget to forget.

When concluding a SST, we may first ask the client if he or she feels that enough has been accomplished in the session to help him or her move on. If the answer is "yes," we may ask for a description of what it was, to encourage lexical encoding, storage, and recall of a useful lesson. At other times, we may prefer to have the client leave with a more diffuse sense that "something" changed or will change soon. In all cases, we let clients know we will remain available on an as-needed basis. We encourage them, however, to take some time on their own (usually 1 to 3 months) to consolidate their gains. We also express a genuine interest in how things turn out for the client and may ask the client to give us a follow-up phone report in a month or two or let them know we might call them in a few months to see how they have been progressing.

Sometimes an SST may conclude relatively uneventfully, with a mutual sense of the work being finished and "all wrapped up." At other times, it is best to stop dramatically after an important piece of work has been partially accomplished, but before all of its ramifications are specifically spelled out. Because we tend to work over "unfinished business" (Perls, 1969) or uncompleted tasks more than completed ones (Zeigarnik, 1938), ending an SST in this fashion allows the patient to continue the work of the therapy on his or her own, realizing the unrealized implications in ensuing weeks and months.

The degree of closure appropriate to a termination covers a wide range and is influenced by the extent to which the therapy was seeking resolution of some issue or attempting to open up new possibilities (Rosenbaum, 1988b). Some clients will need to put the therapist behind them and get on with their lives; others will need to recall the therapist or some words of the therapist with a high degree of vividness. Because some of our SST clients will in the future seek further therapy, it is important to structure the termination in such a way that a decision for more treatment will be seen by the patient as an opportunity for further growth, rather than as an indicator of failure. Whether the termination turns out to be for just a few weeks or forever, though, it still involves saying goodbye to the client, and all goodbyes have some degree of both grief and healing, sorrow and hope.

A young married couple sought consultation, complaining of "communication problems." He referred to his stresses at work, financial frustrations, and sexual dissatisfaction with the marriage. She felt depressed and unable to connect with her husband, worried he would abandon her, and wondered if she should return to her parents' house. They looked reasonably healthy, and neither had any previous psychiatric contact, but both now sat avoiding the other's eyes and appeared depressed. The room grew unpleasantly quiet.

"You look like someone died," the therapist observed aloud. "What happened?"

Previously unmentioned, a painful story was told: A midtrimester pregnancy had miscarried the year before. The couple had tried to bury their grief with the unborn child and had pulled back from one another to avoid the sadness that closeness brought (see Leon, 1987). An hour spent talking, crying, and hugging "unstuck" the grieving/healing process. No further professional psychotherapeutic intervention was needed. (MFH)

Conclusion

Clients often come to psychotherapy having failed to resolve some problem because they have not yet accessed and used all their resources. In a similar fashion, psychotherapies can fail if they do not make use of all the resources at their disposal. Therapists have accumulated an enormous fount of knowledge and range of techniques, the product of nearly a century of work in psychiatry and psychology, plus many centuries' knowledge of human nature afforded by art, philosophy, religion, and common sense. Approaching each meeting as a potential successful SST has convinced us that it is possible to be very helpful with many clients quite quickly so long as we are willing to take an integrated approach to the psychotherapeutic endeavor. When we have attempted to restrict ourselves to the perspectives and techniques of a single therapeutic school, however, or when we have attempted to develop a single theoretical approach to SST, we have had markedly poorer results.

Ideally, therapists should be well trained and skillful with a variety of approaches and techniques, so that they can apply what will be best for a particular client at a particular time. Even if one is theoretically orthodox, the skillful therapist can be *technically* eclectic (Lazarus, 1985; Rubin, 1986) lest every patient be forced into the Procrustean bed of a pet approach or be rejected as "resistant" or "unfit." Often the adherence to a particular therapeutic school does more to cement the personality and identity of the therapist than to resolve problems for the patient (Rosenbaum, 1988a). Therapists need not be "hostages to their early training rigidities" (Lamb, 1988; Wolberg, 1985) but may benefit from an ability to view cases in more than one way, with multiple descriptions. As Bateson (1979) noted, it takes two eyes, each with a slightly different perspective, to provide us with depth vision.

Single-session therapies ultimately work, as any therapy works, by mirroring within the therapy the real-life dilemmas and paradoxes our clients confront. In SST the choices we make as therapists are necessarily based on incomplete information. This, however, is a condition of life, rather than of SST: We cannot ever anticipate all the consequences of our actions until our lives are over and complete (Arendt, 1978). This is what makes Hesse's Magister Ludi, in the quotation prefacing our paper, describe "decisive moments of life" as both "vitalizing *and* painful" (our italics). The necessity to act, without being able to fully anticipate all the consequences of action, creates a mingled "sense of farewell and of setting out on new adventures." Our effort in SST is to create awakenings, a sense that there need be "no more hesitating or lingering." We seek "beginnings [in which] dwells a magic force," whose magic is intrinsic to the very brevity of the intense, mutative moment, in which dwells the experience that the time for change is now:

> time time time time time
>
> —how fortunate are you and i, whose home
> is timelessness: we who have wandered down
> from fragrant mountains of eternal now
>
> to frolic in such mysteries as birth
> and death a day (or maybe even less)
>   —e. e. cummings, "stand with your lover
>   on the ending earth—"

ACKNOWLEDGMENT. Support for this project was partially provided by the Sidney Garfield Memorial Fund (Michael F. Hoyt, principal investigator), administered by the Kaiser Foundation Research Institute. The opinions reported here are those of the authors and do not necessarily reflect any policies of Kaiser-Permanente.

REFERENCES

Arendt, H. (1978). *The life of the mind*. New York: Harcourt Brace Jovanovich.

Bateson, G. (1979). *Mind and nature: A Necessary Unity*. New York: E. P. Dutton.

Bennett, M. J. (1984). Brief psychotherapy and adult development. *Psychotherapy, 21,* 171–177.

Berne, E. (1966). *Principles of group treatment*. New York: Oxford University Press.

Berne, E. (1972). *What do you say after you say hello?* New York: Grove Press.

Bion, W. R. (1967). Notes on memory and desire. *Psychoanalytic Forum, 2,* 271–280.

Bion, W. R. (1970). Attention and interpretation. In W. Bion, *Seven servants*. New York: Jason Aronson.

Bloom, B. L. (1981). Focused single-session therapy: Initial development and evaluation. In S. H. Budman (Ed.), *Forms of brief therapy* (pp. 167–218). New York: Guilford Press.

Breuer, J., & Freud, S. (1944). *Studies in hysteria. Standard edition*, Vol. 2. London: Hogarth Press. (Originally published 1893–1895.)

Budman, S. H., & Gurman, A. S. (1988). *Theory and practice of brief therapy*. New York: Guilford.

Carter, E., & McGoldrick, M. (1980). *The family life cycle*. New York: Gardner Press.

Cermak, L., & Craik, F. I. M. (Eds.). (1979). *Levels of processing in human memory*. Hillsdale, NJ: John Wiley & Sons.

Cummings, N. A., & Follette, W. (1976). Brief psychotherapy and medical utilization. In H. Dorken *et al.* (eds.), *The professional psychologist today* (pp. 165–174). San Francisco: Jossey-Bass.

Davanloo, H. (1986). Intensive short-term psychotherapy with highly resistant patients. I. Handling resistance. *International Journal of Short-Term Psychotherapy, 1,* 107–133.

DeShazer, S. (1985). *Keys to solution in brief therapy*. New York: W. W. Norton.

e e cummings (1958). stand with your lover on the ending earth. from *95 poems*. In *e.e. cummings: A Selection of Poems*. New York: Harcourt, Brace & World, 1963, p. 152.

Frances, A., & Clarkin, J. F. (1981). No treatment as the prescription of choice. *Archives of General Psychiatry, 38,* 542–545.

Frank, J. D. (1973). *Persuasion and healing*. New York: Shocken.

Garfield, S. L. (1978). Research on client variables in psychotherapy. In S. L. Garfield & A. E. Bergin, (Eds.), *Handbook of psychotherapy and behavior change: An empirical analysis* (2nd ed., pp. 191–232). New York: Wiley.

Garfield, S. L., & Wolpin, M. (1963). Expectations regarding psychotherapy. *Journal of Nervous and Mental Disease, 137,* 353–362.

Gould, S. J. (1980). *The panda's thumb: More reflections in natural history*. New York: W. W. Norton.

Goulding, R. L., & Goulding, M. M. (1978). *The power is in the patient*. San Francisco: Transactional Analysis Press.

Goulding, M. M., & Goulding, R. L. (1979). *Changing lives through redecision therapy*. New York: Grove Press.

Goulding, M. M., Goulding, R. L., & Silverthorn, A. I. (1983). Integrators/innkeepers/therapists/trainers/theoreticians. *Voices, 18,* 64–72.

Gustafson, J. P. (1986). *The complex secret of brief psychotherapy*. New York: Norton.

Gustafson, J. (1987). The neighboring field of brief individual psychotherapy. *Journal of Marital and Family Therapy, 13,* 409–422.

Gustafson, J. P., & Dichter, H. (1983). Winnicott and Sullivan in the brief psychotherapy clinic. Part I. Possible activity and passivity. *Contemporary Psychoanalysis, 19,* 624–637.

Haley, J. (1973). *Uncommon therapy: The psychiatric techniques of Milton H. Erickson, M.D.* New York: Ballantine Books.

Haley, J. (1977). *Problem-solving therapy*. San Francisco: Jossey-Bass.

Hesse, H. (1969). *The glass bead game*. Translated by R. and C. Winston. New York: Holt, Rinehart & Winston. (Originally published 1943.)

Hoyt, M. F. (1977). Primal scene and self creation. *Voices, 13*, 24–28.

Hoyt, M. F. (1979a). Aspects of termination in a time-limited brief psychotherapy. *Psychiatry, 42*, 208–219.

Hoyt, M. F. (1979b). "Patient" or "client": What's in a name? *Psychotherapy, 16*, 46–47.

Hoyt, M. F. (1985a). Therapist resistances to short-term dynamic psychotherapy. *Journal of the American Academy of Psychoanalysis, 13*, 93–112.

Hoyt, M. F. (1985b). "Shrink" or "expander": An issue in forming a therapeutic alliance. *Psychotherapy, 22*, 813–814.

Hoyt, M. F. (1987). Resistance to brief therapy. *American Psychologist, 42*, 408–409.

Hoyt, M. F. (1988a). Book review of J. P. Gustafson's "The complex secret of brief psychotherapy." *American Journal of Psychiatry, 145*, 374–375.

Hoyt, M. F. *Teaching and learning short-term psychotherapy: Resistances and phase-specific parallel processes.* Paper presented at the American Psychological Association, 1988b, Atlanta.

Hoyt, M. F. (1989). Psychodiagnosis of personality disorders: A guide for the perplexed. *Transactional Analysis Journal*, forthcoming.

Hoyt, M. F., & Farrell, D. (1984). Countertransference difficulties in a time-limited psychotherapy. *International Journal of Psychoanalytic Psychotherapy, 10*, 191–203.

Hoyt, M. F., & Janis, I. L. (1975). Increasing adherence to a stressful decision via a motivational balance-sheet procedure: A field experiment. *Journal of Personality and Social Psychology, 31*, 833–839. Reprinted in I. L. Janis (Ed.) (1982), *Counseling on personal decisions: Theory and research in short-term helping relationships.* New Haven: Yale University Press.

Hoyt, M. F., & Goulding, R. L. (1989). Rapid resolution of a transference–countertransference impasse using Gestalt techniques in supervision. *Transactional Analysis Journal*, forthcoming.

Hoyt, M. F., Rosenbaum, R., & Talmon, M. *Single-session psychotherapy: Increasing effectiveness and training clinicians.* Paper presented at the American Psychological Association, 1987, New York.

Hoyt, M. F., Rosenbaum, R., & Talmon, M. *Single-session psychotherapy: Increasing effectiveness and training clinicians.* Paper presented at the American Psychological Association, 1987, New York.

Hoyt, M. E., Rosenbaum, R., & Talmon, M. *Single-session psychotherapy: An analysis of 50 attempts.* Paper in preparation.

Keeney, B. P. (1983). *Aesthetics of change.* New York: Guilford.

Kogan, L. S. (1957). The short-term case in a family agency. *Social Casework, 38*, 231–238; 296–302; 366–374.

Lamb, W. (1988). Sources and solutions to affective responses observed in the integration of therapies. *Journal of Integrative and Eclectic Psychotherapy, 7*(1), 37–41.

Lambert, M. J. (1986). Implications of psychotherapy outcome research for eclectic psychotherapy. In J. Norcross (Ed.), *Handbook of Eclectic Psychotherapy* (pp. 436–462). New York: Bruner/Mazel.

Langs, R. (1979). *The therapeutic environment.* New York: Jason Aronson.

Lankton, S., & Lankton, C. H. (1983). *The answer within: A clinical framework of Ericksonian hypnotherapy.* New York: Bruner-Mazel.

Lazarus, A. (1985). The need for technical eclecticism: Science, breadth, depth, and specificity. In J. K. Zeig (Ed.), *The evolution of psychotherapy* (pp. 164–173). New York: Bruner/Mazel.

Leon, I. G. (1987). Short-term psychotherapy for perinatal loss. *Psychotherapy, 24*, 186–195.

Malan, D., Heath, E., Bacal, H., & Balfour, F. (1975). Psychodynamic changes in untreated neurotic patients, II: Apparently genuine improvements. *Archives of General Psychiatry, 32*, 110–126.

Mann, J. (1973). *Time-limited psychotherapy.* Cambridge, MA: Harvard University Press.

Mann, J., & Goldman, R. (1982). *A casebook in time-limited psychotherapy.* New York: McGraw-Hill.

McNeel, J. (1976). The parent interview. *Transactional Analysis Journal, 6*, 61–68.

Pekarik, G., & Wierzbicki, M. (1986). The relationship between clients' expected and actual treatment duration. *Psychotherapy, 23*(4), 532–534.

Perls, F. (1969). *Gestalt therapy verbatim.* Lafayette, CA: Real People Press.

Polster, E., & Polster, M. (1976). Therapy without resistance. In A. Burton, (Ed.), *What makes behavior change possible?* New York: Bruner/Mazel.

Rank, O. (1964). *The myth of the birth of the hero.* New York: Knopf. (originally published 1914)

Rank, O. (1973). *The trauma of birth.* New York: Harper & Row. (originally published 1929)

Rockwell, W. J. K., & Pinkerton, R. S. (1982). Single-session psychotherapy. *American Journal of Psychotherapy, 36*, 32–40.

Rosenbaum, R. *Life-cycle psychotherapies and health maintenance organizations.* Paper presented at American Psychological Association Convention, Anaheim, California, August 1983.

Rosenbaum, R. (1988a). Feelings toward integration: A matter of style and identity. *Journal of Integrative and Eclectic Psychotherapy, 7*(1), 52–60.

Rosenbaum, R. *Musical perspectives on termination.* Symposium presented at the Fourth Annual National Convention of the Society for the Exploration of Psychotherapy Integration, Boston, 1988b.

Rubin, S. S. (1986). Ego-focused psychotherapy: A psychodynamic framework for a technical eclecticism. *Psychotherapy, 23,* 385–389.

Sampson, H. (1976). A critique of certain traditional concepts in the psychoanalytic theory of therapy. *Bulletin of the Menninger Clinic, 10*(3), 255–262.

Selvini-Palazzolli, M., Boscolo, L., Cecchin, G., & Prata, G. (1978). *Paradox and counterparadox.* New York: Jason Aronson.

Shapiro, D. (1965). *Neurotic styles.* New York: Basic Books.

Shectman, F. (1986). Time and the practice of psychotherapy. *Psychotherapy, 23*(4), 521–525.

Sifneos, P. E. (1987). *Short-term dynamic psychotherapy: Evaluation and technique* (2nd ed.). New York: Plenum Press.

Spoerl, O. H. (1975). Single-session psychotherapy. *Diseases of the Nervous System, 36,* 283–285.

Sullivan, H. (1954). *The psychiatric interview.* New York: W. W. Norton.

Suzuki, D. T. (1956). *Zen Buddhism.* Garden City, NY: Doubleday.

Szasz, T. (1970). *The manufacture of madness.* New York: Harper & Row.

Ticho, E. A. (1972). Termination of psychoanalysis: Treatment goals, life goals. *Psychoanalytic Quarterly, 41,* 315–333.

Talmon, M., Hoyt, M. F., & Rosenbaum, R. *When the first session is the last: A map for rapid therapeutic change.* Symposium presented at the Fourth International Congress on Ericksonian Approaches to Hypnosis and Psychotherapy, "Brief Therapy: Myths, Methods, and Metaphors," San Francisco, 1988.

Watzlawick, P., Weakland, H., & Fisch, R. (1974). *Change: Principles of problem formation and problem resolution.* New York: W. W. Norton.

Winnicott, D. W. (1971). *Therapeutic consultations in child psychiatry.* New York: Basic Books.

Winokur, M., & Dasberg, H. (1983). Teaching and learning short-term dynamic psychotherapy. *Bulletin of the Menninger Clinic, 47*(1), 36–52.

Wolberg, L. R. (1980). Catalyzing the therapeutic process: The use of hypnosis. In L. R. Wolberg, *Handbook of short-term psychotherapy* (pp. 190–207). New York: Thieme-Stratton.

Wolberg, L. R. (1985). The evolution of psychotherapy: Future trends. In J. K. Zeig (Ed.), *The evolution of psychotherapy* (pp. 250–260). New York: Bruner/Mazel.

Wolpe, J. (1973). *The practice of behavior therapy.* (2nd ed.) New York: Pergamon.

Zeigarnik, B. (1938). On finished and unfinished tasks. In W. D. Ellis, *A source book of gestalt psychology.* New York: Harcourt, Brace & World, pp. 300–314. Summarized in J. W. Atkinson (1964), *An introduction to motivation.* Princeton, NJ: Van Nostrand, pp. 83–87.

III

Individual Approaches in Brief Psychotherapy

A brief perusal of the theoretical approaches in this section indicates a diverse set of techniques and assumptions concerning how the psychotherapeutic enterprise should be conducted. These range from Worchel's (9) discussion of short-term psychodynamic methods, through cognitive, behavioral, and interpersonal approaches, to the view of crisis intervention as psychotherapy espoused by Ewing (13). This should not be surprising because brief therapy has drawn its knowledge base from the modification and adaptation of traditional open-ended approaches.

However, there are approaches that are absent, and the chapters intentionally do not represent a comprehensive sampling of approaches. Only those approaches that in the editors' opinion have both a solid theoretical and empirical base for effectiveness have been included. This is not to say that theories not included have not been or cannot be effective, but rather the bias is toward a documented history of effectiveness. This bias expresses our hope that both practitioners and policymakers will begin to move toward an empirically based system of delivering services.

Interestingly, the chapter concerning brief psychodynamic therapy might have raised the issue of inclusion based upon effectiveness because considerable doubt has been expressed regarding the efficacy of psychoanalytic approaches. However, the introduction of prearranged time constraints and distillation of theoretical concepts drawing from object relations and ego psychology has created a more parsimonious and focused set of therapeutic operations that has resulted in an approach that cuts to the therapeutic issues with much more sharpness and impact than traditional psychoanalytic therapy. Moreover, unlike the broad field of psychoanalysis, such pioneers in the development of short-term dynamic therapy as Davanloo and Malan, have been particularly noteworthy in encouraging outcome studies and generally exposing their work to empirical scrutiny.

The cognitive approaches included in this section have been developed from their early beginnings with an emphasis upon time limitations and a rigorous approach to researching the efficacy of its methods. Although the cognitive and cognitive-behavioral therapies are separated, they represent more of a difference of emphasis rather than kind. With the increasing recognition in psychology of the critical importance of higher information processing upon learning and the performance of complex tasks, the marriage between cognitive and behavioral approaches was inevitable. Because psychotherapy has as a primary focus the management of negative affect and the development of a set of rational and realistic attitudes that allows persons to fulfill their needs in a responsible manner, the discovery that emotional states are a function of stylistic ways of thinking and that attitudinal change more readily follows behavior change than the reverse (although their relationship is much more recursive) has given cognitive-behavioral therapists effective leverage in the psychotherapeutic enterprise.

Much of the integration of cognitive and behavioral theory was accomplished by social learning theory through its emphasis upon the role of modeling and the reciprocal relationship of organism/environment in the process of learning. The influence of social learning theory is also evident in many of the marital, family, and group approaches described later in this *Handbook*. However, interpersonal psychotherapy for depression represents an integration of attachment theory with an understanding of the critical importance of interpersonal and social reinforcement for emotional well-being. From its original formulation in New Haven to the present chapter by Cornes (12), the recognition of certain specifically problematic interpersonal situations in life—grief, conflict, transition—led to a focused interventive model for the treatment of depression that has combined a solid foundation in psychodynamic theory with a here-and-now focus upon interpersonal clarification and problem solving to improve social functioning. Like cognitive therapy, the interpersonal approach was empirically tested in NIMH's Collaborative Depression Project, and preliminary findings strongly support the effectiveness of both.

Finally, although crisis intervention by definition is time-limited, Ewing's chapter (13) on crisis intervention as psychotherapy reviews crisis theory and therapeutic techniques and emphasizes many common elements of psychotherapy within a framework of a structured, directive, and action-oriented focus. Chapters in later sections of the *Handbook* will draw upon similar theory and technique to expand the notion of crisis response into both the family and group modalities of treatment.

9

Short-Term Dynamic Psychotherapy

Jason Worchel

Introduction

In the past few decades, a number of clinical researchers have conducted systematic studies into short-term dynamic psychotherapy. Their investigations have been enhanced by the advent of audiovisual technology that has allowed for complete documentation of the entire psychotherapeutic process. The three international congresses in short-term dynamic psychotherapy (Montreal, 1975 and 1976, Los Angeles, 1977), all based on audiovisual presentations of actual clinical interviews, demonstrated the effectiveness of several different models of dynamic psychotherapies with regards to criteria for selection, techniques, and outcome evaluations. Over the past decade, a large series of audiovisual symposia and courses in short-term dynamic psychotherapy, especially in North America and Europe, have had a major impact on the field of dynamic psychotherapy.

This chapter begins with the contributions of various schools of brief therapy and then highlights the specific technique of Intensive Short-Term Dynamic Psychotherapy. This form of short-term dynamic psychotherapy has proven effective across the entire spectrum of structural neurosis, from the low-resistant, highly motivated patients to those who are highly resistant and poorly motivated. The importance of the trial therapy model of the initial interview, as the most sensitive method for selection of patients for Intensive Short-Term Dynamic Psychotherapy will be discussed together with the technique of "unlocking the unconscious" (Davanloo, 1984, 1986a,b). Following a discussion of the sequence of phases of several variations of the initial interview based on presenting psychopathology, the chapter will demonstrate, via a detailed case presentation, specific technical and theoretical aspects of Intensive Short-Term Dynamic Psychotherapy. There will be particular attention to the handling of resistance, technique of handling the transference, breakthrough into the unconscious, and analysis of the transference and establishing the psychotherapeutic contract. In addition, specific aspects of the course of therapy, the process

Jason Worchel • American Institute of Short-Term Dynamic Psychotherapy, 2101 Arlington Blvd., Charlottesville, Virginia 21903.

of decathexis, pathological mourning, termination, and outcome evaluation will be highlighted.

SCHOOLS OF SHORT-TERM PSYCHOTHERAPIES

Many forms of Short-Term Dynamic Psychotherapy have been introduced in the past few decades, but this chapter will outline a few schools of brief psychotherapy with a psychodynamic orientation.

I. Franz Alexander

Franz Alexander, in his attempt to shorten the length of the psychoanalytic psychotherapy, advocated the need for flexibility in adapting technique to the patient's psychopathology. Implicit in his writing is that there are a set of criteria for selection. These include the patient demonstrating a high level of ego adaptive capacity, the ability to become actively engaged in the psychotherapeutic process, strong motivation for change, and a positive response to interpretation (Alexander & French, 1946).

II. Brief Psychotherapy—Tavistock System—David Malan

This form of brief psychotherapy was originally developed by Balint's team at the Tavistock Clinic. Malan, a member of Balint's team, gave a comprehensive report of their first series, which consisted of 21 patients, followed by the report of a second report of 39. Malan describes specific criteria for the selection of patients. Their primary focus has been on highly motivated and highly responsive patients. His criteria for selection can be summarized as (1) motivation for insight and change; (2) the capacity to see that their problems are psychological in origin; (3) positive response to interpretation; (4) ability to find a single psychotherapeutic focus, either oedipal or loss; (5) absence of deprivation; (6) good outside relationships; (7) heterosexual experience; and (8) a willingness on the part of the patient and the therapist to become deeply involved and to bear the anxiety that inevitably arises during the course of therapy. Malan describes a set of criteria for rejection that can be summarized as (1) long-term hospitalization, (2) drug addiction, (3) serious suicidal attempt, (4) more than one course of ECT, (5) incapacitating chronic phobic symptoms, and (6) chronic obsessional symptoms. Repeatedly, he emphasized high motivation and high responsiveness. In terms of technical requirements, Malan lists (1) transference reactions are interpreted early, (2) the negative transference must be thoroughly interpreted, and (3) effort should be made to link the transference relationship to relationship with parents' Transference-Past (T-P) interpretation. In terms of termination, he indicated grief and anger about termination must be worked through. Malan sets a date for termination in advance and suggests 20 sessions as an average for the experienced psychotherapist and 30 sessions for those in training (Malan, 1979, 1986).

III. Short-Term Anxiety-Provoking Psychotherapy (STAPP)—Peter Sifneos

This is an effective method of psychotherapy for patients suffering from neurotic disturbances who are highly motivated and highly responsive. Sifneos emphasizes a set of criteria for selection, which is summarized as follows: (1) a circumscribed chief complaint, (2) a meaningful or give-and-take relationship during early childhood, (3) ability to interact flexibly with the evaluator and express feelings appropriately, (4) above-average psychological sophistication, and (5) good-to-excellent motivation for change. He has a set of subcriteria for the assessment for the patient's motivation during the initial interview that can be summarized as (1) ability to recognize the symptoms are of psychological origin, (2) ability for introspection and in giving an honest and truthful account of his or her psychological difficulty, (3) willingness to participate actively in the treatment situation, (4) to have curiosity and willingness to understand oneself, (5) to have willingness to change, and (6) realistic expectation of the result of the therapy and willingness to make a tangible sacrifice. In his criteria, he emphasizes that a specific psychodynamic formulation must be identified by the evaluator and the psychotherapeutic focus must be oedipal in nature.

In terms of the technical requirements in STAPP, they can be summarized as follows: (1) weekly face-to-face interviews lasting 45 minutes, (2) quick establishment of rapport, (3) rapid establishment of a therapeutic alliance, (4) the use of open-ended questions and forced-choice questions, (5) transference feelings for the therapist should be clarified as early as they become manifest, (6) the therapist must actively concentrate on the oedipal focus, (7) repeated use of anxiety-provoking questions and confrontation, (8) avoidance of pregenital chacterological issues that the patient might use defensively, (9) active avoidance of the development of transference neurosis, (10) the therapist should demonstrate to the patient repeatedly his or her neurotic pattern of behavior, (11) the therapist should concentrate on anxiety-laden material, (12) emphasis should be on creating a corrective emotional experience that includes learning new problem-solving skills, (13) the therapist should look for tangible evidence of change in the patient's behavior out of the therapeutic situation to obtain evidence that the more adaptive pattern has replaced maladaptive patterns, and (14) early termination.

The course of STAPP is divided into four major phases: (1) patient/therapist encounter, (2) early phase of therapy, (3) height of treatment, and (4) evidence of change and termination (Sifneos, 1972).

IV. Time-Limited Psychotherapy—Mann

A short-term psychotherapeutic method consisting of 12 interviews was developed by Mann at Boston University. Mann is not explicit in terms of selection criteria, but he definitely rejects patients who are resistant. The essential elements he considers of importance are (1) the patient has a problem that can be focused around a central theme, such as loss or separation, (2) the nature of the problems occurred as a result of a maturational crisis that led to psychological or somatic complaints, (3) the patient can tolerate a quick termination of the therapeutic relationship, and (4) the patient has motivation for insight and change. His rejection criteria can be summarized as acute psychotic state, serious depression interfering with the psychotherapeutic process, and patients incapable of tolerating sustained object relations. The technical requirements described by Mann are summarized as (1) limitation of therapy to 12 sessions, (2) utilization of early positive transference, (3) maintaining the focus on the central issue involving transference and the patient's chronically endured suffering, (4) actively avoiding the development of dependence, (5) repeated clarification of present and past experience, (6) if necessary, actively supporting and encouraging the patient, even possibly providing direct information, and (7) making repeated Transference-Past interpretations. Mann encourages positive identification with the therapist in order to provide a setting where separation can become a maturational event for the patient. In Time-Limited Psychotherapy, the conflicts that are worked through primarily involve (1) unresolved or delayed grief, and (2) independence versus dependence (Mann, 1979; Mann & Godlman, 1982).

All the previously mentioned techniques of Short-Term Dynamic Psychotherapy have attempted to bypass the major problem of resistance by the process of selection. As a result, they apply only to a small proportion of patients suffering from psychoneurotic disturbances.

V. Intensive Short-Term Dynamic Psychotherapy—Davanloo

Davanloo's discovery of the technique of "unlocking the unconscious, with a direct view of the multi-foci core neurotic structure" (1978, 1980, 1984, 1986a,b, 1986–1987, 1987a,b,c) has had a revolutionary impact on dynamic psychiatry. His work has led to the development of a system of psychotherapy termed Intensive Short-Term Dynamic Psychotherapy. The balance of this chapter will focus on Davanloo's technique in terms of the spectrum of patients, evaluation and selection, trial therapy model of the initial interview, indications and contraindications, technique, and the psychotherapeutic process and outcome evaluation.

Type of Patients for Whom the Technique Has Proved Applicable

The technique is effective for the whole spectrum of structural neurosis with the exception of those with severe fragile ego structure. Davanloo divides the structural neurosis into four major categories:

1. Highly motivated, highly responsive patients with relatively simple, circumscribed problems with basically healthy personalities who suffer from mild phobic, obsessional, or depressive symptomatology. They also may have some problems in interpersonal relationships, particularly in heterosexual relationships. In this group, the psychotherapeutic focus is a single one. Typically, it is either an oedipal conflict, or the focus may be concerned with loss. Davanloo places this group to the extreme left of his spectrum.

2. Moderately resistant patients. This category consists of patients in whom the problems are much more complex. They suffer from diffuse psychoneurotic disturbances and characterological problems that often include inability to assert themselves and/or achieve their potential. There are multiple psychotherapeutic foci, and each is complex. Typically these foci consist of a mixture of oedipal conflicts, sibling rivalry, and loss. These conflicts have become embedded in a matrix of characterological defenses (i.e., passivity, compliance) or phobic and obsessional symptomatology.

3. Highly resistant, poorly motivated. These patients suffer from diffuse symptom disturbances as well as character pathology. Their lives and relationships might be severely disrupted by chronic phobic, obsessional, depressive, and other psychoneurotic disturbances. Within this group, Davanloo includes patients suffering from repressive symptomatology, that is, panic disorder, depressive disorder, and functional and somatization disorder. In addition to symptom disturbances, they suffer from character disturbances and severe problems in interpersonal relationships with conflicts over intimacy and closeness. They have an inability to make any true contact with other human beings and maintain distance through passivity, defiance, and sarcasm. Davanloo points out that the core neurotic structure of this group is much more complex. Often persons in this category have a history of severe traumatic experiences in the very early years, multiple losses, severe sibling rivalry, severe oedipal conflicts, and repressed murderous impulses in relation to either or both parents.

4. Highly resistant, poorly motivated with major ego-syntonic character pathology. This category of patients is similar to the preceding group but has an addition to multifoci pathology and severe interpersonal disturbances, and severe ego-syntonic character pathology. This ego syntonicity hides from the patient any awareness or recognition as to the nature or degree of his or her disturbances. In essence, these patients have a total lack of self-perception or awareness of how they impact on others. Of all the groups, members of this group are characterized by a high level of severe, chronic masochism.

Evaluation and Selection

Davanloo, based on a number of systematic research and extensive audiovisually recorded clinical data, has come to the conclusion that selection criteria based on the assessment of major ego functions, such as psychological mindedness, motivation, affective function of the ego, and human relationships are only reliable for those patients who are highly motivated and responsive, namely the left side of the spectrum. He indicates that these criteria cannot be applied to those patients who are highly resistant and poorly responsive as the major ego functions of all these patients on the right side of the spectrum are paralyzed by the forces of resistance. He has developed a comprehensive system of "trial therapy" that is considered the most sensitive method in the selection of patients.

Major Functions of Comprehensive Trial Therapy

The major functions of Davanloo's system of trial therapy can be summarized as follows:

1. A psychodiagnostic tool
2. A sensitive method for selection of patients for Intensive Short-Term Dynamic Psychotherapy
3. Psychotherapeutic intervention
4. Teaching and research

The major function of trial therapy is to provide a comprehensive psychodiagnostic evaluation in terms of clinical diagnosis; psychodynamic formulation; comprehensive biopsychosocial assessment; and formulating a genetic diagnosis as well as psychotherapeutic evaluation and planning. In terms of clinical diagnosis, a comprehensive descriptive, dynamic phenomenological approach to the patient's psychopathology is essential. In this process, a differentiation must be made between structural neurosis vis-à-vis developmental neurosis. A meaningful clinical diagnosis is both descriptive, based on a psychoanalytic classification, as well as a nosologic, based on DSM-III nomenclature. During such an assessment, the clinician must be able to differentiate between ego regression and structural defects of the ego.

As already indicated, all major ego functions can directly be assessed in patients who are highly motivated and highly responsive, but in patients who are moderately to highly resistant, assessment of the major ego function cannot be done in the early part of the trial therapy. Here the therapist must first apply the techniques designed to manage resistance and unlock the unconscious.

The Technique of the "Unlocking of the Unconscious" (Davanloo, 1984, 1986a,b)

This technique applies to all patients who are highly resistant, on the right side of the spectrum. The technical requirements can be summarized as follows:

1. A high degree of activity by the psychotherapist in handling resistance in terms of challenge and pressure to the resistance.

2. Extensive use of the transference. The therapist actively works on two basic psychoanalytic triangles, the triangle of conflict, which consists of impulse/feeling, anxiety, and defense, and the triangle of person. These are illustrated in Figure 1. The triangle of conflict is a theoretical construct that is central to understanding Davanloo's technical intervention. Its foundation is one of the cornerstones of psychoanalytic theory. The triangle of the person depicts the interpersonal sphere in which the intrapsychic conflicts originated and have been perpetuated. The triangle of the person denotes those significant persons in the patient's past life (P) with whom there were unresolved conflicts and those in the patient's current life orbit (C) with whom these conflicts now reside. It also contains the immediate transference relationships with the therapist (T).

3. Free floating attention used in classical psychoanalysis is not sufficient. Davanloo points out that "vigilance" on the part of the therapist is essential.

4. The trial therapy has two major phases, the preinterpretative phase in

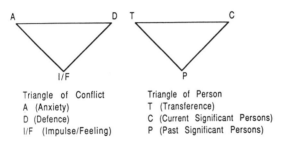

Triangle of Conflict
A (Anxiety)
D (Defence)
I/F (Impulse/Feeling)

Triangle of Person
T (Transference)
C (Current Significant Persons)
P (Past Significant Persons)

FIGURE 1. Basic psychoanalytic triangles.

which the therapist's task is the handling of the resistance and the interpretative phase that starts after the first breakthrough into the unconscious takes place and the unconscious therapeutic alliance has been brought into operation.

The standard technique for handling resistance as developed by Davanloo is summarized as follows:

> Rapid identification and clarification of the patient's defenses in the transference.
> Pressure toward the experience of the impulse/feelings, which leads to a rapid rise in the patient/s complex transference feelings and further intensification of resistance.
> Systematic pressure and challenge to the transference-resistance leading to a further intensification of resistance.
> Head-on collision with the transference-resistance.
> Creation of an intrapsychic crisis with turning of the ego against its own defenses.
> Direct experience of the complex transference feelings—the "triggering" mechanism.
> Mobilization of the unconscious therapeutic alliance and the first unlocking of the unconscious.
> Systematic analysis of the transference to remove the residual resistance and widen the entry into the unconscious. (Davanloo, 1987b, p. 167)

Major derepression of current or recent past (C) and distance past (P) conflicts, leads to a direct view of the dynamic unconscious and multifocal core neurotic structure.

In this group of highly resistant patients following a breakthrough into the unconscious, the process of the trial therapy enters to an interpretative phase. It is now possible for the therapist to complete the descriptive dynamic phenomenological approach, the psychodynamic formulation, the biopsychosocial assessment, the developmental history, and explore for a second time the multi-foci core neurotic structure and its link with the patient's symptom disturbances as well as character disturbances. The final phase is establishing psychotherapeutic planning.

The therapist should take into consideration that this is a guideline and that there are quantitative as well as technical modifications to the trial therapy based on the degree of the patient's resistance and the nature of the patient's psychopathology. Davanloo 1986–1987, 1987b has classified a number of these categories requiring variations to the trial therapy that can be summarized as follows:

1. Highly motivated, highly responsive patient
2. Moderately resistant patient
3. Highly resistant character neurotic

4. Highly resistant patients with major character pathology, chronically depressed with the past history of clinical depression
5. Highly resistant patient suffering panic disorder
6. Highly resistant patient with somatization and functional disorder

Here two major variations in the trial therapy will be outlined.

Highly Motivated, Highly Responsive

Generally, the sequences/phases of the trial therapy are as follows:

1. Descriptive dynamic phenomenological approach
2. Psychodynamic formulation
3. Medical and social history
4. Developmental history
5. Exploring the patient's core neurotic conflict—resistance needs to be handled via the transference
6. Assessment of the patient's response to interpretation
7. Assessment of the patient's motivation and psychotherapeutic planning.

Highly Resistant Patient Suffering from Character Neurosis

With this group of patients, the sequences/phases of the trial therapy will be as follows:

1. Applying the technique of the "unlocking the unconscious and the direct view of the multifoci core neurotic structure"
2. Descriptive dynamic phenomenology approach to the patient's psychopathology
3. Medical and social history
4. Developmental history
5. Further exploration of the multifoci core neurotic structure and its link to the patient's symptoms as well as character disturbances
6. Setting up the psychotherapeutic contract

The technique used in the initial interview is basically the technique used in treatment, and, with the aid of the following case, an attempt will be made to elaborate and highlight some of the important aspects of Intensive Short-Term Dynamic Psychotherapy.

Clinical Material

The patient is a 45-year-old teacher who is self-referred and suffers from a wide range of disturbances: (1) chronic anxiety, (2) episodes of depression, (3) complaints of episodes that he refers to as demoralization and despair, and (4) disturbances of interpersonal relationships with conflict over intimacy and closeness involving both men and women. In relation to women, he has a need to bend over backwards to please and at the same time has difficulty in remaining committed; in his relationship with men he remains detached and superficial; (5) conflict in his marriage and difficulty in remaining committed to it; (6) conflict with his step-children, characterized by detachment, "chronic sense of estrangement"; (7) characterological problem such as detachment, passivity, and compliance which might shift to stubbornness and defiance, episodes in which he has outbursts of temper, shouting, and breaking furniture. He has a self-defeating, self-sabotaging pattern which involves many aspects of his life with need for self-punishment and moving from frying pan to fire. In his job as a teacher, he functions much below his potential; (8) has poor personal hygiene, keeping himself unkempt, almost a compulsion to exercise and bring himself to a state of utter exhaustion.

The first phase of the trial therapy primarily focused on the descriptive phenomenological approach, and he indicated that he had a hard time being married: "I feel like my wife and I have become further apart"; "I deal with her pretty much as I did with my mother." Then he talked about his difficulty of intimacy and closeness with his wife: "I find myself wanting to pull away from her to get involved with other women." He further indicates that he wants to remain in the marriage—"it is my responsibility." He indicated that he has become more and more distanced from his wife Mary and has increasingly become sexually attracted to a number of other women, including one named Sue. During the whole early process of the interview the patient maintains a detached, noninvolved position in relation to the therapist, and the therapist, for the time being, simply "computerizes" the transference pattern of behavior and continues to complete, as much as possible, the patient's area of disturbances.

The Triangle of the Conflict in Relation to His Wife

The patient described an incident in which he was interrupted while completing an application form. His wife had bent a knife in the kitchen and asked for his help to repair it. He did so but indicates that he was seething with anger because his wife had interrupted his concentration. In exploring his anger, it becomes clear he is not able to experience it. He notes that he was seething but there was no sign of affect during the interview, and it is clear that there is a great distance between his affective and cognitive functions with the defense mechanism of isolation being in operation.

The Triangle of the Conflict in Relation to Sue (C): The First Challenge to the Patient's Resistance

Th: Then does this pattern exist with Sue?

Pt: Uh, I don't think so.

Th: So then it is there with Mary but not with Sue?

Pt: No, it feels to me as though, it is not there in as clear and dramatic fashion with Sue. Well, I suppose if I thought about it. . . .

Th: You say "if" and "suppose." Do you notice that you want to leave everything in a state of limbo. That you have difficulty to be definite here with me?

Pt: Uh huh.

Th: Now up until the time you want to leave this in a fuzzy way, it doesn't bring us any clear picture of this particular situation.

Pt: I haven't thought about, about all of this.

Th: But leaving it in a state of limbo doesn't help.

Pt: I don't think it applies to Sue.

Th: Even there you say, "I think."

We saw the first challenge to the patient's resistances. Now the therapist focuses on his relationship with Sue and description of Sue's physical attributes that is anxiety laden with its unconscious implication that intensifies the patient's resistances.

Challenge to "Tactical Defenses"—Davanloo (1986a,b)

Th: You're smiling.
Pt: Pardon me. (Patient is looking away.)
Th: Right away your eyes are going to the wall.
Pt: I guess I'm a little embarrassed.
Th: Guess? Again you want to leave it in a state of limbo.
Pt: I am embarrassed.
Th: What is this feeling of being embarrassed? (Patient is avoiding eye contact and is becoming very psychomotor retarded.) And right away you avoid my eyes again, and do you notice that you are becoming very slow? (The interview is abbreviated, otherwise it is verbatim.)

Intensification of Resistance Leading to Transference Resistance
Intensification of the Resistance

In the preceding passage, the therapist challenged some of the patient's resistances that intensifies the patient's resistance in the transference and the process leads to a phase of systematic challenge to the patient's resistances in the transference. We take up the interview:

Th: How do you feel when I question you about the body of Sue?
Pt: I think (sigh)
Th: A deep sigh.
Pt: I feel embarrassed.
Th: But that is a word. (Patient pauses and looks away.)
Pt: Uh, very . . .
Th: Again you are slow, avoid my eyes and take a deep sigh.
Pt: I am.
Th: And now you are even holding your breath, are you aware of that?
Pt: I am now that you point it out.
Th: Again the smile is there, and actually you are avoiding me with your eyes, too. (Patient shakes his head in agreement.) But agreeing you are avoiding me is still avoiding.
Pt: Yes.
Th: So then let's see how you feel toward me questioning you about the body of Sue? And again your smile is back.
Pt: I guess on some level . . . (Therapist interrupts again.)
Th: Guess? (Patient smiles again.) Still you are smiling and biting your lip.

The preceding passage demonstrates the therapist's systematic challenge to the patient's defenses in the transference and active work on the triangle of conflict in the transference.

Systematic Challenge and Pressure to the Transference Resistance

Th: I am repeatedly asking you how you feel towards me questioning you about the body of Sue and you remain retarded (psychomotor), smiling, avoiding me with your eyes, intellectualizing, holding your breath, and placing a massive wall between you and me. So you want to put a distance between you and me.

Pt: You're a stranger.

Th: So then what you say is that I am a stranger, and you don't want to describe the body of Sue to this stranger. Now what are you going to do about that?

We saw a systematic challenge and pressure to the transference resistance and the therapist focuses on the patient's distancing and his need to erect a wall in relation to him. Concomitantly, he challenges the patient's obsessional defenses as well as his tactical defenses and, as we see, the transference pattern "is similar to the one with his wife." The therapist recognizes this but simply computerizes it as the process has not yet entered into "the interpretative phase of the trial therapy" (Davanloo, 1984, 1986–1987, 1986b).

Further Challenge and Pressure to the Patient's Resistance in the Transference

The therapist continues his active work on the triangle of conflict in the transference; we see a definite rise in the transference feeling.

Pt: (Takes a deep sigh)

Th: Again you take a deep breath and look how slow you have become.

Pt: Yes.

Th: Still you are paralyzed. So what are you going to do about this paralysis and detachment?

Pt: I don't know.

Th: That is a helpless position, and my question is what are you going to do about this helpless position. Now let's look at it; I am here to help you get to the core of your problems, but up until the time you take a remote, detached, helpless position and continue to intellectualize and keep things vague, then how are we going to get there? And still we don't know how you feel towards me questioning you about the body of Sue?

Pt: I feel backed into a corner.

The persistent systematic challenge and pressure to the patient's defenses continues, and the therapist carefully monitors the rise in the "complex transference feeling" (1986a,b, 1987a,b) that, when it reaches a threshold level, will bring about the first breakthrough into the unconscious (1986a).

"Head-On Collision with the Resistance in the Transference"—Davanloo *(1984, 1986a)*

Th: That is intellectualization and rumination. In what way do you experience your anger towards me?

Pt: Physically, I feel like kinda pushing you and saying "back off." (arms thrust outward and voice is raised)

Th: Pushing me how?

Pt: A shove on your shoulders. (again demonstrates with pushing out with both arms)

Th: On my shoulder, you would push me on my shoulders. (patient smiles) and again your smile is back.

Pt: Anger. (Patient makes a chopping motion with his hand.) And that is a word? (good eye contact, no smiling, leaning forward, strong voice)

Th: Angry. What is your internal state when you say you are angry with me, how do you experience this anger, in terms of thought and fantasy, towards me right now?

Pt: The physical expression of it? (hands thrust outward)

Th: If that is in your mind.

Pt: I feel like, that (clench fists thrusting outward, patient is highly charged with feeling. There is a slight tearfulness in his eyes.)

Th: Has there been any time you have really been angry and actually put it out? Can we look to that incident.

Pt: (deep sigh)

Th: You have a tremendous problem with your anger, don't you?

Pt: Yes, yes I do!

Th: Can we look to that incident?

As we saw, there was a definite rise in the patient's transference feeling. The physiological concomitant of anxiety made a major shift to anger in the transference that is being experienced in relation to the therapist. As we will see, the first breakthrough into the unconscious is eminent. Davanloo's technique of trial therapy with patients on the right side of the spectrum has two major phases, a "preinterpretative phase" that consists of pure challenge and pressure to the patient's resistance and an "interpretative phase" that starts after the first entry to the unconscious (1984, 1986a, 1986–1987). At this point, the trial therapy has entered to the second phase.

The First Breakthrough into the Unconscious and the T-C-P Interpretation

He describes an incident involving his brother, mother, and father. His father was an alcoholic. His mother has left the patient to take care of Jim, his younger brother, and Jim was interrupting him. We take up the interview:

Pt: Yes, uh, my brother is 4 years younger than I and he, uh, I was often charged with the responsibility of taking care of him, uh . . .

Th: What was his first name?

Pt: Jim. I had a baseball bat in the living room, and I used to practice my swing in the window, and there was a reflection for practicing the swing and uh, my, Jim, came in once, and I was practicing my swing, and he started getting me angry, doing whatever kids do.

Th: What did he do specifically?

Pt: Uh, I remember his being on the couch, the couch was to my right (patient is totally absorbed in what he is saying, he points to where the couch would be), there was something that he wanted, something that I had to get for him, and my memory is that I had gotten it. I think he wanted some milk, but I had to get it for him because he was unable to get it for himself and my memory is that I not so long ago had gotten it for him already, and I was very irritated, and I was practicing my swing, and he was on the couch and I swung the bat and I hit him.

Th: Where?

As we saw there was a head-on collision with the resistance in the transference that followed a breakthrough into the unconscious, and the patient is fully in touch with his aggressive impulse as well as "repressed unconscious guilt and grief-laden feeling" (1987a,b,c). The following passage shows the interpretative phase and shows that the patient is fully in touch with his most painful feeling, his negative feeling for his brother as well as his positive.

Th: What comes to your mind with these tears?

Pt: What comes to my mind is the feeling of being out of control and angry, I felt as if I could have killed him, and I might have killed him if I had hit him somewhere else on his head or swung harder. I might have killed him! (more sobbing)

Th: So then you are frightened that if you had totally lost control he might be dead.

Pt: I'm very afraid of it (anger). I try to push it down. That time it came out, and it was hurtful and destructive.

Th: And you have a lot of mixed feelings for your brother. If he had dropped dead at that moment in your life, what would have been your reaction?

Pt: I would have had this tremendous self-hatred, self-loathing (patient with great sobbing) . . . oh . . . I was just thinking about that. (more crying)

Th: And what would have been your reaction to your dead brother?

Pt: I would have said, "I'm sorry, I'm sorry, sorry, ooh, I'm sorry, I love you." (another wave of deep sobbing)

Th: There is a lot of mixed feeling for Jim.

Pt: I wanted to take care of him, and I didn't know how.

Th: So then as much as there was anger, there was affection for Jim as well.

Pt: Yes, very much.

C-P

The following passage shows a major fluidity in the patient's unconscious and the operation of the "unconscious therapeutic alliance" (1984), the incident of being interrupted by the wife and his massive rage toward her, and the childhood memory that he was interrupted by the brother with the impulse to murder him, also the triangle of he, his mother, and Jim and major sibling rivalry.

Th: So then what you say is that Jim interrupted what you were doing, and you had to take care of his needs, but then you lost control over the rage.

Pt: Yes, he wanted attention the same as Mary (wife). I feel she needs my attention.

Th: And you said with her you were seething. If you had lost control of your feelings
that day with her, in terms of thoughts and fantasy, what would have happened?

Pt: Oh! I would have slapped her, tell her to leave me alone. (again wave of crying)

Th: How?

Pt: Hard, vigorous.

Th: With which hand?

Pt: That one and this one. (clapping back and forth with both hands)

Th: On which part of her body would you have slapped her?

Pt: Her face.

Th: And with Jim?

Pt: Same way, oh, he turned his head the same way and then he just started crying,
convulsive crying.

Th: Convulsive?

Pt: He cried in a way, hateful, but painful, but unbelieving, hurt, hurt, HURT! At the
point he started crying and sorta doubled over, yes, I thought I had killed him. I
thought he might just cry and then die! (another very painful wave of sobbing)

There is a major change in the therapeutic atmosphere; the patient maintains eye contact
with the therapist. Both conscious as well as unconscious therapeutic alliance is in operation, and the patient is in touch with his most painful feelings.

"Analysis of the Transference" (1986a,b, 1987a) Return to Triangle of Conflict in Transference

Davanloo has developed the technique of "systematic analysis of the transference" following breakthrough into the unconscious. This is a process of systematically recapitulat-
ing for the ego the various aspects of the triangle of conflict within the transference
relationship. The following passage demonstrates some aspects of this technique:

Th: Was there the impulse to lash out at me, if you be honest with yourself?

Pt: Yes, the impulse was to lash out, but I filter it . . . physically it was to push out at
you (demonstrates) and tell you to leave me alone.

Th: Let's look to your relationship here with me. You said there was impulse to lash out
at me, but the way that you dealt with your anger towards me was, you said escape,
which is flight. Then you put all kinds of distance between the two of us. You
became detached and used intellectualizing, vagueness, ruminating, and then
physically you become totally paralyzed and rigid. These are all the mechanisms
you use to deal with your anger. At the same time there was anxiety which you
covered with your smiling.

Pt: Yes.

T-C-P Link

After breakthrough into the unconscious and mobilization of the unconscious therapeutic alliance, the patient comes with fresh memories and incidents that will throw more
light on patient's core psychopathology. It becomes clear that he had allied with the
mother against the father that is then followed by sibling rivalry with his brother. At this

point he comes with a memory that involves his parents—a fight between his mother and father.

Th: What specifically happened in these fights? She complained about his drinking and then what would happen?

Pt: Um, he would, he would sort of pick out something that she had done, like not taking care of the bills, or the housework or his supper wasn't cooked well . . .

Th: He was critical of her and the way she did things?

Pt: Yes, it felt as though . . .

Th: Let's look to a memory of one of those fights.

Pt: Well, this one that keeps coming to mind took place when I was older and with the baseball bat again! I must have been about 14; he had come home that night and he was drunk and our room, my brother and I would sometimes be in the same room and other times we would have different rooms, our room was right next to theirs and he was drunk and they had arguments, the volume would increase.

Th: So you weren't actually in the room, you were listening.

Pt: Yes and my brother would wake up and he'd hear it and he'd start crying and I would just get angry, I would get very, very angry and sometimes I would just holler over to them, you, now, I'd say, "please stop, or please." (patient is very engaged in the memory, hands are moving as he talks)

Th: Let's look to this night, at 14 . . .

Pt: What happened that night was that they wouldn't stop, and I could . . .

The patient described an incident involving a verbal lashing out between his parents. The father was threatening to physically attack the mother when the patient, on over-hearing this, took a baseball bat to attack his father in order to defend his mother. We take up the interview:

Th: If you had hit him in the head the way you felt, what would his skull look like?

Pt: Uh, it would have, uh, oh, it would have had a dent, I have a picture of it having a dent in it.

Th: Uh huh.

Pt: Staggered and he would have fallen to the floor. And blood would be coming out there, so there would be a dent, but sort of a crack and from the crack, blood would be coming out. (patient beginning to get tearful)

Th: So the pain in the neck would be dead, but you don't say how you would feel if that pain in the neck died in your life.

Pt: It's a mixture, I would have felt guilty and relieved. (patient has become increasingly sad)

Th: You're holding all your feelings behind the wall.

Pt: I feel my anger. As soon as he hit the floor, I would have missed him (patient now crying) I would have missed the little bits of affection that he would allow himself, and every now and then he would let me in, there were times when, when my mom worked, and he would show his affection by cooking for me.

What emerges is the murderous impulses toward his father, his guilt, and grief-laden unconscious feeling as well as a craving for close relations with his father. When he was seen the following week he was very positive and hopeful about his treatment, and there was emergence of further fresh memories about his life with his father.

Pt: Physically I felt somewhat cleared out, I, I hadn't cried for a long time, I, I'm, not really sure when I cried last.

Th: First there was sadness and then followed by . . .

Pt: Hopefulness and then a feeling that I wanted to do what, whatever the work was, that I wanted to try to do it.

Th: Were there specific thoughts or anything else that came into your mind?

Pt: Yes, a few things occurred to me as a result of the things that we discussed. And I began to think more about my father and mother, and things occurred to me that I hadn't thought of before, one was that, and it came to me today while I was listening to some tapes my father made, before he died. I asked him to sing some of the old songs into the tape, and he did that for me and I felt today that, wow, I was listening to the tapes and felt that it was a tremendous gift, that he had made me in those tapes.

Th: Is it a long one?

Pt: Oh, goodness, many, many songs . . . they've been there for years.

He talked about his father who had died 5 years ago. During the interview he was very sad and crying. He talked with intense feeling and cried about his life with his father and the focus of the session was on the triangle of the patient, the patient's father, and his mother. He had many memories of a controlling, demanding mother. The pathological grief over the death of his father has now been transformed to active grief that provides an opportunity to work through the unresolved grief over the death of his father. Then the focus of the session is his mother. He comes with memories of a very close warm relationship with his mother in the early years, and the focus of the session is on anxiety-laden, erotized, unconscious feeling for his mother. What follows is the way his alliance with his controlling, demanding mother alienated him from his father. This leads to a pouring out of unconscious guilt and grief-laden feelings in relation to his father, mourning the loss of the father–son relationship. The process of the session then moved to further exploration of the patient's multifoci core neurotic structure and their link to the patient's disturbances, both symptom disturbance as well as character disturbance.

Psychotherapeutic Contract

Having achieved a breakthrough into the unconscious, then the therapist proceeds to complete the comprehensive psychodiagnostic evaluation that, as was mentioned before, includes the following: to complete the descriptive phenomenological approach to the patient's psychopathology to arrive at a clinical diagnosis, psychiatric, medical, and social history; developmental history, and finally setting up a psychotherapeutic contract. The following passage demonstrates the establishment of psychotherapeutic contract:

Th: From what we have accomplished during this 3 to 4 hours, do you feel that if we continued in a much more systematic fashion, since we have been able to only touch the surface of many of these conflicts, it would be of benefit to you?

Pt: I feel that it would.

Th: That from what we have done, we could get to all of your buried feelings and you could make a change in your life?

Pt: I want to try.

Th: So then it has been of help to you?

Pt: Absolutely, I feel in these 4 hours that I have had, at least a glimpse, of where I have to go. And I feel that quite strongly. I feel very charged with the responsibility to do what it takes.

Th: So then with your effort and my help, it would be something that you would like to continue?

Pt: Yes.

Th: I would be willing to take you into therapy. My estimation is that it will take approximately 35 to 40 sessions. It might take less, but that 40 sessions would be the upper limit.

Pt: Thirty-five to 40 sessions? Once a week?

Th: Yes. Each session would last 50 minutes.

Pt: That is fine with me.

Indication and Contraindication

As indicated earlier, intensive Short-Term Dynamic Therapy is highly effective in patients suffering from psychoneurotic disturbances. Davanloo has indicated that for patients suffering from character neurosis, the most important criterion is the patient's response to the initial comprehensive trial therapy. Patients can be treated who demonstrate an ability to withstand the impact of their unconscious, to view their multifoci core neurotic structure (Davanloo, 1978, 1980, 1984, 1986a,b, 1987a,b,c). In terms of contraindications, based on extensive audiovisually recorded clinical research data, Davanloo does exclude the following as contraindications for Intensive Short-Term Dynamic Psychotherapy of 40 sessions duration:

1. Patient suffering from structural neurosis with severe fragile ego structure
2. Developmental neurosis, such as borderline disorder
3. Major affective disorder, that is, bipolar disorder
4. Psychosis—schizophrenic disorder
5. Severe alcoholism or drug abuse
6. Serious sociopathic tendencies
7. Potentially life-threatening psychosomatic conditions like ulcerative colitis.

Technique and Course of Treatment

The technique of Intensive Short-Term Dynamic Psychotherapy is radically different from traditional long-term psychoanalytic psychotherapy and those of psychoanalysis. At the same time, the technical requirement for treating patients at the extreme left of the spectrum are to a major extent different from those on the right side of the spectrum (1986a,b, 1987a,b).

The Technique as Applied to Highly Motivated and Highly Responsive Patients

Briefly, it can be summarized as follows (1980, 1984):

- Establishment of the psychotherapeutic focus
- Concentrating on "the genetically structured central neurotic conflict" underlying the patient's problem
- Rapid establishment of psychotherapeutic alliance
- Actively working on the two-triangle technique of clarification and interpretation
- Therapy from the beginning enters into interpretative phase (no significant preinterpretative phase)
- As soon as the resolution of core conflict is achieved, bring about termination.

Technique as Applies to Highly Resistant Patients

With patients on the right side of the spectrum, the course of the therapy is more complex. As I indicated earlier with this group of patients, central to Davanloo's technique is his systematic management of the resistance and unlocking of the patient's unconscious and the direct view of the multifoci core neurotic structure. Here the highlights of Davanloo's technique as applies to highly resistant character neurosis will be summarized:

1. The technique adheres strictly to psychoanalytic principle but is radically different from psychoanalytic technique.

2. Activity of the psychotherapist in handling resistance in terms of challenge and pressure and bringing about the unlocking of the patient's unconscious.

3. The technique used in the initial interview is essentially the technique used in the therapy with the exception of medical, psychiatric, and social history.

4. As already mentioned, the therapist actively works on two basic psychoanalytic triangles; triangle of conflict and the triangle of person.

5. Davanloo emphasizes that free-floating attention used in classical psychoanalysis is not sufficient; "vigilance" on the part of the therapist is essential.

6. The extensive use of interpretation after "unconscious therapeutic alliance" has been brought into operation.

He classifies interpretation in terms of the triangle of conflict, namely interpretation of impulse/feeling, anxiety, and defense; interpretation that involves the triangle of the conflict in relation to the triangle of the person, such as T-C, T-C-P interpretation. T-C-P interpretation is the interpretation of the impulse/feeling, anxiety, and defense in the transference and linking it with current and past significant people, with the patient experiencing the I/F in the transference. This was clearly demonstrated in this chapter—the case of the man with the baseball bat. Davanloo, in his systematic research, clearly demonstrates that response to T-C-P interpretation, after the unlocking of the unconscious, clearly correlates with the length of therapy.

7. Davanloo's reconceptualization of the analysis of transference is central to his system of Short-Term Dynamic Psychotherapy; the emphasis is on the extensive use of the transference.

8. Handling transference resistance. The therapist actively avoids the development of the transference neurosis. In the very early phase of treatment, when the therapist explores anxiety-laden, guilt-laden unconscious feelings, there is the possibility of the return of the resistance in the transference. Here the therapist must leave the content and rapidly focus on handling resistance in transference (1986a, 1986–1987). In the case of the man with the baseball bat, in the second interview he comes with memories that at night his mother used to lay down next to him at bedtime and make up fairy tales. The therapist had asked him to describe the body of his mother, in an attempt to explore the patient's erotized attachment to his mother. He immediately goes into a state of resistance in the transference. The following passage demonstrates the technique of handling transference resistance:

Pt: Hmm. (patient is tense, face was rigid, blank stare)

Th: Now you are slow, are you aware of that? Your smile is back.

Pt: Huh?

Th: How do you feel when I question you about your disappointment that she does not have large breasts?

Pt: Well, I feel stumped.

Th: Stumped is not a feeling. You are sitting there like a stump but that doesn't say how you feel towards me asking these questions?

Pt: I feel blocked.

Th: You are blocked, but that is still a crippled position.

Pt: I feel like I don't have anything to . . .

Th: Now you are taking a totally helpless, incapable, mute position with me.

Pt: Uh huh.

Th: But agreeing you are helpless is still helpless. What are you going to do about this crippled position you are taking here with me?

Pt: Uh. (smiling and taking a deep sigh)

Th: The smile is back, and you are sitting there totally paralyzed.

Pt: This isn't bad, I'm sitting here the whole time.

Th: Now sarcasm and still you are helpless to declare how you feel towards me asking these questions?

Pt: I feel irritated. (leaning forward)

Th: So you feel irritated. What way do you experience your irritation towards me?

Pt: I just felt the impulse of getting up and overturning your chair. (both hands thrusting out, concentrating on the therapist)

Th: How would you do it, if you put out your anger?

Pt: Just getting up, physically getting up, and grabbing your chair and throwing it.

Th: Throwing it over there. So what would happen to me?

Pt: You would be dumped out.

Th: And then what would happen?

Pt: Then you get up and strike me.

Th: I am going to retaliate against you?

Pt: Yes . . . when you were questioning me about my mother's breasts I felt as though I had no control. . . . There were ways that I was frightened of my father because he could be very, I felt as though he was more, that he was stronger and more defiant, stubborn, and I and uh, if . . .

Th: So with him, you felt he would win?

Pt: Yeah, often there was a battle between the two of us.

Th: Could we look to one of these battles?

Pt: I was scared that he would just blow up.

Th: Blow up and do what?

Pt: In a fit of anger. That he would just scream and get worse.

Th: He was drunk, and if he lost control of himself what was in your mind what might happen?

Pt: I was afraid he would have beaten me for not being . . .

Th: Beaten you with what?

Pt: That he would hit me with the bottle.

Th: So there was a sense that he may retaliate against you. What do you feel right now?

Pt: That memory makes me feel very sad.

Th: So what you say is that he might have struck you with that bottle but then at age 14, you had the club. Hmm? And what would he be saying as he lashed out?

Pt: He'd be saying, "I am the father here, you're not the father. I'm the boss, and you have no right to tell me what to do," and he would be hitting me at the same time. (patient very tearful)

9. Working through of the multifoci core neurotic structure. With the unlocking of the unconscious, fresh memories usually arise that clearly throw light on the whole development of the patient's neurotic conflicts. Fresh memories from earliest childhood experiences appear with the derepression at the C as well as in relation to the person in the patient's early life. There is emergence of complex feelings of rage, guilt, and grief-laden unconscious feelings in relation to the parents, parent substitute, siblings, and other significant persons in the patient's early life. For example, we saw this clearly in the case of the man with the baseball bat, his love and hate relationship with his brother and his father. We saw a process of derepression in relation to his brother, father, as well as his mother.

10. The process of decathexis. During the early and midphase of the therapy the process of decathexis of both positive and negative feelings in relation to parents and siblings takes place. We see the process of fresh memories with dramatic dreams, return of the recurrent dreams that contain the structure of the

patient's infantile neurosis. There is a major decathexis of sadistic impulses, anxiety-laden eroticized sexualized feeling, and guilt and grief-laden uncon-painful feelings.

11. Pathological mourning. In the cases that there is pathological mourning this is actively changed to acute grief reaction, and the first phase of the therapy would focus on the grief work. The case of the man with the baseball bat clearly demonstrates this point. The pathological mourning in relation to the death of his father was actively converted to a normal mourning process in the second interview when he indicated "I began to think more about my father." Becoming very sad and tearful, he talked about the "tape my father made, before he died," "I was listening to the tapes and felt that it was a tremendous gift."

12. Management of repetition compulsion. Davanloo, based on his extensive clinical data, has reformulated the metapsychology of repetition compulsion. He heavily emphasizes the role of punitive superego structure in the genesis and maintenance of neurotic disturbance. The heavy emphasis is on decathexis of the repressed sadism and guilt and grief-laden unconscious painful feeling as well as anxiety-laden erotized unconscious feeling in relation to the infantile object. In patients who show repetition compulsion in their current life, the major focus of the process is breaking through the dynamic forces underlying the forces of repetition compulsion, be it instinctual or arising from punitive superego. Davanloo's data show that the major dynamic force underlying the repetition compulsion arises from a punitive superego structure. The process of decathexis, having the ego experience all the unconscious repressed sadism, guilt-laden erotized unconscious feeling as well as guilt and grief-laden unconscious feeling has an important impact in the restructuring of the punitive superego.

13. The process of mourning. The third phase of the therapy mainly focuses on the process of guilt and grief that also involves mourning, the loss of a major portion of one's life because of neurotic suffering, missed opportunities, mourning the waste of one's life as a result of the repetitive sadomasochistic pattern in life, and finally the process enters to the phase of termination.

Outcome Evaluation

In Davanloo's system of Intensive Short-Term Dynamic Psychotherapy, the outcome of the therapy is validated by a sophisticated technique that involves interviews by both the therapist and an independent evaluator shortly after termination and up to 5 years later. In addition, Davanloo has introduced a specific technique of outcome evaluation (1978), "The Patient as the Evaluator of the Psychotherapeutic Process and Outcome." The patient observes five (randomly selected) of his audiovisually recorded psychotherapy sessions and determines the changes as well as those variables that the patient considers to be of specific importance in the outcome of his treatment. This is done 6 months to 1 year after termination, and the patient does not know about this procedure during the course of his therapy (Davanloo, 1980). Briefly what he considers to be a total psychodynamic change is total resolution of the patient's core neurotic conflict for patients at the extreme left of his spectrum. For patients on the right side of the spectrum, the psychodynamic change involves the total resolution of multifoci core neurotic structure.

In terms of outcome evaluation, Davanloo, in his first series, which involved assessment of 617 patients, demonstrated that 172 (28%) of these patients were candidates for the technique. Malan, in his paper (1986) indicated of the 172 patients, there was a successful outcome with total resolution of the core neurotic conflicts in 143 (83%). In summary, of a large series of patients that presented themselves to a general hospital outpatient psychiatric clinic for treatment, roughly 28% were suitable as candidates for the technique. Of this population, 83% showed positive outcomes judged by the criteria noted above.

Termination

Mann and Melges (1982) have written extensively on how the "timelessness" of long-term therapies becomes a neurotogenic factor, that is, giving the patient the unrealistic expectation that his or her lifetime is timeless. This encourages the magical thinking that time is endless or eternal rather than limited with finite boundaries. Davanloo's system of Intensive Short-Term Dynamic Psychotherapy, with the approximate termination date set at the end of the initial evaluation, forces the patient to recognize the reality that time is limited, separations do occur, and the results of the therapy will be evaluated at a specific time. By about the fifth to eighth psychotherapy session, the psychotherapeutic effect begins to arise. The patient starts to show a clear evidence of change both in his current life as well as in the transference. The therapy is not considered successful unless the patient is not only symptom free, but also the patient's maladaptive character defenses are replaced with adaptive character defenses. At the termination, the patient must have both cognitive and emotional insight into the structure of his pathology. Then the therapist considers termination. Davanloo's data from Intensive Short-Term Dynamic Psychotherapy research indicate that there is a correlation between the type of the patient and the process of termination. In patients with single psychotherapeutic focus of oedipal nature, termination takes place very spontaneously and without any difficulties. In patients where the psychotherapeutic focus is loss, the process of termination may last anywhere from two to three sessions. In patients with a complex multifoci core neurotic structure, termination might last between three to six sessions. Mourning the termination of the relationship with the therapist might become an essential part of the process. In a successful outcome, the patient generally refers to himself as a "free" person, as a "new" person. Dependence on the therapist is rarely a problem.

Summary and Conclusion

This chapter has outlined the contribution of the various schools of short-term dynamic psychotherapy since the contributions of Franz Alexander in the

1940s. The work of a number of clinical researchers, such as Malan at Tavistock Clinic, Sifneos and Mann in Boston, was summarized with particular attention to selection criteria, technical requirements, and phases of therapy. All of these schools have put heavy emphasis on using a process of evaluation and selection of patients that accept for treatment only those patients arriving who are highly motivated and responsive. This represents only a small proportion of those in need of psychotherapy. All of these schools, through their methods of selection, have avoided the problem of resistance in the psychotherapeutic process.

The major focus of this chapter has been on Davanloo's system of ISTDP. Davanloo's discovery of the "unlocking of the dynamic unconscious" is considered a major breakthrough in the field of dynamic psychiatry and in dynamic psychotherapy in particular. One of the major features of his system is his technique of handling resistance that has resulted in its being highly effective across a broad spectrum of the psychotherapeutic population.

ISTDP has application in the whole spectrum of structural neuroses, and this chapter has outlined this spectrum, indicating that on the left, there are the highly motivated/highly responsive, whereas on the right are the highly resistant, poorly motivated group of patients. This chapter emphasized that the major criteria for selection in ISTDP is the patient's response to a comprehensive trial therapy. Furthermore, the major ingredients of a complete psychodiagnostic evaluation have been summarized. With the case material, some of the major ingredients of the technique, such as management of resistance, extensive use of the transference, and handling transference were outlined. Indications and contraindications were briefly presented as were the process of working through, process of decathexis, management of repetition compulsion, and technique of handling pathological mourning. Finally, the chapter outlined the process of termination and highlighted the technique for outcome evaluation.

REFERENCES

Alexander, F., & French, T. M. (1946). *Psychoanalytic therapy*. New York: Ronald Press.
Davanloo, H. (1978). *Basic principles and techniques in Short-Term Dynamic Psychotherapy*. New York: Spectrum Publications.
Davanloo, H. (1980). Short-Term Dynamic Psychotherapy, New York: Jason Aronson.
Davanloo, H. (1984). Short-Term Dynamic Psychotherapy, Chapter 29.11. In H. Kaplan & B. Sadock (Eds.), *Comprehensive textbook of psychiatry* (4th ed., pp. 1460–1467). Baltimore: William & Wilkins.
Davanloo, H. (1986a). Intensive Short-Term Psychotherapy with highly resistant patients. I. Handling resistance. *International Journal of Short-Term Psychotherapy*, 1(2), 107–133.
Davanloo, H. (1986b). Intensive Short-Term Dynamic Psychotherapy with highly resistant patients, II. The Course of an interview after the initial breakthrough, *International Journal of Short-Term Psychotherapy*, 1(4), 239–256.
Davanloo, H. (1986–1987). Core Training Program, International Institute of Short-Term Dynamic Psychotherapy, Montreal.
Davanloo, H. (1987a). Intensive Short-Term Dynamic Psychotherapy with highly resistant depressed patients: Part I—Restructuring ego's regressive defenses. *International Journal of Short-Term Psychotherapy*, 2,(2), 99–132.

Davanloo, H. (1987b). Intensive Short-Term Dynamic Psychotherapy with highly resistant depressed patients: Part II—Royal road to the dynamic unconscious. *IJSTP, 2*(3), 167–185.

Davanloo, H. (1987c). 5th Summer Immersion Course of International Institute of STDP, August.

Davanloo, H. (1988). Unlocking the unconscious. *International Journal of Short-Term Psychotherapy, 3*(2), 100.

Freud, S. (1955). Translated and edited by J. Strachey. Vol. 2. Hogarth: London.

Linderman, E. (1979). *Beyond grief, studies in crisis intervention.* New York & London: Jason Aronson.

Malan, D. H. (1979). *Individual psychotherapy and the science of psychodynamics.* London: Butterworths.

Malan, D. H. (1986). Beyond interpretation, initial evaluation and technique. In *Short-Term Dynamic Psychotherapy* (Parts I & II), *1*(2), 59–106.

Mann, J. (1979). *Time-limited psychotherapy.* Cambridge, MA: Harvard University Press.

Mann, J., & Godlman, R. (1982). *A case book on time-limited psychotherapy.* New York: McGraw-Hill.

Melges, F. (1982). *Time and the inner future, a temporal approach to psychiatric disorders.* New York: John Wiley & Sons.

Said, T. (1986). Characterological depression and Short-Term Dynamic Psychotherapy, *International Journal of Short-Term Psychotherapy, 1*(4), 221–237.

Said, T., & Worchel, J. (1986). *Overview: Intensive Short-Term Dynamic Psychotherapy. International Journal of Short-Term Psychotherapy 1*(4), 281–295.

Sifneos, P. E. (1972). *Short-term psychotherapy and emotional crisis.* Cambridge, MA: Harvard University Press.

Worchel, J. (1986). Transference in Intensive Short-Term Dynamic Psychotherapy, I. Technique of handling initial transference. *International Journal of Short-Term Psychotherapy, 1*(2), 135–146.

Worchel, J. (1986). Transference in Intensive Short-Term Dynamic Psychotherapy. II. Technique of handling initial transference resistance. *International Journal of Short-Term Psychotherapy, 1*(3) 205–215.

10

Cognitive Therapy
Current Issues in Theory and Practice

MARLENE M. MORETTI, LISA A. FELDMAN, AND
BRIAN F. SHAW

The role of cognition in psychopathology has been the subject of considerable controversy during the past decade (Coyne & Gotlib, 1983, 1986; Segal & Shaw, 1986a,b). Not all theoretical models share the view that cognition is significant in the etiology or maintenance of psychopathology, even though negative thoughts and beliefs are widely recognized as important symptoms in several psychological disorders such as depression and anxiety disorder (American Psychiatric Association, 1987). Cognitive models of psychopathology stand in marked contrast to traditional psychodynamic and behavioral schools of thought in this regard.

Psychodynamic models of depression, for example, assume that the direct reports of patients are of limited importance apart from their value as "stepping stones" to underlying dynamic conflicts (Beck, 1976). From this perspective, negative thoughts may reflect transformed or indirect expressions of underlying conflicts, or they may operate as a form of defense to divert attention away from more significant emotionally distressing issues. Consequently, psychodynamic therapists are likely to treat the negative cognitions of depressed patients as secondary rather than primary symptoms of the disorder. Psychodynamic theorists reason that interventions directed at changing negative cognitions in depression are only effective in treating a symptom of the disorder and not the cause. Hence, they predict that such interventions are unlikely to produce lasting clinical improvement.

Behavioral models of depression (Coyne, 1976; Lewisohn, 1974) also contend that the negative thoughts and beliefs that occur in depression are of limited etiological significance. From the behavioral perspective, the negative cognitions experienced by depressed patients reflect the low rate of response-contingent positive reinforcement in their lives. The reduced rate of positive

MARLENE M. MORETTI AND LISA A. FELDMAN • Psychology Department, University of Waterloo, Waterloo, Ontario N2L 3G1, Canada.   BRIAN F. SHAW • Department of Psychology, Toronto General Hospital, 101 College Street, Toronto, Ontario M5G 117, Canada.

reinforcement experienced by depressed patients is thought to be caused by social maladjustment and social skill deficits (Bothwell & Weissman, 1977; Coyne, 1976; Ferster, 1974; Gotlib & Asarnow, 1979; Lewinsohn, 1974; Rounsaville, Weissman, Prusoff, & Herceg-Baron, 1979; Weismann, Paykel, Siegel, & Klerman, 1971). Psychotherapies that have evolved from this hypothesis focus on depressed patients' poor social skills and interactions as the primary targets of intervention. Although behavioral therapies such as thought-stopping techniques (Campbell, 1973; Hays & Waddell, 1976; Stern, 1978) have been developed to directly treat negative cognitions, these methods are based on the assumption that negative thoughts are simply additional behaviors and hold no etiological significance in and of themselves. Behavioral theorists claim that the effectiveness of interventions directly aimed at changing the negative cognitions that occur in depression is due to changes in behavior—that is, changes in cognition are secondary to behavioral alterations (Beidel & Turner, 1986).

In contrast to the psychodynamic and behavioral positions, cognitive models of depression emphasize the significance of negative beliefs and thoughts in the etiology and maintenance of the disorder. The most influential cognitive model of depression was developed by Aaron Beck primarily on the basis of case study and clinical observation (Beck, 1967, 1976). The pivotal assumption of Beck's cognitive model is that depression results from the development of dysfunctional cognitive representations or schemata about the self, the world, and the future. Once triggered, dysfunctional schemata negatively distort the processing of self-relevant information. This process gives rise to negative thoughts and feelings of dysphoria that maintain and exacerbate the depression (Beck, 1967, 1976). Cognitive therapy aims to alter these negative thoughts and beliefs and to help patients regain control over their thought processes (Beck, Rush, Shaw, & Emery, 1979; Moretti & Shaw, 1989).

In this chapter we present an overview of the theoretical basis for cognitive models of psychopathology, with particular emphasis on depression and anxiety disorder. We then review the application and effectiveness of cognitive therapy techniques for depression and make note of the limitations of current research and practice. We conclude with suggested directions for future research that may best advance our understanding of the etiology and treatment of psychopathology.

THE COGNITIVE MODEL: THEORETICAL RATIONALE

> You may say you experience the world directly, but in fact what you experience depends on a model of the world. (Johnson-Laird, 1983, p. 403)

Contemporary models of cognition maintain that in order to understand human functioning, we must recognize not only the role of the environment in directing an individual's experiences but also the role of that individual in interpreting environmental stimuli (Johnson-Laird, 1983; Neisser, 1976). This view departs radically from the position of James J. Gibson (1979), who has proposed that individuals are capable of directly encoding information in the environment without transformation or abstraction. It also differs from earlier models of human cognition that tended to overemphasize the role of perceivers in determining the nature of their experiences (e.g., Neisser, 1967). Rather, contemporary perspectives in cognition tend to stress the ongoing interaction between internal mental representations and external events. The individual is viewed as an active agent operating within a complex environmental context.

A fundamental assumption of cognitive models of psychopathology, then, is that individuals are active information processors. We "construct" our experiences, and these constructions largely determine our emotional reactions to events and future behaviors in similar situations. Our ability to construct internal cognitive representations of our experiences allows us to anticipate events and direct our behavior when confronted with complex environmental circumstances. Thus as Johnson-Laird (1983) points out, the construction of internal representations of the external world has important consequences for survival:

> More advanced organisms . . . do not merely react physically to their immediate environment, but seek to anticipate it since it is advantageous to avoid obstacles before bumping into them. Representations of the world . . . can be used in much the same way that a navigator uses a map to avoid danger and to reach a desired destination in safety. The richer and the more veridical the internal model, the greater will be the organism's chances of survival. (p. 402)

"Interactive" perspectives of this kind have important implications for understanding how individuals experience themselves and interpret self-referent information. In the same way that it is beneficial to develop mental representations of the environment in order to anticipate events and direct one's behavior, it is also advantageous to develop mental representations of the self. These representations are comprised of memories of behaviors, feelings, and interactions with others. The development of self-representations is influenced by events in our lives but once established, these representations begin to influence how we interpret new experiences that are self-relevant.

Self-representations can be useful in anticipating how we might behave and feel in certain situations and what we can expect in our interactions with others. As Johnson-Laird has suggested, however, the advantages offered by a representation depend upon the degree to which it is veridical. In some cases, individuals may develop distorted internal models of the self that are more dysfunctional than functional (Beck, 1967, 1976). Once established, these dysfunctional self-representations may further lead individuals to negatively distort experiences that are self-relevant.

In the next section of this chapter, we discuss cognitive models of psychopathology, the conditions that give rise to the development of dysfunctional cognitive representations, and the impact of these representations on the interpretation of experiences that involve the self.

COGNITIVE MODELS OF PSYCHOPATHOLOGY

The concepts of "cognitive schema" and "schema-driven information processing" are central to Beck's model of depression and anxiety (Beck, 1967, 1976, 1986). Beck adopts the term *schema* to refer to an internal mental representation of information that is relevant to one's understanding of the self, the world, and the future. Self-schemata may contain information about particular events that have occurred in the past, inferences or assumptions that have been made about the self, and rules or beliefs about how one negotiates interpersonal relationships.

Early interpersonal experiences have a direct and powerful impact on the development of self-schemata (Beck, 1987b; Beck & Young, 1985). Because these early experiences form a cognitive filter or guide for the interpretation of subsequent self-relevant experiences, they provide the groundwork for the development of a more elaborate view of the self. Beck (1967, 1976) suggests that if early interpersonal experiences are marked by either real or imagined losses or threats, then negative and dysfunctional schemas regarding the self, the world, and the future are likely to develop. Although these negative self-representations may be relatively inactive and dormant during periods of low stress, they can be primed and become operative during periods of high stress, particularly stress stemming from deprivation, rejection, or threat.

Beck maintains that the activation of negative schemata displaces more appropriate cognitive processes and disrupts processes involved in reality testing and attaining self-objectivity. As a consequence, the processing of self-relevant information is likely to be biased or inaccurate. For example, Beck (1967, 1976) suggests that the activation of negative self-schemata in depression causes depressed patients to negatively bias their interpretation of self-relevant information. These "errors" in cognitive functioning are viewed as distinct from the occasional inaccuracy or inconsistency of everyday cognitive processes because they represent a systematic negative bias with reference to the self.

Beck has identified three classes of cognitive errors that occur in depression: paralogical, stylistic, and semantic. Paralogical errors include drawing conclusions in the absence of evidence, in the face of contradictory evidence, on the basis of irrelevant details interpreted out of context, and on the basis of inadequate or nonrepresentative evidence. Stylistic errors consist of the systematic magnification or minimization of events or information so as to reach negative conclusions. Semantic errors are defined as erroneous or inappropriate labeling of events or outcomes on the bases of affective reactions rather than on the bases of actual intensity or importance of events. These errors in information processing result in extreme and global negative assessments about events that confirm patients' negative expectancies and strengthen their beliefs in the validity of dysfunctional assumptions and attitudes (Beck, 1987b; Beck *et al.*, 1979).

As psychopathology worsens, the processing of self-relevant information becomes increasingly dominated by dysfunctional schemata that have become "hyperactive" (Kovacs & Beck, 1979). Consequently, dysfunctional schemata are evoked in response to more diverse and less logically related information and experiences—that is, "the orderly matching of an appropriate schema to a particular stimulus is upset by the intrusion of these overly active idiosyncratic schemas" (Beck *et al.*, 1979, p. 13). In extreme instances, the processing of information may become dominated by dysfunctional schemata to the extent that patients are insensitive to environmental cues (Beck *et al.*, 1979). In such cases, dysfunctional schemata may be inappropriately used to interpret a wide range of events. Dysfunctional schemata also be applied during early and inappropriate stages of information processing, subsequently giving rise to idiosyncratic, dysfunctional, and inappropriate interpretations of events (Higgins & Moretti, 1988).

It is important to note that the activation of schemata during information processing occurs "automatically" (Moretti & Shaw, 1989). That is, schematic processing can be triggered by environmental stimuli without an individual's intent or awareness. Furthermore, the automatic activation of schemata during information processing may be extremely difficult to inhibit. This is not problematic when schemata are functional and aid in the appropriate interpretation of complex information. However, when dysfunctional schemata are automatically invoked, individuals are likely to be unaware of their operation and the effect that they exert on the interpretation of information. As Moretti and Shaw (1989) have indicated, the automaticity of these processes creates problems for individuals in the detection of error or inaccuracy during information processing. Quite simply, because individuals are unaware of the activation of dysfunctional schemata and their subsequent effects on processing self-relevant information, they are unlikely to doubt the validity of their interpretations.

In summary, a cognitive model of psychopathology such as Beck's emphasizes the interaction between dysfunctional self-schemata and stressful life experiences. Negative interpersonal and self-relevant experiences that occur early in life are seen as the *distal* causes of vulnerability to psychopathology. These experiences contribute to the development of dysfunctional self-schemata that may subsequently be activated by stressful life experiences. Stressful life experiences that activate dysfunctional schemata are seen as the *proximal* causes or precipitators of psychopathology (see Alloy, Abramson, Metalsky, & Hartlage, 1988, for a discussion of the notion of distal and proximal causes in psychopathology). Once activated, dysfunctional schemata displace other cognitive processes and lead to distortions in the processing of self-relevant information. Patients do not question the validity of their interpretations and are unaware of their errors or biases in processing self-relevant information because the operation of schemata during processing is automatic and may be triggered without awareness or intent and because the conclusions and interpretations that they reach confirm their original expectancies.

Cognitive models have been proposed for a large range of disorders including depression (Beck et al., 1979), anxiety disorders (Beck & Emery, 1985), and eating disorders (Garner, 1986; Garner & Bemis, 1984). In addition, recent attempts have been made to extend cognitive formulations to the understanding and treatment of stress-related disorders (Beck, 1984), multiple personality disorder (Caddy, 1985), hypochondriasis (Salkovskis & Warwick, 1986), chronic pain, and psychosomatic disorders (Beck, 1987b). In each case, the cognitive model proposes that the particular content of the dysfunctional cognitive schemata gives rise to the specific affective and behavioral symptoms that characterize the disorder (Beck, 1987b; Beck & Emery, 1985). Because it is beyond the scope of this chapter to review the cognitive formulation and treatment of all these disorders, we have chosen instead to focus on two disorders—depression and anxiety disorder—both of which have received considerable attention from researchers and clinicians adopting a cognitive perspective.

Depression

The essential feature of depression is dysphoric or depressed mood, with a loss of interest and pleasure in almost all activities. Associated symptoms include appetite disturbance, weight fluctuation, sleep disturbance, psychomotor agitation or retardation, energy loss, thinking and concentration difficulties, and recurrent thoughts of death or suicidal ideation (APA, 1987). The cognitive model of depression proposes that many of these symptoms are the result of a chronic negative bias in self-referent information processing (Beck, 1987a). Beck (1967, 1976) has identified three domains of self-referent information processing that are particularly relevant to understanding depression. These include an individual's view of the self, the world, and the future, known collectively as the "cognitive triad" (Beck et al., 1979). Clinical observations led Beck to conclude that the depressed patient's processing of information within each of these domains is marked by a strong negative bias. First, Beck (1967, 1976) noted that depressed individuals view themselves as personally inadequate and helpless. Second, he observed that they tend to misinterpret their interactions with others as representing rejection or deprivation. Finally, Beck found that depressed individuals anticipate that their current suffering will continue indefinitely and, as a consequence, they feel hopeless about the future.

Research clearly supports the contention that depressed persons' self-perceptions are more negative than those of nondepressed persons. Depressed individuals ascribe negative attributes to themselves (Beck, 1967; Derry & Kuiper, 1981; Kuiper & Derry, 1982; Kuiper & MacDonald, 1982; Sacco & Hokanson, 1978) and evaluate their performance as evidence of personal inadequacy and social ineptitude. In contrast to nondepressed persons, they are more likely to predict that they will fail in both achievement and interpersonal contexts (Dobson & Shaw, 1981; Gotlib, 1982; Gotlib & Olson, 1983; Lobitz & Post, 1979; Smolen, 1978; Wollert & Buchwald, 1979; Zarantello, Johnson, & Petzel, 1979), and they are more likely to attribute failure to internal rather than external causes (see Miller & Moretti, 1988, for a review). Furthermore, whereas depressed individuals attribute negative characteristics to themselves, they do not attribute these qualities to others (Hoehn-Hyde, Schlottman, & Rush, 1982; Tabachnik, Crocker, & Alloy, 1982). Depressed persons tend to perceive themselves as unique in their inadequacy and suffering. Conversely, nondepressed individuals estimate that others suffer from more negative experiences and characteristics than themselves.

The validity of the depressed individual's negative self-evaluations is currently a point of debate. Beck (1967, 1976) asserts that depressed persons are unrealistic and negatively biased in their self-appraisals. In opposition, Coyne (1976) contends that depressed individuals may be more accurate than nondepressed individuals in their self-evaluations. He maintains that the depressed patient's negative self-evaluations accurately reflect his or her social experiences. That is, the depressed person's "'distortions' and 'misconceptions' are congruent with the social system in which the depressed person . . . finds himself" (Coyne, 1976, p. 35). Although several studies have produced findings suggesting that depressed persons are accurate in their negative self-perceptions (Alloy & Abramson, 1979; Lewinsohn, Mischel, Chaplin, & Barton, 1980), many of these are flawed by conceptual and methodological problems. The most serious flaw in this research is the failure of investigators to rule out the possibility that the apparent "accuracy" of the depressed individual simply reflects a match between the depressive's negative response bias and the objective rates of negativity in the environment rather than realism or accuracy in perception (for a discussion of this issue, see Coyne & Gotlib, 1983, and Miller & Moretti, 1988).

Regardless of whether the depressed patient's negative self-perceptions are accurate or inaccurate, the motivational and behavioral consequences of these beliefs are clearly negative. For example, indecisiveness, noncommittment to goals, and "paralysis of will" may result from the depressed patient's expectation of and unwillingness to risk failure. Similarly, social withdrawal may stem from the belief that one will be rejected by others. Depressed individuals avoid rather than confront these potentially negative experiences. In doing so, they may create situations that confirm their negative expectancies while reducing the likelihood of experiencing disconfirming events. This cycle of negative expectancy, avoidance, and withdrawal maintains and exacerbates the disorder.

Recent theoretical developments of the cognitive model have focused on identifying individual difference factors that increase vulnerability to depression. In an attempt to explain why individuals differ in their reactions to stressful life events, Beck (1983) has described two personality traits—sociotropy and autonomy—that may predispose individuals to depression in response to specific types of life stressors. Sociotropy (or sociality) refers to "the beliefs, attitudes and goals that draw an individual to other persons" (Beck, Epstein, Harrison, & Emery, 1983, p. 1). Sociotropic individuals place a great deal of importance on interpersonal relationships and judge their self-worth according to the amount of acceptance and affection they receive from others. When confronted with a threat to the stability of interpersonal relationships (e.g., separation, threatened rejection) or an interpersonal loss (e.g., the breakup of a love relationship, the death of a loved one), such individuals are at risk for developing depression (Beck, 1983, 1987a). In contrast to sociotropy, autonomy (or independence) refers to beliefs about and attitudes toward achievement, personal freedom, and control over the environment. Autonomous individuals are likely to evaluate their self-worth in terms of personal accomplishments and control over their environment. When confronted with a threat to independence or autonomy (e.g., loss of a job, failure to achieve a desired goal), such individuals are at risk for developing depression (Beck, 1983, 1987a). Beck has observed that individuals who exhibit a strong tendency toward one or the other personality type are more likely than others to become depressed, although a combination of both types is evident in some depressed individuals. At present, however, it is unclear whether or not these two personality characteristics are causally related to the onset of depression.

In summary, current research investigating the cognitive model of depression supports the contention that the disorder is characterized by a pattern of persistent negative cognitions about the self. It is difficult to determine the veracity of negative self-evaluation in depression, particularly in light of the fact that negatively biased self-evaluations may lead individuals to interact with others in such a way as to elicit responses that confirm their negative expectancies. In addition, even though negative self-cognitions have been shown to co-occur with depression, the role of cognition as a precipitator of depression is less clear (Coyne & Gotlib, 1983). Lewinsohn, Steinmetz, Larsen, and Franklin (1981) investigated the causality of depression-related cognitions over a 1-year period. Contrary to Beck's model, expectancies for positive and negative events were not predictive of depression 1 year later. Furthermore, nondepressed individuals with a history of depressive illness were no more likely to show evidence of negative self-cognitions than were nondepressed individuals with no history of the illness. However, depressed individuals who reported negative self-cognitions tended to experience longer depressive episodes than did individuals who did not report these cognitions.

In reviewing these findings, it is important to note Beck's assertions that negative self-schemata remain inactive during periods of low stress. Thus Beck would not necessarily predict that remitted depressed patients would differ from nondepressed individuals in their thoughts and beliefs about themselves. However, it may be the case that remitted depressed patients process self-referent information in a negatively biased manner under conditions that prime or temporarily activate negative self-schemata. For example, cognitive vulnerability to depression may be apparent in self-referent information processing under conditions of real, or imagined, loss or failure. In addition, it is important for researchers and clinicians to recognize that the cognitive model of depression is an interaction model: Cognitive vulnerability is predicted to interact with life stress to produce depression. Further investigations that take these factors into account will be helpful in clarifying the etiological role of cognition in depression.

Anxiety Disorders

Anxiety disorders include a group of syndromes in which individuals experience subjective anxiety and exhibit avoidance behavior (APA, 1987). The cognitive model of anxiety disorder proposes that anxiety symptoms result from dysfunctional cognitive processes. Although depressive symptoms are believed to arise in response to cognitions of loss and failure, anxiety symptoms are thought to arise in response to cognitions of danger and vulnerability.

As Beck (1986) points out, the accurate detection of threat and danger in the environment has important implications for survival. To facilitate the efficient detection of danger, humans have developed a variety of mechanisms, including the ability to form mental representations of the environment in memory (i.e., schemata), that allow us to anticipate and avoid potentially dangerous situations. Such mental representations help us to quickly and efficiently assess the amount of danger present in a given situation (primary appraisal) and to evaluate our vulnerability and our ability to cope with the event (secondary appraisal).

Several coping strategies have evolved for dealing with perceived threat and danger in the environment, including (1) affective reactions involving the experience of fear; (2) physiological reactions involving activation of the autonomic nervous system (either fight, flight, freeze, or faint reactions); and (3) behavioral reactions involving activation of the somatic nervous system. The mobilization of these systems is experienced as (1) subjective anxiety in response to the fear; (2) physiological sensations associated with sympathetic and parasympathetic nervous system activation (e.g., heart palpitations, nausea, dizziness); and (3) increased or decreased muscular tone.

Fear is experienced when people are exposed to situations that they perceive as dangerous. In such circumstances, an unpleasant emotional state of anxiety ensues. Normally, anxiety has an important protective function in that it forces individuals to attend to potentially dangerous circumstances and to activate coping strategies (Beck, 1986). The adaptiveness of this "alarm" system depends on an accurate appraisal of threat and danger in the environment. When affective, physiological, and behavioral systems are activated in response to inaccurately perceived danger, arousal is no longer congruent with the actual conditions present in the environment and is therefore maladaptive (Beck, 1986).

In most individuals, feelings of fear and anxiety are based on an accurate assessment of the possibility of harm or danger in the environment. Individuals who suffer from anxiety disorders, however, overestimate or magnify the amount of potential danger in certain situations and evaluate themselves as vulnerable to these perceived dangers (Beck & Emery, 1985). It is convenient to think of a person who suffers from anxiety disorder as possessing an "overactive alarm system" where cues from the environment, processed automatically, result in an overwhelming sense of vulnerability (Beck, 1986). Such automatic and dysfunctional systems of processing information leave these individuals "overprepared, overvigilant, and overreactive" (Beck, 1986). The inaccurate appraisal of threat leads to avoidance behavior, which, in turn, prevents these individuals from engaging in activities that would disconfirm their dysfunctional beliefs and expectancies. Anticipatory anxiety, which often appears to maintain and exacerbate an anxiety disorder, can also be understood in terms of this framework. Here, the anticipation or fear of experiencing anxiety and feelings of vulnerability triggers arousal and, ultimately, the anxiety experience.

It is important to note that anxiety disorders are not a homogeneous group of syndromes. Although the experience of the anxiety is common across syndromes, the pattern of associated symptoms differs from disorder to disorder. For example, the predominant symptom in panic disorder and in generalized anxiety disorder is the experience of subjective anxiety, whereas the predominant symptom in phobic disorders and in obsessive–compulsive disorder is avoidance behavior. There has been relatively little attention directed toward understanding the relation between the specific content of vulnerability schemata and the manifestation of one anxiety disorder versus another. It may be that patients who suffer from panic disorder misperceive internal sensations as dangerous and threatening, whereas patients who suffer from generalized anxiety disorder overestimate their vulnerability to many external events. In contrast, people who suffer from phobias may be concerned with their vulnerability to circumscribed, specific external events (Beck, 1986).

Recent theoretical developments have focused on increasing the specificity of the cognitive model for understanding obsessive–compulsive disorder. Beck's (1986) cognitive model of obsessional disorders views pathology as resulting from obsessional thoughts with themes involving danger and vulnerability. A modification to this viewpoint has been forwarded by Salkovskis (1985). He argues that intrusive thoughts with disturbing content, usually involving harm to the self or to others, occur frequently in the experience of normal individuals without leading to serious and long-lasting mood disturbances or obsessive behaviors. Salkovskis further contends that these thoughts lead to severe distress and pathological behavior only when individuals assume personal responsibility for having these thoughts. This perspective is, in many ways, consistent with the notion of "magical thinking," a type of ideation that commonly appears to maintain these disorders. In short, when intrusive thoughts with disturbing content are accompanied by beliefs of personal responsibility, patients are likely to experience feelings of guilt. As a consequence, patients feel responsible for the harm that may come to the self or to others. Because obsessive patients view intrusive thoughts as abnormal and equivalent to engaging in unacceptable behavior, they are led to engage in behaviors that compensate for or undo the imagined consequences of their acts. Salkovskis's view of obsessive patients represents a theoretical reconceptualization of obsessive–compulsive disorder and may have important treatment implications.

Cognitive Therapy

Cognitive therapy adopts a time-limited and highly structured approach to the treatment of emotional disorders. Typically, patients are seen individually on a weekly basis over a period of 20 weeks. However, this basic format has been modified to meet the needs of patients with problems other than depression or anxiety (e.g., Caddy, 1985; Garner, 1986) and to develop other treatment formats such as group therapy (see Beck *et al.*, 1979). Because cognitive therapy adopts a time-limited approach to treatment, it is important that patient characteristics be reviewed prior to initiation of therapy in order to establish a "fit" between patient needs, strengths, and weaknesses, and the cognitive therapy approach. It is also important that therapists establish clear therapy goals at the outset of therapy and work consistently toward these goals in each session. The following discussion focuses on the relevance of these two factors in the cognitive therapy of depression.

Patient Selection

A number of patient factors have been identified as potentially important outcome predictors in cognitive therapy (Safran, Shaw, Segal, & Vallis, 1988). Two factors are the patient's awareness of and ability to report his or her intrusive negative thoughts and the patient's awareness of fluctuations in his or her emotions. To the extent that these thoughts are identifiable by the patients, they will be more readily available for review and evaluation during therapy. On the other hand, patients who are overwhelmed by negative feelings and relatively unaware of internal cognitive processes will be hindered in the process of therapy. For example, a patient, who reports that her feelings of depression are stronger when she thinks about her failings as a mother will be more likely to benefit from cognitive therapy than a patient who reports that feelings of depression fluctuate independently of his, or her, thoughts or life events. Patients who are aware of fluctuations in their feelings can use their feelings as cues to underlying dysfunctional thought processes. That is, they will be able to learn to stop and take notice of their thoughts as their moods fluctuate. These patients are more likely to benefit from cognitive therapy than are patients who are unaware of fluctuations in their emotional state and who may have difficulty identifying the relation between their thought processes and exacerbated negative moods.

These two factors—the ability to identify intrusive negative thoughts and the awareness of emotional fluctuations—will influence the extent to which patients can understand their experiences within a cognitive therapy framework. The greater the congruency between patients' psychological experiences and the rationale for understanding emotional distress provided in cognitive therapy, the more likely they are to benefit from therapy.

There are several additional factors that should be considered in selecting patients for cognitive therapy. One factor is for patients' understanding and acceptance that the focus of cognitive therapy is on contemporary rather than historical factors as precipitators of emotional distress. Although dysfunctional beliefs may stem from experiences in the past, cognitive therapy maintains that an understanding of the source of dysfunctional beliefs is neither necessary nor sufficient to produce change. Patients wishing to focus on issues in their past are more likely to benefit from long-term dynamic psychotherapy than from cognitive therapy. This rule need not be rigidly enforced, however, as a very brief exploration of historical issues may sometimes elucidate a patient's current dysfunctional beliefs.

Another factor to be considered in patient selection concerns the patient's ability to establish a trusting and collaborative relationship with his or her therapist and their ability to assume personal responsibility for change. Patients who require a lengthy period to establish a working relationship with their therapist and have difficulty accepting their role in the change process are unlikely to derive maximal benefit from a brief therapy such as cognitive therapy.

Diagnostic factors also warrant consideration in the process of patient selection. As Beck et al. (1979) point out, the efficacy of cognitive therapy has been established only for unipolar, nonpsychotic, depressed outpatients. Hence, patients suffering from bipolar illnesses or personality disorders that are accompanied by periods of depression (e.g., borderline disorders) may be inappropriate for cognitive therapy treatment. In addition, the therapist should carefully consider the need for pharmacotherapy in conjunction with cognitive therapy in the treatment of severe depressive illness.

Therapeutic Techniques and Goals

A fundamental goal of cognitive therapy is to help the depressed or anxious patient regain control over his or her thought processes (Beck & Emery, 1985; Beck et al., 1979). In order to achieve this goal within 20 sessions, therapists are advised to structure each session by constructing an agenda with the aid of the patient. The first 3 to 4 sessions should focus on assessing the central problems, establishing therapeutic rapport, and explaining the rationale for cognitive therapy to the patient. Following this, therapy should increasingly focus on the identification and modification of dysfunctional thought processes (Beck et al., 1979). The first step in this process is to increase the patient's awareness of his or her dysfunctional thought processes. This can be achieved by asking patients to use their negative feelings as a "cue" to underlying thought processes. For example, depressed patients can be asked to take note of any fluctuation in their feelings, to record external events that occurred at the time of the fluctuation, and to record their own thoughts about the events. This information can be recorded on the Daily Record of Dysfunctional Thoughts (see Beck et al., 1979).

The patient's monitoring of his or her thought processes will often reveal that idiosyncratic and dysfunctional interpretations of life events are important precipitators of negative mood. For example, one patient reported feeling confused and depressed when she came in for her therapy session. The therapist asked the patient to recall when she had first noticed these feelings. The patient reported that she had become extremely dysphoric and confused on the previous day following a friend's compliment on her "informal and easygoing" manner of interacting with others. Initially, her feelings of increased depression and confusion were difficult to reconcile with the objectively positive nature of this interaction. Her feelings made sense, however, when she recalled her thoughts at the time of the "compliment." This patient had interpreted her friend's compliment as a disguised criticism of her lack of social etiquette and sophistication—inadequacies the patient feared she possessed. Once she became aware of her interpretation of this event, the patient was able to discuss her more general belief that she needed to interact with others in a "socially appropriate" way in order to be accepted. This, in turn, led to a discussion of the validity of the patient's rigid beliefs and of what was implied by the term socially appropriate. Not only did the patient reconsider her interpretation of the event that led her to feel distressed, but she also began to reconsider her beliefs about the type of person she needed to be in order for others to accept her. As a result of this process, her feelings of dysphoria and confusion decreased. Her feelings of helplessness and hopelessness were alleviated because she was now able to identify the precipitants of her negative feelings. She could understand the relation between her thoughts and feelings.

Once patients become aware of their self-relevant thoughts and beliefs, they are encouraged to evaluate the accuracy or validity of these cognitions rather than to simply inhibit or replace them. Sometimes merely becoming aware of underlying beliefs and thoughts is sufficient for patients to recognize their lack of evidence and rationality. However, therapists are advised to fully explore the meaning of a patient's dysfunctional belief and the relation of this belief with other self-evaluative beliefs. Whenever possible, patients should be encouraged to "check out" or "test" the validity of their interpretations by setting up "experiments" outside of the therapy session. These experiments should be co-designed by the therapist and the patient, with the former displaying sensitivity to the latter's level of functioning.

As Moretti and Shaw (1989) have suggested, many patients experience difficulties in interrupting dysfunctional thought processes and reviewing their interpretations and beliefs. This problem frequently arises when patients are overwhelmed by emotional distress. In such situations, patients report that although they know their interpretations are biased and inaccurate, they are unable to inhibit or alter them. When this happens, it is important for therapists to help patients understand that the alteration of chronic cognitive processes requires time and practice. Even if patients are unable to identify and alter dysfunctional thought processes as they occur, they are often able to review them shortly thereafter. This can provide relief from negative feelings and the opportunity for patients to consider alternative and more adaptive interpretations of self-relevant events.

In light of the time-limited approach to treatment adopted by cognitive therapy, it is imperative that patients continue to practice techniques during and following the termination of therapy. Patients should be advised that fluctuations in mood are to be expected following termination and that the skills they have learned during therapy can be used to understand and cope with stressful events and periods of dysphoria. "Booster" sessions (Beck et al., 1979) several weeks following termination, and at 3 or 6 months follow-up, can provide patients with useful opportunities to review coping strategies for stressful life events. Such sessions help patients maintain the gains that they have made in therapy.

Efficacy of Cognitive Therapy

Rush, Beck, Kovacs, and Hollon (1977) conducted the first study comparing the efficacy of cognitive therapy for treating depression with that of pharmacotherapy in a clinical outpatient sample. This study randomly assigned patients with clear diagnoses of depression (of at least moderate severity) to 12 weeks of either cognitive therapy or pharmacotherapy (Imipramine up to 250 mg per day). At the end of the 12-week treatment period, the patients who received cognitive therapy had improved significantly more than the patients who received Imipramine. Although the two groups did not significantly differ at 1-year follow-up, patients treated with medication were twice as likely to have relapsed during the year than were patients treated with cognitive therapy (Kovacs, Rush, Beck, & Hollon, 1981). This finding is particularly intriguing given the recurrent nature of major depression (see Keller, Shapiro, Lavori, & Wolfe, 1982).

Since this initial investigation, other studies have examined the relative efficacy of cognitive therapy as compared with other types of psychotherapies and pharmacotherapy. McLean and Hakstian (1979) compared the relative effectiveness of a modified cognitive therapy approach to short-term psychotherapy, pharmacotherapy (Amitriptyline at 150 mg per day), and a relaxation training control group. Their evaluation of 178 patients given primary diagnoses of severe depression revealed a clear-cut advantage of cognitive therapy over the other treatments for depression. Because this study controlled for the amount of therapist contact in each type of treatment, alternative explanations for the greater efficacy of cognitive therapy were ruled out.

Teasdale, Fennel, Hibbert, and Amies (1984) evaluated the addition of cognitive therapy to patients' usual treatment, which consisted primarily of their doctors' choices of antidepressant medication. By the completion of treatment, clinical ratings of symptom severity and self-report measures of depression indicated that patients receiving the combination of cognitive therapy and their usual treatment were significantly less depressed than were those who received only their usual treatment. At a 3-month follow-up, there were no significant differences between the two groups, due mainly to the continued improvement of the usual-treatment group. The most important finding in this study, then, was that the addition of a psychotherapeutic program such as cognitive therapy can have a substantial effect on the rate of recovery of patients with major depressive disorder. Similar results have been reported by Beck, Hollon, Young, Bedrosian, and Budenz (1985) in a 12-week protocol comparison of cognitive therapy alone with a cognitive therapy–amitriptyline combination.

Blackburn, Bishop, Glen, Whalley, and Christie (1981) studied two groups of unipolar, depressed outpatients who received either cognitive therapy alone, or medication alone, or a combination of both. These researchers found that general practice patients treated with cognitive therapy, either alone or in combination with medication, showed a markedly superior outcome to those patients receiving only pharmacotherapy. In their hospital outpatient sample, they found that the combination of cognitive therapy and medication was the most effective treatment, with cognitive therapy alone proving to be only minimally more effective than the pharmacotherapy. Although these results suggest that the effectiveness of cognitive therapy alone or in combination with pharmacotherapy depends on the patient population, they should be interpreted with caution because of several methodological weaknesses in the study. First, there were low numbers of patients receiving pharmacotherapy in the general practice sample. Second, the therapists in the two settings differed, thereby introducing the possibility that the results found were due to differences in therapist, not treatment, efficacy. Hence, the findings of Blackburn *et al.* do not allow us to draw clear conclusions about the relative efficiency of cognitive therapy alone and in combination with other treatments for different patient populations.

Murphy, Simons, Wetzel, and Lustman (1984) conducted a study similar to that of Blackburn *et al.* (1981) but included an additional group receiving a combination of cognitive therapy with a placebo. In contrast to Blackburn *et al.*'s results, Murphy *et al.* (1984) found no differences between their four treatment groups. That is, all patients benefitted to an equal degree, whether they received cognitive therapy alone, cognitive therapy in combination with pharmacotherapy (Nortriptyline prescribed according to carefully monitored blood levels), cognitive therapy in combination with a placebo, or pharmacotherapy alone. Although the patients receiving different treatments did not differ at the end of the treatment period, intriguing results emerged during the follow-up period. Murphy *et al.* reported that, by 1-month follow-up, all treatment groups had maintained their improvements. However, by 1-year follow-up, patients who had received cognitive therapy were significantly less likely to have relapsed than were those treated with Nortriptyline alone (relapse was defined as a return to symptoms or a return to treatment following success in the initial trial). There was no difference in the relapse rates of patients receiving cognitive therapy alone versus those receiving cognitive therapy combined with Nortiptyline. This latter finding is comparable to that found by Beck *et al.* (1985).

Blackburn, Eunson, and Bishop (1986) recently reported a 2-year follow-up of patients from their original 1981 study. Within 6 months of treatment termination, there were significantly more relapses in the pharmacotherapy group as compared with the cognitive therapy groups. Moreover, the number of patients who relapsed within the 2-year period was significantly higher in the pharmacotherapy group than in the cognitive therapy groups. This result suggests again that cognitive therapy has an important prophylactic effect with respect to relapses.

It is important to note that the follow-up studies cited above were "naturalistic" in design and were therefore plagued with methodological difficulties. Such difficulties include the follow-up of patients who are successfully treated, the definition of relapse, and the issue of maintenance medication (i.e., whether or not medication is continued beyond the point of symptom remission). A number of studies have attempted to control for some of these problems, and their results suggest that treatment with cognitive therapy is at least equally effective to treatment with antidepressant drugs (see Covi, Lipman, Roth, Pattison, Smith, & Lasseter, in press; Hollon, Tuason, Weiner, DeRubeis, Evans, & Garvey, 1983; Rotzer, Nabitz, Koch, & Pflug, 1982). The follow-up results of Hollon, Evans, and DeRubeis (1988) are particularly informative in this respect. Although limited by a relatively small sample size (approximately 10 observations per cell), Hollon *et al.* found that patients given cognitive therapy had a 2-

year relapse rate of 20%, whereas those given Imipramine with no maintenance dose had a relapse rate of 50%. These investigators also included a 1-year maintenance Imipramine group and found that providing a maintenance dosage of antidepressant reduced the relapse rate to 30%. This rate of relapse was not significantly different from that of the cognitive therapy group. A relapse rate of 23% was found for those patients given a combination of the two treatments.

There have also been several summary and meta-analytic reviews of the efficacy of cognitive therapy for the treatment of depression. For example, Dobson (in press) completed a meta-analytic review of 20 studies evaluating the efficacy of cognitive therapy for depression. The results of this review indicated that depressed patients treated with cognitive therapy showed greater improvement than did patients treated with behavior therapy or pharmacotherapy or patients who received no treatment. Cognitive therapy also tended to be more effective than other forms of psychotherapy (e.g., interpersonal therapy, nondirective therapy), although not significantly so. These findings are generally consistent with the results of other meta-analytic reviews (Hollon & Beck, 1986; Miller & Berman, 1983; Nietzel, Russell, Hemmings, & Gretter, 1987; Steinbreuck, Maxwell, & Howard, 1983; Weissman, 1979; Williams, 1984) indicating that cognitive therapy is significantly more effective in treating unipolar, nonpsychotic, mild-to-moderately depressed patients than is pharmacotherapy (primarily tricyclic antidepressants) alone. There remains some question, however, as to the efficacy of cognitive therapy for the treatment of unipolar depression relative to that of other forms of psychotherapy (e.g., Klerman, Weissman, Rounsaville, & Chevron, 1984).

The overall results of this research support the efficacy of cognitive therapy in the treatment of unipolar, nonpsychotic, depressed outpatients. More recent work has extended these findings to demonstrate the efficacy of cognitive therapy for elderly depressed patients (see Thompson, Gallagher, & Breckenridge, 1987) and as an adjunctive treatment to the usual inpatient programs (see Miller, Bishop, Norman, & Keitner, 1985; Wright, 1987). Although the research to date generally provides support for the contention that cognitive therapy is effective in treating depression, there are a number of unresolved issues that qualify this support. First, the results indicate that the conclusions investigators reach regarding the effectiveness of cognitive therapy depend on whether they evaluate outcomes immediately following therapy or at follow-ups of 1 or 2 years. Second, researchers need to consider the impact of patient therapy-modality preference on the efficacy of treatment. For example, in the Rush *et al.* (1977) study, there was a marked difference between the dropout rates for patients receiving cognitive therapy (5%) and those for patients receiving pharmacotherapy (32%). This is clearly a significant factor in evaluating the efficacy of different treatments. Finally, it is important that future research address the question of whether or not particular types of treatments are more effective for particular types of patients. An increased understanding of any or all of these factors would be helpful to clinicians in determining the cost-effectiveness of cognitive therapy as opposed to, or in conjunction with, other types of treatments.

SUMMARY

The development of cognitive representations of information pertaining to the self and the environment has important implications for adaptive functioning. Such representations or schemata can help individuals to anticipate environmental and interpersonal events and to activate strategies for coping with stressful or threatening events should they arise. For most individuals, a schematic representation of the self leads to efficient, automatic processing of information and to adaptive responding. However, when schematic representations embody dysfunctional beliefs regarding the self and inaccurate information about the environment, they may produce distortions in the processing of self-relevant information. In the depressed patient these distortions include pervasive negative self-evaluations and perceptions of rejection and disappointment in interpersonal relationships. The activation of dysfunctional schemata in the anxious patient results in exaggerated or magnified estimates of threat and self-perceptions of vulnerability and helplessness.

Cognitive therapy adopts a time-limited and highly structured approach to the treatment of these disorders. Patients who are able to access automatic thoughts and to identify and differentiate their emotional states are most likely to benefit from cognitive therapy. Therapeutic improvement is also more likely to occur for patients who accept personal responsibility for change without self-blame and criticism and are able to establish a trusting and collaborative relationship with their therapist.

The fundamental goal of cognitive therapy is to help patients identify, and change, underlying or core beliefs about the self and dysfunctional patterns of processing self-relevant information. Current research indicates that cognitive therapy is at least as effective as antidepressant medication in the treatment of depression. Moreover, follow-up studies suggest that relapse rates are considerably lower for patients receiving cognitive therapy than for patients receiving pharmacotherapy alone. Although the efficacy of cognitive therapy is clearly supported by treatment trials to date, further research is necessary to overcome methodological flaws of earlier studies and to further establish the role of patient factors as outcome predictors.

REFERENCES

Alloy, L. B., & Abramson, L. Y. (1979). Judgments of contingency in depressed and nondepressed students: Sadder but wiser? *Journal of Experimental Psychology: General, 108,* 441–445.

Alloy, L. B., Abramson, L. Y., Metalsky, G. I., & Hartlage, S. (1988). The hopelessness theory of depression: Attributional aspects. *British Journal of Clinical Psychology, 27,* 5–21.

American Psychiatric Association. (1987). *Diagnostic and statistical manual of mental disorders, third edition—revised.* Washington, DC: American Psychiatric Association.

Beck, A. T. (1967). *Depression: Clinical, experimental, and theoretical aspects.* New York: Harper & Row.

Beck, A. T. (1976). *Cognitive therapy and the emotional disorders.* Madison, Ct: International Universities Press, Inc.

Beck, A. T. (1983). Cognitive therapy of depression: New perspectives. In P. J. Clayton & J. E. Barrett (Eds.), *Treatment of depression: Old Controversies and new Approaches* (p. 265–290). New York: Raven Press.

Beck, A. T. (1984). Cognitive approaches to stress. In R. L. Woolfolk & P. M. Lehrer (Eds.), *Principles and practice of stress management* (pp. 255–305). New York: Guilford Press.

Beck, A. T. (1986). Cognitive approaches to anxiety disorders. In B. F. Shaw, Z. V. Segal, T. M. Vallis, & F. E. Cashman (Eds.), *Anxiety disorders, psychological and biological perspectives* (pp. 115–135). New York: Plenum Press.

Beck, A. T. (1987a). Cognitive models of depression. *Journal of Cognitive Psychotherapy, An International Quarterly, 1*, 5–37.

Beck, A. T. (1987b). Cognitive therapy. In Jeffrey K. Zeig (Ed.), *The evolution of psychotherapy* (pp. 149–163). New York: Brunner/Mazel Publishers.

Beck, A. T., & Emery, G. (1985). *Anxiety disorders and phobias: A cognitive perspective.* New York: Basic Books.

Beck, A. T., & Young, J. E. (1985). Depression. In D. H. Barlow (Ed.), *Clinical handbook of psychological disorders* (pp. 206–244). New York: Guilford Press.

Beck, A. T., Rush, A. J., Shaw, B. F., & Emery, G. (1979). *Cognitive therapy of depression.* New York: Guilford Press.

Beck, A. T., Epstein, N., Harrison, R. P., & Emery, G. (1983). *Development of the sociotropy-autonomy scale: A measure of personality factors in psychopathology.* Unpublished manuscript, University of Pennsylvania.

Beck, A. T., Hollon, S. D., Young, J. E., Bedrosian, R. C., & Budenz, D. (1985). Treatment of depression with cognitive therapy and amitriptyline. *Archives of General Psychiatry, 42*, 142–148.

Beidel, D. C., & Turner, S. M. (1986). A critique of the theoretical bases of cognitive-behavioral theories and therapy. *Clinical Psychology Review, 6*, 177–197.

Blackburn, I. M., Bishop, S., Glen, A. I. M., Whalley, L. J., & Christie, J. E. (1981). The efficacy of cognitive therapy in depression: A treatment trial using cognitive therapy and pharmacotherapy, each alone and in combination. *British Journal of Psychiatry, 139*, 181–189.

Blackburn, I. M., Eunson, K. M., & Bishop, S. (1986). A two-year naturalistic follow-up of depressed patients treated with cognitive therapy, pharmacotherapy, and a combination of both. *Journal of Affective Disorders, 10*, 67–75.

Bothwell, S., & Weismann, M. (1977). Social impairments four years after an acute depressive episode. *American Journal of Orthopsychiatry, 47*, 231–237.

Caddy, G. R. (1985). Cognitive behavior therapy in the treatment of multiple personality. *Behavior Modification, 9*, 267–292.

Campbell, L. M. (1973). A variation of thought-stopping in a twelve year old boy: A case report. *Journal of Behaviour Therapy and Experimental Psychiatry, 4*, 69–70.

Covi, L., Lipman, R. S., Roth, D., Pattison, J. H., Smith, J. E., & Lasseter, V. K. (in press). Cognitive group psychotherapy in depression: A pilot study. *American Journal of Psychiatry.*

Coyne, J. C. (1976). Depression and the response of others. *Journal of Abnormal Psychology, 85*, 186–193.

Coyne, J. C., & Gotlib, I. H. (1983). The role of cognition in depression: A critical appraisal. *Psychological Bulletin, 94*, 472–505.

Coyne, J. C., & Gotlib, I. H. (1986). Studying the role of cognition in depression. Well troden paths and cul-de-sacs. *Cognitive Therapy and Research, 55*, 347–352.

Derry, P. A., & Kuiper, N. A. (1981). Schematic processing and self-reference in clinical depression. *Journal of Abnormal Psychology, 90*, 286–297.

Dobson, K. S. (in press). A meta-analysis of the efficacy of cognitive therapy for depression. *Journal of Consulting and Clinical Psychology.*

Dobson, K. S., & Shaw, B. F. (1981). The effects of self-correction on cognitive distortions in depression. *Cognitive Therapy and Research, 5*, 391–403.

Ferster, C. B. (1974). Behavioral approaches to depression. In R. J. Friedman & M. Katz (Eds.), *The psychology of depression: Contemporary theory and research* (pp. 29–45). Washington, DC: Winston.

Garner, D. M. (1986). cognitive therapy for bulimia nervosa. In S. C. Feinstein (Ed.), *Adolescent psychiatry: Developmental and clinical studies* (Vol. 13, pp. 358–390). Chicago: The University of Chicago Press.

Garner, D. M., & Bemis, K. M. (1984). Cognitive therapy for anorexia nervosa. In D. M. Garner & P. E. Garfinkel (Eds.), *Handbook of psychotherapy for anorexia nervosa and bulimia* (pp. 107–146). New York: Guilford Press.

Gibson, J. J. (1979). *The ecological approach to visual perception*. Boston: Houghton Mifflin.

Gotlib, I. H. (1982). Self-reinforcement and depression in interpersonal interaction: The role of performance level. *Journal of Abnormal Psychology, 88*, 454–457.

Gotlib, I. H., & Asarnow, R. (1979). Interpersonal and impersonal problem-solving skills in mildly and clinically depressed university students. *Journal of Consulting and Clinical Psychology, 47*, 86–95.

Gotlib, I. H., & Olson, J. M. (1983). Depression, psychopathology, and self-serving attributions. *Journal of Personality and Clinical Psychology, 22*, 309–310.

Hays, V., & Waddell, K. J. (1976). A self-reinforcing procedure for thought-stopping *Behavior Therapy, 7*, 559.

Higgins, E. T., & Moretti, M. M. (1988). Standard utilization and the self-evaluative process: Vulnerability to types of aberrant beliefs. In T. F. Oltmanns & B. A. Maher (Eds.), *Delusional beliefs* (pp. 110–137). New York: Wiley and Sons.

Hoehn-Hyde, D., Schlottman, R. S., & Rush, A. J. (1982). Perception of social interactions in depressed psychiatric patients. *Journal of Consulting and Clinical Psychology, 50*, 209–212.

Hollon, S. D., & Beck, A. T. (1986). Psychotherapy and drug therapy: Comparison and combinations. In S. L. Garfield & A. E. Bergin (Eds.), *The handbook of psychotherapy and behavior change* (2nd ed.) (pp. 443–482). New York: John Wiley and Sons.

Hollon, S. D., Evans, M. D., & DeRubeis, R. J. (1988). Preventing relapse following treatment for depression: The cognitive pharmacotherapy project. In T. M. Fields, P. M. McCabe, & N. Schneiderman (Eds.), *Stress and coping across development* (pp. 227–243). New York: Lawrence Erlbaum.

Hollon, S. D., Tuason, V. B., Weiner, M. J., DeRubeis, R. J., Evans, M. D., & Garvey, M. (1983). *Combined cognitive-pharmacotherapy with cognitive therapy alone and pharmacotherapy alone in the treatment of depressed outpatients. Differential treatment outcome in the CPT project.* Paper presented at the Association for the Advancement for Behavior Therapy, Washington, DC, November, 1983.

Johnson-Laird, P. N. (1983). *Mental models.* Cambridge, MA: Harvard University Press.

Keller, M. B., Shapiro, R. W., Lavori, P. W., & Wolfe, N. (1982). Relapse in major depressive disorder. *Archives of General Psychiatry, 39*, 911–915.

Klerman, G. L., Weissman, M., Rounsaville, B. S., & Chevron, E. S. (1984). *Interpersonal psychotherapy for depression.* New York: Basic Books.

Kovacs, M., & Beck, A. T. (1979). Cognitive-affective processes in depression. In C. E. Izard (Ed.), *Emotions in personality and psychotherapy* (pp. 417–441). New York: Plenum Press.

Kovacs, M., Rush, A. J., Beck, A. T., & Hollon, S. D. (1981). Depressed outpatients treated with cognitive therapy or pharmacotherapy. *Archives of General Psychiatry, 38*, 33–39.

Kuiper, N. A., & Derry, P. (1982). Depressed and nondepressed content self-reference in mild depressives. *Journal of Personality, 50*, 67–80.

Kuiper, N. A., & MacDonald, M. R. (1982). Self and other perception in mild depression. *Social Cognition, 3*, 223–239.

Lewinsohn, P. M. (1974). A behavioral approach to depression. In R. J. Friedman & M. Katz (Eds.), *The psychology of depression: Contemporary theory and research* (pp. 157–178). Washington, DC: Winston.

Lewinsohn, P. M., Mischel, W., Chaplin, W., & Barton, R. (1980). Social competence and depression: The role of illusory self-perceptions. *Journal of Abnormal Psychology, 89*, 203–212.

Lewinsohn, P. M., Steinmetz, J. L., Larsen, D. W., & Franklin, J. (1981). Depression-related cognitions: Antecedents or consequence? *Journal of Consulting and Clinical Psychology, 40*, 304–312.

Lobitz, W. C., & Post, R. D. (1979). Parameters of self-reinforcement and depression. *Journal of Abnormal Psychology, 88*, 33–41.

McLean, P. D., & Hakstain, A. R. (1979). Clinical depression: Comparative efficacy of outpatient treatments. *Journal of Consulting and Clinical Psychology, 47*, 818–836.

Miller, D. T., & Moretti M. M. (1988). The causal attributions of depressives: Self-serving or self-disserving? In L. B. Alloy (Ed.), *Cognitive processes in depression*. New York: Guilford Press.

Miller, I. V., Bishop, S. D., Norman, W. H., & Keitner, G. I. (1985). Cognitive-behavioral therapy and pharmacotherapy with chronic, drug-refractory depressed inpatients: A note of optimism. *Behavioral Psychotherapy, 13*, 320–327.

Miller, R., & Berman, J. (1983). The efficacy of cognitive behavior therapies: A quantitative review of the research evidence. *Psychological Bulletin, 94*, 36–51.

Moretti, M. M., & Shaw, B. F. (1989). Automatic and dysfunctional cognitive processes in depression. In J. S. Uleman & J. A. Bargh (Eds.), *Unintended thought: The limits of awareness, intention, and control*. New York: Guilford Press.

Murphy, G. E., Simons, A. D., Wetzel, R. D., & Lustman, P. J. (1984). Cognitive therapy and pharmacotherapy. *Archives of General Psychiatry, 41*, 33–41.

Neisser, U. (1967). *Cognitive psychology*. New York: Appleton-Century-Crofts.

Neisser, U. (1976). *Cognitive and reality: Principles and implications of cognitive psychology*. San Francisco: Freeman.

Nietzel, M. T., Russell, R. L., Hemmings, K. A., & Gretter, M. L. (1987). Clinical significance of psychotherapy for unipolar depression: A meta-analysis approach to social comparison. *Journal of Consulting and Clinical Psychology, 55*, 156–161.

Rounsaville, B., Weissman, M., Prusoff, B., & Herceg-Baron, R. (1979). Marital disputes and treatment outcome in depressed women. *Comprehensive Psychiatry, 20*, 483–490.

Rotzer, F. T., Nabitz, U., Koch, H., & Pflug, B. (1982). Zer Bedeuhing von Attribuierungs - Prozessen bei der Depressionsbehandlung. In L. G. Bericht, *Des 33 Kongresses der Deutschen Gesellschaft für Psychologie*. Mainz, FRG.

Rush, A. J., Beck, A. T., Kovacs, M., & Hollon, S. D. (1977). Comparative efficacy of cognitive therapy and pharmacotherapy in the treatment of depressed outpatients. *Cognitive Therapy and Research, 1*, 17–37.

Sacco, W. P., & Hokanson, J. E. (1978). Performance satisfaction under high and low success conditions. *Journal of Clinical Psychology, 34*, 907–909.

Salkovskis, P. M. (1985). Obsessional-compulsive problems: A cognitive-behavioral analysis. *Behavior Research and Therapy, 23*, 571–583.

Salkovskis, P. M., & Warwick, H. M. C. (1986). Morbid preoccupations, health anxiety, and reassurance: A cognitive-behavioral approach to hypochondriasis. *Behavior Research and Therapy, 24*, 597–602.

Safran, J., Shaw, B. F., Segal, Z. V., & Vallis, M. (1988). Selection criteria for short-term cognitive therapy of depression and anxiety. Research in progress. Clarke Institute of Psychiatry.

Segal, Z. V., & Shaw, B. F. (1986a). Cognition in depression: A reappraisal of Coyne and Gotlib's critique. *Cognitive Therapy and Research, 10*, 779–793.

Segal, Z. V., & Shaw, B. F. (1986b). When cul-de-sacs are more mentality than reality: A rejoinder to Coyne and Gotlib. *Cognitive Therapy and Research, 10*, 813–826.

Smolen, R. C. (1978). Expectancies, mood, and performance of depressed and nondepressed psychiatric inpatients on chance and skill tasks. *Journal of Abnormal Psychology, 87*, 91–101.

Stern, R. (1978). Obsessive thought: The problem of therapy. *British Journal of Psychiatry, 132*, 200–205.

Steinbrueck, S. M., Maxwell, S. E., & Howard, G. S. (1983). A meta-analysis of psychotherapy and drug therapy in the treatment of unipolar depression with adults. *Journal of Consulting and Clinical Psychology, 59*, 856–863.

Tabachnik, N., Crocker, J., & Alloy, L. B. (1983). Depression, social comparison and the false consensus effect. *Journal of Personality and Social Psychology, 45*, 688–699.

Teasdale, J. D., Fennel, M. J. V., Hibbert, G. A., & Amies, P. L. (1984). Cognitive therapy for major depressive disorder in primary care. *British Journal of Psychiatry, 144*, 400–406.

Thompson, L. W., Gallagher, D., & Breckenridge, J. S. (1987). Comparative effectiveness of psychotherapies for depressed elders. *Journal of Consulting and Clinical Psychology, 55*, 385–390.

Weismann, M., Paykel, E., Siegel, R., & Klerman, G. (1971). The social role performance of depressed women: Comparisons with a normal group. *American Journal of Orthopsychiatry, 41*, 390.

Weismann, M. M. (1979). The psychological treatment of depression: Evidence for the efficacy of psychotherapy alone in comparison with and in combination with pharmacotherapy. *Archives of General Psychiatry, 36*, 1261–1269.

Williams, J. M. G. (1984). Cognitive-behavior therapy for depression: Problems and perspectives. *British Journal of Psychiatry, 145*, 254–262.

Wollert, R. W., & Buchwald, A. M. (1979). Subclinical depression and performance expectations, evaluations of performance, and actor performance. *Journal of Nervous and Mental Disease, 167*, 237–242.

Wright, J. H. (1987). Cognitive therapy and medication as combined treatment. In A. Freeman & V. Greenwood (Eds.), *Cognitive therapy: Applications in psychiatric and medical settings* (pp. 36–50). New York: Human Sciences Press.

Zarantonello, M. W., Johnson, J. E., & Petzel, T. P. (1979). The effects of ego involvement and task difficulty on actual and perceived performance of depressed college students. *Journal of Clinical Psychology, 5*, 273–281.

11

An Introduction to Cognitive-Behavior Therapy

ADAM K. LEHMAN AND PETER SALOVEY

HISTORICAL OVERVIEW

Cognitive-behavior therapy has its roots in the resurgent interest in cognition that swept psychology during the late 1960s and early 1970s. This period served as the focal point for a shift in research psychology from a radical behavioral perspective to one emphasizing cognitively mediated processes (Kanfer, 1978; Mahoney, 1974). Broadly speaking, this shift involved the adopting by psychology of the "information-processing" perspective as the dominant metatheoretical approach to research. This perspective emphasizes the higher mental processes such as observational learning, thinking, language use, and problem solving. Within this perspective, humans are understood as actively seeking and processing environmental stimuli, rather than as passive recipients of environmental consequences. Human behavior is seen as originating from the processing of both internal *and* external information (Ingram & Kendall, 1986). Of central importance to the clinician is the impact this model has had on our ability to explore cognitions, affect, and behavior, particularly the interrelationships of these three variables as they contribute to both psychopathology and the therapeutic process.

Contributions from Social Psychology

During the past two decades, psychologists from a wide range of specialty areas have become increasingly interested in cognitive processes and their relation to behavior. Social psychologists, for example, have become fascinated with "schemata," particular types of higher-order knowledge structures. Schemata are cognitive structures containing general information plus examples in some domain and are believed to focus and structure one's experience of a given

ADAM K. LEHMAN AND PETER SALOVEY • Department of Psychology, Yale University, New Haven, Connecticut 06520. Please address reprint requests to Peter Salovey, Department of Psychology, Yale University, P. O. Box 11A, Yale Station, New Haven, Connecticut 06520.

situation (Taylor & Crocker, 1981). The script, a kind of schema, directs and informs one's behavior and expectancies in a variety of clearly defined social situations, such as what one should do upon entering a restaurant (Abelson, 1981; Schank & Abelson, 1977).

Social psychologists have also studied attributional processes, that is, the way in which individuals make inferences about causality. This interest in attribution theory eventually led to the development of "attribution therapy" (Kopel & Arkowitz, 1975; Nisbett & Schachter, 1966; Ross, Rodin, & Zimbardo, 1969; Valins & Nisbett, 1976). The influence of attribution theory on clinical concerns such as depression can be seen in Seligman's work on helplessness (1975) and explanatory style (Seligman, Abramson, Semmel, & von Beyer, 1979). More recent work in this area has focused on the accuracy of depressed versus nondepressed individuals' perceptions of events and control over them (Alloy & Abramson, 1979; Anderson, Horowitz, & deSales French, 1983). Such work exemplifies the attention given to cognitive factors in the etiology and maintenance of psychopathology.

Contributions from Social Learning Theory and Behavior Therapy

During this same period, social learning theorists, who had previously described psychotherapy in predominantly learning theory terms (Bandura, 1961), became increasingly interested in cognitive processes (Bandura, 1969, 1977a,b; Bandura, Adams, & Beyer, 1977). In an attempt to unify what he perceived as two dominant trends in behavior modification, namely the acceptance of cognitive mechanisms and the emphasis on mastery experiences that behavior therapy provides, Bandura (1977) emphasized the importance of self-efficacy in behavioral change. Self-efficacy refers to the individual's belief that she or he has the necessary skills or qualities to carry out a desired behavior. According to Bandura, cognitive processing and appraisal of efficacy information are central to behavior change. Self-efficacy came to be viewed by social learning theorists as a central cognitive antecedent to therapeutic gain and well-being.

Behavior therapists, whose work originally focused on therapy techniques deriving from the principles of classical and operant conditioning (such as systematic desensitization and behavioral contracting, respectively), began to rethink the processes by which these techniques exerted their beneficial effects. Schwartz (1982) describes how Murray and Jacobson's (1971) review of basic learning studies highlighted the inadequacy of strict S-R formulations of learning in understanding the efficacy of behavior therapy. Cognitive factors were required to enhance the explanatory value of this approach to learning. Bregher and McGaugh's (1965) reevaluation of learning theory led some behavior therapists "to greatly expand the framework of behavior therapy to be more compatible with cognitive factors" (Schwartz, 1982, p. 274).

Systematic desensitization, introduced by Wolpe (1958), was originally understood as an application of counterconditioning (learning) principles to behavior therapy. The client learns a new, incompatible response to anxiety (e.g., muscular relaxation). Wolpe's technique involved learning deep muscle relaxation, creating a fear-provoking hierarchy of unpleasant scenes, and imagining these unpleasant fear-arousing scenes while experiencing muscular relaxation. Examination of studies using Wolpe's techniques found that contrary to prior belief, it is not mutual antagonism of muscular relaxation and imagined unpleasant experiences that contribute to systematic desensitization's effectiveness. Rather, central to the effectiveness of systematic desensitization is the cognitive expectancy of therapeutic gain (Brown, 1973; Wilkins, 1971). Additionally, imagining the fear-related scenes in any order was found sufficient in itself to yield therapeutic improvement (Wilkins, 1971).

Increased attention was thus given to the importance of imagination as a central therapeutic element of behavior modification (Singer, 1974, 1979; Singer & Pope, 1978). Imagination, a wholly cognitive process, when allowed to develop freely under controlled therapeutic conditions was thought to be inherently curative (Singer, 1974). By the middle 1970s, inner thoughts or cognitions began to occupy a prominent position in many previously behaviorally oriented clinicians' understanding of the therapeutic process. Private events and internal processes were now viewed as amenable to integration with traditional behavior modification techniques. Ironically, these same processes had been explicitly disparaged by the earliest behaviorists (Watson, 1913).

Cognitive-Behavior Therapy as Integration

Central to cognitive-behavior therapy is its hybrid origins. Some have described it as a resolution between what had been two divergent therapeutic perspectives, namely the behavioral and cognitive/intrapersonal (Mahoney, 1977a) or the behavioral and cognitive/semantic therapies (Meichenbaum, 1977). Many clinical psychologists were moving toward pragmatic eclecticism in the middle 1970s in order to discover effective shorter term treatments (Garfield & Kurtz, 1976). Eclecticism's increased popularity may have stemmed from the humanistic trend of the 1960s, a time when experimentation and variety were more acceptable in psychotherapy. However, another factor that may have contributed to the rise in eclecticism may have been the appearance of cognitive-behavior therapy's now definitive texts (Mahoney, 1974; Meichenbaum, 1977). The emergence of cognitive-behavior therapy at this time can be understood in the context of this integrationist movement in psychotherapy.

Early attempts to integrate psychoanalytic and behavioral viewpoints contented themselves with a simple translation of the concepts from one school into the language of the other. In the 1930s, articles by French (1933) and Kubie (1934) demonstrated that phenomena could be discussed in either a psychoanalytic or learning theory vocabulary. Drawing on his personal experiences, Alexander (1963) cites the extreme conservatism of the psychoanalytic circle as a major contributing factor to the absence of more substantial attempts at integration. Underlying this conservatism was a fear of "excommunication" should one dare to "leave the fold." In 1950, Dollard and Miller published their now classic attempt to unify the psychoanalytic and learning theory traditions, *Personality and Psychotherapy*, dedicating it to both Freud and Pavlov. They explained a wide range of psychoanalytic concepts in learning theory terms. The pleasure principle was understood as reinforcement, repression was interpreted as inhibition, and transference became an example of response generalization. On a broader level, the neuroses were interpreted as faulty learning experiences.

Attempts at integration were not only postulated by learning theorists. The 1940s and 1950s saw a greater emphasis on interpersonal concerns by psychoanalysts. This trend eventually led to a more interpersonal understanding of personality and psychotherapy (Horney, 1950; Sullivan, 1953). Much of the work done by the neo-Freudians balanced the emphasis on the patient's past with equal concern for and interest in the patient's present life. The psychoanalytic emphasis on the reconstruction of the past came to be viewed as residue from a time when research in personality dynamics was seen as a necessary requisite to developing a rational treatment approach (Alexander, 1963).

The early 1960s polarized the psychoanalytic and behavior therapies (Eysenck, 1960; Wolpe & Rachman, 1960), although they were reacquainted in the latter part of the decade (Brady, 1968; Wolf, 1966). For example, in the late 1960s, Weitzman (1967) emphasized the importance of incorporating cognitive processes in behavior therapy. The early 1970s saw further attempts to integrate these two divergent perspectives through combining cognitive factors with behavior therapy techniques (Birk & Brinkley-Birk, 1974; Feather & Rhoads, 1972a,b; Rhoads & Feather, 1974). It was shortly thereafter that the fully developed cognitive-behavioral perspective (Mahoney, 1974; Meichenbaum, 1977) with which we are concerned emerged.

This new form of therapy can be understood as an integration of "internalism" and "externalism." Mahoney (1977a) describes internalism as the view that the central determinants of human behavior lie within the individual. It was Freud who clearly articulated the importance of inner wishes, conflicts, and motivations to the individual's psychological adjustment. Freud's orientation has since been followed and explored in the writings of the neo-Freudians, object-relation theorists, humanists, existentialists, and Rogerians. These perspectives share in common a focus on the inner world of the person as it contributes to their psychological well-being and behavior (Mahoney, 1977a).

The newer perspective is termed "externalism." This view has its roots in turn-of-the-century American behaviorism (Watson, 1913). It takes a more externalized view of what determines human behavior and psychological life. Remaining outside the organism, behaviorists aligned themselves closely with more traditional academic psychology, emphasizing the research component of their work. With time, new therapy techniques were developed based on behaviorist principles (e.g., Skinner, Wolpe, Lazarus, Rachman).

Reciprocal Determinism

Cognitive-behavior therapy adopts as its theoretical base an interactionist perspective regarding the determinants of human behavior and psychological well-being. At the center of this perspective is the belief that the interaction between the individual and the environment continuously determines behavior, cognitions, and affect. Private thoughts and intrapersonal factors act upon the environment. Additionally, environmental factors influence these same intra-personal factors. Further still, intrapersonal factors affect the individual's *perception* of environmental forces. Therefore what emerges is a three-factor model—environment/person/behavior—of person–situation interaction. Band-ura has labeled this *reciprocal determinism* (Bandura, 1978).

One of the earlier proponents of a similar interactionist view was Albert Ellis (1962). Mahoney (1977a) views Ellis as a central figure in the development of cognitive-behavior therapy as a serious alternative to other therapies. Ellis's A-B-C model of behavior and personality disturbance (where A = Activating Events, B = the individual's Belief system, and C = Consequence) stimulated theorists to explore a variety of therapeutic alternatives to unidirectional ther-apies. Cognitions are thought to influence behaviors, which in turn influence the environment, which in turn influence cognitions, and so on. Although this appears tautological, Mahoney (1977a) asserts that it is not. Rather, he views this triad of cognition-behavior-environment as an interactive, or reciprocal, deter-minism. Given the interdependence of these three variables, a variety of possi-ble points of intervention are available to the cognitive behaviorist. Some thera-pists have focused on clients' irrational beliefs (Ellis, 1987), internal dialogues (Meichenbaum, 1977), cognitive distortions (Beck, 1976), perceived contingen-cies (Mahoney, 1977a), images and ongoing thoughts (Singer, 1974), and ob-servable behaviors (Fairburn, 1985; Wilson, 1985). Accepting the principle of reciprocal determinism within the cognitive-behavioral perspective vastly in-creases the range of available therapeutic options.

Summary

Cognitive-behavior therapy stands firmly on an information-processing foundation. More specifically, a belief in reciprocal determinism enhances the cognitive-behavior therapist's sensitivity to a wide variety of data. Cognitive-behavior therapy's close affiliation with research psychology has also promoted its continued development over the years. We will touch on some of these more recent developments toward the end of this chapter. Presently, we will examine processes and variables central to the practice of cognitive-behavior therapy.

GOALS OF COGNITIVE-BEHAVIOR THERAPY

Cognitive-behavior therapy attempts to alter clients' interpretations of themselves and their environments, as well as the manner by which they create these interpretations. The goals of cognitive-behavior therapy can be under-stood as deriving from the sage views of Epictetus, (a first-century Greek philos-opher) who stated that "men are disturbed not by things, but by the views they take of them" (as cited in Meichenbaum, 1974). The views one takes of events are related to the particular meanings one attaches to a given experience. Thus, cognitive-behavior therapy attempts to alter the meaning a client attaches to events (Meichenbaum & Butler, 1980). But, unlike strictly cognitive therapies, it may use behavioral means in order to do so. Over the course of therapy, clients' views of themselves and their environments are challenged by the therapist through a series of specific interventions. Clients are taught new ways of interpreting both themselves and those around them through dialogue, observation, and behavioral experiences. Often these new ways of thinking about themselves involve becoming more accepting of desires, limitations, and strengths. Additionally, clients' new self-concepts are more flexible, enabling them to evaluate aspects of the self in a noncritical manner. Clients who present for therapy stating that "I'm no good, I never do anything right," may come to view themselves as people who usually perform adequately but like everyone else make mistakes from time to time. A cognitive therapist might cause this change by confronting the client with the initial overgeneralization. A cognitive-behavior therapist, however, might also do this, but in addition provide the person with experiences that help solidify the newly acquired and more realistic self-concept.

Cognitive-behavior therapy emphasizes the learning process (Mahoney, 1977b) and encourages clients to acquire new skills during the course of therapy. Coping skills in particular are emphasized; client problems can often be understood as stemming from inadequate coping skills. Mahoney (1977b) has argued that "life is basically a coping process in which a person attempts to react to and influence the complex and ever-changing array of factors which may be of personal relevance to him" (p. 15). New coping skills are intended to increase the client's ability to cope with stressful or problematic situations she or he may encounter outside the therapy. Depending on one's orientation to cognitive-behavior therapy, the skills taught may emphasize the importance of relaxation training (Goldfried, 1977), cognitive coping abilities (Goldfried, 1980), imagery (Crits-Christoph & Singer, 1981), self-efficacy (Bandura, 1982; Goldfried & Robbins, 1982), problem solving and decision making (Kanfer & Busemeyer, 1982), self-instructional methods (Meichenbaum, 1977), irrational beliefs (Ellis, 1987), or automatic thoughts (Beck, 1976).

One of cognitive-behavior therapy's primary goals is providing cost-effective treatment for a wide variety of clinical problems. In the face of increasing health care costs, the provision of affordable treatment has taken on new importance. In this regard, treatment sessions are sometimes limited. Therapists and clients may contract to meet for a certain number of sessions (frequently 15 to 25), with an agreement to renew this contract should both parties feel it necessary. Cognitive-behavior therapy is also concerned with the generalizability of its positive treatment effects. Clients are encouraged to practice skills acquired during a therapy session at home or anywhere else they might be of practical use. One concern is that increased levels of functioning experienced during psychotherapy quickly dissipate once therapy is terminated. Therefore, an effort is made to structurally alter the course of therapy such that responsibility for maintaining improvement is *gradually* shifted from therapist to client. For example, Fairburn (1985), in his work with bulimia nervosa patients, recommends a gradual reduction in the frequency of sessions. In this way, clients come to rely more on themselves as agents of therapeutic improvement over a period of time. The client no longer has to navigate an abrupt ending of the relationship believed to have been responsible for whatever improvements she or he has experienced so far.

Briefly restated, the overarching goals of cognitive-behavior therapy include:

1. Providing cost-effective treatment for a wide range of client problems.
2. Altering clients' *interpretations* of themselves and their environment by changing their behavior, their environment, or their cognitions directly.
3. Increasing clients' available store of coping skills.
4. Increasing the likelihood that therapeutic gain will be maintained once therapy is terminated.

Although these goals are determined by the theoretical orientation of the cognitive-behavior therapist, it is a collaboration between *both* client and therapist that produces the goals of a given course of therapy. Clients present for therapy, often with particular agendas. Therapists listen carefully, drawing upon their experience, and design ways in which clients' needs can be satisfied most effectively and efficiently.

CLIENT ISSUES

In the past 15 years, cognitive-behavior therapies have been used with various client populations including those with interpersonal anxiety (e.g., Goldfried, 1977; Heppner, 1978; Lange & Jakubowski, 1976; Thorpe, 1975), test anxiety (e.g., Denney, 1981; Wine, 1981), writer's block (Salovey & Haar, 1983), uncontrollable anger (Novaco, 1978), depression (e.g., Beck, Rush, Shaw, & Emery, 1979), sexual dysfunction (Rook & Hammen, 1977), schizophrenic symptoms (Meichenbaum & Cameron, 1973), impulsive behavior (Meichenbaum & Goodman, 1971), chronic pain (Turk, Meichenbaum, & Genest, 1983), addictions and substance abuse (e.g., Chaney, O'Leary, & Marlatt, 1978; Marlatt & Gordon, 1980), and eating disorders (e.g., Fairburn, 1985; Wilson, 1985).

Clients bring their own strengths and weaknesses to the therapeutic setting. Some are particularly good at recalling feelings; others focus more on thoughts, and still others relate only their overt behaviors when describing experiences that led them to seek psychotherapy. Given the integrative framework of cognitive-behavior therapy, a therapist working from this perspective should be able to communicate effectively with each of these client types. The cognitive-behavior therapist's attention to *thoughts, feelings,* and *behaviors,* as well as his/her willingness to intervene at any point in the person/environment/behavior triangle allows the therapist to establish a rapport with most clients. Clients who articulate their problems in behavioral terms might be asked to self-monitor their problematic behaviors, whereas those who speak of intrusive or upsetting thoughts might be asked to record their private internal dialogues and eventually challenge them with alternative self-statements. Availability of such varied interventions is one of the attractive features of working within the cognitive-behavioral framework.

Clients vary greatly in the ways they conceptualize their own problems. Some attribute cause for their condition to the environment or significant others ("If only my spouse would stop acting that way, then everything would be fine"); others view themselves as the originating cause for their present troubles ("If I could just stop thinking this way"). The cognitive-behavior therapist is able to work comfortably with both types of clients. In the early stages of therapy, cognitive-behavior therapists adopt the clients' conceptual/explanatory framework; subsequently they expand it to include those parts of the reciprocal-determinism equation that had been overlooked previously. As therapists respond to clients' statements, offering new interpretations of their experiences, they begin to alter clients' conceptualizations of their condition.

As is the case with all psychotherapies, an important variable in the success or failure of a therapy is the theoretical match between therapist and client (Frank, 1961). Given the flexability of the cognitive-behavior orientation, we believe that client–therapist congruity in orientation is quite common. Those clients who are willing to actively participate and enter into a collaborative relationship with the therapist will gain the most from the therapy experience.

Clients seldom enter therapy without having experienced some degree of worry, anxiety, depression, frustration, and preoccupation with their problem(s). Early stages of cognitive-behavior therapy often focus on helping clients articulate their goals for therapy. Clients willing to examine specific areas of their lives that they wish to work on in the course of therapy will benefit from this goal-oriented framework of cognitive-behavior therapy.

Although many clients present for psychotherapy with specific goals, others present for psychotherapy to "learn more about myself" or to "try and understand my past." These clients frequently view psychotherapy as an arena for exploration or education of the self. Even though cognitive-behavior therapy would be of some use to them, these clients could be disappointed by cognitive-behavior therapy's emphasis on the present or recent past and orientation to work on clearly defined problem areas. Additionally, clients who wish to enter into a lengthy relationship with a therapist might also be disappointed by the shorter duration of cognitive-behavior therapy. Clients seeking such a therapeutic experience might well be suited for other forms of treatment such as longer term psychodynamically oriented therapy.

Central to cognitive-behavior therapy is its ability to structure the therapeutic process. Therapy may be structured through the setting of goals, the use of regular "homework" assignments, or a particular spacing of therapy sessions (see Fairburn, 1985, for an example). As such, it might be particularly useful for those clients who seek help in structuring both their lives and inner experience (Meichenbaum & Cameron, 1973).

Cognitive-behavior therapy is compatible with a variety of clients exhibiting a wide range of symptoms. Adults and children, psychotics, and neurotics have all benefitted from cognitive-behavioral interventions (Meichenbaum, 1977).

This ability to be effective with such diverse populations may be related to cognitive-behavior therapy's attention to a wide range of clinically relevant data (e.g., cognitions, affect, and behavior).

ASSESSMENT ISSUES

The Relationship of Assessment to Therapy

Unlike other therapies that have a clearly defined assessment component frequently conducted by someone other than the therapist him/herself, cognitive-behavior therapy assesses the client's functioning throughout the duration of therapy. The assessment phase is inextricably tied to other phases of therapy. Central to cognitive-behavior therapy is the assessment of clients' cognitions and behavior patterns. The behavior therapist often views cognitions that precede maladaptive behaviors as "behaviors" themselves, assuming a continuity between cognition and behavior; the cognitive-behavior therapist does not assume such continuity (Meichenbaum, 1975). Similarly, cognitive therapists focus on clients' irrational beliefs, or thinking styles, believing that clients' problems are due to faulty thought processes. The cognitive-behavior therapist prefers to assess both, the nature of clients' behaviors and accompanying cognitive processes. Particular attention is given to the ways in which these two aspects of the client interact.

Initial Assessment/Intervention Goals

Early stages of assessment, such as the first meeting with a client, should emphasize the client's elaboration of the area or areas of concern that led him or her to seek therapy. This is usually carried out through direct questioning of the client. The therapist should attempt to create a supportive and encouraging atmosphere in which the client feels comfortable disclosing these concerns. Open-ended questions are usually introduced at this time (e.g., "How do you feel?" or "What led you to contact the clinic (or me)?"). In this way, the therapist minimizes any bias introduced by the use of more restrictive questions (e.g., "Are you anxious?"; see Mahoney, 1977b). After gently questioning the client in this way, the therapist may get a sense of why the client is seeking therapy at this time. The therapist may begin to aid the client in voicing goals for the therapy.

In general, the therapist assumes a relatively passive role during this stage of assessment. However, should the client exhibit extreme levels of anxiety or become particularly agitated, the therapist may wish to assume a more active role. An instance when this might be appropriate is illustrated in the following example:

A 33-year-old white male presented himself to a university clinic complaining of "sexual impotence." In the course of the first meeting with his therapist, he reported being unable to sustain an erection when attempting to have intercourse with his girlfriend of 6 months. As he began to describe his condition, he became visibly agitated. Rather than continuing to ask broad, open-ended questions that might serve to increase the client's already agitated state, the therapist chose to ask specific questions about his sexual behavior. By taking a more active role in the questioning of the client and by asking specific closed-ended questions, the client was able to focus more on the task at hand. His agitated state passed, and he was able to provide the therapist with important diagnostic information.

In this case vignette, the therapist made a treatment decision based on the observable behavior of the client. It should be noted, however, that an important assessment opportunity was missed by this therapist. The therapist failed to assess the client's cognitions at the time he became visibly agitated. Later in this first session, once rapport had been established with the client, the therapist returned to this earlier incident. When asked about his cognitive experience at the time, the client became visibly upset (e.g., when asked, "Can you recall any thoughts that were going through your head when you became agitated earlier in the session?", the client reported having thoughts of being "inadequate" as a man). Now informed of both the behavior and cognitions of the client, the therapist was able to interpret the client's faulty generalization of his condition (behavior: inability to sustain an erection ⇒ cognition: I'm a failure as a man). Note that it was important for the therapist to be aware of the client's *behaviors and cognitions* before such an interpretation could be made.

Briefly summarizing, the early assessment phase of cognitive-behavior therapy involves three central goals. First, the therapist needs to understand those cognitions, affects, behaviors, and environmental conditions central to the client's presenting complaints. Second, the therapist should try and understand the manner in which these cognitions, affects, and behaviors interact, causing the client psychological distress. Third, the therapist should try and determine what cognitions, affects, behaviors, and environmental cues are absent from the client's repertoire, which, if present, would help reduce the client's distress and increase his/her coping ability. The therapist needs to be sensitive to both what is present in the client's presentation, and what is absent.

Specific Methods of Assessment and Intervention

Meichenbaum (1975) describes a range of assessment and intervention techniques used by cognitive-behavior therapists. We will therefore only highlight the most important methods currently in use:

1. *The clinical interview.* We have already mentioned the usefulness of a clinical interview in assessing the client's behaviors and cognitions. As is the case with other, more dynamically oriented therapies, the clinical setting is understood as a representation of the client's experiences when not in therapy. Cognitive-behavior therapy takes the position that the process of assessing a given behavior necessarily alters it due to subsequent self-consciousness experienced by the client. Specific instructions designed to enhance the representa-

tiveness of information derived from the client are often incorporated into the clinical interview. For instance, a client who presents for test anxiety might be encouraged to imagine herself preparing to take a test. Through such experiences, problem-related cognitions, affects, and behaviors may be elicited. Once a series of experiences relevant to the presenting complaint is described by the client, the therapist might ask him or her to imagine any other recent situations where these same thoughts, feelings, or behaviors were experienced. In this way, the extent of the client's symptoms can be understood.

2. *Imagery-based techniques.* Meichenbaum (1975) encourages therapists to have the client imagine, or "run a movie through his head," of a recent time when she or he experienced the presenting problem. This technique makes salient certain aspects of the situation that otherwise would have gone unnoticed. This technique is often quite useful when working with clients who might report an affect-laden situation but are unable to recall important details, thus leaving the therapist confused as to the situation's significance for the patient.

A 20-year-old female client reported being in front of the television when her mother began screaming at her. She described in elaborate detail the anger and frustration she felt at her mother. After listening to her affective experience of the incident for a few minutes, the therapist was still puzzled as to why it was that the mother had begun screaming in the first place. When the therapist asked the client this question, the client looked surprised and said she had no idea. Still puzzled, the therapist suggested to the client that, if she felt comfortable enough, she should close her eyes and imagine the circumstances of this unpleasant experience. The client complied and began to imagine herself in the room where the fight with her mother occurred. Shortly thereafter, previously "unretrievable" details returned to her, including the memory of having ignored her mother's repeated request to wash the dinner dishes. The client felt she now understood the series of events that led up to the argument with her mother.

This case vignette illustrates the use of imagery as a tool to increase clients' recall of previously forgotten material. Imagery is also often used to assess those cognitions that accompany clients' behaviors during crucial incidents. As clients imagine these crucial incidents, accompanying cognitions (relevant self-statements, internal dialogues) and feelings return to the clients' conscious awareness. Particular attention should be given to the manner in which clients conceptualize their experience. Do clients experience themselves as passive agents or active participants? Do they consider alternative coping strategies, or was the eventual course of action the only one the client entertained? Using imagery in this way enables therapists to get a more detailed picture of their clients' experiences. In particular, interactions of cognitions, affects, and behaviors may begin to be examined by the therapist.

Cognitive-behavior therapists have long been concerned with clients' internal dialogues. But these self-statements may take a form other than words. Imagery methods are useful in assessing clients' cognitions that take a pictorial form (Meichenbaum, 1975). Clients often carry with them certain core images that represent communications to themselves. These self-images organize clients' experiences and attitudes about themselves. For example, a client who had difficulty asserting herself in relationships repeatedly imagined herself locked in her room. Another client who reported difficulty in sustaining close personal relationships repeatedly saw himself surrounded by concentric circles made of iron. Working from an imagistic framework encourages clients to access such "self-statements" that otherwise, in a purely semantic therapy, may go unnoticed.

Imagery techniques can also be used to assess clients' positive potential. One may encourage clients to imagine themselves carrying out adaptive behaviors or reciting positive self-statements in difficult situations ("covert behavioral rehearsal"). Such a technique allows therapists to examine the boundaries of clients' coping resources. Additionally, this method of assessment emphasizes clients' strengths, as opposed to weaknesses (often examined to the exclusion of their positive attributes during traditional psychotherapy). Other uses of positive images include having clients imagine pleasurable and relaxing images to counteract feelings of anxiety (Singer, 1974).

3. *Behavioral assessment and situational analysis.* Clients who have difficulty working in an imagistic framework may be better able to access cognitions and affects by performing the problematic behavior in those situations in which these behaviors might occur. Performance of the problematic behavior may be either in a realistic setting or through an "enactment" of the behavior during a therapy session. For example, a college student who reported feeling anxious about confronting a roommate was asked to enact the feared confrontation during a session with his therapist. During this behavioral rehearsal, the client was continuously probed about his cognitions and self-statements. The client began to interpret his fears as irrational, and with the therapist's help, he realized that his fear of the confrontation was indicative of a general interactional style. Based on this behavioral assessment, treatment goals were redirected to include general assertiveness training.

Other forms of behavioral assessment include having the client engage in the problematic behavior outside the therapy session. However, the behavior is assessed in a new manner in either an *a priori* or post-hoc fashion. The client may be instructed before performing the behavior to pay close attention to any internal thoughts or dialogue while engaging in the behavior; or the client might be interviewed by the therapist after performing the behavior with an emphasis placed on these same aspects of the client's experience. In both instances, the behavior is conceptualized and evaluated in a new manner. Most importantly, therapists encourage their clients to evaluate their problematic behaviors in such a way as to increase clients' sensitivity to previously hidden, yet important, aspects of the person/environment/behavior triad.

4. *Decision-making and problem-solving strategies.* One of the goals of cognitive-behavior therapy is to help clients acquire skills that will improve their ability to navigate problems that arise during the course of everyday life. Relatively recent interest in problem-solving and decision-making theory and research (reviewed by Turk & Salovey, 1986, 1988) has led to the development of specific psychotherapy interventions aimed at increasing clients' ability to make appropriate

decisions. These procedures teach clients specific problem-solving strategies including how to accurately recognize and define the problem, construct realistic and manageable decision trees, evaluate the costs and benefits of decisions, generate and consider alternatives to problem situations, develop concrete methods of executing a desired decision, and evaluate the outcome of executing the desired decision (Kanfer & Busemeyer, 1982).

Cognitive-behavior therapy strives to make clients aware of new alternatives. Clients who present for psychotherapy feeling overwhelmed by a lack of alternatives and unable to think clearly about their problems may particularly benefit by the problem-solving and decision-making techniques mentioned. These techniques encourage clients to think about their problems in a more "dynamic" manner (Kanfer & Busemeyer, 1982). The goal of problem-solving and decision-making techniques is not to teach clients how to solve a particular problem in a particular situation; rather it is hoped that clients will acquire a set of generalizable skills that may be used to cope with a variety of perceived problem situations.

5. *Self-efficacy training.* Judgments of one's self-efficacy in any given situation are thought to influence one's decisions to engage in and actually perform certain activities. People avoid those activities that they believe exceed their coping abilities and participate in those they are confident of performing capably (Bandura, 1977a, 1982). Additionally, evaluations of one's self-efficacy influences the amount of effort one expends (Bandura, 1982). Building on Bandura's (1977a) belief that psychotherapists can create contexts in which to strengthen self-efficacy expectations, Goldfried and Robbins (1982) outline a series of interventions designed to enhance clients' perceived self-efficacy. The first strategy involves helping the client distinguish between the past and present once progress is made. The past may serve as an anchor against which to measure clients' progress. Highlighting behavioral change in this fashion encourages clients to review their progress (in response to the therapist's questions) and increase their feelings of self-efficacy. For example:

A young woman had been seen in therapy for a few months. She had clearly made progress in controlling her impulses and evaluating her cognitive and affective states. Previously, she had described herself as often being overwhelmed by intense yet nondescript emotions. During one session, the client described being in a particularly difficult situation and being able to "give myself room to step back and think about what I was feeling." The therapist reinforced this positive change and asked the client to "try and compare what you did with what you would have done 3 months ago." The client then recalled her previous and ineffective ways of handling similar situations. In this way, she was able to experience, with her therapist, an acknowledgment of the progress she had made since beginning therapy.

A second strategy outlined by Goldfried and Robbins (1982) is to provide clients with an objective vantage point from which they may more accurately evaluate themselves. Clients, particularly those suffering from depression, often attribute personal successes to an external cause and attribute failures to themselves (Peterson & Seligman, 1984). Therapists can serve as an objective reference point, reminding clients of their personal success experiences, and the aspects of themselves that contributed to these experiences. Therapists may also help clients retrieve past successes and incorporate them into their self-concept. Lastly, therapists can evaluate clients' abilities to evaluate adequately the sequence of events that precede, accompany, and follow opportunities for enhancing self-efficacy. The therapist serves to realign the sequence of expectancies, anticipatory feelings, actual behaviors, objective consequences, and subsequent self-evaluations (Goldfried & Robbins, 1982). Clients often hold inconsistencies between two or more segments in this sequence of events. For instance, clients may possess reasonable expectancies and carry out appropriate behaviors, yet still fail to evaluate themselves accurately subsequent to their successful action. Assessment of clients' anticipatory feelings and thoughts can be accomplished by asking about experiences just prior to engaging in a certain behavior. Similarly, assessment of the subsequent evaluation of the act can be achieved by probing for clients' thoughts and feelings about the self just after engaging in the behavior.

These techniques focus the therapy on issues pertaining to client perceptions of self-efficacy. Through careful consideration of clients past and present experiences (e.g., clients' cognitions, affects, and behaviors), the therapist works with the client to achieve a more accurate and less distorted perception of themselves and their experiences.

6. *Self-monitoring procedures.* A common assessment technique is to use structured self-monitoring sheets designed to assess problematic cognitions, affects, behaviors, or environmental circumstances. Self-monitoring tasks are tailored to meet the needs of specific client populations. For example, Fairburn (1985) describes the use of self-monitoring sheets to assess bulimics' eating patterns. Fairburn's method assesses the cognitive, affective, and behavioral components of the binging process both before and after eating. Therapists differ in the type of monitoring sheets they use. Some prefer that clients construct their own sheets, and others prepare sheets for their clients. Some self-monitoring sheets leave spaces for clients to fill in the blanks, check off boxes, or circle the appropriate responses. Therapist selection/creation of self-monitoring sheets often reflects what they feel will be most beneficial for a particular client. Depressed clients may already be well aware of their feeling states and therefore would benefit from recording their negative self-statements. Other clients, who need to establish greater awareness of their affective responses to situations may benefit by being asked to monitor their feeling states.

Clients vary widely in their capacity to carry out assigned monitoring tasks. Often a clear and concise rationale for a given homework task will increase the chances of a client successfully completing it. Rationales for self-monitoring often include mention of its usefulness in reality testing. Discussion of how clients often underestimate their resources is useful. Homework also serves to sustain the work of therapy in the absence of the therapist, reinforcing the work that occurs during therapy sessions.

After explaining the self-monitoring task to clients, it is important to explore any reasons they might have for thinking they will not be able to carry out the task. Such informal "trouble-shooting" increases the likelihood that clients will actually monitor themselves. Clients' resistances confronted in this fashion are often deflated, becoming less powerful. As clients are taught to recognize their own resistances to change, they become more able to counter these resistances in the absence of their therapist.

7. *Coping skills and stress inoculation training.* Many therapists working from a cognitive-behavioral perspective have adopted the view that therapy should not focus solely on the resolution of specific problems, but rather, more broadly, it should focus on teaching the client a series of effective and generalizable coping skills (Goldfried, 1980). This conceptualization of therapy assumes that members of contemporary society are continually faced with stressful life problems with which they must cope. The transactional perspective of the stress and coping process (Lazarus, Cohen, Folkman, Kanner, & Schaeffer, 1980), like cognitive-behavior therapy, takes a reciprocal-deterministic framework, postulating that individuals both influence and respond to their environments.

The coping skills and stress inoculation approaches to therapy strive to facilitate clients' abilities to respond adaptively to their problems. Particular emphasis is placed on clients' assessing the accuracy of these self-appraisals and the acquisition and rehearsal of effective coping skills. Coping skills frequently addressed in cognitive-behavior therapy include the following:

a. *Taking others' perspectives.* This skill stems from the understanding that "when things are objectively bad, they may seem subjectively worse" (Meichenbaum & Cameron, 1983, p. 135). There are times when clients' ways of viewing their circumstances serve to increase their subjective suffering and distress. Although some clients are able to alter their painful circumstances (e.g., separate from an abusive spouse) others cannot (e.g., mourning the loss of a loved one). Clients suffering from irreversible circumstances are often best treated by exposing them to similar others who are currently coping effectively with a shared experience. For instance, a young mastectomy patient might benefit from exposure to other young women who have had mastectomies. These people may serve to model coping skills that the therapist cannot.

b. *Social support networks.* Clients often present for psychotherapy after their own resources have been exhausted. A client's social support network may be used effectively to sustain them through difficult times. Therapists can encourage clients to engage their friends and relatives in protherapeutic ways. Explaining to clients that their friends are sources of valuable information and aid can often serve to increase interaction with them. Communication and social skills training are often used in conjunction with encouraging clients to seek out members of their social support networks. Central to this type of training is learning to send "clear" messages to others and accurately receive them (Goldfried, 1980).

c. *Relaxation training.* A frequently employed strategy for coping with anxiety is relaxation training. Based on Jacobson's *Progressive Relaxation* (1929), this technique (outlined in Goldfried, 1971), views relaxation training as a specific coping skill. Although it gained its popularity with behavior therapists as a key element in Wolpe's (1958) work on systematic desensitization, relaxation training is currently used widely as a method of promoting general relaxation skills. Outlines of progressive relaxation techniques can be found in Bornstein, Hamilton, Carmody, Rychtarik, and Verold (1977), and Bernstein and Borkovec (1973).

Summary of Assessment and Intervention Techniques

Assessment and therapy are united in cognitive-behavior therapy. Assessment techniques alter clients' conceptualizations of their condition. Whatever form(s) of assessment is (are) selected by the therapist, clients are likely to be encouraged to think of their presenting complaints from a new framework. As clients are sensitized to the interaction of cognition, affect, behavior, and environment, they come to adopt a more flexible attitude toward themselves. What was previously an *automatic* process of thought and behavior is brought to *conscious awareness* through various assessment strategies. To some extent, clients are taught to become their own "action reporters" (Silberstein & Striegel-Moore, 1985), documenting their personal thought and behavior patterns. The metaphor of the "action reporter" serves to underscore the nonevaluative aspect of assessment. Regardless of the techniques employed, the end result should be an increased understanding, for both therapist *and* client, of the client's maladaptive self-statements, behaviors, and any interaction of the two.

Assessment is carried out continuously and inextricably alongside therapy. As clients quietly assimilate their therapists' models of interpreting their experiences, hope is generated within the client, serving a protherapeutic purpose (Frank, 1974). Additionally, with each intervention by the therapist, new data are collected about the client's experience, serving to inform the selection of future interventions. The selection of any given therapeutic technique should be determined, in part, by the therapist's assessment of the client's ability to benefit from it. Thus, a relatively fluid cycle of assessment → intervention selection → further assessment (etc.) emerges, demonstrating the interdependent relationship of these two aspects of cognitive-behavior therapy.

EFFICACY OF COGNITIVE-BEHAVIOR THERAPY

During the 1970s, cognitive-behavior therapy was greeted with excitement by numerous therapists. As was the case with behavior therapy during the 1960s, advocates of cognitive-behavior therapy hoped it would become the single most effective form of treatment for a variety of clinical and nonclinical disorders. To date, a definitive study substantiating this claim has yet to be reported. Attempts to evaluate comparisons among various psychotherapies yield the conclusion that they are all of about equal efficacy and all better than no therapy at all (Luborsky, Singer, & Luborsky, 1975; Smith, Glass, & Miller, 1980).

Miller and Berman (1981) reviewed the literature on the effectiveness of cognitive-behavior therapy. They found that cognitive-behavior therapy's efficacy remained stable across a wide range of diagnostic categories, regardless of whether it was administered in individual or group formats. They also cautioned, however, that cognitive-behavior therapy could not claim to be any more successful than various other modes of therapy. Over the past two decades, practitioners have used cognitive-behavioral techniques with a wide range of clinical and nonclinical disorders and are continuing to do so. Cognitive-behavior therapy is still a relative newcomer to the world of psychotherapy and behavior change. Additionally, it is difficult to make comparisons between various forms of cognitive-behavior therapy because the range of available techniques and interventions is so great.

FUTURE DIRECTIONS OF COGNITIVE-BEHAVIOR THERAPY

Presently, cognitive-behavior therapy is enjoying wide acceptance across a variety of clinical and clinical-health settings. The emphasis on cognition in many of today's therapies has led to a new interest in evaluating the processes of change that occur throughout all forms of therapy. Cognitive structures are relatively amenable to empirical assessment, and as such, attempts have been made to assess the ways in which these structures are altered as a result of psychotherapy. Raz-Duvshnai (1986) found that improvement as a result of analytically oriented psychotherapy was associated with increased complexity in patients' cognitive organizations of the external world. Others influenced by the integrative stance of cognitive-behavior therapy have attempted to relate the integration of affect and cognition to the process of therapeutic change. Greenberg and Safran (1984) suggest that many clinical problems experienced during psychotherapy stem from a breakdown in the synthesis of affect and cognition. They advise that a central element of therapy should be the "integration of different levels of processing involved in the construction of emotional experience" (p. 559).

The future of cognitive-behavior therapy is open to new techniques and approaches. For example, a major thrust of recent writings by cognitive-behavior theorists has focused on the exploration of unconscious processes (Meichenbaum & Gilmore, 1985). More importantly, a new rapprochement between behavioral and psychodynamic perspectives appears to be underway, taking its strength from the integrative approach afforded by cognitive-behavior therapy. Concepts previously left to psychoanalysts and psychodynamically oriented clinicians, such as "countertherapeutic resistance", "repression", "conflict", "transference," and the "unconscious" are presently being examined by cognitive-behaviorists (Goldfried, 1982; Kazdin, 1984; Lazarus & Fay, 1982; Mahoney, 1984; Meichenbaum & Gilmore, 1982, 1985).

Cognitive-behavior therapy will complete its second decade with a healthy flexibility in its theoretical underpinnings and treatment techniques. Continued refinement of cognitive-behavior therapy should encourage further synthesis and integration of its many varied techniques. Clinicians and researchers alike will hopefully continue to adopt the broad perspective of both psychopathology and psychotherapy afforded by this pragmatic yet sophisticated orientation.

Acknowledgment. Preparation of this chapter was supported in part by Biomedical Research Support Grant NIH S07RR07015.

References

Abelson, R. P. (1981). Psychological status of the script concept. *American Psychologist, 36,* 715–729.

Alexander, F. (1963). The dynamics of psychotherapy in the light of learning theory. *American Journal of Psychiatry, 120,* 440–448.

Alloy, L. B., & Abramson, L. Y. (1979). Judgment of contingency in depressed and nondepressed students: Sadder but wiser? *Journal of Experimental Psychology: General, 108,* 441–485.

Anderson, C. A., Horowitz, L. M., & deSales French, R. (1983). Attributional style of lonely and depressed people. *Journal of Personality and Social Psychology, 45,* 127–136.

Bandura, A. (1961). Psychotherapy as a learning process. *Psychological Bulletin, 58,* 143–159.

Bandura, A. (1969). *Principles of behavior modification.* New York: Holt, Rinehart & Winston.

Bandura, A. (1977a). Self-efficacy: Toward a unifying theory of behavioral change. *Psychological Review, 84,* 191–215.

Bandura, A. (1977b). *Social learning theory.* Englewood Cliffs, NJ: Prentice-Hall.

Bandura, A. (1978). The self in reciprocal determinism. *American Psychologist, 33,* 344–358.

Bandura, A. (1982). Self-efficacy mechanism in human agency. *American Psychologist, 37,* 122–147.

Bandura, A., Adams, N. E., & Beyer, J. (1977). Cognitive processes mediating behavioral change. *Journal of Personality and Social Psychology, 35,* 125–139.

Beck, A. T. (1970). Cognitive therapy: Nature and relation to behavior therapy. *Behavior Therapy, 1,* 184–200.

Beck, A. T. (1976). *Cognitive therapy and the emotional disorders.* New York: International Universities Press.

Beck, A. T, Rush, A. J., Shaw, B. F., & Emery, G. (1979). *Cognitive therapy of depression.* New York: Guilford Press.

Bernstein, D. A., & Borkovec, T. D. (1973). *Progressive relaxation training. A manual for the helping professions.* Champaign, IL: Research Press.

Birk, L., & Brinkley-Birk, A. (1974). Psychoanalysis and behavior therapy. *The American Journal of Psychiatry, 131,* 499–510.

Bornstein, P. H., Hamilton, S. B., Carmody, T. B., Rychtarik, R. G., & Verold, D. M. (1977). Reliability enhancement: Increasing the accuracy of self-report through mediation-based procedures. *Cognitive Therapy and Research, 1,* 85–98.

Brady, J. (1968). Psychotherapy in a combined behavioral and dynamic approach. *Comprehensive Psychiatry, 9,* 536–543.

Bregher, L., & McGaugh, J. L. (1965). Critique and reformulation of "learning theory" approaches to psychotherapy and neurosis. *Psychological Bulletin, 63,* 338–358.

Brown, H. A. (1973). Role of expectancy manipulation in systematic desensitization. *Journal of Consulting and Clinical Psychology, 41,* 405–411.

Chaney, E., O'Leary, M., & Marlatt, G. A. (1978). Skill training with alcoholics. *Journal of Consulting and Clinical Psychology, 46,* 1092–1104.

Crits-Christoph, P., & Singer, J. L. (1981). Imagery in cognitive-behavior therapy: Research and application. *Clinical Psychology Review, 1,* 19–32.

Denney, D. R. (1981). Self-control approaches to the treatment of test anxiety. In I. G. Sarason (Ed.), *Test anxiety: Theory, research, and application* (pp. 209–243). Hillsdale, NJ: Erlbaum.

Dollard, J., & Miller, N. (1950). *Personality and psychotherapy.* New York: McGraw-Hill.

Ellis, A. (1962). *Reason and emotion in psychotherapy.* New York: Lyle Stuart.

Ellis, A. (1987). The impossibility of achieving consistently good mental health. *American Psychologist, 42,* 364–375.

Eysenck, H. J. (1960). *Behavior therapy and the neuroses.* New York: Pergamon Press.

Fairburn, C. (1985). Cognitive-behavioral treatment of bulimia. In D. Garner & P. Garfinkel (Eds.), *Handbook of psychotherapy for anorexia nervosa and bulimia* (pp. 160–192). New York: Guilford Press.

Feather, B. W., & Rhoads, J. M., (1972a). Psychodynamic behavior therapy: Theory and rationale. *Archives of General Psychiatry, 26*, 496–503.

Feather, B. W., & Rhoads, J. M., (1972b). Psychodynamic behavior therapy: Clinical aspects. *Archives of General Psychiatry, 26*, 503–511.

Frank, J. D. (1974). *Persuasion and healing*. New York: Schocken Books.

French, T. M. (1933). Interrelations between psychoanalysis and the experimental work of Pavlov. *American Journal of Psychiatry, 12*, 1165–1203.

Garfield, S. L., (1982). Eclecticism and integration in psychotherapy. *Behavior Therapy, 13*, 610–623.

Garfield, S. L., & Kurtz, R. (1976). Clinical psychologists in the 1970s. *American Psychologist, 31*, 1–9.

Goldfried, M. R. (1971). Systematic desensitization as training in self-control. *Journal of Consulting and Clinical Psychology, 37*, 228–234.

Goldfried, M. R. (1977). The use of relaxation and cognitive relabeling as coping skills. In R. B. Stuart (Ed.), *Behavioral self management: Strategies, techniques, and outcomes* (pp. 82–116). New York: Brunner-Mazel.

Goldfried, M. R. (1980). Psychotherapy as coping skills training. In M. J. Mahoney (Ed.), *Psychotherapy process: Current issues and future direction* (pp. 89–119). New York: Plenum Press.

Goldfried, M. R. (1982). Resistance and clinical behavior therapy. In P. Wachtel (Ed.), *Resistance* (pp. 95–114). New York: Plenum Press.

Goldfried, M. R., & Robbins, C. (1982). On the facilitation of self-efficacy. *Cognitive Therapy and Research, 6*, 361–380.

Greenberg, L. S., & Safran, J. D. (1984). Integrating affect and cognition: A perspective on the process of therapeutic change. *Cognitive Therapy and Research, 8*, 559–578.

Heppner, P. P. (1978). A review of problem-solving literature and its relationship to the counseling process. *Journal of Counseling Psychology, 25*, 366–375.

Horney, K. (1950). *Neurosis and human growth*. New York: W. W. Norton.

Ingram, R. E., & Kendall, P. C. (1986). Cognitive-clinical psychology: A paradigm shift without a paradigm. In R. E. Ingram (Ed.), *Information processing approaches to psychopathology and clinical psychology* (pp. 1–21). Orlando: Academic Press.

Jacobson, E. (1929). *Progressive relaxation*. Chicago: Chicago University Press.

Kanfer, F. H. (1979). Self-management: Strategies and tactics. In A. P. Goldstein & F. H. Kanfer (Eds.), *Maximizing treatment gains* (pp. 1–28). New York: Academic Press.

Kanfer, F. H., & Busemeyer, J. R. (1982). The use of problem solving and decision making in behavior therapy. *Clinical Psychology Review, 2*, 239–266.

Kazdin, A. E. (1984). Integration of psychodynamic and behavioral psychotherapies: Conceptual versus empirical syntheses. In H. Arkowitz & S. B. Messer (Eds.), *Psychoanalytic therapy and behavior therapy. Is integration possible?* (pp. 139–170). New York: Plenum Press.

Kopel, S., & Arkowitz, H. (1975). The role of attribution and self-perception in behavior change. *Genetic Psychology Monographs, 92*, 175–212.

Kubie, L. S., (1934). Relation of the conditioned reflex to psychoanalytic technique. *Archives of Neurological Psychiatry, 32*, 1137–1142.

Lange, E. J., & Jakubowski, P. (1976). *Responsible assertive behavior*. Champaign, IL: Research Press.

Lazarus, A. A., & Fay, A. (1982). Resistance or rationalization: A cognitive-behavioral perspective. In P. Wachtel (Ed.), *Resistance* (pp. 115–132). New York: Plenum Press.

Lazarus, R., Cohen, J., Folkman, S., Kanner, A., & Schaefer, C. (1980). Psychological stress and adaptation: Some unresolved issues. In H. Selye (Ed.), *Selye's guide to stress research* (Vol. 1, pp. 90–117). New York: Van Nostrand Reinhold.

Luborsky, L., Singer, B., & Luborsky, L. (1975). Comparative studies of psychotherapy. Is it true that "Everyone has won and all must have prizes"? *Archives of General Psychiatry, 32*, 995–1005.

Mahoney, M. J. (1974). *Cognition and behavior modification*. Cambridge: Ballinger Publishing Co.

Mahoney, M. J. (1977a). Reflections on the cognitive-learning trend in psychotherapy. *American Psychologist, 32*, 5–13.

Mahoney, M. J. (1977b). Personal science: A cognitive-learning therapy. In A. Ellis & R. Grieger (Eds.), *Handbook of rational psychotherapy* (pp. 3–33). New York: Springer.

Mahoney, M. J. (1984). Psychoanalysis and behaviorism: The yin and yang of determinism. In H. Arkowitz & S. B. Messer (Eds.), *Psychoanalytic therapy and behavior therapy. Is integration possible?* (pp. 303–326). New York: Plenum Press.

Marlatt, G. A., & Gordon, J. R. (1980). Determinants of relapse: Implications for the maintenance of behavior change. In P. O. Davidson & S. M. Davidson (Eds.), *Behavioral medicine: Changing health life styles* (pp. 410–452). New York: Brunner/Mazel.

Meichenbaum, D. (1974). *Cognitive behavior modification*. Morristown, NJ: General Learning Press.

Meichenbaum, D. (1975). A cognitive-behavior modification approach to assessment. In M. Hersen & A. Bellack (Eds.), *Behavioral assessment: A practical handbook* (pp. 143–171). New York: Pergamon Press.

Meichenbaum, D. (1977). *Cognitive behavior modification. An integrated approach*. New York: Plenum Press.

Meichenbaum, D., & Butler, L. (1980). Cognitive ethology: Assessing the streams of consciousness and emotion. In K. R. Blankstein, P. Pliner, & J. Polivy (Eds.), *Advances in the study of communication and affect: Assessment and modification of emotional behavior* (Vol. 6, pp. 139–163). New York: Plenum Press.

Meichenbaum, D., & Cameron, R. (1973). Training schizophrenics to talk to themselves: A means of developing attentional controls. *Behavior Therapy, 4,* 515–534.

Meichenbaum, D., & Cameron, R. (1983). Stress inoculation training: Toward a general paradigm for training coping skills. In D. Meichenbaum & M. E. Jaremko (Eds.), *Stress reduction and prevention* (pp. 115–154). New York: Plenum.

Meichenbaum, D., & Gilmore, J. B. (1985). The nature of unconscious processes: A cognitive-behavioral perspective. In K. Bowers & D. Meichenbaum (Eds.), *The unconscious reconsidered* (pp. 273–298). New York: Wiley.

Meichenbaum, D., & Gilmore, J. B. (1982). Resistance from a cognitive-behavioral perspective. In P. Wachtel (Ed.), *Resistance* (pp. 133–156). New York: Plenum Press.

Meichenbaum, D., & Goodman, J. (1971). Training impulsive children to talk to themselves: A means of developing self-control. *Journal of Abnormal Psychology, 77,* 115–126.

Miller, R. C., & Berman, J. S. (1981). *The efficacy of cognitive-behavior therapy: A quantitative review of the research evidence*. Paper presented at the annual meeting of the American Psychological Association, Los Angeles, CA.

Murray, E. J., & Jacobson, L. I. (1971). Cognition and learning in traditional and behavioral therapy. In A. Bergin & S. Garfield (Eds.), *Handbook of psychotherapy and behavior change: An empirical analysis* (pp. 661–687). New York: Wiley.

Nisbett, R., & Schachter, W. (1966). Cognitive manipulation of pain. *Journal of Experimental Social Psychology, 2,* 227–236.

Novaco, R. W. (1978). Anger and coping with stress: Cognitive-behavioral interventions. In J. P. Foreyt & D. P. Rathjen (Eds.), *Cognitive behavior therapy: Research and application* (pp. 135–173). New York: Plenum Press.

Peterson, C., & Seligman, M. E. P. (1984). Causal explanations as a risk factor for depression: Theory and evidence. *Psychological Review, 91,* 347–374.

Raz-Duvshnai, A. (1986). Cognitive structure changes with psychotherapy in neurosis. *British Journal of Medical Psychology, 59,* 341–350.

Rhoads, J. M., & Feather, B. W. (1974). The application of psychodynamics to behavior therapy. *American Journal of Psychiatry, 131,* 17–20.

Rook, K. S., & Hammen, C. L. (1977). A cognitive perspective on the experience of sexual arousal. *Journal of Social Issues, 33,* 7–29.

Ross, L., Rodin, J., & Zimbardo, P. (1969). Toward an attribution therapy: The reduction of fear through induced cognitive-emotional misattribution. *Journal of Personality and Social Psychology, 12,* 279–288.

Salovey, P., & Haar M. D. (1983). *The efficacy of cognitive-behavior therapy and writing process training for alleviating writing anxiety*. Paper presented at the meeting of the American Education Research Association, Montreal, Quebec.

Schank, R. R., & Abelson, R. P. (1977). *Scripts, plans, goals, and understanding*. New York: Halsted.

Schwartz, R. M. (1982). Cognitive-behavior modification: A conceptual review. *Clinical Psychology Review, 2,* 267–293.

Seligman, M. E. P. (1975). *Helplessness: On depression, development, and death*. San Francisco: Freeman.

Seligman, M. E. P., Abramson, L. Y., Semmel, A., & von Baeyer, C. (1979). Depressive attributional style. *Journal of Abnormal Psychology, 88,* 242–247.

Silberstein, L. R., & Striegel-Moore, R. H. (1985). *Bulimia: A feminist and therapeutic challenge*. Paper presented at the meeting of the Association of Women and Psychotherapy, New York, New York.

Singer, J. L. (1974). *Imagery and daydream methods in psychotherapy and behavior modification*. New York: Academic Press.

Singer, J. L. (1979). Imagery and affect in psychotherapy: Elaborating private scripts and generating contexts. In A. A. Sheikh & J. T. Shaffer (Eds.), *The potential of fantasy and imagination* (pp. 27–39). New York: Brandon House.

Singer, J. L., & Pope, K. S. (1978). The use of imagery and fantasy techniques in psychotherapy. In J. L. Singer & K. S. Pope (Eds.), *The power of human imagination* (pp. 3–34). New York: Plenum Press.

Smith, M. I., Glass, G. V., & Miller, T. I. (1980). *The benefits of psychotherapy*. Baltimore: Johns Hopkins University Press.

Sullivan, H. S. (1953). *The interpersonal theory of psychiatry*. New York: Norton.

Taylor, S. E., & Crocker, J. (1981). Schematic bases of social information processing. In E. T. Higgins, C. P. Herman, & M. P. Zanna (Eds.), *Social cognition: The Ontario symposium in personality and social psychology* (pp. 89–134). Hillsdale, NJ: Erlbaum.

Turk, D. C., Holzman, A. D., & Kerns, R. D. (1989). Treatment of chronic pain: Emphasis on self-management. In K. A. Holroyd & T. Creer (Eds.), *Self-Management in health psychology and behavioral medicine* (pp. 441–472). New York: Academic Press.

Turk, D. C., Meichenbaum, D., & Genest, M. (1983). *Pain and behavioral medicine*. New York: Guilford Press.

Turk, D. C., & Salovey, P. (1985). Cognitive structures, cognitive processes, and cognitive-behavior modification: I. Client issues. *Cognitive Therapy and Research, 9*, 1–17.

Turk, D. C., & Salovey, P. (1986). Clinical information processing: Bias inoculation. In R. E. Ingram (Ed.), *Information processing approaches to psychopathology and clinical psychology* (pp. 305–323). Orlando: Academic Press.

Turk, D. C., & Salovey, P. (Eds.). (1988). *Reasoning, inference and judgment in psychotherapy*. New York: Free Press.

Valins, S., & Nisbett, R. (1976). *Attribution Processes in the Development and Treatment of Emotional Disorders*. Morristown, NJ: General Learning Press.

Wachtel, P. L. (1977). *Psychoanalysis and behavior therapy: Toward an integration*. New York: Basic Books.

Watson, J. B. (1913). Psychology as a behaviorist views it. *Psychological Review, 20*, 158–177.

Weitzman, B. (1967). Behavior therapy and psychotherapy. *Psychological Review, 74*, 300–317.

Wilkins, W. (1971). Desensitization: Social and cognitive factors underlying the effectiveness of Wolpe's procedures. *Psychological Bulletin, 76*, 311–317.

Wilson, G. T. (1985). *The treatment of bulimia nervosa: A cognitive-behavioral perspective*. Division 12 presidential address presented at the 93rd Annual Convention of the American Psychological Association, Los Angeles.

Wine, J. (1981). Cognitive-attentional theory of test anxiety. In I. G. Sarason (Ed.), *Test anxiety: Theory, research and application* (pp. 349–385). Hillsdale, NJ: Erlbaum.

Wolf, E. (1966). Learning theory and psychoanalysis. *British Journal of Medical Psychology, 39*, 1–10.

Wolpe, J. (1958). *Psychotherapy by reciprocal inhibition*. Stanford: Stanford University Press.

Wolpe, J. & Rachman, S. (1960). Psychoanalytic "evidence": A critique based on Freud's case of Little Hans. *Journal of Nervous and Mental Disease, 131*, 135–148.

12

Interpersonal Psychotherapy of Depression (IPT)

Cleon Cornes

Historical Background

Among the forms of short-term psychotherapies, IPT is a relative newcomer. It has evolved over the past 15 to 20 years and has been used primarily in carefully controlled studies. However, the technique and principles of short-term IPT are based on a long-standing tradition and practice of interpersonal psychotherapy. Two of Freud's early colleagues, Ferenczi and Rank (1925), were interested in developing techniques to shorten the course of psychoanalysis. Ferenczi suggested a variety of more active techniques, and Rank focused on the effects of traumatic events (particularly the trauma of birth). Later at the University of Chicago, Alexander and French (1946) developed a shorter form of psychoanalysis in which they narrowed the scope of treatment by focusing primarily on the present and developing the concept of a "corrective emotional experience." Thomas French (1958) also introduced the term *focal conflict* that was utilized and studied further by Michael Balint and his colleagues in Great Britain (Balint, Ornstein, & Balint, 1972). Their work clearly demonstrated the value of organizing the treatment around one or two specific areas of conflict.

Several American psychiatrists have been particularly important in the development of an interpersonal approach to psychotherapy. The first of these was Adolf Meyer (1957), who was perhaps the most influential professor of psychiatry in the United States. His work at Johns Hopkins University was the beginning of the Baltimore–Washington group of interpersonal therapists, and he educated many excellent psychiatric residents who subsequently developed their own training programs throughout the country. Meyer's approach, which was called psychobiology, focused on details of patients' life history, their experiences during each stage of development, and the impact of these life events on feelings and behavior. He conceptualized psychopathology in terms of these

Cleon Cornes • Western Psychiatric Institute and Clinic, 3811 O'Hara Street, Pittsburgh, Pennsylvania 15213.

"reactions" (depressive reaction, schizophrenic reaction, etc.), and his approach continued to have a pervasive effect on our nomenclature until the development of DSM-II in 1968.

A student of Meyer, Harry Stack Sullivan, continued to develop and apply an interpersonal approach to the treatment of different types of patients, including those with schizophrenia. Sullivan (1956) and Frieda Fromm-Reichman (1960) have been the leading exponents in the field of interpersonal psychiatry, and the major publication describing IPT (Klerman, Weissman, Rounsaville, & Chevron, 1984) is sprinkled liberally with quotations from Sullivan's writings. Another member of the Baltimore–Washington group was Mabel Blake Cohen and colleagues (1954) who had a major interest in the treatment of depression and utilized an interpersonal approach in the treatment of patients with manic-depressive illness.

THEORETICAL AND EMPIRICAL FRAMEWORK

The emergence of short-term Interpersonal Psychotherapy of Depression (IPT) occurred in the early 1970s in the New Haven–Boston Collaborative Depression Research Project as a psychological treatment designed specifically for the needs of depressed patients. "It is a focused, short-term, time-limited therapy that emphasizes the current interpersonal relations of the depressed patient while recognizing the role of genetic, biochemical, developmental, and personality factors in the causation of and vulnerability to depression" (Klerman et al., 1984, p. 6). These authors describe the clinical experience and research evidence that indicate that psychotherapeutic interventions directed at an interpersonal context will facilitate recovery from an episode of depression and possibly have preventive effects against relapse and recurrence. The recognition that multiple factors may contribute to the cause of depression has led to the use of IPT as a single modality of treatment and also in combination with antidepressant medication. The rationale and technique of IPT was initially described in a training manual developed for research projects and subsequently published in the form of a textbook (Klerman et al., 1984).

The IPT approach, as described in the previous paragraph, is based on a specific view of the concept of depression. The term *depression* generally has three meanings—a mood, a symptom, and a syndrome. As a mood, it is a universal phenomenon associated with life experiences that lead to feelings of disappointment, frustration, and sadness. It is usually a mild, transient state, lasting a few hours or at most a few days, and requiring no treatment. Depression can also be a symptom that commonly occurs in patients suffering from a variety of medical and psychiatric disorders. The depression may be a symptom or a result of the illness itself (for example in association with a viral infection, schizophrenia, diabetes, thyroid disease, etc.), or it may be a complication of the medication used to treat various illnesses (antihypertensive drugs, antipsychotic drugs, etc.). Depression is also often a symptom in people who abuse drugs or alcohol. In all of these situations in which depression is a secondary manifestation of another illness, the treatment should be focused on the underlying or primary disorder. When we define depression as a syndrome, however, we are referring to a collection of specific symptoms that persist over a considerable period of time and are severe enough to produce significant impairment or disability. One example of this definition of depression would be the criteria for major depression in the current *Diagnostic and Statistical Manual of the American Psychiatric Association* (APA, 1987). When we view depression as a syndrome or illness, we begin to think of specific forms of treatment directed toward reducing or eliminating the symptoms associated with that depression, and short-term IPT is one such specific and effective treatment.

In addition to the theoretical framework for IPT, there is an empirical basis for understanding depression in an interpersonal context, springing from several divergent sources, including developmental studies of children as well as clinical and epidemiological studies of adults. Observations made during these studies have led to a theory of attachment bonds that suggests that the most intense human emotions are associated with the formation, disruption, and renewal of these bonds (beginning a friendship or romance, marriage, divorce, remarriage, etc.). Bowlby (1969) studied early mother–child relationships and found that a disruption of these attachment bonds led to depression and despair. He suggested that a number of psychiatric disorders could result from a person's inability to make or maintain these emotional bonds. Bowlby (1977) also proposed a system of psychotherapy designed to help patients see the connections between these early attachments and their current interpersonal relationships. Rutter (1972) extended Bowlby's work to other relationships, demonstrating that deprivation and the disruption of attachment bonds are related to the onset of depression. Henderson and his colleagues (1982) found that depressed patients have fewer friends and relationships, less support, and fewer pleasant interactions with others. Brown *et al.* (1977) studied a group of women living in London and found that the presence of an intimate, confiding relationship with a man was the most important protection against developing a depression in the presence of a variety of stressful life events. A number of investigators have attempted to evaluate the impact of current social stress, and the work of Paykel (1978) at Yale appears to be most relevant to becoming depressed. He found that "exits from the social field" occurred more frequently in the 6-month period prior to the onset of depression and that marital friction was the most common event reported by patients before they became depressed. Similar results were reported by Ilfeld (1977) who studied 3,000 adults in Chicago and found that depressive symptoms were closely related to stresses in marriage and parenting. Weissman and Paykel (1974) observed that depressed women are more impaired in all aspects of their social function, with close family relationships being most severely affected by hostility and poor communication. Most of these patterns improved when the women recovered from their symptoms of depression. Thus it seems to be true that close and satisfactory interpersonal relationships are quite important in the prevention of depression, and the disruption of those attachments plays a major role in the development of depression.

SELECTION OF PATIENTS

As noted previously, IPT has been designed primarily to treat patients with a major depression. Klerman *et al.* (1984) have recommended that it only be used to treat patients who are suffering from a nonpsychotic, nonbipolar depression and who are not in need of inpatient care and treatment. Because most of the reported experience with IPT has been in the context of carefully designed research studies, those recommendations have usually been followed. In most protocols, the age range for patients has been between 18 and 65 years. As with most effective forms of treatment, however, the boundaries for its application have begun to expand. Rounsaville and colleagues (1983) has reported on his efforts to use IPT with a group of patients whose primary problem was drug abuse. He did not find IPT to be as effective with that population as it is with depressed patients. Sholomskas and his colleagues (1983) completed a pilot project in which they used IPT to successfully treat a group of older patients with depression. We have recently developed a protocol in Pittsburgh in which we plan to evaluate the effectiveness of IPT in treating depressed patients aged 60–80 and maintaining them in a euthymic state.

IPT has been clearly established as an effective form of treatment for younger and middle-aged adults experiencing an episode of major depression, unipolar type. Its efficacy is currently being evaluated in Pittsburgh in a slightly modified form called Maintenance Interpersonal Psychotherapy (MIPT) through a long-term study with patients who have experienced recurrent episodes of major depression. The acute episode of depression is treated with a combination of IPT and imipramine. When a remission of symptoms occurs, patients are randomly assigned to maintenance treatment for several years with IPT, imipramine, placebo, or their combinations. One goal of this protocol, presently being conducted by our Depression Prevention Program with David Kupfer as principal investigator, is to demonstrate whether MIPT is effective in helping to prevent future episodes of depression.

If IPT continues to be applied to different populations of patients in the future, it would seem to be most appropriate to study its effectiveness in patients in which symptoms of depression predominate. These could be older or younger patients with depression, patients experiencing adjustment disorders with depressed mood, patients with dysthymic disorders, and the like. We should probably continue to exclude patients with bipolar depressions because of their cyclical, recurrent features that seem to be more biologically determined and not so clearly related to the major problem areas that have been the focus of IPT. We should also continue to exclude patients with a psychotic depression because they are too disorganized and regressed and would require more structure than IPT can provide.

TIME LIMITS

When IPT was initially developed as a specific treatment for depression, between 12 and 20 weekly sessions were found to be effective in achieving the therapeutic goals. Thus, the preferable duration was set at approximately 16 sessions over a 4-month period of time. Extra sessions can be added to deal with a crisis or to complete the therapeutic work in a more satisfactory manner. Occasionally the major problem areas seem to be resolved more quickly leading to termination of the therapy before 16 weeks. In the maintainance therapy modification (MIPT), patients are seen weekly for 12 weeks, biweekly for 2 months, and monthly thereafter throughout the course of treatment (2 to 3 years).

IPT sessions are usually 45 to 60 minutes in length. They are closer to 45 minutes when IPT is used alone and closer to 60 minutes when it is used in combination with medication (allowing for review of symptoms and side effects, discussion of medical issues, writing prescriptions, etc.). The rationale for the time limits is based on developing a more narrow focus for the therapy and concentrating on one or two major problem areas. Empirical observations in pilot projects and carefully controlled studies have supported the continued use of these time limits.

ASSESSMENT TECHNIQUES

Because most of the reported experience with IPT has been in a research setting, rather elaborate assessment techniques have been used to assure that patients have a major depression. Rating scales such as the Hamilton, Raskin, and Beck have been utilized, with minimum scores for entry into a protocol. Many of the research programs use an extensive evaluation such as the Schedule for Affective Disorders and Schizophrenia (SADS) to determine the presence or absence of major depression and to rule out other disorders. In those settings, the initial assessment is often performed by a clinical evaluator skilled in administering the instruments necessary to assure a homogeneous population for the study. After patients have been evaluated and selected for the research, they are then seen by the treating clinician to begin a course of IPT.

However, as IPT comes into more general clinical practice, less intensive methods of assessment are being developed. The first several sessions (the initial phase) are designed to review the symptoms of depression, determine the interpersonal context at the onset of the depression, and conduct an interpersonal inventory. It is quite reasonable to expect the therapist to assess the symptoms and determine if the criteria for major depression are present. The criteria in DSM-III-R can be evaluated using traditional observation and clinical interviewing techniques, or more structured assessments could be included if desired. In addition to making a diagnosis of depression, the therapist would need to assess the patient's ability to describe the onset and course of the illness in an interpersonal context and to discuss the impact that important relationships are having in his or her current life. IPT is not wedded to a specific etiologic theory of depression but is based on the belief that psychopathology is manifest in the interpersonal sphere. Thus a major effort is made to understand how problems in interpersonal relations contribute to the symptoms and how psychosocial events are correlated in time with the onset of the depressive illness. The patient should be able to participate actively in this process, and the therapist encourages a collaborative relationship as an important part of the therapeutic process.

GOALS OF THE THERAPY

The goals of IPT are partly determined by viewing depression as having three component processes: symptom formation, social and interpersonal relations, and personality patterns. The symptoms include a depressed mood, decreased pleasure and interest in usual activities, changes in sleep and appetite, decreased energy and motivation, feelings of worthlessness and guilt, difficulty with concentration and memory, and thoughts about death or suicide. Social and interpersonal relations may be affected by tendencies to withdraw and become more irritable, to be critical and pessimistic, to base current expectations on earlier experiences, to develop low self-esteem that interferes with personal mastery and competence and to have difficulty dealing with feelings associated with loss or other major life events. The patient's personality may contribute to the depression through enduring traits such as inhibited expression of anger, poor patterns of communication, persistent feelings of guilt and low self-esteem and so forth. IPT attempts to intervene in the first two processes but is not intensive enough or long enough to have a marked impact on enduring aspects of personality.

The first goal (reduction of depressive symptoms) is achieved by helping patients understand that their vague and confusing experiences are part of a depressive syndrome, which is well understood and quite common. Patients are told that the syndrome responds to a variety of treatments and that the prognosis for alleviating the depressive symptoms is quite good (70%–80%). IPT is described as one of the successful treatment approaches, and the patient is encouraged to begin to explore the factors that may contribute to the depression. The second goal is to help the patient develop more successful patterns for dealing with current social and interpersonal problems that were associated with the onset of depression. The major problem areas that have been commonly associated with the onset of depression are (1) delayed or distorted grief reactions, (2) interpersonal role disputes, (3) role transitions, and (4) interpersonal deficits (Klerman et al., 1984). This is achieved by determining which of the four common problem areas are present and focusing the therapy around one or two of those problem areas, leading to a more complete mastery of current social roles and resolution of interpersonal conflicts.

CASE ILLUSTRATIONS

Before considering a number of clinical examples, it seems appropriate at this point to briefly summarize the course of IPT. There are three phases in the treatment. The initial sessions (1–3) are utilized to obtain a history of the depressive illness, explain the rationale and intent of IPT, complete an interpersonal inventory, identify the major problem areas, and agree on a focus and plan for the treatment. The middle phase (sessions 4–13) focuses primarily on the one or two problem areas that have been identified as related to the depression, using the goals and strategies that are pertinent to each problem area. During this phase, the therapist helps the patient maintain the focus while attending to his or her feelings and uses the therapeutic relationship to further the goals of the treatment. In the termination phase (sessions 14–16), the course of therapy is reviewed, and the progress is reinforced. There is explicit discussion about the end of treatment, which is acknowledged as a time of loss and possible grieving. There is increasing recognition of the patient's competence, ability to function independently, and acquisition of new capacities to reduce vulnerability to depression in the future.

Delayed Grief Reactions

Freud (1917) described normal and abnormal grief reactions in his paper entitled *Mourning and Melancholia*. The process of mourning involves recalling the memories of the events associated with the person who died, experiencing the feelings associated with those events, and a gradual weaning from those experiences that frees the mourner to participate more fully in new experiences and relationships in the future. Resolving ambivalent feelings about the lost person is often an important part of the grieving process. The normal process of mourning may be adversely affected by fear of the pain involved, strong feelings such as anger and guilt, or holding on to narrow or rigid attitudes about the relationship. This kind of interference in the grief process seems to make people more vulnerable to developing an episode of depression. The brief description of the following case will illustrate a pattern of abnormal grief in a patient who became depressed and was treated with IPT:

The patient was a 35-year-old married woman who has two sons (ages 1 and 3 years) and had worked in the past as a nurse.[1] She complained of increasing depression over the past year, becoming worse in the last few months. Her symptoms included dysphoric mood, decreased energy and interest, feelings of sadness and hopelessness, decreased sleep and appetite, feelings of guilt and resentment, and social withdrawal. Her clinical picture was consistent with a diagnosis of major depression, single episode. Her depression began shortly after the death of her father and the birth of her younger son. She described conflicted feelings and more difficulty caring for this child than she had with her first son. Her husband was described as an ambitious college professor, who "works all the time and frequently is away from home." She stated he has been less supportive of her and the children in the past year, and there has been increased conflict in their relationship.

When I attempted to evaluate the patient's reaction to her father's death, she indicated an inability to grieve, partly due to the fact that his death occurred during her pregnancy, and she was fearful that a strong emotional reaction might lead to a miscar-

---

[1]To ensure confidentiality, descriptive details about each patient have been modified in ways that should protect their identity but not interfere with the value of the cases as examples of the major problem areas of IPT.

riage. She also tended to describe her father in entirely positive terms and to be more critical of her mother. It was my impression that she had been unable to resolve her ambivalent feelings about her father, had been unable to adequately mourn his death, and had subsequently become depressed, directing her feelings of anger and resentment toward her younger son, husband, and mother. We agreed to focus primarily on the major problem areas of delayed grief and interpersonal conflict.

During the middle phase of treatment, we reviewed the circumstances around her father's death and her reaction to it. Although she "went through the motions" during his funeral, she stated she did not feel the same sense of loss and sadness she had experienced with earlier deaths in her family. She recognized that after the funeral she did not periodically think about her father and become tearful as she had expected she would. Instead she gradually became more irritable, angry, and depressed. When I suggested it might be important and helpful to review her experiences and feelings regarding his death she said, "I was afraid of that." However, she was able to do that very well in sessions 5 through 8, with overt expressions of grief and a reduction in her symptoms of depression. She became more resistant in sessions 9 and 10 as I encouraged her to recall more feelings of anger or disappointment toward her father. The anger was directed toward me, and she threatened to discontinue the treatment. With support from her husband (who told her she was improving), she was able to discuss her feelings with me, recognize the presence of ambivalent feelings in her relationship with her father prior to his death, and agree that these feelings have been displaced onto other people— including me—since his death. That was followed by further improvement of her depression and an ability to focus more directly in the therapy on the feelings of resentment toward her son and the conflict with her husband. She realized that in some strange way she had blamed her son and his birth for her father's death and blamed her husband for abandoning her when her father died.

During the last 5 weeks of the treatment, she began to enjoy spending more time with her son, was able to communicate more directly with her husband, and her mood returned to normal along with her energy level and interest in usual activities. During the termination phase, we reviewed the course of the treatment, discussed the gains she had made, and attempted to anticipate some aspects of her life in the future. She expressed concern about needing more treatment but agreed to "try it on my own" for a while. She was evaluated at 6-month intervals for 18 months and continued to do well. There was no return of depressed symptoms, and she did not seek further therapy.

This case illustrates a number of goals and strategies that are an important part of an IPT approach to dealing with depression in the context of an abnormal grief reaction. Two of the goals were "to facilitate the delayed mourning process, and to help the patient reestablish interests and relationships that can substitute for what has been lost" (Klerman et al., 1984, p. 97). The treatment strategies include nonjudgemental exploration of the feelings associated with her father's death, reassurance that those feelings are natural and will not destroy her, reconstruction of important facets of the relationship leading to new awareness of its impact on her life, and encouragement to improve the quality of current relationships and develop new and meaningful ones in the future.

Interpersonal Role Disputes

The second major problem area commonly associated with the onset of a depressive episode is the presence of interpersonal role disputes. Social roles develop within the family, at work, in the neighborhood, and in a variety of friendly and intimate relationships. These roles can be described according to the current patterns of interaction, the history of the developing relationships, and the thoughts and feelings that each person has about his or her respective roles. There are many factors that can lead to changes in social roles and possibly to interpersonal disputes. Some of the more common ones are illness, financial problems, job loss, aging, developmental delays, psychodynamic conflicts, societal expectations or pressures, cross-cultural differences, and so forth.

An interpersonal dispute occurs when the patient and at least one other significant person develop nonreciprocal expectations about their relationships. The therapist will focus on these disputes if they seem to be important in contributing to the onset or maintaining the episode of depression. This frequently happens when the disputes are stalled or repetitious with little hope for improvement, leading to a loss of self-esteem, belief that the dispute can no longer be controlled, and fear of losing the relationship and what it provides. Role disputes are perpetuated by a sense of demoralization, poor patterns of communication, and irreconcilable differences.

The persistence of these disputes can lead to depression that is appropriately treated with IPT. The therapist should first help the patient to identify the disputes that are related to the early feelings of depression. Then a plan can be developed to deal with the dispute, modify patterns of communication, and reassess expectations about the relationship. In developing this plan, the patient and therapist need to identify the current stage of the dispute—renegotiation, impasse, or dissolution. In the renegotiation stage, there is awareness of the differences and active attempts to talk about the problem, even if there has not been success in changing or resolving it. An impasse occurs when discussion has stopped and smoldering feelings of anger and resentment persist. Dissolution indicates that the relationship has been permanently damaged and cannot be reestablished. The following case will illustrate the use of IPT with a patient who became depressed in the context of several role disputes:

The patient, a 27-year-old married woman, described increasing symptoms of depression over the past 6 months, which she related primarily to the many difficulties she had working as an assistant manager in a restaurant. She spent most of the first session angrily complaining about how she was mistreated by her fellow workers, causing her to quit her job several weeks ago. Her current symptoms included dysphoric feelings, loneliness, constant worry, feelings of guilt, religious preoccupations, poor self-esteem, pessimistic feelings about the future, and suicidal thoughts (but no plan or intent). She also complained of hypersomnia, increased appetite, weight gain, anhedonia, and anergia and irritability that were both worse in the morning. She related in a defensive, histrionic style, and was often vague and diffuse. My diagnoses were major depression and histrionic personality. We agreed on a 16-week course of interpersonal psychotherapy.

In the remainder of the initial phase of treatment we reviewed the important relationships in her life. Her father suffered from alcoholism and depression and died 5 years ago. She impulsively married a man with the same first name shortly after her father's death. Her husband left after a year of marriage, and she experienced her first episode of depression that lasted for 6 months without treatment. Her mother was described as a demanding and controlling woman "who is still trying to run my life for me." She attended the college that was chosen for her by her mother and did not learn to drive a car until she was 25 years old. She continues to have frequent contacts with her mother that often lead to arguments or disputes about their respective roles in each other's lives. She married her second husband 2 years ago and describes him as supportive but unhappy about her decision to quit her job. We agreed that the numerous interpersonal conflicts might have contributed to her depression and developed a plan to try to understand more about those disputes and attempt to resolve them.

We began the middle phase of therapy by reviewing the problems with her cowork- ers that led to the loss of her job. She described her boss (the owner of the restaurant) as a chauvinistic man who was constantly putting her down in ways that were reminiscent of her father's treatment of her in the past. She became tearful as she recalled becoming a sharpshooter on the rifle team and going fishing with her father as part of her unsuc- cessful efforts to please him, "to be a son for him" (she is an only child). She poignantly described planning a fishing vacation for him shortly before his death, which he refused to take. We talked about how some of her disappointment and anger in relation to her father, as well as her mixed feelings about wanting to please him, may have gotten displaced onto her relationships at work thus contributing to some of the disputes. She also described the manager of the restaurant as overly critical and demanding, which we discussed as similar to her perception of her mother.

Because she quit her job before seeking treatment, it was not possible to work further on resolving the disputes at work, so we focused mostly on her current relationships with her mother and husband. As she began to express her feelings (particularly anger and sadness) more directly about these conflicts, her depressive symptoms began to improve. We talked about possibilities for renegotiating some of the role disputes with her mother, and she made some efforts in that direction. We also focused more specifically on the disagreements she was having with her husband and were able to identify two of her major concerns: that he resents her making more money than him and that he will grow tired of her and leave if she does not support him financially. It was clear these expecta- tions were derived directly from her parents' behavior and from her experience in her first marriage. She began to communicate these and other concerns more directly to her husband, and they began to make some progress in clarifying their respective roles and feelings toward each other.

Around sessions 8 and 9, she became more defensive and resistant to continuing our work. She "forgot" to come for one session, arrived late for the next one, and spent most of that session talking about her difficulty controlling her weight since childhood. We discussed these reactions as possibly being related to increasing anxiety about her recent successful efforts to express her feelings more directly, behaving in a more autonomous and independent manner, and anticipating my upcoming vacation. She continued to work on these issues, her depression improved, and she dealt with my absence quite well. While I was away, she and her husband made plans for their own vacation this summer. We talked about how she seems to be making choices other than repeating the patterns of disappointment, anger, avoidance, and depression that she had observed in her parents' relationship and that had persisted in her own relationships until recently.

During the termination phase, the patient obtained a new job as an assistant buyer in a clothing store. Clothes have always been quite important to her, and she enjoys her current employment in that area. We reviewed the course of treatment, agreeing that her depressive illness had developed in the context of her difficulties with relationships at work and in her family. I reinforced the progress she had made in expressing feelings more openly and dealing with interpersonal disputes more directly. She expressed some concern about needing more therapy in the future but agreed to try and see how things go "on her own" for a while. She seems to understand how she can be more influential in shaping her interpersonal relationships, which may help her avoid future depressive episodes. She feels more hopeful about the future and was able to express her appreciation for my help. She continued to do well during the 18-month follow-up period.

The case illustrates the problem of interpersonal disputes that led to a dissolution in her relationships at work prior to seeking treatment. She was helped to put those relationships in perspective, understand how unrealistic expectations led to conflict, mourn the loss of those relationships, and go on with her life. We were also able to focus on two important continuing relationships and help her more calmly attempt to resolve disputes within them. We explored the anxiety and resentment associated with nonreciprocal role expectations, worked on improving patterns of communication, and succeeded in resolving some conflict. The same process occurred to some extent in the interpersonal relationship of the patient and therapist, leading to a working through of some resistance to the therapy. The resolution of these disputes led to improvement of her depression and the decision to start a new job with the prospect of less conflict and more pleasure.

Role Transitions

The third major problem area associated with the onset of depression is role transitions. Patients often become depressed when they have difficulty coping with life events that require changes in their usual roles, and these changes are most likely to lead to impairment in social function when they are experienced as a loss. Role transitions frequently occur as a person develops from one stage to another in the human life cycle. They are also a part of common experiences such as moving, changing jobs, getting married or divorced, becoming ill, having children, letting them go, and so forth. Difficulty coping with these transitions is associated with the loss of familiar supports and attachments, intense feelings such as anger and fear, the need for new social skills, and diminished self-esteem. The task of therapy with depressed patients experiencing role transitions includes evaluation of the importance of the old role, exploration of the feelings elicited by the change (including mourning the loss of the old role), learning new social skills to cope with the changes, and developing a new social support system. The next case illustration describes a patient who became depressed in response to changes in his life that required difficult role transitions:

In this instance the patient was a 29-year-old married man who had become increasingly depressed over the past 2 years. He described symptoms of dysphoric mood, apathy, reduced energy, loss of interest, libido, and motivation to work, decreased sleep and appetite, a 15-pound weight loss, fear of the future, and suicidal thoughts. He related the onset of his depression to the loss of his job in a steel mill and his inability to find another similar job. He described a previous episode of depression 10 years ago after graduating from high school and having difficulty obtaining work. His recent unemployment and subsequent depression have led to increased conflict with his wife, and he has been more critical of the fact that she has not become pregnant. He initially explained his depression as "an illness that results from situations in my life and leads to chemical changes in my body." He was disappointed that he would not be treated with medication but agreed to a trial of short-term psychotherapy.

The patient described a good relationship with his parents except for some conflict related to his rebellious behavior during adolescence. He had experienced some competitive feelings and disputes with an older brother and stated that his older sister is "quite depressed but will not seek treatment." His wife and his parents had remained supportive during his illness and his decision to seek treatment. We agreed that the depression might be related to his difficulty coping with the loss of his job, his inability to establish a new and meaningful role for himself, and his subsequent conflict with his wife (partly due to not achieving his desired role as a parent). It is interesting to note that his previous episode of depression occurred in the context of a role transition as well—from being a high-school student to difficulty finding employment. We talked about how his self-esteem is clearly related to being successfully employed and how losing a job might make him vulnerable to depression.

In the middle phase of treatment, his symptoms of depression gradually improved. We talked about losing his job, his subsequent feelings of inadequacy and shame, and his increasing social withdrawal as he became more depressed. He was slowly able to mourn the losses associated with his unemployment (including a familiar support system) and began to express some anger about being laid off. We agreed that some of his anger had been inappropriately directed toward his wife in the past. By the seventh session, his affect was brighter, he seemed more energetic and was beginning to talk more optimistically about the future. Within a week, he obtained a part-time job and began to socialize with his "buddies" at work. We then began to focus more on his relationship with his wife. His sexual interest had improved, and they resumed their efforts to have a child, leading to considerable anxiety. We discussed the possibility of consulting a fertility specialist and also their feelings about adopting a child in the future. He and his wife decided to take a 2-week vacation together, and there was an increase in anxiety and depressive symptoms prior to leaving. We discussed his reactions in relation to some continuing discomfort about his role as husband, sexual partner, and potential father, and also in anticipation of ending our therapy in 4 weeks.

He returned from vacation feeling "great." He talked enthusiastically about the time he and his wife spent together at the seashore and felt rested and ready to begin in earnest to look for a full-time job. He found one within a week. Our last two sessions were spent reviewing the course of therapy, supporting and consolidating the gains that were made, and reemphasizing his understanding of how role transitions have been difficult for him, leading to a loss of self-esteem, feelings of anger, and vulnerability to depression. If his increased understanding of that sequence of events enables him to anticipate the pattern and deal with it more quickly, he may be less vulnerable to developing a major depressive episode in the future.

Interpersonal Deficits

The fourth problem area that is occasionally present in patients who become depressed is interpersonal deficits. These patients lead lonely, isolated lives and have great difficulty establishing and maintaining meaningful relationships. They may have never established intimate or lasting relationships as adults. A major goal of the treatment is to reduce the patient's social isolation. The tasks involved in IPT with patients having interpersonal deficits include reviewing the positive and negative aspects of previous relationships, exploring the maladaptive patterns that have resulted from those experiences, and focusing the discussion more directly on the therapeutic relationship as a model for other relationships currently or in the future. The following case illustrates the treatment of depression in a patient with interpersonal deficits:

The patient was a 25-year-old single woman who complained of depression for the past year with an increase of symptoms 3 months ago. She described a dysphoric mood, poor self-esteem, social withdrawal, pessimistic and suicidal thoughts, mild sleep disorder, decreased motivation and concentration. She has been able to work regularly but did not feel satisfied with her position and recently began a volunteer job "to fill up some of the empty hours." She lived alone and described regular phone contacts and occasional visits with her parents and older sister. In the past several years, she had been involved in unsatisfying relationships with two men. She said she is still in love with one of them who is "in the process of getting a divorce." She described long-standing patterns of shyness, poor self-esteem, and self-critical behavior; and stated her parents have always been critical of her in many ways. She was not very spontaneous in our sessions, tending to relate in a rather passive and dependent manner. As I attempted to learn more about her current interpersonal relationships, she described a lonely and isolated life-style with no real meaningful or satisfying friendships.

I talked with her about how the loneliness and isolation may be contributing to her depression. She agreed and described the gradual disintegration in her most recent romantic relationship as a typical pattern in her life. She also recognized that her own insecurity and poor self-esteem interfered with her ability to deal more actively with problems as they developed in those relationships. We agreed to establish several goals for the treatment: to gain a better understanding of her negative views of herself and attempt to modify them; to learn more about the factors that contribute to unsatisfactory relationships; and to improve her ability to relate in more meaningful ways.

By the fifth session, she seemed better able to participate actively in the therapy, was recognizing some of her maladaptive patterns, and seemed less depressed. She described increasing anxiety in the past as her relationships became closer and more important to her and said "that probably won't happen in here since we only have a couple of months left." We talked about how her lack of a solid sense of self and self-esteem made her feel more vulnerable in a close relationship. I also pointed out that she has some control over the intensity and distance in our relationship, as well as in other situations in her life. She compared and contrasted my comments with recent conversations with her father who seemed to be putting pressure on her to apply for a new job. She continues to see him as overly critical and controlling and does not feel that she gets much help from her mother. We talked about how some of her own passivity and dependence was similar to her mother's behavior, and she agreed to try dealing with both her parents more actively. She described a pattern of responding to anxiety by becoming more passive and withdrawn, feeling helpless, and waiting for someone to rescue her. She also tends to communicate strong feelings in a nonverbal way. I suggested some more active verbal strategies for her to consider when strong feelings arise in her relationships outside the therapy and in our sessions as well. That led to some increased resistance, with her feeling that I was (like her father) attempting to control her behavior. She recalled being very submissive to her parents during childhood, with some rebelliousness as a teenager leading to many family disputes. Since then, it has been difficult to feel good about her relationship with her parents. I reminded her that she is now an independent adult, living alone, supporting herself, with much more control of her life than she had in the past.

By the tenth session she was much less depressed and began to spend more time visiting with her parents. In fact, she and her mother decided to take a trip to Florida together, and we spent several sessions trying to anticipate what might happen, how she could use it as a chance to improve their relationship, and how she might avoid self-critical patterns of behavior that could destroy her own opportunities for pleasure during the vacation.

In the fourteenth session, she described their experiences. She was able to try some of the patterns of relating and communicating we had talked about, for the most part got along well with her mother, and was able to enjoy the trip. She went back to work feeling more interested and enthusiastic about her job. The last three sessions were devoted primarily to the process of termination. She admitted that it would be difficult to say good-bye to me, said she was surprised about that, and would like to avoid talking about it. But we did review the course of the treatment, the progress she has made, and how that might be helpful to her in the future. She was able to express some positive feelings about her work with me but less able to explore her feelings of disappointment or anger. We agreed about the importance of developing some new relationships in the near future, in which she can continue to practice some of the patterns she has learned in her recent interactions with her parents and me, and that might reduce her vulnerability to depression.

This fourth problem area is more closely related to a long-standing personality disorder and is therefore more difficult to treat successfully with a short-term approach. We did make some progress in understanding repetitive maladaptive patterns, and she was able to modify them to some extent in her existing relationships. She feels more optimistic but still has a lot of work to do in the future to reduce her social isolation, experience more pleasure from interpersonal contacts, and develop some close and meaningful relationships.

Clinical Issues with IPT

I would like to present one more case to illustrate some of the difficulties involved in using IPT. The patient, a 33-year-old single white woman, sought treatment for anxiety and depression. Her symptoms of depression included a dysphoric mood, decreased energy and motivation, irritability, decreased sleep and appetite, difficulty with concentration and memory, agitation, and thoughts of committing suicide by taking an overdose of pills. She stated the depression and anxiety began several months ago after breaking up with her boyfriend. She lost her job 6 months ago after repeated arguments and disputes with her boss and coworkers. There was a history of several previous episodes of depression in the past 5 years leading to suicidal attempts and brief hospital admissions. She had been treated with antidepressants and minor tranquilizers that she took sporadically. Her father died from alcoholism 6 years ago. She lived alone but talks to her mother for several hours every day on the phone, "when we're not fighting." She was currently not speaking to her mother after an argument about money. Her boyfriend lived with her "off and on," but they were currently separated "because of his drinking and running around."

We agreed that the major problem area was role disputes and began IPT. She missed several appointments during the first phase of treatment. During that time she made up and broke up again with her boyfriend and had repeated arguments with her mother. Her mood was quite labile; at times appearing depressed, or anxious, or angry. We attempted to focus on the repetitive patterns of behavior that were manifest in her role disputes, and she seemed to recognize them as maladaptive and possible contributors to her depression. After the fifth session, she had another fight with her boyfriend, got drunk, took an overdose of pills, and was hospitalized.

In retrospect, the patient was not a good candidate for IPT. Although she met the criteria for major depression, her symptoms seemed more labile and highly reactive to interpersonal disputes. Rather than being part of a primary depression, the symptoms were more likely secondary to a severe personality disorder. The patient was aware of her behavior patterns and her painful mood states but was unable to begin making some changes that might be helpful. Instead she acted in an impulsive and self-destructive manner. She will probably need long-term treatment in a more structured setting to help her reduce her impulsive and maladaptive behavior while learning to contain and cope with intense affect.

TECHNIQUES AND TRAINING

As indicated in the clinical examples, the techniques used in IPT are not unique. This psychotherapeutic approach relies on familiar techniques such as reassurance, clarification of emotional states, improvement of interpersonal communication, and reality testing of perceptions and performance. The emphasis is on current problems and feelings as they are experienced in an interpersonal context. Unconscious factors and early childhood experiences are recognized as important but do not become the focus of the therapy, which remains in the "here and now." Likewise, transference reactions are noted but not dealt with directly unless they threaten to disrupt the therapy. The main thrust of IPT is to intervene at conscious and preconscious levels, working predominantly on current issues, to reduce symptoms, and improve social adjustment and interpersonal relations.

IPT was designed for experienced therapists who have demonstrated competence in some form of dynamic psychotherapy. Their previous training has usually been at the master's or doctoral level in the fields of social work, nursing, psychology, or psychiatry. The skills required to conduct IPT are most readily learned by professionals who have had 2 or 3 years of experience treating patients with depression in an outpatient setting. The training has usually included the use of the IPT manual, 20 hours or more of didactic seminars, and careful supervision of two or more training cases. The sessions with these patients have been videotaped and reviewed by the supervisor. Now that the book *Interpersonal Psychotherapy of Depression* (Klerman *et al.*, 1984) has been published, it has replaced the training manual. But nothing can replace the careful attention to training and supervision that has been a part of the history of IPT from the beginning.

EVALUATION OF OUTCOME

The evaluation of outcome using IPT has been quite extensive. Because it has been utilized primarily in research protocols, specific instruments have been used to demonstrate reduction of depressive symptoms, social adjustment, and the like. Most of these studies have included follow-up periods of 1 to 2 years. The initial clinical trials that demonstrated the effectiveness of IPT were carried out by Klerman, Weissman, and their colleagues (Klerman *et al.*, 1984). A large multicenter collaborative study has recently been completed that showed that IPT was as effective as imipramine and cognitive therapy in treating depression. Several more clinical trials are currently underway, including efforts to demonstrate the efficacy of maintainance IPT in preventing future episodes of depression. In my opinion, IPT has proven to be a useful, efficient, and effective form of short-term psychotherapy for patients suffering from depression and can now be justifiably used in more general clinical populations in the future.

REFERENCES

Alexander, F., & French, T. M. (1946). *Psychoanalytic theory, principles and application.* New York: Ronald Press.

American Psychiatric Association (1987). *Diagnostic and statistical manual of mental disorders* (3rd ed.–Revised). Washington, DC: Author.

Balint, M., Ornstein, P. H., & Balint, E. (1972). *Focal psychotherapy.* Philadelphia: Lippincott.

Bowlby, J. (1969). *Attachment.* New York: Basic Books.

Bowlby, J. (1977). The making and breaking of affectional bonds: II. Some principles of psychotherapy. *British Journal of Psychiatry, 130,* 421–431.

Brown, G. W., Harris, T., & Copeland, J. R. (1977). Depression and loss. *British Journal of Psychiatry, 130,* 1–18.

Cohen, M. B., Baker, G., Cohen, R. A., Fromm-Reichman, F., & Weigert, E. A. (1954). An intensive study of twelve cases of manic depressive psychoses. *Psychiatry, 17,* 103–137.

Ferenczi, S., & Rank, O. (1925). *The development of psychoanalysis.* New York: Nervous and Mental Disease Publication Company.

French, T. M. (1958). *The integrations of behavior* (Vol. 3). Chicago: University of Chicago Press.

Freud, S. (1917). Mourning and melancholia. In J. Strachey (Ed.), *Standard edition of the works of Sigmund Freud,* Vol. 14. London: Hogarth Press.

Fromm-Reichman, F. (1960). *Principles of intensive psychotherapy.* Chicago: Phoenix Books.

Henderson, S., Byrne, D. G., & Duncan, P. (1982). *Neurosis and the social environment.* Sydney: Academic Press.

Ilfeld, F. W. (1977). Current social stressors and symptoms of depression. *American Journal of Psychiatry, 134,* 161–166.

Klerman, G. L., Weissman, M. M., Rounsaville, B. J., & Chevron, E. S. (1984). *Interpersonal psychotherapy of depression.* New York: Basic Books.

Meyer, A. (1957). *Psychobiology: A science of man.* Springfield, IL: Thomas.

Paykel, E. (1978). Recent life events in the development of depressive disorders. In R. A. Depue (Ed.), *The psychobiology of depression disorders: Implications for the effects of stress* (pp. 245–262). New York: Academic Press.

Rounsaville, B. J., Glazer, W., Wilber, C. H., Weissman, M. M., & Kleber, H. D. (1983). Short-term interpersonal psychotherapy in methadone maintained opiate addicts. *Archives of General Psychiatry, 40,* 629–636.

Rutter, M. (1972). *Maternal deprivation reassessed.* London: Penguin Books.

Sholomskas, A. J., Chevron, E. S., Prusoff, B. A., & Berry, C. (1983). Short-term interpersonal therapy with the depressed elderly. *American Journal of Psychotherapy, 37,* 552–566.

Sullivan, H. A. (1956). *Clinical studies in psychiatry.* New York: Norton.

Weissman, M. M., & Paykel, E. S. (1974). *The depressed woman: A study of social relationships.* Chicago: University of Chicago Press.

13

Crisis Intervention as Brief Psychotherapy

Charles Patrick Ewing

A telephone "hotline" worker takes a call from a depressed teenager contemplating suicide. A social services caseworker follows up on a teacher's complaint that a father has been abusing his 5-year-old son. An emergency room nurse counsels a rape victim. A police officer calms the disputants in a domestic violence call. A hospital chaplain consoles the grief-stricken wife of a man who just died on the operating table. A psychologist in a child guidance clinic advises the parents of a preschool child who has suddenly begun having nightmares. A psychiatrist evaluates a patient with chronic schizophrenia who has stopped taking his medications, decompensated, and may need to be hospitalized against his will.

Every one of these scenarios, as well as numerous and diverse others, might be described as "crisis intervention." In a generic sense, *crisis intervention* has come to mean virtually any effort to help another person cope with some particularly stressful life event or situation. More specifically, however, the term *crisis intervention* is perhaps most often used to describe a particular form of short-term psychotherapy derived from the principles of crisis theory. Without questioning the therapeutic value of other kinds of "crisis intervention," this chapter deals exclusively with what has been called "crisis intervention as psychotherapy" (Ewing, 1978, 1982).

For purposes of this chapter, then, crisis intervention may be defined as "the informed and planful application of techniques derived from the established principles of crisis theory, by persons qualified through training and experience to understand these principles, with the intention of assisting individuals or families to modify personal characteristics such as feelings, attitudes, and behaviors that are judged to be maladaptive or maladjustive" (Ewing, 1978, pp. 6–7, paraphrasing Meltzoff & Kornreich, 1970). This definition, although somewhat general, clearly limits the scope of this chapter. As conceived here, "crisis intervention involves a relatively structured and planned encounter be-

CHARLES PATRICK EWING • Faculty of Law and Jurisprudence, State University of New York at Buffalo, Buffalo, New York 14260.

tween client and therapist in which both are aware of and agreed upon the therapeutic nature and aims of their relationship" (Ewing, 1978, p. 7). By intent, this definition excludes many other less planned and less structured helping efforts that have been loosely denonimated "crisis intervention."

Historical and Conceptual Background

Describing crisis intervention as a form of psychotherapy makes sense not only in practical terms but also historically and conceptually. Crisis intervention and the theory upon which it is based have both evolved largely from the early psychotherapeutic work of a group of practicing clinicians (e.g., Caplan, 1964; Lindemann, 1944; Rapoport, 1962). Both crisis intervention and crisis theory have their earliest roots in the work of Erich Lindemann (1944), a psychiatrist who reported on the evaluation and treatment of 101 victims and/or close relatives of victims of Boston's Coconut Grove nightclub fire, a tragedy that claimed nearly 500 lives in 1942. Laying the cornerstone for what was to become the theoretical and clinical understanding of human crises (i.e., crisis theory and crisis intervention), Lindemann observed that the acute grief experienced by these survivors was "a normal reaction to a distressing situation." Additionally, and also of great theoretical and clinical significance, Lindemann noted that these reactions presented what appeared to be a remarkably uniform, distinct, and identifiable syndrome.

These normal grief reactions, Lindemann found, were generally acute, had identifiable onsets, and endured for only relatively brief periods. Moreover, these reactions usually followed a predictable course with specific, identifiable stages. Although these reactions might eventuate in serious psychopathology, Lindemann was convinced that the reactions, themselves, were not pathological but normal struggles to master difficult situations. Finally, and perhaps of greatest clinical importance, Lindemann posited that the possibility of psychopathological sequelae could be minimized through appropriate and timely intervention aimed at helping the person identify, understand, and master the tasks posed by the stressful situation. There can little doubt that this approach, which Lindemann called "preventive intervention," is the theoretical and practical forerunner of modern crisis intervention as psychotherapy.

Lindemann's pioneering efforts with acute grief reactions led him and his colleagues to begin examining the potential of preventive intervention for dealing clinically with other acute reactions to stress. Lindemann's principal colleague in these later efforts was Gerald Caplan, a psychiatrist and public health expert. Building upon the foundation laid by Lindemann, Caplan erected what might be called the framework of crisis theory, the essential theoretical basis for modern crisis intervention practice.

Caplan's (1964) crisis theory is grounded in the concept of homeostasis. People are continually confronted with situations that threaten to upset the consistent pattern and balance of their emotional functioning. Ordinarily these threats are short lived; the threatening situation is mastered by habitual problem-solving activity. Although the person is in a state of tension during the period prior to successful mastery, this tension is generally minimal because the period is relatively brief and the person knows from past experience that mastery is forthcoming. In some instances, however, the threat is such that it cannot be readily mastered by resort to habitual problem-solving methods. It is then, according to Caplan, that the person begins to experience "crisis."

According to Caplan, *crisis* refers to the person's emotional reaction, not to the threatening situation itself. Thus the perception of crisis clearly depends to some extent upon the psychological makeup of the person. Still, Caplan was able to identify numerous situations commonly of sufficient threat as to precipitate a state of crisis—for example, loss of a loved one, loss or change of job, social role or status, or entry into a new developmental life stage such as adolescence, adulthood, marriage, or parenthood.

In Caplan's view, regardless of whether the precipitant is "accidental" or "developmental," the essential factor that determines the occurrence of a crisis is an imbalance between the perceived difficulty and significance of the threatening situation and the resources immediately available for coping with that situation. If the person perceives a situation as threatening the satisfaction of some fundamental need(s) and circumstances are such that habitual problem-solving methods are inadequate for mastery within a reasonable period of time, his/her reaction will be one of crisis.

As described by Caplan, the typical crisis has no more than four progressive phases. Initially the person confronted with a threatening situation responds to the increased tension by calling forth habitual problem-solving methods in an effort to resolve the problem and restore emotional equilibrium. If habitual methods fail and the threat persists, tension increases, functioning becomes disorganized, and the person resorts to trial and error in efforts to master the threatening situation. With continued failure of problem-solving efforts, tension rises further and serves to mobilize emergency and novel problem-solving measures. From this point on, one of several outcomes is possible. The person may redefine the problem to make it fit with past experience; she or he may set aside certain aspects of the problem as impossible but irrelevant; she or he may resign her-/himself to the problem; or, as a result of this mobilization of effort, she or he may resolve the problem and restore emotional equilibrium. If, however, the problem continues and cannot be resolved, surmounted or avoided by any means, tension mounts beyond what Caplan calls the "breaking point," and major personality disorganization ensues.

Caplan acknowledges that many people who suffer from mental disorders have apparently undergone significant personality decompensation during relatively brief periods of crisis. Yet he maintains that crisis, itself, is not a pathological state but rather a normal struggle for adjustment and adaptation in the face of problems that seem for a time to be insoluble. Indeed, according to Caplan, crisis presents at once not only an increased vulnerability to psychopathology but also an opportunity for significant personality growth. Depending upon how a person deals with a crisis, she or he may emerge from it more or less mentally healthy than she or he had been prior to its onset.

Finally, Caplan identified four other aspects of crisis that are particularly relevant to therapeutic intervention. First, crises are generally self-limiting and are resolved for better or worse within 5 weeks. Second, antecedent factors, such as the nature of the problem and the individual's personality or experience, may "load the dice" one way or the other, but the actual outcome of a crisis depends chiefly upon the actions of the person and the intervention of others. Third, during crisis, people not only experience but signal to others an increased desire to be helped by them. Fourth, people in crisis are also much more open and amenable to outside intervention than they are at times of more stable functioning.

Since Caplan first described his theory of crisis, others have attempted to articulate it more fully, expand upon it, and in some instances modify it. For example, numerous authors have asserted that the basic unit of analysis in understanding a crisis is not the individual but rather "one or more of the social orbits of which he [or she] is a member" (Klein & Lindemann, 1961). In particular, the role of the family has been singled out for attention. For example, Parad and Caplan (1960) pointed out that families experience crises much as individuals do. And just as Caplan described the individual as more susceptible to external intervention, so families in crisis have been described by others (e.g., Kaffman, 1963; Rapoport, 1962; Waldfogel & Gardner, 1961).

Others, such as Rapoport (1962) agreed with Caplan that crisis represents an emotional reaction to a present threat but also pointed out that a crisis may be rooted in, or at least directly affected by, the person's past experience with threats to his/her basic needs. In Rapoport's view, a present threat is frequently linked symbolically with previous threats and is thus likely to "reactivate unresolved or partially resolved unconscious conflicts." A person's past failure to resolve threatening situations may place him or her at a particular disadvantage in confronting current but similar threats. On the other hand, current crises may provide a person with what Rapoport called a "second chance" in that by dealing adaptively with a present threat, the person may be able to "correct earlier faulty problem solving."

Additionally, Rapoport spelled out a pattern of responses she saw as necessary for an individual or family to resolve a crisis adaptively. According to Rapoport, a resolution that strengthens an individual's or family's adaptive capacity requires (1) an accurate cognitive appraisal of the situation creating the crisis; (2) appropriate management of affect, including the identification and expression of feelings in ways that allow for tension reduction but do not interfere with mastery of the situation; and (3) a willingness to seek and accept the help of others in attempting to master the situation.

GENERAL PRINCIPLES OF CLINICAL PRACTICE

Although Lindemann, Caplan, and others provided a comprehensive and coherent theory of crisis useful to clinical practitioners, these theorists did not, for the most part, articulate specific modes of interventions. The actual clinical practice of crisis intervention as psychotherapy has developed over the past few decades out of the work of various clinicians. Although the techniques and clinical principles developed by these clinicians have generally been grounded in crisis theory, most appear to have developed rather independently, primarily through pragmatic efforts to serve particular client populations more effectively.

Today, although there are an almost infinite variety of approaches to the practice of crisis intervention as psychotherapy, most of these approaches have in common a number of features that may be regarded as general principles of crisis intervention practice.

1. *Crisis intervention is readily available and brief.* In keeping with Caplan's theory that crises are self-limiting, endure for only brief periods, and are marked by a heightened openness to external influence, it is generally maintained that, to be effective, crisis intervention must be readily available. Availability of crisis intervention within 24 hours of the client's initial application seems optimal (McGee, 1983; Patterson & O'Sullivan, 1974; Wolberg, 1980). It has been suggested that a delay of 2 or more weeks in seeing a client in crisis often results in a loss of his or her "spontaneously generated receptivity" to treatment (Kardener, 1975).

Interestingly, some clinicians believe that crisis intervention may benefit clients with chronic, deeply entrenched problems as well as those with more acute difficulties and who are currently "in crisis." What little research has been done on this question is about evenly split between studies finding support for the requirement of immediate intervention and those finding no support for that requirement (see Ewing, 1978; McGee, 1983).

Although opinion is split as to the need for immediate intervention, there seems to be virtually universal agreement that crisis intervention must be time limited. Crisis intervention practitioners frequently point to the role that time limits play in enhancing and maintaining client motivation. Actual time limits vary among clinicians, some expressing these limits in terms of weeks, others in terms of number of sessions, still others in terms of both. For example, Phillips (1985) suggests that crisis intervention last no more than 5 or 6 weeks. Wolberg (1980) and McGee (1983) advise crisis therapists to terminate with clients within six sessions.

Regardless of the specific time limits, several points are especially worth noting. If time limits are to play an important role in crisis intervention, they need to be set explicitly and from the start of the intervention. Therapists need to be aware, however, that crisis intervention clients can and often do terminate therapy abruptly and without notice. Some crisis clinicians believe that many crisis intervention clients benefit appreciably from even a single psychotherapy session (e.g., Bloom, 1981; Duggan, 1984; Ewing, 1978). Nevertheless, given the often high rate of early attrition among crisis intervention clients, all crisis clinicians would do well to heed Butcher and Maudal's (1976) advice that "all crisis psychotherapy sessions should be conducted as though they may be the last contact with the patient."

2. *Crisis intervention deals not simply with individuals but with families and social networks.* Many crisis clinicians have emphasized that a crisis is rarely experienced by an individual alone but is usually felt also by the person's family and significant others. Thus it has become virtually standard procedure, wherever possible and appropriate, to seek family and other interpersonal involvement in the actual treatment process (Ewing, 1978, 1982; McGee, 1983; Wolberg, 1980).

3. *Crisis intervention addresses no single definition of crisis but rather a wide range of human problems.* Some clinicians believe that crisis intervention should be reserved for those clients who are clearly "in crisis," strictly defined (e.g., Butcher & Maudal, 1976; Kaplan, 1968; LaVietes, 1974; McGee, 1983). Yet the trend in clinical practice has long been and continues to be toward a significant broadening of the concept "in crisis" (Duggan, 1984; Ewing, 1978, 1982). Indeed, many crisis psychotherapists take the position that anyone requesting mental health services is *ipso facto* "in crisis" (e.g., Ewing, 1978; Lang, 1974; Newman & San Martino, 1969; Schwartz, 1978; Wolkon, 1972). There remains, of course, the question of which clients are appropriate or at least most appropriate for crisis intervention as psychotherapy. That question is explored in more detail later in this chapter.

4. *Crisis intervention is focused on present problems.* Regardless of how one defines "in crisis," it is generally agreed that crisis intervention must be directed toward current problems, particularly those that precipitated the client's request for help (Ewing, 1978, 1982; Kolotkin & Johnson, 1983; Phillips, 1985). Indeed, crisis intervention as psychotherapy generally begins with what has been called "uncovering the precipitant" (Hoffman & Remmel, 1975). The therapist asks the client in many different ways, "Why now?" What is "the straw that broke the camel's back" (Kardener, 1975)?

Many crisis clinicians have stressed not only delineating but also maintaining such a narrow focus throughout the intervention. Crisis clinicians do not ignore other problems identified by the client, "but the brief time available must be clearly allocated to helping the client deal with the specific issues that led to treatment. The intervention must maintain this narrow focus if the therapeutic effort is to be utilized most efficiently" (Ewing, 1978, pp. 2–25).

5. *Crisis intervention aims not only to resolve the present problem or "crisis" and to relieve symptoms but also to help clients develop more adaptive ways of coping with future problems and crises.* Despite this clear focus on present problems, crisis therapists seek to provide their clients with a basis for the adaptive resolution of other difficulties confronting or yet to confront them. At a minimum, the crisis therapist tries to "utilize the crisis situation to help [the client] not only to solve present problems but also to become strengthened in mastering future vicissitudes by the use of more effective adaptive and coping mechanisms" (Parad, 1965, p. 2). Thus, in a sense, the crisis therapist tries to help the client develop coping skills useful not only in the present situation but throughout the rest of his or her life.

It should be noted, however, that some clinicians view the likely results of crisis intervention even more optimistically. In addition to helping the client resolve the current problem or crisis and develop long-term coping skills, these clinicians "expect and strive to bring about lasting personality changes in their clients" (Ewing, 1978, p. 25). Whether such optimism is warranted is an open question. But, as is discussed later, there is good reason to believe that effective crisis intervention may pave the way for additional longer term psychotherapy that clearly has the potential for bringing about durable personality changes.

6. *Crisis intervention is reality oriented.* Crisis therapists, like all psychotherapists, must be accepting, empathic, and emotionally supportive. At the same time, however, the nature of crisis intervention requires them also to be realistic, even confrontational. Specifically, crisis intervention generally involves taking active measures to keep clients focused not only on the realities of their current situations but also on their role in creating and maintaining those situations. Such measures include discouraging the use of denial, avoidance, or projection (McGee, 1983; Schwartz, 1971), confronting the client with the unrealistic nature of his/her current goals, life-styles, or belief systems (Butcher & Maudal, 1976), giving the client realistic, factual information (Cadden, 1964; McGee, 1983; Pasewark & Albers, 1972); and avoiding false reassurance (Cadden, 1964; McGee, 1983).

It should be kept in mind, of course, that such confrontation needs to be given in "manageable doses" despite the time constraints of crisis intervention—the crisis therapist "must have an empathic sense of how much the client can take at one time, and be prepared to discontinue and resume later if confrontation becomes too painful" (McGee, 1983, p. 114, citing Cadden, 1964).

7. *Crisis intervention requires psychotherapists to assume nontraditional roles.* Unlike the traditionally passive, nondirective analytically oriented therapist, a crisis therapist must expect to play an active, direct, and involved role in the intervention. As Butcher and Maudal (1976, p. 27) suggested, "traditional attitudes of therapists such as 'objective' (aloof), 'disinterested' (noninvolved), and 'nondirective' (inefficient) are not appropriate in the crisis context."

Moreover, whatever their clinical orientations, crisis therapists must be pragmatic and willing to use any resources leading to healthier adjustments for their clients (Kaffman, 1963). Specifically, "the crisis therapist must feel comfortable playing such non-traditional roles as educator, advisor, partner and model . . . and be able to take the view—'almost antithetical' to traditional insight therapy—that changes initiated in behavior can lead to increased understanding, self-awareness, and self-esteem" (Ewing, 1978).

8. *Crisis intervention may help prepare the client for additional treatment.* As noted earlier, the likelihood that crisis intervention will result in durable personality changes is an open question. There is, however, little question that crisis intervention may help pave the way for such changes by helping to prepare clients for additional, longer term treatment capable of bringing about lasting personality changes (Ewing, 1978, 1982; Phillips, 1985). The "sense of success and accomplishment" often engendered by a positive experience with crisis intervention frequently encourages clients to undertake additional, more extensive, psychotherapy (Kardener, 1975; cf. Kolotkin & Johnson, 1983). And when that

happens, these clients often seem to respond more favorably to long-term psychotherapy than do clients without such prior experience (see, e.g., Ewalt, 1973; Ewing, 1982).

METHODS AND TECHNIQUES IN CLINICAL PRACTICE

As indicated earlier, the actual methods and techniques of crisis intervention have been developed largely on an ad hoc basis. What methods and techniques are used in a given case is usually determined pragmatically—that is, in response to how the therapist conceives of the client's specific needs. Moreover, many if not most of these methods and techniques are not unique to crisis intervention but are common aspects of psychotherapeutic practice in general. Crisis intervention therapists are generally eclectic in their practices, selecting methods and techniques from a variety of therapeutic approaches. In short, they often do what seems to work in any given case.

Nevertheless, it does seem possible to sketch a general model for the practice of crisis intervention as psychotherapy. This model—which is, of course, simply one of many that have been offered over the years (see, e.g., Cadden, 1964; Wolberg, 1980)—portrays crisis intervention as encompassing six essential stages: (1) delineating the problem focus, (2) evaluation, (3) contracting, (4) intervening, (5) termination, and (6) follow-up. For purposes of discussion, these stages will be treated separately and as though they were sequential. In actual practice, however, they overlap and converge frequently throughout the intervention.

Delineating the Problem Focus

Given the extremely brief nature of crisis intervention, it is generally essential for the therapist and client to quickly define a fairly specific problem toward which the intervention will be directed. Occasionally a client is readily able to articulate clearly such a specific problem focus. More often, however, clients present multiple difficulties, have only relatively vague ideas about what is troubling them, or, for reasons conscious or unconscious, avoid mentioning their real concerns. Thus in the "typical" case, a good deal of time will be spent initially exploring the client's problems in an effort to find an appropriate problem focus.

To that end, crisis therapists generally question clients and encourage them to explain why they are seeking treatment now. The key to an appropriate problem focus is almost always found in the client's description of the event(s) or situation(s) that precipitated his or her call for help. Although time is of the essence, crisis clinicians still need to be sure to develop the kind of rapport the client needs in order to feel comfortable discussing his or her problems in such a direct fashion. Here, as in all other forms of psychotherapy, there is no surefire approach to rapport and no such thing as instant rapport. It has been suggested, however, that rapport building, and thus delineation of the problem focus, may be expedited in the crisis context by beginning therapy with a quick sketch of what the client can expect. Obviously, the realities of the situation dictate what is actually said, but the client may be told something such as:

> As you already know, we generally see people here on a short-term basis only. We feel that most people who come in for help are not mentally ill, but simply have problems they can't cope with right at the moment. Our major concern is to help get things going smoothly again as quickly as possible. I'll be available to meet with you (and your family) for up to X hours over the next few weeks, if you feel that would be helpful. A little help at the right time is what most people seem to need, but if later you decide that you want more help than this, I may be able to help arrange that, too. (Ewing, 1978, pp. 96–97)

This sort of message, if conveyed with sincerity, lets clients know that they will not be viewed as mentally ill or rejected by the therapist, that they can expect to helped relatively quickly, and that the therapist is interested in them and believes that they can be helped.

Once a reasonable degree of rapport has been established, probably the easiest way to begin the search for an appropriate problem focus is to ask the client (in a variety of ways) "Why now?" or "What has led you to seek help at this particular time?" Often these inquiries will provide leads to a potential problem focus. Where they do not, it is often useful to conduct a review of various aspects of the client's recent life experience (e.g., work, family and social relations, sexual functioning, etc.). In conducting this review, which is analogous to a physician's "systems review," the therapist is interested in learning of life changes, events, or situations temporally related to the client's presenting complaints or symptoms. Usually such a review will quickly uncover a significant problem or concern with which the client has been struggling and that can be designated as the problem focus.

For example, a college student consulted a crisis clinician complaining that she had suddenly begun drinking heavily and having suicidal thoughts. She claimed to have no idea why. A quick review of her recent life suggested no specific traumatic events or situations. In reviewing her relationships, however, it became clear that the student had long been having serious difficulties with her boyfriend. Discussion of these difficulties revealed that the student had been raped about 1 year earlier and had never discussed the details of the assault with anyone, including her boyfriend, whom she felt "would not want to hear the details." Further discussion revealed that her current symptoms had developed around the time she had been given a written course assignment dealing with criminal violence. Preparing the assignment, she finally recalled, had brought back memories of the rape that made it impossible for her to complete the assignment. As a result, she was failing the course in question. In turn, she had become so obsessed with passing that course, despite her problems, that she had fallen behind in, and was now at risk of failing her other courses.

Although the client's symptomology seemed directly related to the rape trauma, it was decided that her most pressing problem at the moment was how to get through the remaining few weeks of the semester without "flunking out." Thus, although acknowledging that the client needed (and later should seek) help dealing with her feelings about the rape, both client and therapist agreed that a more realistic problem focus for the intervention would be the client's pressing academic difficulties.

Evaluation

Crisis therapists rarely feel the need to bother with the formal diagnostic classification of clients, but they do, indeed must, always strive to evaluate carefully, though quickly, the client and the client's life situation. Evaluation is a continuing process that begins the moment therapist and client meet and continues until the intervention, including follow-up, is complete. The therapist's initial efforts at delineating a problem focus are, themselves, a major aspect of evaluation. But generally, adequate evaluation in the crisis context requires additional data regarding the client and his or her history and functioning.

At a minimum, the crisis therapist needs to have basic demographic data about each client as well as a brief history of each client's mental health and medical treatment. To save time in collecting such data, crisis therapists often find it helpful to use preprinted questionnaires, which clients can fill out before their first session. Demographic data (such as employment, marital status, number of children, education, place of residence, etc.) provide important clues as to the kinds of stresses a client faces as well as the sorts of resources available to him or her.

The client's treatment history is important for several reasons. Prior long-term treatment may be indicative of the sort of pathology or chronic problems that could make successful crisis intervention unlikely if not impossible. Such history also provides clues as to the client's level of commitment; some would-be crisis intervention clients turn out to be "doctor shoppers" who rarely make any real commitment to treatment, certainly not the kind required to make a brief regimen of crisis intervention successful. Additionally, the client's history helps establish whether he or she suffers any physical conditions or is taking any medications (psychotropic or other) that might influence (e.g., hinder) his or her response to crisis intervention.

Finally, treatment history should indicate whether or not the client is currently in ongoing treatment elsewhere. It is not unusual for crisis clinicians to see clients who are already in psychotherapy with other clinicians. In general, crisis clinicians should avoid establishing treatment contracts with clients already being seen by other mental health professionals. If a client insists on changing therapists, the crisis clinician should make every effort to fully understand the client's motives and, as a rule, be sure to consult with the other therapist or agency before agreeing to treat the client.

In addition to data gathered in delineating the problem focus and through questions or forms dealing with demographic data and treatment history, crisis therapists should also assess the mental status of every client during every session. A formal full-scale mental status examination is rarely necessary, desirable, or even feasible, but the therapist should always strive to carefully observe and evaluate the client's appearance and behavior, speech, thought and perception, affect, mood, and both suicidal and homicidal ideations, noting both current status and changes over time.

Assessment of affect, mood, and suicidal and homicidal ideations is especially critical in dealing with clients in crisis. To begin with, many clients in crisis are depressed, but depression that is severe and/or has no apparent roots in loss, setback, or other recent trauma may not respond well to, indeed might even be exacerbated by, crisis intervention. Second, where a client is in imminent danger of harming self or others, crisis intervention may be an appropriate treatment choice but not by itself. In these cases, there is clearly a need for the therapist to take appropriate action to prevent the client from injuring or killing him-/herself or anyone else.

Finally, in every case, crisis clinicians need to assess the client's precrisis adjustment and degree of motivation for change. Because a major goal of crisis intervention is to restore the client to his or her precrisis level of functioning, the clinician must have at least some notion of the client's previous adjustment. Thus, at least briefly, the clinician has to depart from the immediate "here-and-now" focus of the intervention and seek a fair amount of historical data about the client's prior functioning and adaptation. A review of the client's treatment history is helpful in this regard, but the clinician should also question the client as to his or her perception of and response to earlier life crises, both accidental and developmental. The client's work and school history, family relationships, and experiences with drugs, alcohol, and crime will also provide important clues as to previous functioning.

Assessment of the client's motivation is, of course, essential in all forms of psychotherapies but especially so in crisis intervention. The brevity and narrow focus of crisis intervention demands the client's active participation and precludes extensive working through of resistance. Both research and clinical experience suggest that positive client motivation is directly and significantly related to positive outcome in crisis intervention as psychotherapy.

Client motivation may be assessed in a number of ways. Generally, however, it is important to determine what if anything the client has already done to resolve the crisis on his or her own and to what extent he or she has been pressured by others to seek psychotherapy. Obviously, clients who have already made active efforts to resolve their problems are likely to be more highly motivated than those who have reacted passively and given little thought to possible adaptive resolutions. Likewise, clients who seek professional help of their own accord are more likely to be highly motivated than those who have been pressured by others to seek help.

There is no acid test either for motivation or for the amount of motivation needed for successful crisis intervention. Each case is unique and calls for the clinician to exercise clinical judgment, keeping in mind the time-limited and highly focused nature of the intervention. Generally, by the end of the initial session with the client, the crisis clinician will have gathered enough data to determine whether the client's motivation is sufficient to make further sessions worthwhile. Where there is doubt about the client's motivation, this is an issue that should be addressed immediately and resolved before going any further with the intervention.

Contracting

Once a problem focus has been delineated and agreed upon and the clinician has concluded that the client may benefit from crisis intervention, clinician and client should negotiate a treatment contract. Such a contract may be written or verbal but should always be explicit with regard to the problem focus, the time limits, and the responsibilities of clinician and client. Properly executed, such a contract structures the limited time available, reinforces the time-limited and highly focused nature of the intervention, offers the client a realistic notion of what to expect, and often helps motivate the client to succeed.

The problem focus should be stated with particularity and in terms of specific goals—for example, not "we will work on your academic problems" but "we will develop a more efficient and realistic study schedule." Time limits should be spelled out in terms of available therapy hours, number of therapy sessions, or both. Scheduling can be left somewhat flexible, but a clear limit should be set with regard to duration of the intervention—for example not "a month or so" but "6 weeks, from now until July 8th." Client and clinician responsibilities should also be spelled out with care. Clients are to keep appointments, work actively to explore their problems honestly and openly, attempt to develop and implement realistic and adaptive solutions, and strive to avoid behavior that creates, maintains, or exacerbates problems. The clinician will keep appointments, be available to the client as agreed, and help the client understand his or her problems and resources, see the consequences of his or her behaviors, become aware of alternatives, and develop realistic solutions.

Intervening

Obviously, all of these described "steps" are, in themselves, important interventions. Virtually everything the crisis clinician does with the client is part of the intervention. There are, however, a number of frequently employed crisis intervention tactics worth mentioning specifically. Experienced clinicians will note that these tactics are used throughout the course of crisis intervention and that none of these tactics is unique to crisis intervention as psychotherapy.

1. *Listening.* Given the great premium placed upon time in crisis intervention and the related need for crisis clinicians to take a rather active role in such psychotherapy, it is worth reminding even experienced crisis clinicians of the therapeutic importance of listening. It is essential to keep the intervention "on track," maintain the problem focus, and adhere to agreed upon time limits. Thus crisis clinicians must actively direct the course of treatment and strive to minimize needless digressions. But, at the same time, crisis clinicians have to be sensitive to clients' needs to express feelings, offer ideas, and play a substantial role in shaping adaptive solutions to their problems.

2. *Utilizing interpersonal resources.* Crises rarely, if ever, occur in a social vacuum. Almost invariably, others close to the client are touched by, if not directly involved in, the client's crisis. Indeed, many if not most crises are rooted in significant interpersonal relationships. Thus crisis therapists often seek to utilize the input, influence, assistance, and encouragement of significant others on the client's behalf. Crisis therapists also encourage clients to seek and make use of the help of such significant others. Indeed, where appropriate and feasible, it is helpful to include certain of the client's closest friends and/or relatives in the actual treatment process.

3. *Utilizing institutional resources.* Many clients require services and/or information that crisis clinicians cannot provide directly. For example, in order to resolve their crises, some clients may need financial assistance, debt counseling, job placement, birth control information or services, legal advice, medical treatment, child care services, or other kinds of help the clinician is not equipped to provide. For such clients, referral to appropriate institutions in the community is an important aspect of crisis intervention.

4. *Advocacy.* With regard to interpersonal and institutional resources, crisis clinicians need to recognize that in some cases a major part of the client's problem lies in the failure of certain individuals or institutions to respond to his or her needs. Generally it is desirable, if not essential, to encourage such clients to use alternative resources or to develop more effective ways of dealing with the unresponsive parties. But, in some instances, the client's need is not only legitimate but urgent, and the crisis clinician will have to assume, at least temporarily, the role of advocate, directly intervening with the recalcitrant individual or institution on the client's behalf.

5. *Confrontation.* Often without realizing it, many clients in crisis play a major role in creating and/or maintaining their own problems. For example, they persist in self-defeating behavior, cling to unrealistic attitudes and beliefs, and overutilize defense mechanisms. In long-term psychotherapy, therapists have the luxury of working in subtle ways to help clients understand how they contribute to their own difficulties. In crisis intervention, however, time is generally too precious to allow such subtlety. The crisis therapist must move swiftly to confront clients with maladaptive aspects of their behavior and attitudes. Sometimes pointed questioning and interpretation are sufficient, but if not, the crisis therapist should not hesitate to comment directly and critically upon the client's maladaptive, self-defeating, or unrealistic ways. Additionally, crisis therapists may find it helpful to predict for clients the ultimate, sometimes dire, consequences of persisting in such behavior and/or attitudes.

6. *Giving information.* In many cases, a client's maladaptive behavior appears to be based, at least in part, on some form of misinformation. The client is acting on an assumption that, unknown to him or her, has no factual basis. Often the therapist is perceived by the client as a knowledgeable, authoritative source and can be quite helpful by simply providing accurate, factual information. In some instances, however, it may be appropriate for crisis therapists to refer clients to other more specialized and/or knowledgeable sources of information.

7. *Exploring alternative coping mechanisms.* Clients in crisis often come to

treatment with the explanation that they have "tried everything." Only rarely is this actually so. Most often, the client has overlooked or prematurely dismissed some potentially adaptive mechanism for coping with or resolving his or her problem(s). In every case, a primary therapeutic task is to enable the client to become aware of and give careful consideration to all reasonable alternative coping mechanisms.

A major part of the evaluation in crisis intervention lies in exploring what the client has already "tried"—that is, what steps he or she has previously considered and/or taken to cope with or resolve his or her current difficulties. In some cases, it will also prove helpful to explore strategies the client has used in coping with or resolving previous problems. This kind of detailed exploration of coping strategies, by itself, often leads clients to become aware of, articulate and try new alternatives, or to modify alternatives tried earlier without success.

If exploration of recent and past coping strategies fails to yield potentially viable coping efforts, the crisis therapist should encourage clients to "brainstorm"—that is, think of and verbalize as many alternative strategies as possible. The therapist may then focus upon, clarify, and reinforce those strategies that seem most promising. Alternatively, or additionally, in some cases it may be necessary to suggest specific alternatives to the client.

8. *Advice and suggestion.* Advice and suggestion, though frowned upon by many traditional psychotherapists, are not only appropriate but often necessary in crisis intervention. Many clients in crisis need to be nudged, if not pushed, in the right (or at least a potentially right) direction. Still, crisis therapists should keep in mind the risks involved. Some clients will respond to advice as though they have been given "the answer." These clients often terminate prematurely and fail to achieve any sense of personal mastery. Others may resist advice and repeatedly respond that they have "already tried that and it doesn't work." Worse yet, still others will take the therapist's tentative suggestions as commands only to find that they are inappropriate, unworkable, or even damaging. Given these risks, crisis therapists should use advice and suggestion sparingly and cautiously with all clients and probably not at all with clients who are especially resistant or who seem to be looking for easy, pat answers to complex problems.

9. *Behavioral task assignment.* Related to and yet distinct from advice and suggestion is the assignment of specific behavioral tasks to be performed by the client outside of treatment. These tasks, behavioral prescriptions, or "homework" assignments are not presented as "solutions" but rather as opportunities to practice certain adaptive coping skills that may ultimately help the client resolve his or her problem(s). For instance, the parents of an unruly adolescent may be directed to practice saying "no" to—and not backing down in the face of—his unreasonable demands. Such parental behavior will not, by itself, resolve the problem (i.e., the adolescent's unruly conduct), but it does provide the parents with a useful coping skill that may ultimately help resolve the problem.

Like advice and suggestion, task assignment has risks and should be used with caution. Clients should always be warned of possible adverse consequences, be prepared to deal with such consequences, and advised that tasks are assigned for practice in developing coping skills, not as direct solutions to the client's problem(s).

Termination

Given the explicit time limits imposed from the start, termination of crisis intervention should come as no surprise. That does not mean, however, that termination is always a routine or easy task requiring little thought or effort. Termination of any therapeutic relationship may evoke strong sentiments, and the relationship between crisis therapist and client, though brief and highly focused, is no exception. Crisis therapists should begin planning termination as soon as they begin treatment. Explicit specification of time limits is, of course, a major part of this planning. Specific reactions to termination vary among clients and generally dictate the specific ways in which the therapist handles the issue.

With clients who view termination with a sense of accomplishment, mastery, independence, and optimism, crisis therapists need do little more than reinforce the client's positive feelings, wish them well, and casually point out that further help is available should the need arise. Unfortunately, not all crisis clients react so positively to termination, and in some cases, termination is perhaps the most difficult part of the intervention.

For example, some clients see termination as a serious threat to their needs; they develop and express acute feelings of dependency, sadness, fear, even dread. Often these clients seek, consciously or unconsciously, to prolong the intervention by raising new problems or regressing at the last minute. In dealing with such clients at termination, the crisis therapist should focus attention and energy on the client's underlying feelings rather than the newly raised problems or regressive behavior. First, the therapist should remind the client of the time-limited nature of the intervention and the previously agreed-to time limits but at the same time recognize and help the client recognize and verbalize his or her desire to prolong the intervention. Next, the therapist needs to empathize with the client (perhaps sharing his or her own emotional reactions to termination), accentuate the accomplishments of the intervention, express appropriate optimism, schedule a follow-up contact some weeks or months in the future, and/or, if warranted, offer to refer the client to another therapist or agency for additional help. In all cases, however, the crisis therapist should enforce the treatment contract and, absent extreme circumstances (e.g., a suicidal or homicidal client), terminate as scheduled.

Other clients who pose particular termination problems are those who react to impending termination with utter indifference and those who terminate unilaterally, early in the intervention. In dealing with indifferent clients, crisis therapists need not force the issue but should resist the temptation to "leave well enough alone"—that is, to allow the client to terminate without any real discussion of termination and termination-related sentiments. The brevity of crisis intervention precludes extensive efforts to get the indifferent client to deal with termination, but the therapist usually can act quickly and effectively to facilitate at least some discussion of termination and the client's feelings about it.

Probably most difficult of all are those cases in which the client terminates prematurely, unilaterally, and without notice. In all such cases, the crisis therapist should strive to contact the client and determine why he or she has left treatment. If the client feels he or she has already benefitted or that his or her life has taken a sudden turn for the better, the therapist need only point out that further help is available if and when the need should arise. Even where the client can articulate no reason for terminating, this kind of therapeutic contact is also appropriate. In some instances, however, the client's "termination" is really little more than a "test" of the therapist's concern or commitment. In these cases, a brief telephone contact is often sufficient to reassure the client and facilitate further treatment.

Follow-Up

No matter how a client terminates, the crisis therapist should strive to determine the client's condition and progress sometime after termination. A follow-up telephone call a month or two after termination serves important evaluative, educational, and clinical functions. Such follow-up (1) offers at least a minimal assessment of the efficacy of the intervention; (2) provides feedback helpful to therapists in sharpening their crisis intervention skills; and (3) enables the therapist to reinforce especially significant aspects of the intervention, discover whether referrals have been acted upon, and reevaluate the client's need for additional treatment or referral.

THE EFFICACY OF CRISIS INTERVENTION

Despite its widespread use as a form of brief psychotherapy and many published anecdotal claims regarding its effectiveness with a variety of clients and problems, crisis intervention has been the subject of relatively few real outcome studies (i.e., studies designed to assess the efficacy of this treatment modality) and virtually no recent ones.

Not only were virtually all outcome studies of crisis intervention conducted more than a decade ago (see Kolotkin & Johnson, 1983), but most of them "have been so thoroughly plagued with problems of control and other methodological difficulties as to preclude any unequivocal interpretation of their findings" (Ewing, 1978, p. 64). For example, many of these studies "suffer from methodological weaknesses such as failure to employ adequate control groups, failure to clearly specify the treatment procedures, failure to clearly define the client population, and failure to clearly define meaningful outcome criteria" (Kolotkin & Johnson, 1983, p. 142).

Although there is certainly a need for more and better research on the effectiveness of crisis intervention as psychotherapy, the evidence from these early studies at least "suggests that crisis-oriented therapies produce positive results" (Kolotkin & Johnson, 1983). Overall, existing outcome data indicate measured improvement in 70% to 80% of clients treated with crisis intervention;

when only the best designed studies are considered, however, measured improvement is found in 60% to 70% of such clients (Butcher & Koss, 1978; Kolotkin & Johnson, 1983).

Thus, although there is reason for continued optimism about crisis intervention as psychotherapy, that optimism must be tempered with the recognition that the general efficacy of this treatment modality remains to be demonstrated. The lack of scientifically demonstrated efficacy, however, seems unlikely to undermine the continued and growing importance of crisis intervention as psychotherapy.

In an age marked by a growing and legitimate demand for evaluation and accountability in professional practice, more and better research on crisis intervention must be encouraged and supported. Yet what seemed to be the case a decade ago still seems true today:

> There is no doubt that substantial positive research findings may enhance future acceptance and utilization of crisis intervention as psychotherapy. In the long run, however, it seems unlikely that evaluative research or the lack of it will "make or break" crisis intervention or any other psychotherapeutic approach. More likely, such research will lead to refinements in clinical procedures and to a better understanding of the applicability of crisis intervention. (Ewing, 1978, p. 89)

REFERENCES

Butcher, J. N., & Koss, M. P. (1978). Research in brief and crisis-oriented therapy. In S. Garfield & A. Bergin (Eds.), *Handbook of psychotherapy and behavior change* (pp. 627–670). New York: John Wiley & Sons.

Butcher, J. N., & Maudal, G. R. (1976). Crisis intervention. In I. B. Weiner (Ed.), *Clinical methods in psychology* (pp. 591–648). New York: John Wiley & Sons.

Cadden, V. (1964). Crisis in the family. In G. Caplan (Ed.), *Principles of preventive psychiatry* (pp. 288–296). New York: Basic Books.

Caplan, G. (1964). *Principles of preventive psychiatry.* New York: Basic Books.

Duggan, H. A. (1984). *Crisis intervention: Helping individuals at risk.* Lexington, MA: D. C. Heath & Co.

Ewalt, P. L. (1973). The crisis treatment approach in a child guidance clinic. *Social Casework, 54,* 406–411.

Ewing, C. P. (1975). *Family crisis intervention and traditional child guidance: A comparison of outcome and factors related to success in treatment.* Unpublished doctoral dissertation, Cornell University.

Ewing, C. P. (1978). *Crisis intervention as psychotherapy.* New York: Oxford University Press.

Ewing, C. P. (1982). Crisis intervention: Helping clients in turmoil. In P. Keller & L. Ritt (eds.), *Innovations in clinical practice* (Vol. I, pp. 5–15). Sarasota, FL: Professional Resource Exchange.

Hoffman, D. L., & Remmel, M. L. (1975). Uncovering the precipitant in crisis intervention. *Social Casework. 56,* 259–267.

Kaffman, M. (1963). Short term family therapy. *Family Process, 2,* 202–219.

Kaplan, D. M. (1968). Observations on crisis theory and practice. *Social Casework, 49,* 151–155.

Kardener, S. H. (1975). A methodologic approach to crisis therapy. *American Journal of Psychotherapy, 29,* 4–13.

Klein, D. C., & Lindemann, E. (1961). Preventive intervention in individual and family crisis situations. In G. Caplan (Ed.), *The prevention of mental disorders in children* (pp. 283–306). New York: Basic Books.

Kolotkin, R. L., & Johnson, M. (1983). Crisis intervention and measurement of treatment outcome.

In M. Lambert, E. Christensen, & S. DeJulio (Eds.), *The assessment of psychotherapy outcome* (pp. 132–159). New York: John Wiley & Sons.

Lang, J. (1974). Planned short-term treatment in a family agency. *Social Casework, 55,* 369–374.

LaVietes, R. L. (1974). Crisis intervention for ghetto children: Contraindications and alternative considerations. *American Journal of Orthopsychiatry, 44,* 720–727.

Lindemann, E. (1944). Symptomology and management of acute grief. *American Journal of Psychiatry, 101,* 141–148.

McGee, R. K. (1983). Crisis intervention and brief psychotherapy. In M. Hersen, A. Kazdin, & A. Bellack (Eds.), *The clinical psychology handbook* (pp. 759–781). New York: Pergamon Press.

Meltzoff, J., & Kornreich, M. (1970). *Research in psychotherapy.* New York: Atherton.

Newman, M. B., & San Martino, M. (1969). Therapeutic intervention in a community child psychiatric clinic. *Journal of Child Psychiatry, 8,* 692–710.

Parad, H. J. (1965). Crisis intervention: Selected readings. New York: FSAA.

Parad, H. J., & Caplan, G. (1960). A framework for studying families in crisis. *Journal of Social Work, 5,* 3–15.

Pasewark, R. A., & Albers, D. A. (1972). Crisis intervention: Theory in search of a program. *Social Work, 17,* 70–77.

Patterson, V., & O'Sullivan, M. (1974). Three perspectives on brief psychotherapy. *American Journal of Psychotherapy, 28,* 265–277.

Phillips, E. L. (1985). *A guide for therapists and patients to short-term psychotherapy.* Springfield, IL: Charles C. Thomas.

Rapoport, L. (1962). The state of crisis: Some theoretical considerations. *Social Service Review, 36,* 22–31.

Schwartz, S. L. (1978). A review of crisis intervention programs. *Psychiatric Quarterly, 45,* 498–508.

Waldfogel, S., & Gardner, G. E. (1961). Intervention in crises as a method of primary prevention. In G. Caplan (Ed.), *The prevention of mental disorders in children.* New York: Basic Books.

Wolberg, L. R. (1980). *Handbook of short-term psychotherapy.* New York: Grune & Stratton.

Wolkon, G. H. (1972). Crisis theory, the application for treatment, and dependency. *Comprehensive Psychiatry, 13,* 459–464.

IV

Family and Marital Brief Therapies

There is a curious juxtaposition between the overall field of brief treatment and the family and marital approaches—some have even considered the two to be identical. Yet there is no question, as the overview chapter at the beginning of this volume recounts, that the family therapy movement played a important role in stimulating the development of brief psychotherapy and, to this day, most of the family and marital treatment methods are practiced within a time-limited context. Certainly no volume on brief therapy could be considered truly comprehensive if it did not include them.

The chapter on family crisis therapy by Pittman, Flomenhaft, and DeYoung (14) reunites the clinical team that played such a significant role, 25 years ago, in the development of this approach. Their chapter blends concepts drawn from crisis theory with the techniques and strategies of family intervention, to create a highly effective clinical approach in which the family is seen as both a frequent source of crisis and as the major resource for its resolution. The well-designed research study that substantiated this approach was one of the first empirical examinations of brief family intervention.

Two similar, yet contrasting, approaches to marital therapy are outlined in chapters by Whisman and Jacobson (15), and Segraves (18), respectively. The former update the findings of behavioral marital therapy to incorporate the cognitively flavored stance now characteristic of almost all the behavioral interventions; the latter chapter presents a uniquely cognitive approach to the conjoint treatment of conflicted couples, integrating theory and technique in a comprehensive manner.

Strategic psychotherapy has evolved through the work of such luminaries as Jay Haley, Milton Erickson, and Don Jackson, and its present-day proponents continue to offer a vigorous, sometimes idiosyncratic approach to therapeutic treatment. Rosenbaum's (16) chapter is particularly successful in capturing the fascinating combination of simplicity of goal and sophistication of intervention that characterizes the best work of the strategic school.

The well-publicized methods for the treatment of sexual dysfunction pioneered by Masters and Johnson, almost 25 years ago, were formulated within a time-limited context from their very beginning. Beck's chapter (19) reviews these methods in the light of contemporary sexuality research and in relation to outcome studies more sophisticated than Masters and Johnson's own work, affirming the continued usefulness of brief sex therapy in treating a vital area of human functioning.

Finally, it is worth noting that at least two of the family methods described in this section represent powerful interventions with the social, emotional, and behavioral problems experienced by children and adolescents. For example, much of the clinical work in Epstein *et al.*'s problem-centered family therapy (17) has focused on resolving such problems by strengthening and stabilizing family resources. In addition, Szapocznik and his colleagues (20) in their one person family therapy, offer a highly innovative, yet well-validated method of treating the pervasive problems of substance abuse affecting so many adolescents in this country. Both of these approaches have evolved in the context of carefully designed clinical research projects where the development of treatment techniques goes hand in hand with the generation of outcome data.

Throughout these chapters the reader will find a refreshing openness of viewpoint and an absence of polemic. Family therapists no longer find it necessary to present their work in a spirit of competiveness and advocacy. Indeed, in both Rosenbaum's chapter on strategic psychotherapy, and in Szapocznik *et al.*'s description of one person family therapy, much of the intervention is in an *individual* modality, though conceptualized in relation to the family system.

14

Family Crisis Therapy

FRANK S. PITTMAN, III, KALMAN FLOMENHAFT, AND
CAROL D. DEYOUNG

Family crisis therapy, the treatment of families in crisis, began as an effort to find an alternative to psychiatric hospitalization for families containing a member who was acutely and severely symptomatic and dysfunctional. Family Crisis Therapy developed by blending crisis theory, emergency psychiatry, and family therapy and has roots in each of those developments.

Family crisis therapy, like community mental health and family therapy, emerged during the early 1960s in reaction to a period of discouragement in the treatment of mental illness. It is hard now, a quarter of a century later, to appreciate the situation then. Mental illness was severely stigmatized. Society wanted to believe that there was a sharp, clear division between those who were crazy and those who were sane. There should be a high stone wall separating the insane from the sane. Those who were crazy could be isolated from the rest of us, rounded up and put in asylums where they could stay as long as necessary, perhaps forever. The treatment provided in these asylums consisted mostly of separation from the rigors of the real world. The violently insane might be given shock treatment, electric or insulin convulsions, or even put in "snake pits." Tranquilizers were fairly new and still rather suspect.

In sharp contrast to these crude methods of dealing with psychosis, psychoanalysis was on the ascendancy for the treatment of neurosis. The Freudians and post-Freudians took Freud's methods and expanded them, so that the process of psychoanalysis now lasted for many years, even a lifetime. Psychoanalysis was attempted with psychotic patients in very expensive private asylums where the patients were kept out of contact with their families. They were not given any medication, no matter how impressive the research that showed that the phe-

FRANK S. PITTMAN, III • 960 Johnson Ferry Road, N. E., Suite 543, Atlanta, Georgia 30342.   KALMAN FLOMENHAFT • Health Science Center at Brooklyn, State University of New York, Brooklyn, New York 11203.   CAROL D. DEYOUNG • Colorado Department of Health, 4210 East 11th Avenue, Denver, Colorado 80222. Much of this discussion has been adapted from an article, "Evaluating the Family in Crisis," by Frank S. Pittman, III, published in Serge Henao and Nellie Grose (Eds.), *Principles of Family Systems in Family Medicine* (New York: Bruner/Mazel, 1985), and from Frank S. Pittman, III, *Turning Points: Treating Families in Transition and Crisis* (New York: W. W. Norton, 1987).

nothiazines were a dramatically effective treatment. Instead they were psycho-analyzed. It did not work, but it did have a certain prestige. The failure of psychoanalysis with psychoses was largely overlooked because the success of the treatment was considered far less important than the purity of the method. All mental illness, neurotic or psychotic, from infantile autism to xenophobia, was considered rooted in early childhood trauma in the relationship with the parents. Even the traumatic neuroses of war were related back to imperfect parenting, while psychotic patients were thought to have gotten that way be-cause the parent–child traumata were earlier and more subtle. There was not one whit of evidence to support any of this, or to demonstrate any benefits from a treatment program based on these theories. Nonetheless that was the state of the art in the early 1960s.

The professions knew better. The phenothiazines had been introduced and tested and had demonstrated their dramatic effect on schizophrenia. Anti-depressants had been tested and were shown to be about as effective as shock treatment for depression. There were soon to be reports of lithium salts with the ability to prevent manic episodes. We knew how to treat psychoses well e-nough, but we did not know how to package those techniques effectively enough to avoid the engulfing forces of the psychiatric hospital and the repul-sion of these people by society. Treatment was still hospital rather than commu-nity based and between the hospital and the community stood the family. Both the asylums and psychoanalysis had determinedly left the family out of the treatment, and they now lacked the theoretical comfort to bring the family back in.

FAMILY THERAPY

Family therapy was new in 1964. Ackerman had written a book, in 1958, in which he described changing the child guidance model—a separate therapist for each family member—to a model in which a therapist saw the whole family together. This was considered perverse and dangerous by some of the mainline textbooks of the day. At the same time, Bowen (1957) and others were studying schizophrenic families at NIMH, Satir was doing discharge planning at a mid-western VA hospital, and Whitaker (1958) was putting outpatients through an experiental process. All were seeing the family members in the same room with the patients. In Palo Alto, Bateson, Jackson, Haley, and Weakland (1956) were investigating communication patterns in psychotic families. Lidz, Cornelison, Fleck, and Terry (1957) and Singer and Wynne (1965) were studying communica-tion styles. The journal *Family Process* started in 1962. A second family therapy book appeared in 1964 by MacGregor and his colleagues describing multiple impact therapy with families, another variation on the old child guidance, multi-disciplinary team approach. Still, family therapy was in an experimental phase and was highly suspect. There was no real data to support its effectiveness, and its theory was splintered. Ackerman, Bowen, Haley, Satir, and Whitaker would have had a hard time—and did—coming to agreement about much of anything, so it was hard to define family therapy. Haley and Hoffman (1967) studied and contrasted the various schools of family therapy in the 1960s and included our Denver Group.

EMERGENCY PSYCHIATRY

The usual approach toward psychiatric emergencies had been simple enough—it consisted of sedation, physical restraint, and straight jackets as the patient was brought under control and locked into the asylum. That changed, largely as a result of experience providing practical treatment for the traumatic neuroses of war during World War II.

Valuable lessons were gained from military psychiatrists during World War II and the Korean War. The military psychiatrists (Glass, 1953) found that large numbers of soldiers were lost to military duty when they were treated in hospitals, distant from the front lines. A few days of rest and treatment provided immediately while close to the front lines could get soldiers back on duty effectively. There were far fewer long-range casualties.

After the war, Europe was forced to make do and discovered the advantages of treatment that was less drastic, total, and isolating. Postwar Holland had lost its psychiatric hospitals, so the Dutch were compelled to find alternatives to psychiatric hospitalization. Querido (1956), a Dutch psychiatrist, discovered that there were advantages to treating people without access to a psychiatric hospital. He found that the family was more available, that the family issues could be dealt with. The Dutch home treatment program was quite effective in reducing the numbers of patients admitted to hospitals.

The British (Carse *et al.*, 1958) in a similar situation, found that treating acute psychotic patients in their home districts, rather than in distant mental hospital, was more efficient and more effective in getting people quickly back to functioning.

In 1963, President Kennedy signed the Community Mental Health Center Act, which required that both inpatient and outpatient mental health services be made available to the general public. The goal was to provide bolstering for families and communities and an end to the reliance on psychiatric institutions. The Denver grant to study family therapy as an alternative to psychiatric hospitalization was part of Kennedy's Community Mental Health thrust.

CRISIS THEORY

Our attention was first drawn to crisis theory by Erich Lindemann (1944) in his classic study of the acute grief reactions of survivors of the Coconut Grove Fire. From his psychoanalytic viewpoint, the crisis was seen as reviving childhood conflicts. Since then, we have assumed that a characteristic process follows stress; whatever the stress, a crisis follows a predictable pattern.

A few years later, Gerald Caplan (1956) began publishing his extensive investigations of crisis, and he identified the typical phases of crisis resolution. After a stress, according to Caplan (1956), a system will attempt its traditional problem-solving mechanisms. If these do not resolve the stress, the crisis will become more intense. Thus the system will be mobilized to do something outside its usual range and repertoire. The mobilization either works and resolves the stress or fails and leads to disruption of the system or such intense pressure on the one person to change that the individual becomes symptomatic and creates new stresses. Caplan observed that if some resolution does not take place within 6 weeks, the disequilibrium will become a way of life. Caplan (1964) also expanded the concept of crisis from an individual phenomenon to a family situation.

Erik Erikson's theory of development (1959) highlighted each stage of growth as a crisis that must be successfully resolved by each individual. Although Erikson focused on the individual, his exposition of the stages of development and the human life cycle became vital underpinning for family theory, too.

David Kaplan, who had worked with Gerald Caplan, studied such specific stresses as the premature birth of a child (Kaplan & Mason, 1960), and he described acute emotional upsets (Kaplan, 1962). Kaplan and others expanded the family focus, moving from a psychoanalytic framework to one of systems. They described crisis behavior as more related to the specific nature of the stress or hazard rather than just to the premorbid personality. The sociologist Reuben Hill (1958/1965) provided the only truly family-based theory in crisis intervention literature. Hill clearly viewed the whole family as the "locus" of the crisis and explained family crisis in terms of the complex interplay of various factors within the family. The resolution of each situation can be conceptualized as a series of tasks. If the family can be encouraged to engage in these tasks, they can successfully master the situation.

CRISIS AND SYSTEMS

A crisis is the state of things at a time of impending change. It is the turning point at which things will get better or worse, the intersection of events at which change is possible. Crisis and change are related concepts. It is possible to have a crisis that does not result in change, although that would require that everyone remain very still and in place and that no one do or say anything new. But, as a matter of definition, it is not possible to have change without crisis.

When a stress comes to bear upon a system, the system is thrown into a state of crisis that can be resolved by change in the system or by removal of the stress. To define four words: A *stress* is a force that tends to distort; a *system* is a set of interacting parts; a *crisis* is a state of impending change; and a *change* is a new or unaccustomed action outside one's usual repertoire.

Systems in general—families, individuals (each person is a system, too, of course), or other groups—have certain qualities that affect their crisis response. One characteristic of a system is that anything that affects one part of the system will affect the other parts, too. If one member of the family is in trouble, changes his or her functioning, or is concealing a secret, the shock waves will be felt throughout the immediate and extended family, and someone else may develop symptoms.

Another characteristic of a system is its inherent resistance to change. Families may even overlook or misinterpret stresses to avoid responding because response might mean change. These two qualities of systems make family members exquisitely sensitive to changes in one another, yet highly resistant to outside forces. The family may grow tighter and closer the harder the world tries to change it. Thus the requisite unit of crisis response, and therefore of change, is the family. It could be assumed that the treatment of the family in crisis would effectively prevent psychiatric hospitalizations and promptly return individuals in crisis to their usual level of functioning. The experience in Denver confirmed just that.

THE DENVER EXPERIENCE

In 1964, Dave Kaplan joined psychiatrist Donald G. Langsley in Colorado to organize a study of the basic assumptions of community mental health. They got an NIMH grant, with which they brought together the three of us (Pittman, Flomenhaft, and DeYoung) as a clinical team to develop a pilot treatment program of crisis-oriented family therapy as an alternative to psychiatric hospitalization. We were asked to devise techniques by which we could provide an alternative to psychiatric hospitalization for acutely psychotic patients. Psychologist Pavel Machotka was later added to the team to direct the follow-up evaluations of the experimental and control groups. The experience of this project and its results were published widely and were highly influential at the time in giving credence and direction to the developing community mental health movement. This project also provided the first concrete demonstration that family therapy worked.

The theoretical framework of the project rested on the assumption that the request for psychiatric hospitalization of a family member represented an effort to solve a family crisis. On one level, the project tested the effectiveness of family therapy as an alternative to psychiatric hospitalization. On a second level, the project developed techniques of crisis therapy. On still another level the project tried to explore the relationship between family crisis and serious mental illness. In its simplest form, the theory was that a stress comes to bear upon a family system, throwing it into a state of crisis, which the family may attempt to resolve by hospitalizing one of its members (Langsley, Kaplan, Pittman, Machotka, Flomenhaft, & DeYoung, 1968).

We took a random sample of voluntary patients who had been evaluated by the emergency room psychiatrist and were determined to require immediate psychiatric hospitalization. Each of the 150 patients lived with some adult relative within an hour's drive of Denver's Colorado Psychopathic Hospital. One-third of the patients were suffering from acute psychoses, another third were suicidally depressed or had made suicide attempts, and the rest were in manic states, had organic brain conditions, were in alcohol withdrawal, were adolescent runaways, or had school phobias or other disorders. We prevented the hospitalization in all these cases, offering crisis-oriented family therapy and appropriate medication, visiting the home, making collateral contacts, and arranging appropriate outpatient follow-ups. The group was compared to a matched group of hospitalized controls and followed for several years.

The results (Flomenhaft, 1974; Flomenhaft, Kaplan, & Langsley, 1969; Langsley, Pittman, Machotka, & Flomenhaft, 1968; Langsley, Machotka, & Flomenhaft, 1971) revealed that essentially all patients with families could be treated outside the hospital, with less interruption of functioning, less disruption of families, and no increase in suicides or other disasters. What's more, family crisis therapy cost about one-sixth as much as the average 28-day hospital stay. All experimental patients were kept out of the hospital initially, and only about 15% went on to subsequent hospitalizations, whereas 40% of those hospitalized initially had subsequent hospitalizations. Most strikingly, later hospitalization of the experimental patients were not only far less frequent but also far briefer than those of the controls. In the follow-up, the cumulative days in hospital of the comparison group was much greater than that of the experimental. It was clear that family crisis therapy was not postponing hospitalization but, by preventing this hospitalization, was teaching families and patients a more efficient way of using mental health services to handle their crisis.

FAMILY CRISIS AND FAMILY THERAPY

The widely reported data from the Denver project had considerable influence on the community mental health movement. The destructiveness of psychiatric hospitalization—its tendency to encourage chronicity—may result from removing the problem from the family. This removal of one member prevents the family from learning how to solve its own problems and makes mental illness seem more mysterious and difficult than it needs to be. One retrospective conclusion from the study might be that in general, it may not help psychotic people to remove them from a hospital, but it does hurt them to remove them from their family in a time of crisis. The family's involvement is an important part of the treatment of serious mental illness, if there is no family, the prognosis is worse. If the family is not involved in treatment, the treatment will be more costly, less efficient, and more likely to lead to chronicity or disruptive recurrence. The Denver project's conclusion was that any treatment that does not involve the family bypasses the core of the problem. No family and no patient are too crazy for family therapy. Because family therapy is the treatment of choice for acute psychosis, the presence of a psychotic member, acute or chronic, hospitalized or at home, is certainly no contraindication to family therapy for family crisis.

Freeman and Simmons, in *The Mental Patient Comes Home* (1963), found that patients did better if the family was tolerant of symptoms but intolerant of nonfunctioning. By contrast, society in general and the medical profession in particular have tended to regard cessation of functioning as an appropriate response to symptoms. Anxious or depressed people are seen as suffering from excessive functional stress and encouraged to take it easy, take time off from work, give up productive activity, tranquilize themselves, get out of conflictual relationships, or even horror of horrors, go on disability. This may be appropriate for a day or even a week but not for long. People's lives cannot be protected by sacrificing their functioning. There are rare exceptions to this but, generally, a stressful, even a stark raving mad family should not be avoided. A misguided effort by family members undercuts the therapy more if they are uninvolved than if they are involved in the treatment. The more mysterious and isolated the treatment process, the more likely the family will be to misunderstand what is therapeutic about it and thus to sabotage it quite inadvertently. We cannot protect families from their patients without damaging the patients, and we cannot protect patients from their families. The best protection we can offer comes from requiring them to live with the results of their effects on one another and to take responsibility for driving one another crazy or sane.

When we are presented with a symptomatic individual, we must assume that he or she represents a family in crisis, even if the family crisis may be no more than a helpless reaction to the symptomatic member. As often as not, our first contact with a family is with a relative who is concerned about another family member's behavior. It is insufficient to focus our evaluation solely on the person with symptoms or only the one concerned about the person with symptoms. We must evaluate the system, the context in which the problematic behavior occurs.

EVALUATING THE FAMILY SYSTEM

Several papers from the Denver group explored the techniques of family crisis therapy (Pittman, Langsley, Flomenhaft, DeYoung, Machotka, & Kaplan, 1971; Pittman, 1984). Others outlined the process of evaluating the family in crisis (Pittman, 1973). And of course there were papers describing the application of this approach to specific family crises. Langsley, Pittman, and Swank (1969) compared schizophrenic and nonschizophrenic families, Machotka, Pittman, and Flomenhaft (1967) looked at incest. Flomenhaft and Kaplan (1968) explored maladaptive intergenerational patterns of families in crisis, Pittman, Langsley, and DeYoung (1968) looked at school and work phobias, and Pittman and Flomenhaft (1970) treated the Doll's House marriage.

Central to all of this is the effort to define the family crisis and specifically to answer two questions: "Why now?" and "What, above all, does this family not want to change?" In answering these questions, there are elements we need to consider about each family. Each family system has certain characteristics that influence its crisis proneness and crisis response. These characteristics determine how families differ from one another even while facing the same stress or undergoing a similar crisis.

Boundaries

Each family has a set of members. Some belong to the immediate family, others to the extended family, and some are merely relatives. The degree to which they are included in the family functioning, family activities, and, perhaps most importantly, in family decision making varies. The relatives are included in ceremonial occasions, may have the right to visit informally, may exchange appropriate favors, and may be privy to family business. Aunts, uncles, and cousins are sometimes treated like siblings or parents, sometimes like friends, sometimes like duties. Siblings, and even parents, are sometimes treated like duties and seen only on ceremonial occasions or not at all. Most families, however, have some extended family members who are involved in essentially all decisions and many activities. Families with close functional ties to many extended family members are more resistant to sudden change and are cushioned through life's crisis. On the other hand, families with close functional ties to only one extended family member may be somewhat immobile and dependent. Loose boundaried families, in which the members have close relationships to outsiders but little closeness to one another, may lack the mechanisms for subtle changes in functioning and tend to drift apart rather than change in response to crisis. By contrast, families with tight boundaries may intensify internal conflict and pressure on one another more easily than call for help from outside.

In evaluating a family in crisis, we must know whether someone else—another family member or someone outside the family—needs to be consulted for change to take place. The appropriate questions here are: How do the others react to the problem? Who can help with this? Whom do we need to talk to about doing things differently? Who else sees it as a problem? Whom do you talk to about it?

It is not unusual for the family to have undergone boundary changes before the request for professional help. Some family members may have moved out or been sent away. Members of the extended family may have moved in for a time. Close friends, even casual ones, may have been brought in, too. We must know who is included as stabilizers for the family during the crisis and who is part of the usual family structure. We cannot assume that the members of the household and the members of the functional family are the same.

Some people, even when they marry, maintain strong boundaries between themselves and their spouses, treating a wife or husband much as an adolescent treats parents—as a functional necessity but a threat to individuality. Bigamists, male chauvinists, people who are having affairs, or those who are in psychoanalysis may similarly leave a spouse out of decision making. Somewhat more common are marriages that are too tightly bound to admit any third person, even a child. Some couples have children but keep their life secret from them. The parents may even divorce and remarry without considering the children or even explaining the situation to them.

At the opposite end of the spectrum are those couples who use their children as marriage counselors and referees in marital battles. Occasionally a parent will go so far as to let one of the children know the details of an affair that is being kept secret from the other parent. It is probably healthier for parents to air their differences around the children than to pretend the children do not or should not notice. But for one parent to conspire with a child to keep secrets from the other parent can only be destructive; it gives far too much power and responsibility to the child, who needs to know that the parents are more or less together as security and stability for the family. Subgrouping across generations is a major cause for crisis proneness.

Subgrouping occurs also when one spouse conspires with a parent, a sibling, a friend, a lover, or a therapist to keep problems secret from the other spouse. In family decisions, such alliances may outvote or overpower the other spouse, and they can certainly outmaneuver the left-out spouse, who is then trapped behind enemy lines. The domestic devastation produced by a secret affair is well known, as are the more insidious effects of a conspiring in-law.

Anyone who crosses family boundaries to champion one party of a domestic dispute can be just as destructive. This is true even if the championed party appears to the outsider to be an abused child, a battered husband or wife, or the misunderstood mate of a paranoid person. It is characteristic of families in crisis to loosen their boundaries and cry for outside help. The police officer, the divorce lawyer, the mother-in-law, the hairdresser, and the family therapist may all cross the boundary at the same time, and all may be equally destructive if they see their function as protecting one family member from another one. Speck and Attneave (1973) expanded the locus of the identified patient's network to include not only immediate and extended family but all significant others in the neighborhood and community as the means for understanding and resolving the crisis. For example, they will ask a family to bring 40 people to the next interview, who can assist in understanding the problem and can be a resource in it solution. These 40 people may include relatives, neighbors, friends, lawyers, gas attendant, postman, and so on.

Clearly, a parent who abuses a child must be reported to the legal authorities. Yet clinical experience has shown that when the therapist sides with the child against the parent or if the emphasis is mainly on protecting the child, the child is endangered even more. The therapist must recognize the child's guilt-producing effects and convey to the parent the message that he or she will also be protected from the child. The function of the intruder in the family crisis—the therapist—is to respect and protect power alignments sufficiently to help stabilize the family.

Roles

Each family assigns roles to its members. Some roles are functional (breadwinner, cook, banker, dumper of the kitty litter); others are emotional (jester, family doctor, etiquette adviser, family problem). Functional role assignments are generally quite clear and obvious, although they may be conflictual. Rigidity in roles is a frequent source of crisis proneness. Well-functioning families provide some degree of backup for a member whose role is not being performed. Some families, though, assign roles based on gender, which prevents the flexibility necessary to adapt to change. As repugnant as it is to most of us, the "me-Tarzan,-you-Jane; me-hunt,-you-cook" arrangement is as workable as any other if both parties agree. But if Tarzan cannot cook and Jane cannot hunt, either would starve if the other one ceased to function. The male need to be served can get bizarre. Phyllis Rose (1983, p. 9) in an analysis of five Victorian marriages notes: "Happy marriages seem to me those in which the two partners agree on the scenario they are enacting, even if the couple's own idea of their relationship is totally at variance with the facts." One man inspected the faucets each evening to be sure his wife had polished them as his mother would have. Another man could be sexually aroused only by the sight of his wife on her knees scrubbing the floor. By contrast, there are women who actually believe that they should never have to hold a paying job outside the home and therefore never prepared themselves for a career. Such people, when called upon to perform roles they consider inappropriate for their gender, may feel quite oppressed. It seems difficult to maintain a family that contains a prince or princess who feels too special to do the work that needs to be done. And when such a person also usurps a full-time emotional role, such as family critic or family patient, without also becoming "the family problem" and therefore the one to be changed, the family's range becomes greatly limited and crisis prone.

Crisis proneness is not just the result of functional or emotional rigidity. It can also result from functional looseness. Some families prefer to ignore certain roles, as if they are not really necessary. There are families in which no one cleans up, pays the bills, oversees the schedule, or determines the appropriateness of other people's behavior. Thus, when the power is cut off, or the garbage blocks access to the kitchen, or various members drift away, a crisis occurs. The situation is treated as unique, and the member who expressed dissatisfaction is seen as the problem.

Families can become crisis prone, too, when the more emotional roles go unperformed. Not only must the family members be loved and encouraged and comforted, they must also be criticized. It must be someone's job to comment on the appropriateness of behavior. When that job is not done, behavior may become bizarre and offensive. Politeness is not necessarily helpful in family living. Someone treating a family in which someone behaves inappropriately should realize that no one may ever have noticed or complained before.

In some families, one person, perhaps an adult, perhaps one of the children, is defined as vulnerable—as one who cannot help it but must always be obeyed and catered to. Asthmatic children who could stop breathing if upset, alcoholic parents who could start drinking if angered, or those defined as mentally ill are prime candidates for this role. If anyone questions the vulnerability of the family patient, it is the questioner who becomes the family problem—the one whose behavior must be changed. The family gives its highest priority to protecting the family patient from becoming self-sufficient.

It takes at least two people to produce a family patient, but they also produce a crisis-prone family. Other emotional roles may stifle families. If the father must always know best, if the second child must always be at fault, if the child marked for success must always be blameless in his failures, if mother's actions must always be seen as love, if anyone must always be anything, then nothing can ever be understood, and no change can take place. Three-generation families are particularly vulnerable in this way where a grandmother will frequently sabatoge and undercut her daughter's parenting role with a grandchild.

Family Rules

Just as family roles determine who does what, family rules determine who cannot do what. Family rules are even more ubiquitous than family roles and often just as bizarre. Crisis proneness results when rules prohibit the family from functioning, or from having friends outside the family, when the rules interfere with normal socialization and development of the children, or prevent awareness and discussion of problems that require change. The possibilities for stifling growth are limitless, but they seem proportional to the degree with which the family fears the world around them. Some families protect themselves from adolescent sexuality by prohibiting normal adolescent socialization. A rule commonly taught young girls is that any man who wants sex with a girl does not respect or love her, which means she must marry a man who is not attracted to her. Men may fear their wives' adultery or rape to such a degree that they keep them in a virtual chastity belt, preventing them from working, driving at night, or going out with friends. Other families have rules against any alcohol use because they fear alcoholism. Rules against language are not uncommon. One old woman had a large sign over the mantle spelling out the four letter words that could not be spoken in her house. Recently arrived immigrant families from the West Indies and Asia experience considerable difficulty and strain when the parents apply strict rules of social behavior and curfew to their adolescent children, particularly daughters.

Rules for protecting the home can become incompatible with comfortable living. Joan Crawford's rule against wire hangers is well known. Some families have rooms tended like museums, which no one may enter, and yards too well kempt to permit children to play in.

Few rules are more explosive than those involving infidelities. Although most people agree at marriage to remain faithful, and a majority actually do, occasional adultery is common, and continual adultery not at all rare. A few couples negotiate the conditions under which extramarital sex will be permitted or even encouraged, and therefore the adultery is open and shared and seen as not quite an infidelity, at least in theory. In practice, it may be surprisingly stimulating, or it may be unsettling. More often, people move around furtively and compound their infidelities with lies or even efforts to blame the cuckolded spouse for some deficiency that drove the other spouse to do it. Such an infidelity tears at the heart of the marriage by the insult, desertion, rivalry, insecurity, and sudden loss of trust; the results may be devastating. Yet people who want to have affairs and intend to do so may find it hard to negotiate openly about their intentions because they would prefer that their partner follow the rule of fidelity. Some couples permit extramarital sex while physically separated or on a trip. Affairs may be more permissible with prostitutes, with members of the same sex, or with strangers. One man, an artist, insisted that he had never been unfaithful "except with ex-wives and models and they didn't count." His wife saw it otherwise and left him. The rules on such an emotionally charged issue must be clear. Many women assume all men are adulterous, and some men assume it of all women. If a marriage is conducted under the assumption of infidelity, a faithful spouse may be kept at a distance with little opportunity for intimacy to develop.

Rules against open communication stifle problem solving. Early family researchers spent years analyzing fragments of family conversations to delineate the rules about who speaks after whom. These rules, about who can say what to whom, and about what and when, are usually subtle and uncodified and may not even be apparent to the family members. Many family fights ignore content entirely and focus exclusively on whether people are speaking respectfully or have a right to say what is being said. The most basic job of a family problem solver is to cut through this and let the family members deliver the necessary messages and opinions.

Communication rules may always be in conflict. When a man from a diplomatic, silent family marries a woman from a noisy, conflict-loving family, both spouses may be continuously uncomfortable. When a liberated child decides to open communication with a closed family, or a cautious, sneaky child enters a stormy family, the child's style may trigger a crisis.

Goals and Values

Some people never question their reasons for believing as they believe. Those who are not very bright remember only the first thing they learn about any subject and reject any subsequent information that does not seem compatible with it. As a result, their belief and value system may be strongly held, yet never examined. It has been said that people are not fit for life until they realize that their parents were stark raving mad and everything they've been taught is dangerously suspect and must be continuously reexamined until they are sure it is a belief of their own choosing and therefore changeable in the face of new data. Families that constantly reexamine their goals and values become more interesting and more flexible. Of course, families with no long-range view of themselves and their place in the world have little ability to inspire their children. The result could only be children who are either as nonconflictually complacent as their parents or who show unexpected, but unprotested, talents and ambitions.

Crisis proneness results from unachievable goals and values; some goals and values are innately at odds with one another. We know, for instance, that popularity of junior high-school students results from social comfort—the unquestioned assumption that people will like them. Parents' anxious efforts to keep children constantly alert to rejection or to potentially offensive aspects of their behavior or appearance can only result in the social anxiety antithetical to such popularity. Some goals and values are simply incompatible with the nature of the human animal or with that of the individual family member. Any effort to rid oneself of normal or even abnormal feelings only increases those feelings. Still, parents may set for their children the goal of not feeling certain things. Mothers who spank small children for crying in grocery stores, invariably cause their children to cry harder. When anxious, some people attempt to appear calm, which surely increases their anxiety. Similarly, guilt over sexual attraction can remove the pleasure of the attraction while turning it into an obsession, which then takes on far more importance than it deserves.

Some families try to avoid certain experiences. Their goal is to get through life without any member's having a divorce, abortion, affair, imprisonment, psychiatric hospitalization, or even a failing grade or any overt acknowledgment that all has not gone ideally well. Occasionally one sees in the newspaper the story of a couple who have lived through 50 years of marriage without an unkind word or of a child who had not missed Sunday school in 15 years. Most of us realize that life is a comedy, not a tragedy, and no one gets through it without an occasional pie in the face. Yet families who must have only ideal experiences may believe that there is no recovery from a bad one. The failing grade, the abortion, or the adultery marks the individual and the family for life, an ineradicable blot on the family that makes further efforts pointless because the primary goal of avoiding these unpleasant but common experiences is unachievable. Some families feel little will to continue after a child becomes illegitimately pregnant, fails in school, or goes to jail or a hospital. Divorce is common after a rape or the death of a child, even eat when there is no blame or distrust—just a sense of unachievable perfection. Less traumatic experiences, even minor slights, have also sufficiently dispelled the magical perfection to bring a particular family to grief.

Issues from the Past

Every family has certain unresolved issues that are kept in storage for an uproar whenever needed. These past conflicts fall into two categories; those that are secret or lied about, and those that are open, symbolic, and past. Obviously, any real issue has to be handled in some way as it occurs, with some people taking action and others at least accepting or tolerating that action. But secret issues cannot be resolved to anyone's satisfaction, and symbolic issues exist for the primary purpose of remaining unsolved.

Secrets usually involve past rule breaking. Someone has an affair, lies about it, and offers no explanation for his or her changed behavior, leaving everyone vaguely confused. The mystery may continue to disorient the family for years, postponing solution of the problems. Much energy may go into protecting a secret item of past history—a degree not earned, a debt not reported, a child given up, a marriage not acknowledged, a dread secret from the family of origin. The secret may affect behavior and decisions only slightly most of the time but, like a lightly mined field, may make a few areas hazardous. Suspicious people may know there is a secret and become increasingly uncomfortable around the person who holds the secret but do a terrible job of guessing what the secret is. In the treatment process, the therapist has to weigh carefully whether or not to have the family communicate about the secret. Most family secrets are known to every member, but there is a sanction against revealing and discussing them. Exposing secrets can seem terribly dangerous, as people fear great harm will come if they are understood by one another.

Tension

Tension is the family members' awareness of one another; it may be seen as a measure of the members' fears of displeasing one another or of the degree to which they experience one another's pain. Tension may be so low that no one feels involved in anyone else's life. One 14-year-old girl lived at home through a 9-month pregnancy without her parents noticing she was pregnant. Adolescents may develop severe drug habits, young adults may have affairs, or older ones deteriorate as a result of Alzheimer's disease, before anyone is aware of anything unusual.

A more visible problem is a family with a high level of tension, in which everyone bounces off everyone else, and it is unclear where each emotion begins or who owns any problem. There are enmeshed families—"smothering mothers," *folies a deux*, "gruesome twosomes," and other relationships in which the emotional tension is so intense that one person's feelings are felt instantly by other family members and seem owned by the reactor rather than the originator. Some people even experience other's physical sensations or think they can do so. One theory concerning anorexia nervosa suggests that the anorexic person may be reacting to parental efforts to feed her when the parents experience hunger, a process that goes on so long that she never learns to experience hunger on her own. Likewise, obesity has been seen as a result of the child's learning to when the parent is anxious. By contrast, paranoid people seem more aware of other people's anger than of their own, failing to notice their attacks on others but being acutely aware of the other person's response to their unrecognized attack. This leaves them, inexplicably, feeling attacked. When tension is high, symptoms and emotions are transmitted rapidly.

Some years ago in Colorado, John McDonald (1968) set aside a ward of the hospital for patients who had threatened to kill others. Because there were too few people who had made such threats, the ward was not filled, and other patients were housed there. The anxious staff knew it was the "threat to kill ward" and lived with acute sensitivity to the possibility of violence. Soon, even the depressed little old women were threatening murder in order to use the telephone or get their PRN medication.

Stress

A stress is a force that tends to distort. What is stressful for one family may not be stressful for another; stresses are specific to the system in question. The death of a spouse or bankruptcy might be considered more stressful than a fistfight with neighbors or Christmas, but there are families in which a bankruptcy or the pregnancy of an unmarried daughter would be routine, whereas a family gathering would constitute a crisis. In many marriages a husband's death is far less stressful than his retirement. The degree of stress depends on the family's values and expectations and on the nature of its relationships.

Stress might be categorized according to whether a stress is overt or covert, whether it is unique or habitual, permanent or temporary, real or imagined, and whether it is seen as structural or situational.

Overt/Covert

In general, overt stress creates fewer problems. In a misguided effort to avoid embarrassment, pain, blame, or change, many people keep secrets, compounding the confusion created by an event that affects one family member for reasons not understood by the others. If a stress is overt (the house burns down), then the family can band together, and outsiders can offer help. If it is covert (a secret affair or loss of money), then no one knows how to help.

Habitual/Unique

Response to habitual or recurrent behavior is different from response to unique behavior. One episode of drunkenness is quite different from chronic alcoholism. One lost job is different from recurrent job instability. Many family battles occur over the question of whether a stress is unique or habitual, and the distinction is significant. The sixth failed grade, affair, arrest, suicide attempt, or episode of violence becomes obnoxious rather than alarming to the family. A person called in to help may be shocked by the irritated complacency of families who have been through such an episode many times. The same helper, on the other hand, may be surprised later when the family reacts to the next episode in the series as if it had never occurred before. Determination of habitual versus unique requires accuracy by all concerned.

Temporary/Permanent

Families may also battle over whether a certain stress is temporary or permanent. The family member pushing for change may concentrate on the permanent effects and stigmatas of an abortion, an arrest, a failing grade, or an affair, even if a more permanent baby, imprisonment, expulsion, or divorce did not occur. Likewise, people who resist change may see only the temporary impact and downplay long-range consequences. The mother who did not want her son to wear an earring treated the pierced ear as if it were permanent like a tattoo, rather than temporary like a hairdo. Many adolescents, dropping out of college, insist that they will return to school in the fall. One young man, marrying for the seventh time, had nothing more permanent in mind than the dental work his prospective father-in-law could perform.

Real/Imagined

Sometimes it is not clear whether or not a stress is real. Incest may be reported by a child when it did not actually occur, or it may have happened and been denied by the accused parent. The same thing is true of infidelities. Sometimes people destroy their children to prevent incest from becoming known, and they often convince everyone of a spouse's insanity to keep an affair secret. Yet, from the standpoint of a therapist, whether or not the act occurred may not matter as much as the reality of the disturbed relationships and high tensions. It is not uncommon for a child to report an act of incest by a new step-parent who is actually intrusive in nonsexual ways. An imagined affair may not yet be sexual but may accurately identify the direction of someone's attentions. Emotional reality may take priority over physical reality. Emotional accuracy is enormously important, even if the physical details are fuzzy.

Situational/Structural

Stresses may arise from within the structure of the family, or a family may find itself in a stressful situation brought on by outside forces. In facing an enemy, it helps to know, as Pogo did, whether or not it is us. Families in whom the blame is always externalized may feel no need to change the behavior that is causing the stress. Parents of failing children may blame the school system, addicts blame doctors or Vietnam, blacks blame whites, men blame women, and everyone blames parents, whereas nobody takes the responsibility for change. On the other hand, it is equally unhelpful to internalize each stress and blame a favorite defect in the family structure for whatever comes up. Children of a divorcing family may blame their poor school grades or messy rooms for the marriage problems. Battling couples may blame everything that happens on an ancient affair, an unpleasant in-law, or some old offense. Depressed people may blame any crisis on some internal defect, constantly asking, "How have I failed?" By doing that, they miss the opportunity to appropriately assign responsibility within the family or to escape or understand difficult realities.

If these parameters can be properly evaluated and defined, the stress, its characteristics, effects, and sources can be understood clearly enough to point the way to change. When the stress is clearly understood, the crisis can be minimized. When the stress is confusing, the crisis extends unnecessarily and amplifies uncontrollably.

Crisis

A crisis results when a stress bears upon a system and requires change outside the system's usual repertoire. The state of crisis is marked by nonspecific changes in the system. The boundaries are loosened, which enables a therapist or anyone else to enter and influence the way the system operates. Rules and roles become confused. Both expectations and prohibitions become relaxed. Goals and values lose importance and may even be lost altogether. Unresolved conflicts are revived and become the focus of much attention; tension between family members rises. A therapist observing a family in crisis may find the family disorganized, nonfunctional, directionless, battling over long-dead issues. One may assume the family is far sicker than it is, may assume the revived conflicts to be the real issues, and may overlook the stress entirely. By this time, the family may want to dump its stress in some way that will reduce tension without solving the problem. Members may decide to dissolve the family, ship someone off, get a divorce, have an affair (the loosened boundaries permit this), or put someone in a hospital. On a vulnerable family member, the pressure may reach a level sufficient to bring forth symptoms, even psychosis. The scapegoating of one member may become the focus of everyone's attention and that person may isolated or punished or treated. To an observer who does not understand the stress, this may appear perfectly appropriate.

Perhaps each crisis is unique, but most crises fall roughly into four categories. The first, simplest, and least common is the "bolt from the blue." The stress here is overt, unique, real, and situational. Someone may die, the house may burn down, the economy may collapse, the plumbing may overflow just before the guests arrive, the sweepstakes ticket may win, or the child may be kidnapped. If everyone can pull together to define the stress and the changes required, the crisis may not destroy the family; functional changes will vary with the duration of the stress. Bolts from the blue are obvious, clearly arising from forces outside the family. The stress is real, it could not have been anticipated, it has not happened before, and it is unlikely to happen again. Neither soulsearching nor blame are appropriate or helpful, though they occur. Anticipating a recurrence would be a mistake, though such anxiety is almost universal. Most of the family's attention can be directed to the regrouping necessary to keep the family going.

Obviously, bolts from the blue are as likely to occur in well-functioning families as in families with all manner of problems, but old problems and the new crisis may become confused. One example is a house burning down around a family in which there was incest, drug abuse, alcoholism, and a matriarchal, intruding grandmother. The fire, however, caused the family to focus on a young child's hyperactivity, which had been ignored in the large house, but became intolerable in the motel where the family lived temporarily.

The danger of bolts from the blue lies in the search for blame—the effort to find something someone could have done to prevent the disaster. This attempt will undoubtedly uncover all sorts of personal and structural deficiencies to which responsibility for the crisis becomes attached. As a result, the real task of pulling together and adapting to the situation is bypassed in favor of attack and defense.

Developmental crises are expectable. They are overt but may have a few covert features. Instead of temporary phases, they represent permanent changes in status and function that clearly arise from the nature of biology or society, not the family structure. They are real, even as they provoke fantasies and expectations that may not be real. There is nothing unique about developmental crises, and, above all, they cannot be prevented. The usual developmental crises include marriage; birth of children; children starting school, going through puberty, becoming independent, and leaving home; and parents growing older, retiring, and dying. Teenage sexual activity and pregnancy, drug use, or school deficiencies are not true developmental crises, but they are so prevalent that they might as well be. Infidelities, midlife crises, and divorce seem to be on the verge of becoming expectable crises in society. Children born to unmarried mothers, jail terms, unemployment, and addiction may be almost as common, but these remain abberations that are preventable if the people involved are aware of choices as they make them. Preventable crises are characteristic at each stage of development; knowing they are expectable may help to keep them from being inevitable.

More subtle developmental crises occur in marriage. One is the cooling of romantic love that occurs during the first year or so as mates see each other more clearly. When the honeymoon is over, it is usually replaced by a far more mature partnership. Another marital crisis is the cooling of sexual interest in the 30s as the sexual drive becomes less hormonally urgent and more dependent on the relationship. During the 40s, awareness of patterns of career success or failure emerges, and a rethinking of goals takes place.

Subtle developmental stages occur also in child raising. Two-year-old children learn to say *no*, 6-year-olds work to please, 12-year-olds become aware of parents' deficiencies. Fourteen-year-old adolescents ignore their parents' values in search of the assurance of popularity from their cruel peers and find manifold deficiencies in themselves. Sixteen-year-olds want freedom; 18-year-olds are afraid of it.

At each developmental stage a crisis of some sort is inevitable. Problems arise when one part of the family tries to prevent the crisis rather than define and adapt to it. A common developmental crisis centers on adolescent sexuality. Parents may go to amazing extremes to prevent their children, especially their daughters, from being actively sexual. One mother cut off her 16-year-old daughter's hair to make her less sexually attractive; another mother tried to have breast reduction surgery performed on her 14-year-old daughter. A parent's intervention into a child's sexuality may go as far as incest or voyeurism. Someone must tell frightened parents what is normal, and they certainly will not take the adolescent's word for this.

Adolescent sexuality cannot be dictated. One pair of parents who were proud of their liberality, allowed their 15-year-old daughter to acquire birth control devices, required her to drink and smoke marijuana with them, and encouraged her to have "experiences." They objected only to cigarettes as bad for asthma. She refused "experiences" and sat in her room sullenly smoking. The parents had overlooked the cardinal rules of developmental crises: They cannot be stopped, they cannot be produced prematurely; they can only be understood and thereby dampened and coordinated with all the other forces that operate in the family.

Caretaker crises occur when a family has an inherent defect that makes them dependent unilaterally on some power outside the family. Although the family's structure may be faulty, the stresses arise from forces outside its control. The structural defect may be permanent; the stress may be overt or covert, but it is often habitual and represents a situation of chronic dependency. Families subject to caretaker crises include those dependent on outsiders for financial support, like families supported by welfare payments, trust funds, alimony, or the kindness of strangers.

Similarly, families with a chronically ill member are unable to control their destiny, as the treatments, orders, and restrictions leave everyone helplessly dependent upon the physicians—who may be caring, sensitive, and communicative, but are still outside the give and take of equal relationships. Families dependent on a psychotherapist are in the same situation, with the added mistrust created by a vague air of mystery and a definite air of secrecy.

Another situation of dependence arises when a single parent has an affair with a married person. No matter how much a married man or woman may love the other person, he or she spends all holidays with the spouse, and that is not negotiable.

Some chronic psychiatric illnesses also create conditions outside a family's influence. Manic depression seems to be a predominantly chemical, genetic disease the patient and family cannot control. The family's efforts are unlikely to influence its course and are usually destructive, encouraging the manic-depressive patient to control his or her emotions. Schizophrenia, which probably is at least partially chemical in origin, often becomes recurrent or chronic and is incompletely influenced by the individual's or family's efforts. The family's attempts to find a once-and-for-all "cure" may prevent acceptance of the chronic or recurrent nature of these conditions. Schizophrenia is often managed and stabilized without invalidism, but it may well require long-term medication and therapy. The family's resistance to continuing treatment frequently results in the patient's relapse. In these situations, the recent introduction of psychoeducational programs appears to offer much promise of managing and maintaining the schizophrenic within the family community (Anderson *et al.*, 1980).

In all caretaker situations, the family must assess the need for continuing dependence on the caretaker. If dependence cannot be avoided, the family must establish a relationship with the caretaker in which the family is being considered. Equally important may be the family's understanding of the nature of the dependence, the purpose of the caretaker, and the rules of the relationship. If the modus operandi of the caretaker is mysterious to the family, the relationship loses any semblance of predictability. Caretaker crises occur when the caretaker's rules change and do not seem negotiable, or when the caretaker makes decisions without explaining them.

Structural crises are those that exacerbate struggles within the family. They may occur without any perceptible external stress but seem like an earthquake that arises periodically from underground forces. Unless the first crisis in the series is handled well enough to resolve the internal problem structural crises are likely to recur, caused perhaps by an overt, but more likely by a covert stress. And if a real stress does not trigger the next structural crisis, then an imaginary one will. These crises have nothing to do with stress and are not an effort to avoid, understand, or change anything. They are the most difficult crises to treat because they represent an effort to prevent the change. Families with an alcoholic member, violent families, and adulterous families all fall into this category. So do families in which a member intermittently uses divorce, suicide attempts, job changes, running away, or creating an uproar as reactions to ordinary stresses. Because of the excessive, nonspecific quality of the typical structural family crisis, the family may never deal effectively with the stresses it encounters, putting all its energy into avoiding the usual crisis. Therefore, nothing ever changes.

Alcoholic families are especially difficult. Nothing should be easier to resolve than alcoholism: Do not drink. But an alcoholic may be a joyless, difficult person without alcohol, so the family may not require or even tolerate his or her sobriety. Of course, even if the family objected, the alcoholic might not completely control the drinking, but the family does not have to tolerate it if it chooses not to. Nor do people have to tolerate violence with its guilt-producing remorse, adultery with its disorienting lies, or suicide attempts with their threat of eternal guilt. Yet families do choose to retain such members. The crisis pattern itself seems to be its own reward, keeping reality from being considered and deficiencies from being dealt with rationally.

In treating families of this kind, the therapist must shift the focus from the current crisis and isolate the problem from the surrounding chaos. We are always astounded to see people take responsibility for having caused someone else's recurrent outlandish behavior. One must find out how anyone got the idea someone else is not responsible for his or her own behavior. What is so frightening about rationality? Families who tolerate bullies (and suicide attempters are no less bullies than alcoholics, adulterers, and husband or wife beaters) are not victims but accomplices. If the bully unilaterally stops the chaos, he or she may destroy the raison d'être of the family.

One common pattern of structural crisis occurs in marriages in which one partner recurrently threatens divorce. He or she may believe the marriage is unworthy of him or her, that the marriage belongs to the other spouse who uses it tyrannically. Taking little responsibility for making the marriage work, such a person does not leave but from time to time precipitates a crisis in which the other spouse must prove commitment to the marriage by some tolerance or sacrifice.

Treating Families in Crisis

The treatment of families in crisis is conceptually quite simple. In psychoanalytically oriented psychotherapy of either individuals or families, the definition of the problem is made increasingly subtle and complex. Crisis therapists—whether they are psychiatrists, family physicians, family counselors, or family therapists—above all, simplify. Essentially, the following treatment techniques rest on the premise that the family is both the vehicle by which to understand and resolve problems.

The format developed by the Denver group is easy to follow and provides sufficient structure to keep us oriented in even the most chaotic family or the wildest array of intersecting crises. The format has a simplicity and logic unusual in psychiatry. There are seven steps. The therapist should enter the situation with an air of calmness but urgency, convey a clear sense of how things work, be impatient but not unkind with people who seem to prefer chaos to change, and be optimistic that obstacles can be hurdled if one knows what is going on. Sympathy is out of place, as is a passive interest in understanding people's feelings better, disapproval of behavior on moral rather than practical grounds, or a protective willingness to join in conspiracies. The therapist's central posture is that of the friendly, impartial, sensible expert. Where one is encountering an acutely psychotic and suicidal individual, the therapist may need to be a part of a crisis team in order to make rapid assessments and interventions and to be available around the clock in a demanding and volatile situation.

Emergency Response

This means we must respond right away, within days certainly, preferably within hours. Perhaps our being there, calm and interested, is enough to prevent the family from doing something drastic to relieve the tension. The first therapeutic person on the scene is admitted into the loosened boundaries of the family and granted great power and influence. He or she may have more power to bring about the second step than any therapist subsequently. He or she can take over some of the family's administrative functions during the crisis, an action that would have been resisted a few days before and will be resisted a few weeks later. The therapist has to arrive quickly and work fast. A few minutes when all hell is breaking loose are worth more than hours of work later on.

FOCUS ON THE FAMILY SYSTEM

This second step is usually easy for us to bring about, especially after the other family members have been made aware of the crisis. We bring together whomever needs to be involved in understanding and solving the problem. If the member crying for help is not involving the others, we may have to call them.

Ordinarily in a crisis, the family will choose an individual to be changed so that the rest of the family will not have to do so. If family members are sufficiently concerned, they will be willing to be involved. But the therapist must be willing to start with whomever shows up. As Anderson and Stewart (1983) said, someone who treats families is in the position of the salesman who "must be willing to agree to anything that will get his foot in the door." Once started, we involve the others as quickly as possible by whatever means we can. A telephone call to the missing members may be sufficient, but sometimes a home visit is required. The home visit conveys a strong interest in assisting the family with their problem and the opportunity to understand the actual context of the crisis. The guiltier people feel about their involvement, the more frightened they are of seeking help. A friendly, competent voice on the telephone may seem sufficiently tolerant to offer some protection. Even on those rare occasions when a family member refuses to come in or talk, he or she can be included in the formulations. He or she can be sent a specific message explaining the situation and suggesting actions. The absent member must, however, be protected from blame.

Small children need not be included, but all other family members must be involved, particularly those who have the power to sanction or prohibit change. At the onset of the treatment, it is well to interview the whole family, including younger children because they may provide information not easily derived from the adults. How parents relate to infants and toddlers during the interview can provide important diagnostic clues on the family's functioning. When other caretakers have been involved with the family (e.g., ministers, physicians, social workers, probation officers, etc.), they are immediately contacted and involved and urged to continue their relationship with the family after crisis therapy.

Defining the Problem

This step is crucial and complex; it involves finding out why the crisis is happening now. The past needs to be explored only far enough to identify the points of crisis, when things went so wrong that the family felt the need to call for help. The step is complex because the family may already have defined the problem so unhelpfully that their efforts were futile or destructive. Every family has collected a lifetime of extraneous information and many unresolved problems that are being connected to the current crisis. When we treat families in crisis, we must wade through all that and focus everyone's attention on the current problem.

In the midst of the chaos, as everyone blames everyone else and digs for the roots of the problem in the past, in the stars, in the society, the therapist's small voice keeps repeating, "Why now"? The information the therapist is given is not incorrect or irrelevant, and it will be helpful later on. But without the understanding of why the crisis has happened now, the other information can be misleading.

If this crisis is a bolt from the blue, the therapist may be told quickly, but the information may not apply to the family's functioning before the crisis. In a caretaker crisis, the information also surfaces rapidly. In a developmental crisis, the information may be distorted, most likely being the story of one person's troublesome or psychopathic behavior, although the person described may not be the one forcing the change from one developmental stage to another. The individual identified may be the one opposing the development or contributing to its distortion. With persistence and patience, the practitioner should be able to figure out who is changing.

Structural crises are the misleading ones. No matter how often the same crisis has occurred, a family member will describe it as unique and brought on by external circumstances, or as a caretaker crisis, in which one person has a chronic defect outside his or her control and the world has not been supportive enough. The blame may be put on another member's development.

If the focus is sharply on the question, Why now?, and it turns out the crisis is one of a series, it has been caused by a structural problem no matter how much the current episode may be related to other stresses. So, in addition to asking, Why now?, the therapist must ask if this has happened before and explore the past deeply enough to find out when the family was last functioning well enough not to need help. There are pitfalls in getting the story because people tell the history according to the way their family looks at things.

A classic example is: "The whole problem is me. I've never been good at anything. Just ask my parents. They'll tell you." Or, "Everything was OK until she started dating. That was when my husband began to drink. So I helped her sneak out of the house. When he found out about it he beat me up and that was when I took all those pills."

If the information is put together in such a way as to explain the interaction and everyone's part in it, then the symptomatic behavior seems to be an understandable, if not necessarily a reasonable, reaction to the situation. Until it makes sense, the therapist must keep on probing and act as though he or she does not understand the situation yet. The "one-down" position outlined by Fisch, Weakland, and Segal (1982) is a powerful one; it requires patients to come up with coherent explanations rather than resisting the diagnosis.

General Prescription

As soon as the crisis is defined, efforts can be made to calm everyone in preparation for some sensible action. Someone or everyone may need to take sedative medicine for a day or so, or the therapist's reassurance that he or she now understands the situation and knows what to do about it may be tranquilizing enough. If someone's hospitalization cannot be avoided, this should be done now or later, never before the family situation is clear. Simplistic as it may sound, we have found that chamber music, refreshments, and an air of confidence calm everyone as much as putting someone in the hospital. Yet calming the situation should not interfere with the therapeutic effort of solving the problem. The family may have to remain upset until the problem is clearer. Abating the family tension too quickly may remove the impetus for a more constructive solution.

Specific Prescription

This step flows directly from the definition of the problem and, in its simplest form, is an act of logical, practical reality testing. We tell the family to do something sensible that will either solve the problem or symbolize a change that will solve it eventually.

The therapist must describe the situation without blaming anyone, but with the unshakable conviction that everyone wants to do something sensible and is perfectly capable of doing so. Family members may object to the formulation, but they are less likely to reject it if the therapist is supportive. With some families, vagueness about some aspects of the problem is permissible, but vagueness about the solution is not. The therapist tells them what sensible people would do under the same circumstances. This step cannot be faked; it marks the difference between helpful helpers and unhelpful ones.

The prescription may be quite simple: "Stop drinking. If you're not an alcoholic, it should be easy. If you are, Antabuse will help." "Stop the affair, at least for now. You can call him from here. I'll call if you're embarrassed to." "Do not commit suicide tonight. We'll find other alternatives tomorrow." "Go on to school/work, they'll help you if you need it." "Stay home tonight. The family needs to be together."

The prescription should also be directed towards the symptom in question. When such simple directions are given, they are usually joined with instructions to the other family members to either talk or not talk about the issue and to help in various ways to perform the prescribed task.

If there is conflict about who is to do what, separate prescriptions can be given to each member of the "you-go-ahead-and-hunt-and-you-go-ahead-and-cook" variety. For example, "You job hunt tomorrow, and she'll write the letter to your mother." Each person's task performance must be independent of the others', so that one person cannot avoid the task because someone else did: "You are to hunt, whether or not he cooks."

In bolts from the blue, simple structure is usually sufficient—returning to normal functioning in most areas and doing the special tasks produced by the crisis. In caretaker crises, the therapist has already done the job by becoming the new caretaker, but he or she must now assign an end to the dependence or an acceptance of it. The therapist tells the unemployed to look for a job and work, the manic-depressive patient to resume taking lithium. In developmental crises, if the crisis-producing change is in a child, the therapist supports the parents' authority but then allies himself/herself with the developmental phase, asking the parents to accept it while they maintain control and the child demonstrates responsibility in going through it. In adult developmental changes, the therapist must support the family's authority as the adult adapts his new goals and patterns to the family. In structural crises, the bully is defined as responsible for his or her behavior, and the tasks involve a cessation of bullying and encouragement of the family to protect itself from it, whereas the issues are negotiated from positions of greater equality. If the therapist has been skillful in defining the crisis as one in which all are players, then this should not be difficult. Everyone is given a task, even if it is only to oversee someone else's task. Then the meeting ends, perhaps with the admonition that the therapist knows that perhaps not everyone will do their work—and that is OK because, if they do not, the real problem will surface. The tasks are not only realistically useful, but they have symbolic value and are tests of cooperation. The carrying out of a task may be abetted through a home visit. And above all, the therapist maintains a therapeutic intensity during the first several days by scheduling frequent visits and telephone contracts.

Negotiating the Resistance to Change

The family has been gathered quickly, the chaos reduced, the problem defined as a solvable one, and everyone told some simple things they can do to help solve it. Sometimes they will do those things. When they do not, we must explore their reasons for not doing the things that would solve the problem. This may take time and require further explorations into the innate peculiarities of the family, but if we keep everyone's attention on the solution of the presenting crisis, the process has a focus.

In this sixth step, which usually takes place at the second session with the family, the therapist will learn much more about the family than during the first meeting. Most likely, the person protecting the family from change is not the initially identified patient.

New tasks, new explorations, and even revisions of the original definition are in order. Bolts from the blue will be resolved quickly. Caretaker crises will return rapidly to the point at which the last caretaker ran away, so that the therapist may discover that the previous caretaker misjudged the problem and the therapist can now solve it. Developmental crises always require some negotiation but usually not many sessions before the family will accept objective wisdom from an outsider.

Families in structural crises often resist change. They may drop out of the treatment process early, try to send only one member, or play a touch-and-go game. It is these families who need therapy most, but they are most resistant to it. It is these families about whom the family therapy books are written.

Do not expect them to change quickly because when one member improves, another may sabotage the improvement. The family members are accustomed to doing the opposite of what they are told, so one technique may be for the therapist to admit helplessness and defeat, at which point the family may change to keep the therapist involved. But if the therapist can persuade just one person that change is possible, that the bully is competent, that the victims are free to escape the pattern, the impasse will be broken, and change will become possible. The question at this stage is: "What, above all, do you not want to change?" The answers are often amazing.

Termination

The seventh step is the last, although not all problems will be solved. Appropriate referrals are made, and they may be accepted or not. Either way the family has a resource available for the subsequent crises that are inevitable in all families.

The people who need psychotherapy least want it most, and those who need it most resist it most stubbornly. The biggest crises are the fastest to treat. In treatment of family crises, change, if it occurs, is achieved quickly and, whether the change occurs or not, the crisis is over in a few weeks.

Let families experiencing bolts from the blue go gracefully, and they will be back when they need a therapist. If these families do not terminate quickly enough and if the therapist gets lost in the situation, then the families should be encouraged to try getting along on their own and check in later.

In certain caretaker crises, especially those involving schizophrenic and manic-depressive patients, someone may have to manage the patient's medication indefinitely. That is not enough though; the family also needs a therapist as these situations involve important family work. The family of a manic-depressive patient taking lithium must learn that the danger is over, and there is no need to protect the patient from emotions. With schizophrenic persons, the converse is true, in that a low level of emotionality seems helpful, as are firm expectations of functioning. Schizophrenics, once past the acutely psychotic episode, benefit from associations with groups and other opportunities for learning to be normal. Family protectiveness from normality should be stopped, even if the schizophrenic must leave home to accomplish this.

Structural crises often end quickly and return in time, the second round of treatment often being more helpful. Eventually, families who have recurrent structural crises may become amenable to serious family psychotherapy to prevent the crises, rather than use the crises to prevent therapy.

There is a limit to how much saving any of us can offer to families who do not want to be saved from their problems. But each family crisis is an opportunity for the family and the therapist to learn more about how people can get through life without driving one another crazy.

Family crisis therapy is fun for the therapist. It is lively, and it works, but the demands are intense. Assessments and interventions have to be made rapidly, under great pressure, sometimes in the face of acutely psychotic, suicidal, even violent individuals, and always in the face of conflicting family opinions. There is much to be said for doing this sort of work as part of crisis team, a group of colleagues with whom you can share responsibility, distribute assessment and treatment functions, and divide all those things that have to be going on all at the same time. A well-functioning crisis team nurtures and cushions one another, and permits each member a certain well-earned craziness in a safe setting—like a family does when it is working right.

REFERENCES

Ackerman, N. W. (1958). *The psychodynamics of family life*. New York: Basic Books.
Anderson, C. M., Hogarty, G. E., & Reiss, D. J. (1980). Family treatment of adult schizophrenic patients: A psychoeducational approach. *Schizophrenia Bulletin* 6(3), 490–505.
Anderson, C., & Stewart, S. (1983). *Mastering resistance*. New York: Guilford Press.
Bateson, G., Jackson, D. D., Haley, J., & Weakland, J. D. (1956). Toward a theory of schizophrenia. *Behavioral Science, 1,* 251–264.
Bowen, M., Dysinger, R H., Brodey, W. M., & Basarmania, B. (1957). *Study and treatment of five hospitalized families each with a psychotic member.* Paper presented at the American Orthopsychiatric Association, Chicago, March.

Caplan, G. (1956). An approach to the study of family mental health. *U.S. Public Health Reports, 71* (10). Washington, D C: U.S. Government Printing Office.

Caplan, G. (1964). *Principles of preventive psychiatry.* New York: Basic Books.

Carse, J., Panton, N. E., & Watt, A. (1958). A district mental health service: The Worthing experiment. *Lancet, 2*(1), 39–41.

Erikson, E. H. (1959). Identity and the life cycle. *Psychological Issues, 1,* 1–171, New York: International Universities Press.

Fisch, R., Weakland, J. H., & Segal, L. (1982). *The tactics of change: Doing therapy briefly.* San Francisco: Jossey-Bass.

Flomenhaft, K. (1974). Outcome of treatment for adolescence. *Adolescence,* (Spring), 57–66.

Flomenhaft, K., & Kaplan, D. M. (1968). Clinical significance of current kinship relations. *Social Work, 13,* 68–75.

Flomenhaft, K., Kaplan, D. M., & Langsley, D. G. (1969). Avoiding psychiatric hospitalization. *Social Work, 14,* 38–45.

Freeman, H., & Simmons, O. (1963). *The mental patient comes home.* New York: Wiley.

Glass, A. J. (1953). Psychiatry in the Korean campaign: A historical review. *U.S. Armed Forces Medical Journal, 4,* 1563–1583.

Haley, J., & Hoffman, L. (1967). *Techniques of family therapy.* New York: Basic Books.

Hill, R. (1965). Generic features of families under stress. In H. J. Parad (Ed.), *Crisis intervention: Selected readings* (pp. 32–52). New York: Family Service Association of America. (Original work published 1958)

Kaplan, D. (1962, April). A concept of acute situational disorder. *Social Casework, 7,* 15–23.

Kaplan, D., & Mason, E. (1960). Maternal reactions to premature birth viewed as an acute emotional disorder. *American Journal of Orthopsychiatry, 30,*(3).

Langsley, D., Kaplan, D., Pittman, F., Machotka, P., Flomenhaft, K., & DeYoung, C. (1968). *The treatment of families in crisis.* New York: Grune & Stratton.

Langsley, D. G., Pittman, F. S., Machotka, P., & Flomenhaft, K. (1968). Crisis family therapy: Results and implications. *Family Process, 7,*(2), 145–168.

Langsley, D. G., Pittman, F. S., & Swank, G. (1969). Family crises in schizophrenics and other mental patients. *Journal of Nervous & Mental Disease, 149,*(3), 270–276.

Langsley, D. G., Machotka, P., & Flomenhaft, K. (1971). Avoiding mental hospital admissions. *American Journal of Psychiatry, 127,* 1391–1394.

Lidz, T., Cornelison, A., Fleck, S., & Terry, D. (1957). Intrafamilial environment of schizophrenic patients II: Marital schism and skew. *American Journal of Psychiatry, 114,* 241–248.

Lindemann, E. (1944). Symptomatology and management of acute grief. *American Journal of Psychiatry, 101,* 141–148.

MacGregor, R., Ritchie, A. M., Serrano, A. C., Schuster, F. P., McDonald, E. C., & Goolishan, H. A. (1964). *Multiple impact therapy with families.* New York: McGraw-Hill.

Machotka, P., Pittman, F. S., & Flomenhaft, K. (1967). Incest as a family affair. *Family Process, 6,*(1), 98–116.

McDonald, J. (1968). *Homicidal threats:* Springfield, IL: Charles C Thomas.

Pittman, F. S. (1973). Managing acute psychiatric emergencies: Airing the family crisis. In D. Bloch (Ed.), *Techniques of family psychotherapy: Seminars on psychiatry, 5,*(2), 219–227. New York: Grune & Stratton.

Pittman, F. S. (1984). Wet cocker spaniel therapy: An essay on technique in family therapy. *Family Process, 23,*(1), 1–9.

Pittman, F. S. (1985). Evaluating the family in crisis. In S. Henao & N. Grose (Eds.), *Principles of family systems in family medicine.* (pp. 347–371). New York: Bruner/Mazel.

Pittman, F. S. (1987). *Turning points: Treating families in transistion and crisis.* New York: W. W. Norton.

Pittman, F. S., & Klomenhaft, K. (1970). Treating the Doll's House marriage. *Family Process, 9*(2), 143–155.

Pittman, F. S., Langsley, D. G., & DeYoung, C. D. (1968). Work and school phobias: A family approach to treatment. *American Journal of Psychiatry, 124,*(11), 93–99.

Pittman, F. S., Langsley, D. G., Flomenhaft, K., DeYoung, C. D., Machotka, P., & Kaplan, D. M. (1971). Therapy techniques of the family treatment unit. In J. Haley (Ed.), *Changing families: A family therapy reader* (pp. 259–271). New York: Grune & Stratton.

Querido, A. (1956). Early diagnosis and treatment services. In *Elements of a community health program* (pp. 158–169). New York: Millbank Memorial Fund.

Rose, P. (1983). Parallel lives: Five Victorian marriages. New York: Alfred A. Knopf.

Singer, M. T., & Wynne, L. C. (1965). Thought disorder and family relations of schizophrenics, IV: Results and implications. *Archives of General Psychiatry, 12,* 201–212.

Speck, R. V., & Attneave, C. (1973). *Family networks.* New York: Pantheon Press.

Whitaker, C. (Ed.). (1958). *Psychotherapy of chronic schizophrenic patients.* Boston: Little, Brown.

15

Brief Behavioral Marital Therapy

Mark A. Whisman and Neil S. Jacobson

Introduction

An impressive body of evidence has accumulated in recent years implicating marital problems with physical health problems (Kiecolt-Glaser *et al.*, 1987; Levenson & Gottman, 1985) and a variety of major psychiatric disorders, including depression, agoraphobia, alcoholism (Jacobson, Holtzworth-Munroe, & Schmaling, 1989), and behavior problems in children (Emery, 1982; Margolin, 1981b). Marital disruption is one of life's most stressful events (Bloom, Asher, & White, 1978; Holmes & Rahe, 1967), and individuals who are experiencing marital difficulties are more likely to report a family history of marital problems (Overall, Henry, & Woodward, 1974). Thus the cost of marital distress to society is enormous, and it is therefore not surprising that there has been great effort spent on developing interventions and techniques designed to alleviate marital distress.

For the past 20 years, clinical researchers have been developing, evaluating, and refining a treatment program for distressed married couples based upon social-learning (Jacobson, 1983a,b; Jacobson & Holtzworth-Munroe, 1986; Jacobson & Margolin, 1979; Wood & Jacobson, 1985) and cognitive principles (Baucom & Lester, 1986; Berley & Jacobson, 1984; Jacobson, 1984b; Jacobson & Margolin, 1979; Schindler & Vollmer, 1984; Weiss, 1980, 1984). This treatment has collectively come to be known as behavioral marital therapy (BMT). BMT has been evaluated in a number of controlled studies, and not only is it the most thoroughly researched approach to marital therapy, but it is also the only approach with a substantial body of experimental research (reviewed recently by Baucom & Hoffman, 1986, and Hahlweg & Markman, 1988). In this chapter, we first describe the social-learning-based model of marital distress and then outline the stages of therapy based upon these principles. We then discuss strategies to overcome treatment noncompliance and outline therapist characteristics necessary for the practice of marital therapy. Finally, we provide a summary of the

Mark A. Whisman and Neil S. Jacobson • Department of Psychology, University of Washington, Seattle, Washington 98195.

empirical evidence for the efficacy of therapy, along with a brief description of new directions in the behavioral treatment of marital discord.

SOCIAL-LEARNING-BASED MODEL OF MARITAL DISTRESS

BMT involves the application of social psychological exchange theories and learning principles derived from social and experimental psychology to the problems of distressed marital relationships. Behavioral research on marital exchange has elucidated a number of parameters that differentiate happy from unhappy couples. These research findings have contributed to the theoretical model of marital distress as well as to the treatment model that has come to be known as BMT. These studies have shown that distressed couples reward each other less and punish each other more frequently and reciprocally (e.g., Birchler, Weiss, & Vincent, 1975; Gottman, 1979; Jacobson, Follette, & McDonald, 1982; Levenson & Gottman, 1983; Margolin, 1981a; Margolin & Wampold, 1981; Vincent, Weiss, & Birchler, 1975), are more emotionally sensitive to immediate relationship events (e.g., Jacobson et al., 1982), and disagree significantly more often about what events occur in the relationship (e.g., Jacobson & Moore, 1981) than do their nondistressed counterparts. In general, distressed couples seem to rely upon aversive behavior control techniques and consequently appear deficient in a number of skills necessary for the effective functioning of a relationship (Weiss, 1980). These deficits are especially striking in the areas of conflict resolution and communication. Thus helping couples acquire the process skills they lack upon entering treatment is an important part of BMT.

The focus of BMT is also on the content of spouses' presenting problems. Marital distress occurs not only because of performance or skill deficits but also because many spouses in long-term relationships gradually become unable or unwilling to provide those behaviors that the other needs in order to feel satisfied with the relationship (Jacobson & Margolin, 1979). Consequently, another focus of BMT is on increasing the frequency of positive exchanges between spouses.

Finally, compared to nondistressed couples, spouses in distressed relationships endorse more unrealistic beliefs and expectations regarding marital relationships (Eidelson & Epstein, 1982) and make more destructive attributions for their partners' negative behaviors and less benign attributions for their partners' positive behaviors (e.g., Fincham, 1985; Fincham, Beach, & Baucom, 1987; Fincham, Beach, & Nelson, 1987; Fincham & Bradbury, 1987; Fincham & O'Leary, 1983; Holtzworth-Munroe & Jacobson, 1985; Jacobson, McDonald, Follette, & Berley, 1985). These findings have resulted in incorporating techniques within BMT designed to challenge unrealistic beliefs and relabel attributions.

As is generally true of behavior therapy approaches, BMT focuses on current rather than historical determinants of behavior, emphasizes overt behavior change, specifies treatment procedures in order to potentiate replication, and carefully specifies treatment goals so that the efficacy of treatment can be evaluated in a rigorous, objective manner. In addition, weekly homework assignments are an integral part of therapy, to ensure that skills learned in therapy sessions transfer and generalize to the home environment.

DESCRIPTION OF TREATMENT PROGRAM

The core BMT treatment package is based upon a treatment manual published by Jacobson and Margolin (1979) and supplemented by a variety of additional perspectives (e.g., Barbach, 1984; Gottman, Markman, Notarius, & Gonso, 1976; Greenberg & Johnson, 1988; Guerney, 1977; Jacobson, 1983a,b, 1984b, 1989; Weiss, 1980, 1984; Wile, 1981). The basic treatment package has been gradually refined and modified over the last 10 years in response to data from a number of controlled studies.

BMT is a suitable treatment for most maritally distressed couples, although there are several client characteristics that may make therapy particularly difficult. These factors include couples who have one spouse suffering from severe behavioral or emotional problems, have different agendas regarding the desirable outcome of therapy, refuse to buy into the philosophical underpinnings of the treatment, have little reinforcing value for each other, have incompatible life goals, have a large discrepancy in the amount of intimacy desired in their relationship, are abusive or who engage in other malicious or painful behavior, or have a long history of marital distress (Jacobson, Berley, Melman, Elwood, & Phelps, 1985). Several recent investigations have attempted to empirically identify client variables that are predictive of positive outcome to BMT—the results of these studies will be presented later under the discussion of the effectiveness of treatment.

BMT usually involves 2 to 3 sessions devoted to assessment, followed by 12 to 17 weekly treatment sessions, all of which last between 60 to 90 minutes. In a recent analysis comparing a 20-session structured treatment regimen with a flexible treatment regimen where the number of sessions was determined by therapists based upon their assessment of the couple's needs, the short-term program was found to be as effective as the open-ended treatment, although the latter averaged over twice the number of sessions (Jacobson et al., 1989). Consequently, we endorse the use of short-term marital therapy as a more cost-effective treatment program.

A typical treatment session involves (1) setting an agenda for the session in collaboration with the couple, (2) reviewing the previous homework assignment and discussing any difficulties the couple encountered in completing it, (3) reviewing the progress of the couple and the content of the last several sessions, (4) presenting new material, and (5) assigning new homework for the upcoming week.

From the first session through the end of therapy, spouses are asked each day to rate their satisfaction with themselves, their marriage, and 11 relationship domain areas (e.g., consideration, affection, communication) on a 10-point Likert scale. Therapists either contact the couple the night before the session to obtain these daily ratings, or they ask the couple to bring their ratings to the session with them. These ratings are then averaged for the week, with each average being plotted on a chart. The charts can then be shown to the couple periodically to provide visual feedback regarding the progress made in therapy. They can also be used to assess whether interventions targeted at specific relationship domain areas are having the intended effect.

Assessment

The first two to three sessions of BMT are devoted to assessment and evaluation, with the goal of identifying variables that are contributing to marital problems and thereby enabling the selection of appropriate therapeutic interventions (Whisman & Jacobson, in press). Spouses are informed that the purpose of the assessment period is to determine the appropriateness of marital therapy and that their actual commitment to therapy will not be required until the end of the assessment period. Furthermore, because couples often enter therapy with the expectation of immediate changes in their relationship, they are informed not to expect changes in their relationship during this assessment phase. However, the structure of the evaluation process maximizes the likelihood of improvement. In fact, building positive expectancies and trust in the couple as well as actually providing them with some relief is just as important in the early stages of therapy as is gathering assessment information (Jacobson & Margolin, 1979).

From the initial interview throughout the course of therapy, BMT attempts to achieve a balance between the positive and the negative aspects of the couple's relationship. This balance is maintained in the initial sessions by assessing relationship strengths as well as weaknesses. One way to limit a couple's hopelessness and despair about their relationship is to limit the scope of their problems by asking them about the immediate precipitants of their decision to seek therapy at the present time. This focus circumvents a typical pattern displayed by many couples who dredge up a long history of marital problems. As an additional counterbalance to their discussion of their current relationship difficulties, therapists should attempt to elicit positive information about the relationship. One technique involves obtaining a developmental history of their relationship (Jacobson & Margolin, 1979). For many couples, discussing the early stages in their relationship helps to focus their attention on pleasant memories and illustrates that the relationship has not always been plagued with problems. Questions commonly asked to elicit positive memories include: (1) How did you meet? (2) What was it that initially attracted you to your partner? (3) What was the initial dating period like? (4) How and when did you decide to marry (or live together)? (5) What was your wedding (and honeymoon) like?

In addition to identifying immediate precipitants in seeking therapy and obtaining a developmental history, therapists should provide couples with a brief introduction to therapy. This introduction should include an explanation of the time-limited nature of therapy, its orientation to current marital problems, the importance of complying with homework assignments, and information regarding treatment outcome. Spouses should leave the first appointment having had an opportunity to engage in positive interactions with each other and with the therapist, which ideally will lead them to view their relationship more positively and therapy more optimistically.

In addition to meeting with the couple together, the therapist will often spend one assessment session meeting with each spouse individually to explore individual histories (including individual problems, prior dating/marital relationships, and relationships with the family of origin), prior therapy experience, current and past involvements in extramarital affairs, and sexual satisfaction and adjustment. Furthermore, spouses also complete a number of self-report questionnaires at home during the assessment phase to provide information regarding marital satisfaction (e.g., Dyadic Adjustment Scale; Spanier, 1976; Marital Satisfaction Inventory; Snyder, 1979), behaviors in which change is requested of the partner (e.g., Areas of Change; Weiss, Hops, & Patterson, 1973), divorce intent and ideation (Marital Status Inventory; Weiss & Cerreto, 1980), sexual behaviors and satisfaction (Sexual Interaction Inventory; LoPiccolo & Steger, 1974), and observations of their partners behaviors (Spouse Observation Checklist; Patterson, 1976; Weiss & Perry, 1979). Detailed information about these and other assessment instruments is provided elsewhere (cf. Jacobson, Elwood, & Dallas, 1981; Margolin, Michelli, & Jacobson, 1988).

Once the therapist has evaluated the couple, they are presented with an assessment of the strengths and weaknesses in their relationship. Included in this relationship assessment is an emphasis on the reciprocal responsibility of each spouse in maintaining his or her current strengths and weaknesses. Furthermore, the therapist encourages each partner to adopt a "collaborative set" about their marriage. That is, both persons are encouraged to acknowledge reciprocal responsibility for their marital problems and commit themselves to adopt those attitudes and behaviors that foster a cooperative effort in working together toward building a better relationship. This orientation to relationship difficulties runs counter to the typical approach to marital problems: Most couples initially blame the partner for the problems in the marriage and rarely present the relationship as the cause of their problems. Therefore, it is critical that the therapist inform the couple that each spouse must focus on his or her own behavior if therapy is to be beneficial. Even if the couple does not believe the therapist's presentation of the reciprocal nature of their problems, they must agree to act as if it is true for therapy to proceed.

After presenting the couple with their relationship assessment, the therapist outlines the proposed treatment plan (Whisman & Jacobson, in press). Spouses provide feedback on this plan, and necessary modifications are made. Once the therapist and spouses have agreed upon a treatment plan, the therapist asks the couple to commit to therapy and to collaboratively work together (i.e., focus on changing one's own behavior, adhere to the agenda of each therapy session, and comply with homework assignments). Once this commitment is obtained, any future rule violations can be enforced by referring back to this commitment.

Behavior Exchange Techniques

Most couples present for therapy at a time when both spouses are deriving little satisfaction from their relationship and are focusing most of their attention on perceived deficits in their partner. Our initial goal is not to focus on changing these undesirable behaviors but rather to identify and increase the occurrence of those behaviors that would enhance each partner's satisfaction through a strategy labeled *behavior exchange* (BE). There are several reasons for employing this strategy. First, focusing on and removing negative relationship events does not guarantee that positive events will occur. Second, undesirable behaviors in one's spouse tend to diminish over time, even if they are not specifically targeted for change. Third, such a focus reinforces the idea of changing one's own behavior and thereby helps to reverse the typical pattern of waiting for the partner to change first. Fourth, this strategy tends to provide an immediate increase in each spouse's satisfaction, thereby enhancing their positive expectations regarding therapy and preparing them for later demands for greater change. Finally, because couples often enter therapy with the belief that there is nothing they can do to improve the relationship, these techniques are also designed to increase each person's perception of control over daily changes in marital satisfaction. Therapists should take care to point out, however, that they are well aware of the major problems in the relationship and ensure the couple that they will be working on these problems later in therapy.

The primary goal of BE is to teach each spouse how to become more effective at providing behaviors that make the partner more satisfied with the relationship. Consequently, the cardinal rule of this phase is for the spouses to focus on their own behavior, as opposed to changes they would like from their partner. A secondary goal of BE is to teach the couple that maintaining a happy marriage requires daily attention by each spouse.

Both partners are first taught to pinpoint specific behaviors that would result in a more satisfying relationship for their spouse. The most straightforward way of doing this is to ask the partners to generate a list of behaviors they *could* do (not necessarily that they would do) that they believe would make their partner more satisfied with the relationship. The therapist should forewarn the couple that their lists are likely to have different items on them, which in no way implies that they are incompatible. Both persons are then asked to choose some of the items from their list and increase the frequency of these behaviors during the week, with the underlying goal of increasing the daily satisfaction of the partner. The only stipulation on this assignment is that they not engage in any behavior that they would subsequently resent doing. Allowing the giver to choose the content and frequency of behaviors they engage in during the week decreases the likelihood of resistance. Furthermore, by having both spouses make their own list and choose which items they perform on any given day undermines the common criticism that "she only did that because you told her to." If this criticism is raised, therapists can point out that, although the therapist asked both spouses to increase their rate of positive behaviors, it was the spouse who chose the particular items. The therapist can also relabel the intent of doing the behaviors from following the therapist's directive to that of attempting to improve the relationship (Jacobson, 1984b).

If spouses are unable to generate lists of behaviors they could do to improve the relationship, the therapist can provide them with a copy of the Spouse Observation Checklist, which consists of 409 hypothetical relationship behaviors. Each spouse can then choose items from this list to do during the coming week.

In addition to engaging in independent activities, it is also recommended that the therapist encourage the couple to engage in activities together to build a greater sense of companionship into the relationship. For example, therapists may suggest that spouses participate in joint activities (e.g., hiking, skiing, shopping) that they used to engage in but no longer share. In addition to activities the couple have done together in the past, therapists are encouraged to assist the couple in identifying and creating situations that create an unfamiliar or novel situation for them or that involve risk taking, in an attempt to heighten the couples' affective and emotional experience.

During subsequent sessions, both spouses can be asked what they observed their partner doing during the week and the impact these behaviors had on their feelings about the relationship. In addition, therapists can show them the graphs of their weekly averaged marital happiness ratings to illustrate the effects that their behaviors are having on the other person's satisfaction with the relationship. Both spouses can also be asked how they would like their partner to show appreciation for the things that they have done. For example, the husband may not appreciate it when his wife thanks him profusely for doing the dishes if he doubts her sincerity. Instead, he may be more satisfied with a simple "thank you." On the other hand, spouses are likely to become discouraged with doing things to please the partner if that person never acknowledges the things that have been done. Ensuring that the occurrence of these pleasing interactions are adequately reinforced will help to guarantee that such behavior will continue after therapy.

Session time can also be devoted to having both spouses make requests for specific behaviors from their partner. Care should be taken to make sure that these requests are given in a nondemanding, yet assertive manner. Recommended formats include "I would like you to . . ." or "Would you please . . . ?" Statements such as "You never say you love me" or "You always leave a mess wherever you go" should be restated by the partner. Couples often complain that the partner "should know what I like" since they have been married several years. This provides an opportunity for the therapist to challenge the basis of this unrealistic belief (cf. Epstein, 1982).

By the time a couple begins to focus on high-cost behavior change in latter stages of therapy, the momentum derived from the earlier, less demanding format will prepare them for the collaboration necessary to negotiate the changes in these difficult areas.

Communication Training

According to a survey of marital therapists, communication problems are the most commonly reported problem of couples seeking therapy, with approximately 82% of couples identifying communication as a problem in their relationship (Geiss & O'Leary, 1981). Communication problems have been shown to be related to global measures of marital distress (Gottman, 1979; cf. Boland & Follingstad, 1987) and daily changes in marital satisfaction (Jacobson & Moore, 1981). Furthermore, they have been shown to longitudinally predict relationship satisfaction in married couples (e.g., Gottman & Krokoff, 1989; Levenson & Gottman, 1985) and couples planning marriage (Markman, 1981). It is no small wonder then that so many marital therapies place an emphasis on communication training. What separates BMT from many other approaches to marital therapy, however, is the use of direct teaching strategies to promote positive communication.

The BMT approach to communication training has been influenced by the work of Guerney (1977) and Gottman *et al.* (1976). It involves three components, all of which have been identified as necessary conditions for effective training (Jacobson & Anderson, 1980). These components include (1) didactic instructions from the therapist; (2) practice by the couple both within and between sessions; and (3) the therapist's feedback regarding the practice sessions. The goal of training is to teach couples good communication skills to promote not only the clear transmission of information but also to enhance closeness and intimacy (Margolin, 1983). Furthermore, it establishes the groundwork for future discussion about problem areas in their relationship.

During communication training, the communication process is divided into "listening" and "expressive" skills. The therapist first models the skills and then allows the couple to practice them, giving feedback as to their performance. Communication training often begins humorously, with the therapist modeling negative verbal (e.g., interrupting, changing the subject) and nonverbal (e.g., yawning, looking away) listening skills in an exaggerated manner. The couple then is asked to identify the inappropriate behaviors. Following this, the therapist models positive nonverbal listening skills (e.g., making eye contact, leaning forward, and occasionally nodding the head) and asks the couple to point out how these behaviors differ from the negative example.

Particularly salient to the discussion of nonverbal skills is Gottman's (1979) distinction between intent and impact of a message. Although studies have shown that distressed and nondistressed spouses do not differ in the intent of statements they make to their partners, distressed couples rate these statements as having less positive impact than do nondistressed couples (Gottman, Notarius, Markman, Bank, Yoppi, & Rubin, 1976). Gottman (1979) concludes this is due to a difficulty distressed couples have in reading their partners' nonverbal behaviors (cf. Noller, 1980). Thus, although training in nonverbal listening skills may seem trivial to some couples, it is an important facet of communication training.

Following this discussion of positive nonverbal behavior, the therapist teaches spouses how to paraphrase each other, checking to be sure that the paraphrase is accurate: "So you feel angry when Jim comments on the work that Sally does because you feel like you are the one who should be recognized, is that correct?" Each spouse then practices listening and paraphrasing, first with the therapist and then with each other, discussing pleasant (e.g., positive experiences from BE, pleasant memories) or neutral activities (e.g., eating lunch, playing tennis).

Once the couple has mastered paraphrasing and active listening skills, the focus of communication training shifts to expressive skills. Spouses are first taught to use "I statements" (e.g., "I really enjoy it when you rub my shoulders after dinner") and then are asked to identify and communicate their feelings by linking events with emotions. Because some individuals have difficulty doing this, we often use a structured format when first starting out: "I feel Z in situation Y" (e.g., "I felt relieved when I finished cleaning out the garage"). This format can be modified to include feeling statements about the behavior of others (including the spouse): "When you do X in situation Y, I feel Z" (e.g., "When I came home from work today and you put down your paper and asked me about my day, I felt really special"). Because sharing thoughts and feelings has been identified as a fundamental aspect of intimacy in marriage (Waring, Tillman, Frelick, Russell, & Weisz, 1980), and because distressed spouses commonly close off their partners from their inner feelings, having them open up to each other and talk about their emotions builds intimacy and sensitivity in the relationship. Furthermore, having spouses paraphrase these statements of emotion builds trust in the relationship as each partner learns that the marriage can be a safe environment for sharing inner feelings (Margolin, 1983).

It is recommended that the couple first talk about positive or neutral subjects when practicing listening and expressive skills because the skills are difficult enough for many couples, in and of themselves, without the negative emotions associated with conflictual subjects. However, to ensure generalization of these skills and to prepare the couple for problem solving, each spouse should have an opportunity to discuss negative emotions as well.

Once both spouses have mastered listening and expressive communication skills within session, they are asked to continue practicing them at home. It is important, however, to make sure that both spouses have mastered these skills during the session before they are asked to practice them at home.

Markman and Kraft (1989) have suggested that men and women may experience intimacy through communication in different ways because of different socialization histories and that these differences may contribute to marital conflict. Although women may place a premium on face-to-face communication, men may prefer interaction in the context of an activity. Consequently, therapists may want to assign homework that will meet both spouses' needs for intimacy by suggesting that they not only interact with one another face to face but that they also link communication exercises with companionship activities (e.g., talking while driving or engaging in some sporting activity together).

Problem-Solving Training

Following general communication training, couples are taught (through practice, instructions, and feedback from the therapist) a variety of skills that have been associated with effective conflict resolution. Couples are first given a problem-solving manual to read at home (see Jacobson & Margolin, 1979, pp. 215–251) to provide them with the format to be used during treatment. When beginning problem-solving training, it is often helpful to ask spouses to spend a few minutes within the session and attempt to resolve a moderate-sized problem in their relationship. The therapist can look for idiosyncratic communication problems or deficits during this brief interaction and can tailor problem-solving training to meet the specific needs of each couple.

Our approach to problem solving is divided into two stages: problem definition and problem solution. During problem definition, the goal is emotional expression and validation, not generating solutions to the problem. Couples are taught to follow specific guidelines in defining their problem. First, they are to begin problem definition with an expression of appreciation. This expression of appreciation, which is ideally related to the behavior being criticized, should be genuine and not just a perfunctory precursor to a criticism. It is easier to acknowledge the statement "you are a very organized and conscientious person, but recently you haven't been writing down the amount of the checks that you have been writing" than the statement "there you go again, always forgetting to write down the amount of the check."

Second, the problem should be defined in specific behavioral terms, specifying situations in which the undesirable behavior occurs. Distressed spouses often make global statements about their partner's personality, rather than specific statements about a particular aspect of their behavior. Statements such as "you are an inconsiderate slob" are better presented as "when you fix yourself something to eat after I have just cleaned the kitchen, you leave the food and kitchen utensils on the counter."

Third, because something about the other person's behavior is upsetting to the individual defining the problem, these feelings should be expressed. Such expressions of feeling tend to reduce the defensiveness in the receiver and thereby promote collaboration: "When you do not kiss me goodbye, I feel unloved."

Finally, the definer of the problem should acknowledge ways in which he or she contributes to the problem. Acknowledging reciprocal responsibility for the problem is difficult for many spouses, but it is an effective way of reducing the receiver's defensiveness and promoting collaboration. Once the speaker has defined the problem, the listener is then asked to paraphrase the definition.

As an illustration of these guidelines, consider the case of John and Terry, a couple in their mid-30s. John had recently gone back to graduate school part-time, to receive his master's degree in engineering so that he could get a promotion at work. Before going back to school, both he and Terry enjoyed spending time together with each other and with other couples. However, since starting school, most of his free time was spent studying, and Terry was upset about the amount of time they spent together. Terry's initial statement of the problem was "all you care about is your job and your classes, John—you don't care anything about me." During therapy, this problem was restated as follows: "John, I am really proud of how well you are doing in your classes and how hard you have been working toward getting that promotion (Guideline 1), but when you spend your weekend nights studying rather than spending at least an hour each night with me (Guideline 2), I feel bored, unloved, and insecure (Guideline 3). I realize I contribute to the problem by waiting until the weekend to discuss our weekend plans (Guideline 4)." Once the problem has been clearly defined and both spouses understand it (which is ensured by having the listener paraphrase the definition), discussion moves on to problem solution.

During the problem solution phase of problem solving, discussion is focused on factors designed to rectify the problem. First, spouses are asked to brainstorm as many possible solutions to the problem as they can think of, without regard to the quality of the solutions. This last caveat is included for two reasons. We encourage couples to come up with ridiculous and comical suggestions to add humor to what is potentially an emotional subject. Furthermore, encouraging spouses to suggest anything that comes to mind dispels the reluctance a partner may have about raising a solution that he or she feels the spouse would immediately reject. Spouses are encouraged to suggest a solution that would involve changes in their own behavior first, in order to show their willingness to make changes to overcome the problem.

In the previous mentioned example of Terry and John, the following suggestions were generated:

- Terry could help type John's papers so that he would have more free time.
- John could cancel his midweek luncheon and spend the time studying.
- Terry could spend more time socializing with others.
- John could drop out of graduate school and/or quit his job.
- Terry could enter the same graduate program so that she would see more of John.
- John could spend weekend nights with Terry and then take No-Doze and study all night.
- Terry could initiate discussion of their weekend plans earlier in the week.

Once the couple has a list of solutions, the next step is to go through and examine each one. They first ask, "Is the solution absurd?" If both spouses agree it is, the solution is discarded. They then ask, "If we implemented this solution, would it solve or help in any way to solve the problem?" Both partners have to agree that it would not help to solve the problem before the solution is discarded. Finally, if the proposed solution is not absurd and would help to solve the problem, the pros and then the cons of the solution are delineated. Beginning with the proposed benefits of each solution keeps the discussion upbeat and helps to promote optimism that the problem can be solved. An item is discarded only if both partners agree that there are more drawbacks than benefits, and that no modifications can be made to improve the solution. Thus, a proposed solution is discarded only if (1) both partners agree it is absurd; (2)

neither one thinks the solution would help to solve the problem; or (3) both agree that the drawbacks outweigh the benefits.

The final stage in problem solution is combining the solutions that remain into a change agreement that both spouses can agree upon. Like the problem definition, the change agreement should be very specific and spelled out in clear, descriptive behavioral terms. Because unforeseen difficulties with an agreement may appear once it has been implemented, spouses are encouraged to set a date to review the contract and make any modifications on it that are warranted. It is also recommended that these change agreements be recorded in writing. A written agreement can help to avoid unnecessary disagreements at a later date about what each person agreed to do or not to do.

In the preceding example of John and Terry, the following change agreement was reached:

> By Wednesday of each week, Terry will ask John about his weekend plans. John will spend at least one weekend night with Terry. If Terry wants to do something socially on a night that John has to study, she will get together with friends. John will cancel his midweek luncheon and use that time to study so that he will have one weekend night free. John and Terry will meet on the last day of the month to renegotiate the contract.

Because there are several steps to problem solving, training is usually spread out over several weeks. For example, during one session, the couple may work on problem definition of one or two problems. During the next session, they may work on brainstorming and going through the pros and cons of each proposed solution. Finally, during the third session, they may work on writing a final change agreement. Homework assignments mirror what is done in therapy; therapists should not assign homework that goes beyond that which was covered in session. Thus a couple may be working on one problem in session and a second problem at home. We commonly ask couples to tape all home sessions so that the therapist can provide feedback about their performance. Once a change agreement has been made, compliance is reviewed briefly during subsequent therapy sessions.

Couples first practice problem-solving skills on minor complaints before using them to tackle major problems in their relationship. Because many couples have a long-standing pattern of either avoiding conflict or handling conflict poorly, focusing on minor problems that are easier to solve enhances their confidence in their problem-solving abilities. As these skills are mastered, the content shifts to more central relationship problems. The goal of problem solving is to have couples not only resolve current problems in their relationship but also to acquire skills that are generalizable to problems that may occur subsequent to the termination of therapy.

A few cautionary notes regarding problem solving should be raised. First, it should be made clear to each spouse that problem solving is a specialized, structured form of communication. Thus they should set aside a special time and place (where the couple is alone and free from distractions) for their problem-solving sessions. Second, spouses should not attempt problem solving when they are angry at one another. Furthermore, it should be stressed to the couple that there may be occasions when a partner has a complaint that he or she may simply want to talk about, without attempting problem solving. During those times, the partner can best assist the discontented spouse by being supportive through empathic listening, rather than through generating solutions. To avoid unnecessary disagreement, the therapist should help the couple learn how to discriminate between requests for support and acknowledgment and requests for problem solving.

Modifying Characteristic Interaction Themes

Although BMT has traditionally been interested in altering molecular aspects of couple's communication patterns, there has been a recent trend toward the development of techniques designed to modify more molar, characteristic patterns (cf. Jacobson, 1989). The emergence of these techniques has been stimulated by the works of Greenberg and Johnson (1988) and Wile (1981).

Couples often display repetitive interaction patterns that manifest themselves in a variety of situations. One of the most common interaction themes involves one partner requesting more intimacy and closeness, whereas the other partner is seeking greater autonomy and distance.

The first step in modifying molar interaction patterns is to immerse the couple in the issues that they are disagreeing about. The easiest way to do this is to have the couple continue a typical argument within the session until the therapist understands its content. The therapist then stops the argument and allows both persons to explain their perspective ("develop their position"; Wile, 1981), while the other person is asked to sit and listen. The therapist's goal is to elicit each spouse's (1) cognitions and attributions about their partner's behavior (i.e., "What is it about X that is upsetting you?"), and (2) their affect about their partner's behavior (i.e., "How do you feel when your partner does X?"). These cognitions and emotions are made more accessible by first having the couple recreate the argument in session. By allowing each person to develop his or her perspective, both spouses gain additional understanding of what is truly bothering their partner. Thus, the argument is replaced with a new experience of the underlying emotional experience, from which both spouses can view their actions and the actions of their spouse with more acceptance and compassion (Greenberg & Johnson, 1988).

Once both partners have developed their perspective, the therapist has several options. First, the therapist might go through the disagreement step by step and ask each spouse what could have been done differently to stop the escalation of the argument (Wood & Jacobson, 1985). Second, the therapist can show the couple that they are both trapped by the situation in that each is trying to get something from the other in ways that are unlikely to be successful (Wile, 1981). For example, an individual who wants more intimacy tries to get it by asking for more, which pushes his or her partner further away; the individual who want more autonomy tries to get it by withdrawing, which pulls his or her partner closer. Thus the therapist can provide a detailed description of the roles both spouses play in their characteristic interaction and how these roles are contributing to their problem. Third, the couple can self-monitor their interaction pattern at home and then debrief these patterns after they have occurred. Each person can discuss his or her own role in the pattern, which increases the couple's resiliency and opens up communication after an argument. Finally, the therapist can work with the couple in rewriting their interaction pattern. Usually this involves each person taking a different, uncharacteristic role. For example, the person who wants autonomy may be asked to initiate sex or another act of intimacy, whereas the person who wants more intimacy is asked to reject this advance.

Sexual Enrichment

A majority of couples seeking marital therapy also report sexual problems. Most marital therapists assume that if nonsexual marital problems are dealt with in therapy, sexual problems will resolve themselves. Improvement in sexual relations is very rare, however, even if other relationship areas do show improvement (Melman & Jacobson, 1983). Consequently, we routinely include a "sexual enrichment" component in our treatment program.

Sexual enrichment is extremely individualized. If the couple has a sexual dysfunction, techniques pioneered by Masters and Johnson (1970) have been shown to be beneficial. If, as is more common, the major problem is a disorder of sexual desire or generalized dissatisfaction with the quantity or quality of sexual activity, then a variety of treatment strategies are utilized (cf. Barbach, 1984; Melman & Jacobson, 1983). Common areas of focus include nongenital and genital sensate-focus exercises oriented toward increasing sensitivity and providing information; communication training in which spouses provide specific information regarding sexual preferences and turnoffs; explicit agreements regarding the rituals of initiation and refusal; and discussion regarding the conditions that enhance sexual satisfaction for each spouse. Many couples also benefit from learning how to discriminate nonsexual affectionate behavior from affection given prior to sexual activity.

Generalization and Maintenance

During the last phase of BMT, sessions are specifically oriented toward maintaining treatment gains after therapy is completed. One goal is to ensure that couple continue to communicate with each other and work on conflict areas in their relationship. To accomplish this goal, couples need to have a comfortable format for solving their problems. Many couples like the problem-solving format described here and choose to follow it just as they have learned it. Other couples, however, feel that this format is too structured, in which case it may need to be tailored to meet their particular needs. One way to accomplish this is for the therapist to go through the format with the couple, asking which parts they feel are necessary—anything which *either* spouse identifies as important is retained and incorporated into a revised problem-solving format. The goal is to develop a format that the couple will use after therapy to continue to work on their areas of disagreement.

In addition to individualizing the problem-solving format to maximize the likelihood that couples will continue these problem-solving exercises subsequent to the termination of therapy, couples are taught to meet regularly for "state-of-the-relationship" meetings. It is typical for many couples to stop paying attention to their relationship when therapy ends, thereby allowing it to deteriorate. These meetings, which substitute for regularly scheduled therapy sessions, ensure that spouses continue to communicate and work on their relationship on a regular basis (even when there are no apparent conflicts). During thee sessions, prior change agreements are evaluated, problem-solving sessions are conducted when necessary, and overall relationship strengths are discussed, including compliments and other statements of appreciation for each other and the positive things each spouse has been doing for the relationship. The therapist works with the couple to form a general agenda to be followed during these meetings as well as to determine their frequency and duration.

Maintenance and generalization of treatment gains are also promoted during the last few phase of BMT by increasing the interval between sessions. By limiting contact with the therapist, the couple gets used to functioning autonomously. In addition, session time is spent summarizing the events of therapy and the progress the couple has made so that they gain a perspective on their accomplishments. Finally, during this last phase, the therapist asks the couple to anticipate future problems and discusses with them how these problems can be either prevented or overcome should they occur.

HOMEWORK COMPLIANCE

As stated earlier, homework is an integral part of our treatment program to ensure that the skills learned in session are maintained and generalized to the home environment. Two recent investigations (Holtzworth-Munroe, Jacobson, DeKlyen, & Whisman, in press; Whisman & Jacobson, 1987) have illustrated the importance of homework compliance to positive treatment outcome. Because homework compliance is imperative, any incident of noncompliance must be dealt with immediately and directly. Consequently, a number of methods for dealing with noncompliance have been developed (cf. Wood & Jacobson, 1985).

In contrast to many treatment approaches that deal with noncompliance after it has occurred, we employ a number of methods to ensure that noncompliance does not occur in the first place. First, we use the term *between-session task* with couples to avoid resistance individuals may have with the phrase *homework assignment*. Second, the importance of the task is stressed to the couple. Third, the therapist elicits from each spouse a commitment to do each task. Fourth, the therapist asks the couple to anticipate anything that may interfere with completing the task, in an effort to eliminate potential excuses in advance. Finally, if the task is complicated, the couple is asked either to write it down or repeat it back to the therapist to ensure that it is understood. In addition, completion of each task is reinforced by spending time at the beginning of each session debriefing the past week's assignment, with the therapist praising its completion.

A basic underlying assumption of BMT is that most couples who request therapy genuinely want to change their marriage. This does not mean, however, that couples always comply with homework assignments designed to elicit such changes. These tasks are aversive to many couples because they require time and effort in the short run, whereas the benefits of an improved relationship are delayed. Thus, even after employing the previously mentioned strategies, some couples will not complete their homework. Should this occur, the therapist should not reinforce this behavior by continuing with the next session as planned. Instead, the therapist discusses with the couple what interfered with homework completion and what they could do differently to ensure that the task is completed the coming week. If the assignment was inappropriate for some reason, it is modified. The (modified) task is then given to the couple to complete during the coming week, and the session is postponed until the following week. An alternative strategy for noncompliance is to have the couple do their homework within the session itself. These strategies give the couple the clear message that noncompliance is not tolerated. Usually, only one such experience is necessary for couples to maintain compliance throughout the duration of therapy. If the couple continues to not do their homework, the therapist should assess for any underlying reasons or extenuating circumstances. The couple may have decided that the cost of improving their relationship is greater than the benefits of an improved relationship, in which case the focus of therapy may need to be shifted to helping the couple adjust to their current relationship or reconsidering their decision to remain married.

THERAPIST CHARACTERISTICS

A common criticism leveled at behavioral approaches to therapy is the exclusive focus on technology, without any consideration given to characteristics of the therapist. It is our belief, however, that there are a number of therapist characteristics that are necessary for marital therapy to be successful (cf. Jacobson, Berley, Melman, Elwood, & Phelps, 1985).

The first set of characteristics necessary for successful BMT are structuring skills. Therapists need to structure time efficiently both within sessions, to ensure that the material for the session gets covered, as well as across sessions, to ensure that each of the couple's presenting problems is addressed. In addition, therapists need to interrupt spouses' destructive behaviors to maintain a positive focus and ensure that the agenda for the session is followed. Asking spouses "why am I stopping you?" when they transgress session rules helps spouses learn not only how they are violating rules but also assists them in monitoring their own behavior.

Second, the successful BMT therapist possesses instigative skills, whereby the techniques couples acquire in therapy are transferred to the home environment. To foster the collaboration, spouses need to work together on their relationship, and the therapist must work towards building a collaborative set with the couple (see the previous section on assessment). Another way of instigating skills learned in therapy is to have the couple practice them during homework assignments. Furthermore, although it is necessary for BMT therapists to direct spouses during skill acquisition, they also need to fade their directiveness once skills are acquired. This generalization of skills is ensured later in therapy by having couples meet less frequently, instigating "state-of-the-relationship" sessions, and tailoring structured formats (such as problem solving) to meet the individual needs of each couple.

The third set of characteristics necessary for successful BMT are teaching skills. Because BMT is a skills acquisition program, effective teaching is essential. As with any skilled teacher, the therapist must be clear and concise, presenting material with a minimum of psychological jargon. Furthermore, every effort should be made to link specific examples of the principles being taught in therapy to the general principles themselves. Finally, the skilled therapist will repeat rules and guidelines as needed and will not assume that the couple will process this information the first time it is given. To ensure that the couple is learning the material covered in therapy, the therapist may have each spouse paraphrase the material covered during the session and periodically summarize the course of therapy up that point in time.

Fourth, the skillful BMT therapist possesses skills necessary to induce and maintain positive expectancies regarding therapy. It is important for the therapist to exhibit optimism regarding the outcome of therapy, which can be supported by referring to the experimental evidence of the efficacy of BMT. However, these optimistic statements about outcome should be tempered with the information that treatment gains come about through the effort of each spouse. In addition, because progress in therapy is rarely linear, it is important for the couple to expect that changes in their satisfaction with the relationship may be erratic. Consequently, therapists should make sure to predict relapses and setbacks over the course of therapy. When embarking on interventions that are not likely to lead to immediate changes in satisfaction (e.g., during assessment or during the onset of problem solving), these warnings are particularly important. Otherwise the couple is often demoralized when relapses occur. Finally, to induce and maintain positive expectancies, it is crucial that the therapist conveys excitement about the therapeutic approach, conducting therapy in an upbeat manner to maintain vitality within sessions and thereby mitigate the common negative reactions elicited during discussion of marital problems. This vitality can be maintained and enhanced by utilizing humor, to help spouses recognize the lighter side of their problems.

The final set of skills necessary for successful BMT are skills in providing emotional nurturance. It is important for partners to talk about their emotional response to the treatment program and to their spouse over the course of therapy. The effective therapist will periodically ask spouses about their emotional involvement in therapy, as well as their reaction to changes that they see occurring. If feelings that run counter to the assumptions of therapy are expressed, the therapist needs to show that these feelings are understood but that they are not allowed to serve as an excuse for noncollaborative behavior.

Treatment Effectiveness

BMT has been evaluated in a number of controlled studies and is not only the most thoroughly researched approach to marital therapy but also the only one with a substantial body of experimental research. In their exhaustive review of marital therapy outcome research, Baucom and Hoffman (1986) provide the following conclusions regarding the effectiveness of BMT: (1) BMT results in decreases in negative communication assessed in the therapy setting, decreases in reported problem areas and requests for behavior change, and increases in overall marital adjustment relative to waiting list controls; (2) BMT has been found to be more effective than nonspecific treatments in altering communication and other specific behavior of concern to the couple; (3) few significant differences have been found between BMT and other treatment approaches; and (4) there are no major differences in the effectiveness of different BMT treatment procedures when used as a combined package, when used in isolation, or when the order of presentation is varied.

In a recent meta-analysis of BMT outcome studies, Hahlweg and Markman (1988) report that the average couple receiving BMT was better off at the end of treatment than 83% of the couples receiving either no treatment or nonspecific treatment. Similarly, several studies (e.g., Baucom & Lester, 1986; Jacobson & Follette, 1985; Jacobson, Follette, Revenstorf, Baucom, Hahlweg, & Margolin, 1984) have examined the clinical significance of treatment changes and have concluded that approximately 67% of couples exhibit statistically reliable improvement following therapy (i.e., the magnitude of change exceeds that which could be expected based on measurement error alone), whereas 50% improve to the point where they are no longer distressed by the end of treatment.

Recently, clinical researchers have begun to examine several parameters of the treatment approach, including comparing the effectiveness of the treatment package with one or more of its components in isolation (e.g., Baucom, 1982; Jacobson, 1984a; Jacobson, Follette, Follette, Holtzworth-Munroe, Katt, & Schmaling, 1985; Jacobson, Schmaling, & Holtzworth-Munroe, 1987) or comparing a standard treatment with an additional cognitive component (e.g., Baucom & Lester, 1986; Margolin & Weiss, 1978); comparing structured versus clinically flexible treatments (Jacobson et al., 1989), and group versus individual treatments (e.g., Hahlweg, Revenstorf, & Schindler, 1982; Wilson, Bornstein, & Wilson, 1988); comparing outcome of therapy provided by experienced versus inexperienced therapists (Jacobson et al., 1989) or individual versus co-therapists (Mehlman, Baucom, & Anderson, 1983); and examining the effects of offering immediate versus delayed treatment (Mehlman et al., 1983). Varying these parameters has had little impact on treatment effectiveness.

Several investigations have been conducted to identify variables predictive of positive treatment outcome. To date, these have included younger couples, less educated couples, couples who were less likely to be thinking of and acting toward divorce prior to treatment, couples who reported greater satisfaction with their communication and who had observable negative communication before treatment, and couples in which the wife's self-reported level of femininity was high (reviewed by Baucom & Hoffman, 1986). Similarly, positive outcome has been found to be related to couples who endorse more depressive symptomatology and who do not reflect traditional affiliation/independence patterns (i.e., highly affiliative wife and highly independent husband) (Jacobson, Follette, & Pagel, 1986). However, it should be noted that several variables that have been found to predict outcome in one study have not been replicated in other studies.

There is a noticeable lack of research examining the long-term effects of marital therapy (Baucom & Hoffman, 1986). In their review of 17 published outcome studies of BMT, Hahlweg and Markman (1988) report that 8 studies had follow-ups of between 3 to 6 months, whereas only 5 studies had follow-ups of between 9 to 12 months. Results of their meta-analysis of these studies suggests that BMT produces long-lasting stable effects. Results from longer term follow-up (Jacobson, Follette, Follette, Holtzworth-Munroe, Katt, & Schmaling, 1985; Jacobson et al., 1987) suggest that 70% of couples who initially improve in treatment maintain their treatment gains for 2 years. These findings, combined with findings that suggest that approximately two-thirds of the couples who enter treatment initially improve, suggest that approximately 50% of couples who enter BMT will benefit and maintain those benefits for 2 years (Jacobson, 1988). The influence of therapy can be extended for a period of time by focusing on prevention of future problems and training couples in the communication skills that enable them to function as their own therapist subsequent to termination. However, given the myriad of stresses and life transitions associated with marriage (Markman, Floyd, Stanley, & Lewis, 1986), the effects of any brief marital treatment, no matter how powerful, might be expected to diminish over time. In fact, life stress is the only variable that has been found to predict relapse in couples 2 years after receiving BMT (Jacobson et al., 1987).

NEW DIRECTIONS IN MARITAL THERAPY

As research methods become more sophisticated and experimental questions more refined, researchers have become increasingly aware of the limitations as well as the strengths of the approach. This awareness has led to several recent clinical innovations, including the use of booster maintenance sessions and the application of marital therapy for psychological problems other than marital distress.

Booster Maintenance Sessions

To enhance the long-term effects of our treatment program, we are currently in the process of evaluating several clinical innovations. Foremost among these is the use of booster maintenance sessions following the termination of the initial phase of treatment. Instead of an intensive, short-term treatment program with a formal termination, we are beginning to adopt a new model of marital therapy, one in which the therapist and couple form a long-term relationship but only meet periodically following the end of weekly sessions. Much like the dentist or the accountant, the marital therapist serves as a person with whom the couple has an ongoing relationship, meeting either in times of crisis or for regular "marital checkups."

For couples who are maintaining treatment gains, the primary focus of maintenance sessions is to reiterate the skills taught in therapy and to accentuate the reasons for the smooth relationship functioning that has occurred since therapy ended. For those couples who have not been particularly successful in maintaining their treatment gains, an attempt is made to identify the problem areas that have occurred since therapy so the skills learned in therapy may be applied to them. Thus these sessions are really condensed versions of the treatment program, which serve as refresher courses of the skills taught in therapy.

The booster session concept is well-suited for BMT, as it represents a perspective on psychotherapy that is more consistent with contemporary notions as to how psychosocial interventions work. A social-learning view emphasizes the power of the social environment in influencing behavior, which leads to the expectation that continued contact with a therapist would lead to greater generalization and maintenance of treatment-induced changes, as well as mitigate the negative impact of life stress on the marital relationship. Maintenance sessions are believed to benefit couples by (1) decreasing the trauma of termination for couples; (2) extending the stimulus control of the therapy regimen into the environment of the couple, increasing the likelihood that they will implement the skills acquired during therapy; and (3) aiding in the consolidation of skills learned during therapy, thereby facilitating their maintenance (Jacobson, 1988).

Marital Therapy for Selected Psychological Disorders

A second clinical innovation in BMT is the use of marital therapy for psychological problems that have been traditionally conceptualized as individual problems (Jacobson, Holtzworth-Munroe, & Schmaling, 1989). In particular, we have been evaluating the effectiveness of BMT singly and in combination with cognitive therapy (Beck, Rush, Shaw, & Emery, 1979) as a treatment of depression because marital problems have been identified as a vulnerability factor, a precipitant, a concomitant, and a consequence of depression (Coyne, Kahn, & Gotlib, 1987). Preliminary results indicate that BMT is an effective form of treatment for depression for spouses who are in distressed relationships (Whisman, Jacobson, Fruzzetti, Schmaling, & Dobson, 1988). Other researchers have also been studying BMT as a treatment of depression (Beach & O'Leary, 1986), as well as examining marital therapy techniques derived from social-learning theory in the marital treatment of alcoholism (McCrady et al., 1986; O'Farrell & Cutter, 1984; O'Farrell, Cutter, & Floyd, 1985) and agoraphobia (Arnow, Taylor, Agras, & Telch, 1985; Barlow, O'Brien, & Last, 1984).

In this chapter we have attempted to provide the reader with an overview of the social-learning-based model of marital distress and therapy, with an emphasis on the unique integration of theory and technique. This field has greatly expanded over the past two decades; we anxiously await to see what developments are in store for the next two.

ACKNOWLEDGMENTS. Preparation of the chapter was supported by National Research Service Award 5 F31MH09684-02 and Grant 5 R01MH33838-08 from the National Institute of Mental Health, awarded to Mark A. Whisman and Neil S. Jacobson, respectively. Special thanks to Judy M. Torkelson for her helpful comments on an earlier draft of this chapter.

REFERENCES

Arnow, B. A., Taylor, D. B., Agras, W. S., & Telch, M. J. (1985). Enhancing agoraphobia treatment outcome by changing couple communication patterns. *Behavior Therapy, 16,* 452–467.

Barbach, L. (1984). *For each other.* New York: New American Library.

Barlow, D. H., O'Brien, G. J., & Last, C. G. (1984). Couples treatment for agoraphobia. *Behavior Therapy, 15,* 41–58.

Baucom, D. H. (1982). A comparison of behavioral contracting and problem-solving/communications training in behavioral marital therapy. *Behavior Therapy, 13,* 162–174.

Baucom, D. H., & Hoffman, J. A. (1986). The effectiveness of marital therapy: Current status and application to the clinical setting. In N. S. Jacobson & A. S. Gurman (Eds.), *Clinical handbook of marital therapy* (pp. 597–620). New York: Guilford.

Baucom, D. H., & Lester, G. W. (1986). The usefulness of cognitive restructuring as an adjunct to behavioral marital therapy. *Behavior Therapy, 17,* 385–403.

Beach, S. R. H., & O'Leary, K. D. (1986). The treatment of depression occurring in the context of marital discord. *Behavior Therapy, 17,* 43–49.

Beck, A. T., Rush, A. J., Shaw, B. F., Emery, G. (1979). *Cognitive therapy of depression.* New York: Guilford.

Berley, R. A., & Jacobson, N. S. (1984). Causal attributions in intimate relationships: Toward a model of cognitive-behavioral marital therapy. In P. Kendall (Ed.), *Advances in cognitive-behavioral research and therapy* (Vol. 3, pp. 1–60). New York: Academic.

Birchler, G. R., Weiss, R. L., & Vincent, J. P. (1975). A multimethod analysis of social reinforcement exchange between maritally distressed and nondistressed spouse and stranger dyads. *Journal of Personality and Social Psychology, 31,* 349–360.

Bloom, B. L., Asher, S. J., & White, S. W. (1978). Marital disruption as a stressor: A review and analysis. *Psychological Bulletin, 85,* 867–894.

Boland, J. P., & Follingstad, D. R. (1987). The relationship between communication and marital satisfaction: A review. *Journal of Sex & Marital Therapy, 13,* 286–313.

Coyne, J. C., Kahn, J., & Gotlib, I. (1987). Depression. In T. Jacobs (Ed.), *Family interaction and psychopathology* (pp. 509–533). New York: Pergamon.

Eidelson, R. J., & Epstein, N. (1982). Cognition and relationship maladjustment: Development of a measure of dysfunctional relationship beliefs. *Journal of Consulting and Clinical Psychology, 50,* 715–720.

Emery, R. E. (1982). Interparental conflict and the children of discord and divorce. *Psychological Bulletin, 92,* 310–330.

Epstein, N. (1982). Cognitive therapy with couples. *The American Journal of Family Therapy, 10,* 5–16.

Fincham, F. D. (1985). Attribution processes in distressed and nondistressed couples: 2. Responsibility for marital problems. *Journal of Abnormal Psychology, 94,* 183–190.

Fincham, F. D., & Bradbury, T. N. (1987). The impact of attributions in marriage: A longitudinal analysis. *Journal of Personality and Social Psychology, 53,* 510–517.

Fincham, F. D., & O'Leary, D. K. (1983). Causal inferences for spouse behavior in maritally distressed and nondistressed couples. *Journal of Social and Clinical Psychology, 1,* 42–57.

Fincham, F. D., Beach, S. R., & Baucom, D. H. (1987). Attribution processes in distressed and nondistressed couples: 4. Self-partner attribution differences. *Journal of Personality and Social Psychology, 52,* 739–748.

Fincham, F. D., Beach, S., & Nelson, G. (1987). Attribution processes in distressed and nondistressed couples: 3. Causal and responsibility attributions for spouse behavior. *Cognitive Therapy and Research, 11,* 71–86.

Geiss, S. K., & O'Leary, K. D. (1981). Therapist ratings of frequency and severity of marital problems: Implications for research. *Journal of Marital and Family Therapy, 7,* 515–520.

Gottman, J. W. (1979). *Marital interaction: Experimental investigations.* New York: Academic.

Gottman, J. M., & Krokoff, L. J. (1989). Marital interaction and satisfaction: A longitudinal view. *Journal of Consulting and Clinical Psychology, 57,* 47–52.

Gottman, J., Markman, H., Notarius, C., & Gonso, J. (1976). *A couple's guide to communication.* Champaign, IL: Research.

Gottman, J., Notarius, C., Markman, H., Bank, S., Yoppi, B., & Rubin, M. E. (1976). Behavior exchange theory and marital decision making. *Journal of Personality and Social Psychology, 34,* 14–23.

Greenberg, L., & Johnson, S. (1988). *Emotionally focused therapy for couples.* New York: Guilford.

Guerney, B. (1977). *Relationship enhancement.* San Francisco: Jessey-Bass.

Hahlweg, K., & Markman, H. J. (1988). Effectiveness of behavioral marital therapy: Empirical status of behavioral techniques in preventing and alleviating marital distress. *Journal of Consulting and Clinical Psychology, 56,* 440–447.

Hahlweg, K., Revenstorf, D., & Schindler, L. (1982). Treatment of marital distress: Comparing formats and modalities. *Advances in Behaviour Research and Therapy, 4,* 57–74.

Holmes, T. H., & Rahe, R. H. (1967). The social readjustment rating scale. *Journal of Psychosomatic Research, 11,* 123–128.

Holtzworth-Munroe, A., & Jacobson, N. S. (1985). Causal attributions of married couples: When do they search for causes? What do the conclude when they do? *Journal of Personality and Social Psychology, 48,* 1398–1412.

Holtzworth-Munroe, A., Jacobson, N. S., DeKlyen, M., & Whisman, M. A. (in press). The relationship between behavioral marital therapy outcome and process variables. *Journal of Consulting and Clinical Psychology.*

Jacobson, N. S. (1983a). Clinical innovations in behavioral marital therapy. In K. Craig & R. J. McMahon (Eds.), *Advances in clinical behavior therapy* (pp. 74–98). New York: Brunner/Mazel.

Jacobson, N. S. (1983b). Expanding the range and applicability of behavioral marital therapy. *The Behavior Therapist, 6,* 189–191.

Jacobson, N. S. (1984a). A component analysis of behavioral marital therapy: The relative effectiveness of behavior exchange and problem solving training. *Journal of Consulting and Clinical Psychology, 52,* 295–305.

Jacobson, N. S. (1984b). The modification of cognitive processes in behavioral marital therapy: Integrating cognitive and behavioral intervention strategies. In K. Hahlweg & N. S. Jacobson (Eds.), *Marital interaction: Analyses and modification* (pp. 285–308). New York: Guilford.

Jacobson, N. S. (1988). *The maintenance of treatment gains following social learning-based marital therapy.* Manuscript submitted for publication.

Jacobson, N. S. (1989). The politics of intimacy. *Behavior Therapist, 12,* 29–32.

Jacobson, N. S., & Anderson, E. A. (1980). The effects of behavior rehearsal and feedback on the acquisition of problem solving skills in distressed and nondistressed couples. *Behaviour Research and Therapy, 18,* 25–36.

Jacobson, N. S., & Follette, W. C. (1985). Clinical significance of improvement resulting from two behavioral marital therapy components. *Behavior Therapy, 16,* 249–262.

Jacobson, N. S., & Holtzworth-Munroe, A. (1986). Marital therapy: A social-learning cognitive perspective. In N. S. Jacobson & A. S. Gurman (Eds.), *Clinical handbook of marital therapy* (pp. 29–70). New York: Guilford.

Jacobson, N. S., & Margolin, G. (1979). *Marital therapy: Strategies based on social learning and behavior exchange principles.* New York: Brunner/Mazel.

Jacobson, N. S., & Moore, D. (1981). Spouses as observers of the events in their relationship. *Journal of Consulting and Clinical Psychology, 49,* 269–277.

Jacobson, N. S., Elwood, R., & Dallas, M. (1981). Assessment of marital dysfunction. In D. H. Barlow (Ed.), *Behavioral assessment of adult disorders* (pp. 439–479). New York: Guilford.

Jacobson, N. S., Follette, W. C., & McDonald, D. W. (1982). Reactivity to positive and negative behavior in distressed and nondistressed married couples. *Journal of Consulting and Clinical Psychology, 50,* 706–714.

Jacobson, N. S., Follette, W. C., Revenstorf, D., Baucom, D. H., Hahlweg, K., & Margolin, G. (1984). Variability in outcome and clinical significance of behavioral marital therapy: A re-analysis of outcome data. *Journal of Consulting and Clinical Psychology, 54,* 497–504.

Jacobson, N. S., Follette, V. M., Follette, W. C., Holtzworth-Munroe, A., Katt, J. L., & Schmaling, K. B. (1985). A component analysis of behavioral marital therapy: 1-year follow-up. *Behaviour Research and Therapy, 23,* 549–555.

Jacobson, N. S., Berley, R. A., Melman, K. N., Elwood, R., & Phelps, C. (1985). Failure in behavioral marital therapy. In S. Coleman (Ed.), *Failures in family therapy,* (pp. 91–134). New York: Guilford.

Jacobson, N. S., McDonald, D. W., Follette, W. C., & Berley, R. A. (1985). Attributional processes in distressed and nondistressed married couples. *Cognitive Therapy and Research, 9,* 35–50.

Jacobson, N. S., Follette, W. C., & Pagel, M. (1986). Predicting who will benefit from behavioral marital therapy. *Journal of Consulting and Clinical Psychology, 54,* 518–522.

Jacobson, N. S., Schmaling, K. B., & Holtzworth-Munroe, A. (1987). A component analysis of behavioral marital therapy: Two year follow-up and prediction of relapse. *Journal of Marital and Family Therapy, 13,* 187–195.

Jacobson, N. S., Holtzworth-Munroe, A., & Schmaling, K. B. (1989). Marital therapy and spouse involvement in the treatment of depression, agoraphobia, and alcoholism. *Journal of Consulting and Clinical Psychology, 57,* 5–10.

Jacobson, N. S., Schmaling, K. B., Holtzworth-Munroe, A., Katt, J., & Wood, L. F., & Follette, V. M. (1989). Research-structured versus clinically flexible versions of social learning-based marital therapy. *Behaviour Research and Therapy, 27,* 173–180.

Kiecolt-Glaser, J. K., Fisher, L. D., Ogrocki, P., Stout, J. C., Speicher, C. E., & Glaser, R. (1987). Marital quality, marital disruption, and immune function. *Psychosomatic Medicine, 49,* 13–34.

Levenson, R. W., & Gottman, J. M. (1983). Marital interaction: Physiological linkage and affective exchange. *Journal of Personality and Social Psychology, 45,* 585–597.

Levenson, R. W., & Gottman, J. M. (1985). Physiological and affective predictors of change in relationship satisfaction. *Journal of Personality and Social Psychology, 49,* 85–94.

LoPiccolo, J. & Steger, J. C. (1974). The Sexual Interaction Inventory: A new instrument of assessment of sexual dysfunction. *Archives of Sexual Behavior, 3,* 585–595.

Margolin, G. (1981a). Behavior exchange in happy and unhappy marriages: A family cycle perspective. *Behavior Therapy, 12,* 329–343.

Margolin, G. (1981b). The reciprocal relationship between marital and child problems. In J. P. Vincent (Ed.), *Advances in family intervention, assessment and theory* (Vol. 2, pp. 131–182). Greenwich, CT: JAI.

Margolin, G. (1983). Behavioral marital therapy: Is there a place for passion, play, and other non-negotiable dimensions? *Behavior Therapist, 6,* 65–68.

Margolin, G., & Wampold, B. E. (1981). Sequential analysis of conflict and accord in distressed and nondistressed marital partners. *Journal of Consulting and Clinical Psychology, 49,* 554–567.

Margolin, G., & Weiss, R. L. (1978). Comparative evaluation of therapeutic components associated with behavioral marital treatments. *Journal of Consulting and Clinical Psychology, 46,* 1476–1486.

Margolin, G., Michelli, J., & Jacobson, N. S. (1988). Assessment of marital dysfunction. In M. Hersen & A. S. Bellack (Eds.), *Behavioral assessment: A practical handbook* (3rd ed.), (pp. 441–489). London: Pergamon.

Markman, H. J. (1981). Prediction of marital distress: A 5-year follow-up. *Journal of Consulting and Clinical Psychology, 49,* 760–762.

Markman, H. J., & Kraft, S. A. (1989). Men and women in marriage: Dealing with gender differences in marital therapy. *Behavior Therapist, 12,* 51–56.

Markman, H. J., Floyd, F. J., Stanley, S. M., & Lewis, H. C. (1986). Prevention. In N. S. Jacobson & A. S. Gurman (Eds.), *Clinical handbook of marital therapy* (pp. 173–196). New York: Guilford.

Masters, W. H., & Johnson, V. E. (1970). *Human sexual inadequacy.* Boston: Little-Brown.

McCrady, B. S., Noel, N. E., Abrams, D. B., Stout, R. L., Nelson, H. F., & Hay, W. N. (1986). Comparative effectiveness of three types of spouse involvement in outpatient behavioral alcoholism treatment. *Journal of Studies on Alcohol, 47,* 459–467.

Mehlman, S. K., Baucom, D. H., & Anderson, D. (1983). Effectiveness of cotherapists versus single therapists and immediate versus delayed treatment in behavioral marital therapy. *Journal of Consulting and Clinical Psychology, 51,* 258–266.

Melman, K. N., & Jacobson, N. S. (1983). The integration of behavioral marital therapy and sex therapy. In M. L. Aronson & L. R. Wolberg (Eds.), *Group and family therapy* (pp. 238–251). New York: Brunner/Mazel.

Noller, P. (1980). Misunderstandings in marital communication: A study of couples' nonverbal communication. *Journal of Personality and Social Psychology, 39,* 1135–1148.

O'Farrel, T. J., & Cutter, H. S. G. (1984). Behavioral marital therapy couples groups for male alcoholics and their wives. *Journal of Substance Abuse Treatment, 1,* 191–204.

O'Farrell, T. J., Cutter, H. S. G., & Floyd, F. J. (1985). Evaluating behavioral marital therapy for male alcoholics: Effects on marital adjustment and communication from before to after treatment. *Behavior Therapy, 16,* 147–167.

Overall, J. E., Henry, B. W., & Woodward, A. (1974). Dependence of marital problems on parental family history. *Journal of Abnormal Psychology, 83,* 446–450.

Patterson, G. R. (1976). Some procedures for assessing changes in marital interaction patterns. *Oregon Research Institute Bulletin, 16*(7).

Schindler, L., & Vollmer, M. (1984). Cognitive perspectives in behavioral marital therapy: Some proposals for bridging theory, research, and practice. In K. Hahlweg & N. S. Jacobson (Eds.), *Marital interaction: Analysis and modification* (pp. 309–324). New York: Guilford.

Snyder, D. K. (1979). *Marital Satisfaction Inventory.* Los Angeles: Western Psychological Services.

Spanier, G. B. (1976). Measuring dyadic adjustment: New scales for assessing the quality of marriage and similar dyads. *Journal of Marriage and the Family, 38,* 15–28.

Vincent, J. P., Weiss, R. L., & Birchler, G. R. (1975). A behavioral analysis of problem-solving in distressed and nondistressed married and stranger dyads. *Behavior Therapy, 6,* 475–487.

Waring, E. M., Tillman, M. P., Frelick, L., Russell, L., & Weisz, G. (1980). Concepts of intimacy in the general population. *Journal of Nervous and Mental Disease, 168,* 471–474.

Weiss, R. L. (1980). Strategic behavioral marital therapy: Toward a model for assessment and intervention. In J. F. Vincent (Ed.), *Advances in family intervention, assessment and theory* (Vol. 1, pp. 229–271). Greenwich, CT: JAI.

Weiss, R. L. (1984). Cognitive and strategic interventions in behavioral marital therapy. In K. Hahlweg & N. S. Jacobson (Eds.), *Marital interaction: Analysis and modification* (pp. 337–355). New York: Guilford.

Weiss, R. L., & Cerreto, M. C. (1980). The Marital Status Inventory: Development of a measure of dissolution potential. *American Journal of Family Therapy, 8,* 80–85.

Weiss, R. L., & Perry, B. A. (1979). *Assessment and treatment of marital dysfunction.* Eugene: Oregon Marital Studies Program.

Weiss, R. L., Hops, H., & Patterson, G. R. (1973). A framework for conceptualizing marital conflict, technology for altering it, some data for evaluating it. In L. A. Hamerlynck, L. C. Handy, & E. J. Mash (Eds.), *Behavior change: Methodology, concepts and practice.* Champaign, IL: Research.

Whisman, M. A., & Jacobson, N. S. (1987, November). *Homework compliance in behavioral marital therapy: Client, therapist, and outcome variables.* Paper presented at the annual meeting of the Association for Advancement of Behavior Therapy, Boston.

Whisman, M. A., & Jacobson, N. S. (in press). The treatment of marital distress: Matching client characteristics with treatment strategies. In A. M. Nezu & C. M. Nezu (Eds.), *Clinical decision making and judgment in the practice of behavior therapy: A problem-solving perspective.* Champaign, IL: Research.

Whisman, M. A., Jacobson, N. S., Fruzzetti, A. E., Schmaling, K. B., & Dobson, K. S. (November, 1988). *Treating the couple versus the depressed spouse alone: The short- and long-term effects of cognitive behavior therapies for depression.* Paper presented at the annual meeting of the Association for Advancement of Behavior Therapy, New York.

Wile, D. B. (1981). *Couples therapy: A nontraditional approach.* New York: Wiley.

Wilson, G. L., Bornstein, P. H., & Wilson, L. J. (1988). Treatment of relationship dysfunction: An empirical evaluation of group and conjoint behavioral marital therapy. *Journal of Consulting and Clinical Psychology, 56,* 929–931.

Wood, L. F., & Jacobson, N. S. (1985). Marital distress. In D. H. Barlow (Ed.), *Clinical handbook of psychological disorders* (pp. 344–416). New York: Guilford

16

Strategic Psychotherapy

ROBERT ROSENBAUM

INTRODUCTION

By choosing to read this book, you show a willingness to entertain new ideas, expand your therapeutic knowledge, and generally enjoy the fruits of curiosity and enquiry. Since beginning a new chapter has certain uncertainties, it's important to read critically to pick out certain ideas you may find new or valuable. You may already be anticipating what valuable knowledge you will rediscover here that you already know, or you may be looking forward to learning something new and useful. Perhaps you would like to make yourself comfortable before you get absorbed in this chapter; you might want to start as soon as you are ready to absorb whatever is most useful from the experience, or just have an absorbing beginning from the start.

Strategic therapy teaches that clients' problems contain the seeds of beginning a new chapter in their lives. People find turning over a new page can be an effortful pleasure or a pleasurable effort; you know how you have had experiences where you were already well underway with a project almost before you realized how you began it, and then were surprised at how easy it was; it is especially helpful to realize you can continue as long as you wish, then stop, then come back to the task when it makes the most sense to you.

I don't know how well the preceding two paragraphs worked for you, or what you made of them, but they contain many elements of a strategic approach. In effect, the "*in*(tro)*duction*" to this chapter constitutes a kind of indirect hypnotic *induction*. I began the chapter this way because strategic therapy owes much to hypnosis, specifically Ericksonian hypnosis, as a progenitor. I cannot know what effect something like this has in print, and since the essence of the strategic style is to match interventions to patient responses and patient messages which reflect the client's model of the world, this can be only a metaphor. Strategic therapists tend to like using metaphors, though, and I think it would be worthwhile discussing here how the paragraphs were crafted, to give you some sense of some of the elements of strategic therapy.

ROBERT ROSENBAUM • Department of Psychiatry, Kaiser-Permanente Medical Center, Hayward, California 94545-4299.

The strategic therapist always begins by acknowledging the assets and strengths a patient has that are often obscured by the "tunnel vision" patients acquire as they focus on their complaints. Thus I began this chapter with an acknowledgment of the efforts you are making. Subsequently, any "resistance" the patient may exhibit is utilized in the service of the treatment, rather than removed or analyzed. Thus, to the extent you approach this chapter skeptically, I invite you to "read critically," but I phrased it so that the critical faculties are devoted not to searching out flaws but rather to seeking the "valuable new ideas you will encounter." Notice here that already there is a presupposition of a positive change experience: I do not speak of new ideas you *may* encounter, but those you *will* encounter. Similarly, suggesting that you "make yourself comfortable *before* getting absorbed" indirectly implies that you will get absorbed; the implication is not open to question because it is not stated directly.

The presentation of such strong positive presumptions can, however, paradoxically lead to doubt. You may ask, how can the author be certain I'm going to encounter new ideas? I can be certain you will discover new ideas because your mind is *always* generating new ideas; even if I do not present you with any information you have not encountered before, you are bound to generate some new associations or perspectives on the material yourself. Strategic therapists believe that clients carry their answers within them. Rather than attempt to convince you of that directly, however, the introductory paragraph attempts to depotentiate your skepticism by using a certain amount of confusion: it talks of "certain uncertainties" while simultaneously seeding the inevitability of change: you are "beginning a new chapter" (taking something which is actually happening currently, and letting this imply something valuable will also occur in the future). Finally, at the end of the paragraph you are presented with an illusion of alternatives: whether you choose to "rediscover valuable information you already know," or choose to "learn something new and useful," you will be entering a positive learning set. The next sentence uses a non sequitur which is phrased to seem to follow logically (" . . . new and useful. You can start something new . . .") but really contains a whole new thought and suggestion: "You *can* start something new" (reading this chapter, contemplating a new way of therapeutic practice, etc.), again providing a positive indirect suggestion, utilizing an illusion of alternatives so that the choice becomes one of *how* to start, rather than *whether* to start.

At this point, I began to worry I would lose your attention if I did not adopt a more "conventional" chapter beginning. All strategic therapists make it a point to meet clients at the start at the level of the clients' world-view, rather than the therapist's world-view. Thus the second paragraph begins conventionally with "Strategic therapy teaches . . . " but again uses "chapter" and "page" wording to make it applicable to you even while ostensibly talking of someone else. Strategic therapy tends to address its targets indirectly. Thus the paragraph shifts pronouns from "people" to "you" in a colloquial manner which facilitates your involvement without asking for it directly (and thus giving you less of a chance to decline). Strategic therapists also want to utilize past successful experiences to reframe current experiences and orient them toward a successful future. I therefore appeal to experiences I can be reasonably sure you have already had (the experience of being in the middle of something) which match what you are currently experiencing (being already involved in reading the introduction), and pair it with a suggestion of its being easy.

With all of the suggestions and framings in this in(tro)duction, I am careful to give you the control of the experience, by suggesting you go at your own pace, stopping when necessary; notice that "resistant" stopping then becomes compliance, and even here there is a suggestion that when you come back, it will make sense to you. Strategic therapists are extremely respectful of the client's resources and ability to make the best choices they can for themselves at any given moment, but they attempt to shift the focus of the choices available even while delimiting that range to the more helpful alternatives.

Finally, after all these carefully framed directives, and apparently when the "*introduction* to the reader" is completed, there is one last task: to take a "one-down" stance so as not to alienate you or put you off by taking an overly powerful role. Thus the above explanation begins by my confessing the truth: I don't now how well this worked for you, and can't know what you made out of it all. I can feel confident, however, that you had *some* reaction, and if this were a therapy—which it's not—I would base my further actions on your reactions thus far.

DISTINGUISHING CHARACTERISTICS OF STRATEGIC THERAPY

Strategic therapy traces it sources back to the work of Milton Erickson (Erickson, 1967; Haley, 1973). A voluminous amount of literature has appeared in the last decade on Erickson (cf. Erickson, 1980; Erickson, Rossi, & Rossi, 1976; Lankton & Lankton, 1983), but he labored in comparative anonymity for several decades until, in the 1950s, coincidental with a rising disenchantment with traditional psychodynamic therapies and a growing interest in systems theory and cybernetics, numerous clinicians and theoreticians began finding their way to Phoenix to study Erickson's methods.

At the same time that interest in hypnotherapy was reviving, "systems thinking" was promoting the growth of the family therapy movement. In addition to its roots in hypnotherapy, strategic therapy has rich interconnections with the family therapy movement and systems thinking in general (cf. Fraser, 1986; Roberts, 1986). In 1956 Gregory Bateson, Don Jackson, Jay Haley, and John Weakland published a seminal paper, "Toward a Theory of Schizophrenia" (reprinted in Bateson, 1972), which brought systems thinking to the attention of the clinician. The Mental Research Institute in Palo Alto, California, many of whose founders had studied with Erickson, grew out of this research; many of the most prominent people in the development of strategic therapy have been associated, at one time or another, with MRI. The MRI group, many of whom had studied Erickson's hypnotherapy, developed a theory of change based on communications and systems concepts and coupled it with a symptom-focused, brief treatment approach. The MRI group contributed theoretical underpinnings of strategic therapy as set forth by Watzlawick and his associates (Watzlawick, Beavin, & Jackson, 1967; Watzlawick, Weakland, & Fisch, 1974; Watzlawick, 1983, 1984), as well as pragmatic methods of strategic therapy in a seminal paper (Weakland, Fisch, Watzlawick, & Bodin, 1974) and a subsequent book (Fisch, Weakland, & Segal, 1982). At the same time, strategic and problem-solving approaches were being set forth by Haley (1973, 1976), Madanes (1980), further developed by De Shazer (1985) and De Shazer *et al.* (1986), and a growing number of others (cf. Efron, 1986; Bergman, 1985).

So far, I have been talking rather cavalierly of "strategic therapists," as if there were some fraternity or sorority that clearly set forth a body of rules defining the field of strategic therapy and classified people as being or not being strategic therapists according to how well they went by the rules. This is not the case. Strategic therapy is not a particular approach or theory (Haley, 1973, 1976; Madanes, 1980). It rather refers, in its broadest sense, to any therapy in which the therapist is willing to take on the responsibility for influencing people and takes an active role in planning a strategy for promoting change (De Shazer, 1985; Fisch *et al.*, 1982; Madanes, 1980; Papp, 1980; Weakland *et al.*, 1974). In this sense, any therapist who actively plans his or her treatment with a hope to effecting certain ends is a strategic therapist. When a psychoanalyst decides to interpret resistance in order to encourage development of the transference, the analyst is engaging in strategic behavior. When a behaviorist decides to work on relaxation exercises before assertiveness training, so that the client has the necessary tools for coping with any anxiety created by being more assertive, the behaviorist is involved in strategic behavior. This broad formulation of strategic therapy has important implications for the field of psychotherapy integration. First, though, it is important to study the major distinguishing characteristics of strategic therapy as it is usually conceptualized. These characteristics are each discussed next:

1. *Therapists are in the business of influencing people.* This was noted before as the single most distinctive characteristic of strategic therapy, yet one to which therapists of many different schools subscribe, to varying extents. Clinicians who identify themselves as strategic therapists differ from others, however, in that they do not see their responsibility to influence the client as an option that is exercised occasionally at their discretion. Instead, influencing the client is seen as an inevitability. Strategic therapists tend to subscribe to general systems theory, in which all behavior is seen as essentially interactional. As soon as client(s) and therapist(s) sit down together, they are creating a therapeutic *system* in which the behaviors of all parties are inevitably linked in multiple feedback loops. In such human systems, one cannot *not* communicate (Bateson, 1972, 1979; Watzlawick *et al.*, 1967); silence or refraining to communicate is itself a communication. In a systems view, mutual influence is an inevitability: The therapist cannot *not* influence the patient (and vice versa). Systems therapists take the approach that, as long as they are fated to influence their clients, they may as well do so in a planned manner that will maximize its beneficial effects.

2. *Strategic therapists meet the client at his or her view of the world.* Strategic therapists do not believe they, or anyone, can have a "correct" grasp of what is

the "actual reality" of the patient's experience (Watzlawick, 1984). This is based partly on a profound respect for the patient and partly on the adoption of a systemic epistemology in which "reality" is seen as a series of multiple recursive descriptions (Keeney, 1983; Watzlawick, 1984).

Meeting the patient at his or her view of the world (Lankton & Lankton, 1983) is an intensely empathic approach. It means accepting *all* the client's behavior, without labeling any of it as pathological. It is also humbling, for we must accept that we do not have a "better" world view to offer the patient; we do not have more wisdom than the patient; all we have to offer is a different perspective. This different perspective, however, can prove crucial. Although we *meet* a client at his or her view of the world, that does not mean we *adopt* his or her view; we may enter into his or her house for a visit, but we will not live there. Our value to the client lies not only in our ability to put on their spectacles but also in our ability to take them off. Because we can visit but not stay in their world view, we do not have any need to label any parts of it as good or bad; we can accept the facticity of all parts of their experience, without drawing judgmental distinctions or falling into the pathognomic errors clients make, when they either deny parts of their experience or insist their experience "should" be a certain way (Watzlawick *et al.*, 1974). Accepting *all* of a client's experience allows us to draw different distinctions than the client does, to reframe their experience and modify it.

Clients will believe you more if you talk their language. If you try to convince them of a different set of values or attitudes, it is easy for them to turn you off. If, on the other hand, you take their own attitudes but recombine them in a different way, it is harder for them not to listen.

A classic example of meeting the client at their view of the world is given in Haley's description of a case of Erickson's. An overweight client came in to Erickson who had extreme self-loathing; she described herself as a "plain, fat slob." Rather then be sympathetic, Erickson validated the patient's view of herself as worthless:

> You are *not* a plain, fat, disgusting slob. You are the fattest, homeliest, most disgustingly horrible bucket of lard I have ever seen, and it is appalling to have to look at you. . . . To put it simply—you are a hideous mess. But you do need help. I'm willing to give you this help. I think you know now that I won't hesitate to tell you the truth. (Haley, 1973, p. 116)

This is a radical step to take, and many people object to it as being unempathic and manipulative. I would argue, rather, that this kind of statement is extremely empathic: It does not offer sympathy or reassurance, which is useless, but speaks directly to what the client *knows* is the case, and then uses that to insert a little seed of a new concept that can transform his or her life. The strategic therapist looks for a seed within the client's realm of experience that can be nurtured to transform the experience.

An alcoholic man who had been on the wagon for 2 years came in to our crisis group after a 1-night relapse. During that time, he had gone to a bar, gotten a ride home with some strangers from the bar who waylaid him, committed homosexual rape on him, assaulted and beat him severely, and robbed him. He had intrusive images of the rape and the assault, feeling it was his fault; he was agitated and on the verge of a panic attack. Group members repeatedly reassured him over several days he hadn't "asked for" the rape; although this was true, it only led to the patient becoming more agitated. I finally turned to the patient and told him harshly he was right: the assault and the rape was his fault, if he hadn't stopped taking the Antabuse, this never would have happened. I asked him what he was going to do about it. The patient stated he was never going to stop his Antabuse again. He immediately experienced a lessening of his symptoms, which progressively resolved. The group was dismayed that I was being too rough on him, but the patient heard me talking his language: He *knew* he was guilty, and nothing would dissuade him from that. The intervention, however, changed him from a *passive* guilty victim, fated to suffer his symptoms as an atonement, to a *responsible* guilty party, who could choose some constructive actions (maintaining Antabuse) as a "penance."

In regard to whether this is manipulative, it is necessary to take some time here to talk a bit about epistemology because strategic therapy looks very different depending on what epistemology you employ. To the extent you employ the linear, causal epistemology in common use, strategic therapy can look manipulative and controlling. Once you realize, using systemic epistemology, that there is no such thing as unidirectional control, strategic therapy begins to look more like a creative, cooperative dance between therapist and client.

3. *Strategic therapists work with a systemic epistemology.* Numerous books have been written on the subject of cybernetic/systemic epistemology, and it is beyond the scope of this chapter to elaborate overmuch on this topic. Leaving it out, however, would be like leaving out the concept of "self" from a discussion of Kohutian psychoanalysis; without an appreciation of the epistemology involved, strategic therapy becomes a bag of tricks that *will not work as effectively* when employed in an inappropriate epistemology. I will attempt to give a brief sense of the "flavor" of systems thinking here: For fuller expositions, I highly recommend reading any of Gregory Bateson's (1972, 1979) works or, more recently, the excellent treatment by Bradford Keeney (1983).

Epistemology is the study of how we know what we know. *How* one thinks is inseparable from *what* one knows. It is impossible not to have an epistemology, but it is quite possible—in fact, it is the norm—to be unaware of what it is. Epistemology involves the whole set of our (usually unexamined) assumptions about what the world is and how it works. It is thus more fundamental than what we do: Whatever action we perform, our epistemology then tells us what we have done.

To take a simple example: most of us will say, at bedtime, "I'm going to sleep now." This usually involves a set of epistemological assumptions: that there is an "I" which actively initiates and controls, with willful intent, an action: "going to sleep." There is also an implication here that this "I" manages and controls the body, directing what it is to do, and that this "I" is somehow separate from or superordinate to the body. Anyone who has ever had insomnia, however, knows that if the "I" starts consciously willing to body to go to sleep on command, this will usually produce intense wakefulness. Different epistemological framings are possible, such as: "Dream-self is waking up."

Notice that in this framing, the experience of the body need not be included: "dream-self" may wake up with the eyes open or shut, with the body fatigued or alert, in a bed or while driving. In this framing, it is not that there is no mind-body separation; there isn't any *relevant* body, period. There will be different elements in a system, depending upon how it is framed. As an exercise, the reader might want to find other framings, e.g., one in which the body is seen as separate from but superordinate to (i.e., controlling) the mind, one in which there is no body–mind separation.

The above example, it is hoped, begins to indicate some of the differences between a systemic and a traditional linear epistemology. Linear epistemologies consist of discrete elements that are assumed to have existences of their own, independent of the relationships and contexts in which they appear. Causality is linear and unidirectional: One atomistic element acts on the other to produce an effect that starts and stops. In contrast, systemic epistemologies see patterns and relationships that alter in different contexts: there is no ultimate essence or identity separate from how it is framed by its participants. This framing is in turn recursive: The way something is framed then acts on the framer to alter the framing. This is a rather radical notion: It means there is no ultimate "I" separate from the relationships I am engaged in, which define me even as I define them. More interesting yet, this definition is *arbitrary* even as it is *inevitable*. There is no "accurate" description. It is not "wrong" to say, "I am going to sleep," and "right" to say, "the bed calls and the light wants to be turned out so it can rest"; either one is a possible framing of a continuous flow of experience, and both are incomplete but potentially useful in certain contexts (the latter framing is useful for saving on electric bills!).

We live in a continuous flow of sensory experience. Our first epistemological act that makes sense of that experience, by representing it psychologically, is to draw a distinction. It is not possible to not draw distinctions, just as it is not possible to not communicate. Saying "A" is different from "B" draws a boundary and delineates a system, but we can draw these boundaries in many different ways. For example, we are used to saying the therapist is different from the client, and we tend to look at the distinctions between the two. Many people do not do this, however. For example, much of the lay public lumps both therapist and client together as "two crazies sitting in a room doing crazy stuff." Clients tend to make a distinction between their symptom—"not me"—and their "usual selves," whereas therapists tend to see the symptom as an integral part of the client.

The important thing to realize here is that the kind of distinction one makes presupposes the kinds of descriptions that will follow. If you distinguish between pathological and healthy behavior, you will then devote much of your time to seeing pathology. Strategic therapists therefore attempt to avoid making this kind of distinction. The kind of data you collect helps create the "reality" being investigated, which in turn influences the kinds of data you look for. If you ask questions about whether patients wake up in the middle of the night, you will "discover" numerous endogenous depressions which must be treated with antidepressants, and this will lead you to ask more patients about their sleep habits. Before antidepressants were available, therapists rarely inquired about sleep habits: antidepressants, by offering a solution, also helped create the problem. (This is not to say the problem is "not real" nor that it "is real", but merely to point out the recursiveness of the data-gathering procedure.)

Often, we make errors in the level of abstraction in which we frame and describe "reality." Crying, staying in bed, not eating are all items of action: Depression describes a *category* of actions. It is easier to alter items than it is to alter categories. We can confuse our observations, our immediate sensory experiences, with our conclusions about our experiences. We may see a patient with a certain facial expression, and then classify it as fright, but we should always be aware that "fright" is an interpretation, a classification of a higher order logical type than the series of muscle actions we saw in the first place. We sometimes treat our categories as if they had the same factual basis as actions, but categories are only abstr-actions, not actions. It is also easy to create dormitive principles if we repackage a description as an explanation. We may categorize an unhappy, not-sleeping not-eating person as depressed, but this does not *explain* what the person is doing, and if we think it does, we will stop looking for useful interventions. It is important to note that the framing of a problem can worsen it. If you label unhappiness as *depression*, it can be much more difficult to deal with because if you think you are depressed, then you think you have an illness that can linger on and on. If you think you are unhappy, you can see this as a condition of life that comes and goes, partially dependent on your actions, partially dependent on the vicissitudes of random fortune.

The question you ask implies the kinds of answers you will accept: How often does a client ask the therapist, "Doc, I'm so nervous, what's wrong with me?" Obviously, this presupposes that something is wrong. If the therapist answers, "There's nothing wrong with you," in an attempt at reassurance, you run the risk that the client will think you do not know what you are talking about. If, however, you state, "what's wrong with you is that you haven't figured out yet what valuable signals your nervousness is sending you about when you need to be careful, and I think our first task is to have you pay attention to which part of the body gets nervous first, while all the rest of your body is staying relaxed," then you are meeting the client at his or her view of the world even while altering, expanding, and reframing it.

It is worth noting here that making distinctions can involve punctuating sequences of behaviors as well as assumptions about who does what to whom. Looking at our distinctions in a new light can lead to some interesting turn-arounds in our ideas. Keeney (1983) cites Pavlov as an interesting example. Pavlov thought he had proved that pairing a ringing bell with meat made the bell a "conditioned stimulus" for the dog. Recently, however, we've learned that if you remove the clapper from the bell, the dogs still salivate. It appears that in the classic conditioning experiments, the ringing bell was a conditioned stimulus (i.e., one with meaning to be attended to) for Pavlov but not for the dogs; the dogs do not seem to be attending to the atomistic elements Pavlov did but rather learn generalized contexts for making discriminations (i.e., "in a laboratory, look for stimuli that presage food").

On a more clinical note, we frequently see couples who punctuate a series of events at different starting points. The wife will say, "he withdraws, so I have to nag him to get him to do anything." The husband says, "she nags me, so I withdraw to get away from it."

The clinician sees an ongoing cycle of nag-withdraw/withdraw-nag punctuated arbitrarily by its participants. The wife's view is not more correct than the husband's; the husband's is not more correct than the wife's; and the therapist's overarching view is not more correct that the individual's. Systemic epistemologies stress the usefulness of obtaining *multiple descriptions* of events, and that collating these multiple descriptions results in a richer, more flexible (and thus, less problematical) sense of the reality. Just as each of our eyes sees a slightly different visual perspective and lets our brain combine them to obtain depth vision, so therapist and patient participate in a process of mutual redefining of each others' views to obtain a final perspective different from what either one started out with alone.

When a strategic therapist offers a different framing of experience to a patient, the therapist is not hoping the patient will go off and have a *particular* experience anticipated and predicted by the therapist. Rather, the therapist is throwing something new into the therapist–client ring and seeing what happens. Very often outcomes in strategic therapy are rather different from what either party anticipated originally. All therapies involve a repunctuation and reframing of experience (cf. Frank, 1973); strategic therapy makes this a central point of its work but does not offer a "correct" punctuation or explanation of reality. Rather, strategic therapy seeks to initiate *any* difference in the client's current framing of the "reality" of his or her problem because *any* difference can be the difference that makes a difference.

The adoption of this kind of systemic epistemology has certain immediate consequences that lead to further distinguishing characteristics of strategic therapists.

4. *Strategic therapy focuses on problems and their solutions.* Usually, clients come to therapy concerned about a particular problem, rather than for a generalized experience of "growth." Strategic therapists focus on the client's presenting problem, especially the overt behavioral complaints, because this allows them to meet the client at his or her view of the world. At the same time, focusing on the presenting problem offers concrete avenues for intervention on specific behaviors and allows a clear assessment of when changes occur or do not occur.

Insight is not seen as particularly necessary or even useful for change. The term *insight* presumes there is a "correct" view of the problem the patient must recognize: "the truth shall set you free." In a systemic epistemology, however, we cannot point to "truth." As discussed before, problems are a function of their punctuation. Furthermore, in line with the idea that clients make the best possible decisions from the choices available to them, at times it would be disrespectful to the client to "give them insight." *Insight* could force the client to think consciously about an issue he or she may have unconsciously decided to not think about, and this may not be useful, but merely upsetting, unless there is an attractive alternative choice available. As mentioned, strategic therapy has strong roots in Ericksonian hypnosis, which assumes that unconscious decisions are generally wise. In hypnosis, it is sometimes better to create or maintain amnesia for certain events or problems patients are not ready to review consciously. Thus sometimes insight is to be actively avoided.

Case example: A patient, a Vietnam veteran, was seen as an inpatient after he had attacked his brother-in-law with a hammer following a flashback of his experiences in Vietnam. In an effort to gain insight, therapy focused on uncovering and "ventilating" his experiences as a member of the body detail in which the patient was responsible for going to battlefields and removing dismembered pieces of corpses, piling them on a truck. The more the patient remembered of this, the more agitated he became. In an effort to "provide him with insight into his conflicts over his aggressive impulses," the therapy linked his distress with the anger he had felt being beaten up by his father as a child. This led to an uncovering of an incident in which the patient had participated in a "fragging" in which an officer who had been mistreating the patients regiment was murdered by his men. Recall of this incident led to profound agitation, depression, and the patient breaking off therapy.

Exploring and reviewing the causes of a problem creates a punctuation that implies that the problem is, "in fact," a problem; this then helps to create and maintain the problem. In strategic therapy, the very existence of whether there is a problem requires a reframing. It is usually not effective to reframe with words and ideas, though; strategic therapists prefer to give patients a new experience of the world. This is best done by taking the specific behaviors and putting them in new contexts, with behavioral enactment playing a key role.

Strategic therapists do not view problems as products of "inner" forces that must be brought to the light of insight. If we live in a continuous flow of experience whose meaning is produced by our punctuations and framings, then the psychodynamic framing is one view among many. Strategic and psychodynamic viewpoints have very different assumptions, each providing a perspective on experience but neither being "correct." Strategic therapists often have a rather negative attitude toward psychodynamics, which they see as overly reductionistic, acontextual, and committed to dormitive principles that serve to further entrench the problems they purport to explain. This is an oversimplified attitude, particularly in view of recent efforts to reformulate psychodynamic theory in systemic or information-processing terms (cf. Horowitz, 1979b; Peterfreund & Schwartz, 1971; Schaefer, 1976). As we have noted, the recursive epistemology associated with systems theory is not more accurate than the linear epistemology associated with classical behaviorism or psychoanalysis, although it does allow the creation of an extra dimension on the problem. Systems theory lets us see that insight is not *necessary* for change; because punctuation of experience is arbitrary, there is no "correct" insight a patient must achieve. Any new *structuring* of experience will recursively lead to a new subjective *sense* of the experience.

Strategic therapy is nothing if not pragmatic, and this pragmatic approach extends to the issue of insight. If we take an integrated approach and define strategic therapy as any therapy in which the clinician actively matches treatment technique to specific client needs, then strategic therapy includes the insight therapies. For that small subset of clients who want to find out about the historical antecedents of their condition or who come to therapy asking for "insight," a strategic therapist would not suggest a behavioral manipulation. Instead, a strategic therapist has several options in how to meet clients at their view of the world. One would be to offer a fairly standard short-term dynamic psychotherapy, with historical "insights" and "transference interpretations," but to do this from a systemic viewpoint where there is no "correct" formulation that a patient must get insight about, the strategic therapist will help clients obtain insights into their behavior from multiple perspectives, and by so doing, the therapist changes the meaning of insight, and helps clients move away from a "single explanation" world view that is maintaining the problem. There are also multiple other options: The therapist can join with the patient in achieving insight into how they have started to change or can congratulate patients on their wisdom for realizing they must not change too much too fast but should think things over first, or can offer an "insightful explanation" that leads to a behavioral prescription.

Because we can draw the boundaries of a system in whatever way is most useful, strategic therapists tend to frame problems as behavioral acts with communicational meanings occurring in an interpersonal network. This framing of problems creates many opportunities for intervention. Bits of behavior are of a lower level logical type than the internal descriptions clients generate of their behavior: It is easier to change discrete behaviors directly than to alter internal maps with insights. By not focusing on patients' "inner" experiences, which by definition are not directly accessible to the therapist, strategic therapists can work on bits of behavior that, displayed and discussed between the therapist and client, can be reframed and restructured with equal value by either participant. Any alteration in patients' attempted solutions can change the behavioral loop, and because systems are generally unstable and require effort to maintain the status quo, the creation of a difference produces feedback situations in which further change tends to be augmented.

In order to maintain stability, you must make constant small adjustments and changes: If you want to steer a sailboat in a constant direction, you must constantly be adjusting your sails and rudder. In therapy, the client has taken a new, temporary passenger (the therapist) into the boat: This will change the ballast of the boat and require the client to make different kinds of changes and adjustments. Making these new adjustments in the sails and rudder makes the possibility of changing the course of the boat rather likely: It will take considerable active effort to keep the boat on its old, constant course. Ultimately clients may decide they want to maintain the boat on the old course; if clients decide to maintain their old course, this will be a change; now the course (the symptom) is voluntary, whereas before, it was seen as out of control. Strategic therapists do not take symptoms away from clients; they respect their clients' right to have their symptoms. The act of coming to the therapist makes a change for the client: The strategic therapist helps the client pursue the change profitably. The strategic therapist tends to be less interested in theories of celestial navigation than in helping clients who are sailing in circles move their rudder, pull on their sheets, or lean over the side of the boat.

Although strategic therapists work on problems and their solutions and see change as inevitable, there are some subtle issues regarding goal setting in strategic therapy. In an effort to speak clients' language and meet them at their view of the world, the therapist adopts clients' problems as the central focus for the therapy. However, if the therapist joins overmuch with the client, the therapist will not be able to effect to change. It will not help clients if we are so empathic that we adopt their view that the problem is awful and insoluble. The trick in strategic therapy is to join with the client's world view while maintaining a differing world view that will alter the client's framing. For example, Watzlawick (1983) will take the attitude that a client's problems are hopeless (thus joining with the client) but not serious (offering a new perspective).

In setting up the goals for a therapy, strategic therapists join with their clients by agreeing to work on the problem as described by the client: They will differ from the client by not agreeing with the client's proposed solutions. Using a case example described in Fisch *et al.* (1982), therapist and client can agree to work on solving the problem defined as a fear of playing the violin in public. The client may think this implies the goal is to help him fearlessly play the violin without making mistakes in public. The therapist, however, will recognize that this is just another version of the client's attempted solution (repeatedly confronting his fear in situations likely to lead to failure); this actually prevents the resolution of the problem. The therapist's goal is not the patient's: The patient wants a specific kind of performance, but what the patient wants usually precludes his obtaining it. The therapist, in contrast, simply wants something different to happen, so that the patient's experience of the world changes.

A successful therapy may not involve the client attaining the original goal but may involve the client discovering a different perspective on his or her original desire that makes the nonattainment of the original goal cease to be a problem. Sometimes, this then leads to the attainment of the original goal. In the preceding example, the therapist may work toward having the client play the violin fearfully in public, or fearlessly privately, or have the client play fearlessly in public while making many errors. In the course of doing any of these, the client may start to punctuate his or her experience differently. Perhaps the client will become less concerned about achievement; perhaps the client will decide that being anxious while playing does not indicate cowardice or ineptness but rather "courage in the face of fear." There are many possible outcomes, and the "proper" outcome *cannot be anticipated in advance by either therapist or client.*

De Shazer (1985) has a "crystal ball" technique, during part of which the client in the current session imagines himself telling the therapist at a future session how he solved the problem. Although this technique is often effective, usually the actual means by which the client solved the problem turns out to be different from the means he or she envisioned. Predicting the future is viewed by cognitive-behavioral therapists as a kind of irrational thought (Ellis & Harper, 1975), simply because it is not possible to predict the future with any certainty. All client problems involve some rigid predictions of the future; usually these involve a narrow set of catastrophic expectations combined with idealized happy endings. It is a distinct mistake to try to help clients achieve their "happy ending," because the happy ending depends on playing out the unhappy fairy story in a stereotyped manner. It is the strategic therapist's task to create more degrees of freedom, more possible alternatives.

If we cannot anticipate the outcome of the therapy in advance, how can we set goals for a strategic therapy? The solution here is simple: The treatment contract is to work on making the problem "no longer a problem;" that is, to resolve the patient's complaint. This can sometimes occur through finding a "solution," one different from those attempted before, and this can lead to the client's envisioned desired outcome. The problem can also cease to be a problem through a reframing of experience; clients sometimes report "the same events are occurring, but somehow I'm no longer bothered by them." In this latter case, the therapist will often want to see some behavioral change that has occurred, which if maintained is incommensurate with simultaneously maintaining the symptom. What a patient does always has more weight than what a patient says. When a patient starts feeling that the original problem is no longer bothersome, though, this often leads to a change in events. For example, an acting-out teenager who finds his or her parents are no longer so upset by his or her misbehavior often gets bored and stops acting out. Whether resolution occurs through achieving a certain goal or from an alteration in the attitude toward the presenting difficulty, treatment is regarded as successful when the client is no longer defining the problem as a problem.

5. *Strategic therapists tend to see client problems as maintained by their attempted solutions.* We have alluded to this before and so will only mention a few points briefly here. Clients' problems are usually presented as discrete entities, but strategic therapists see the problem as one segment of a larger loop of behavior in which the client's "solution" figures prominently. Generally these are positive feedback loops, in which more of the "solution" leads to more of the "problem." Examples are legion: The obsessive perfectionist who attempts to avoid anxiety attendant on making mistakes by scrutinizing for tiny imperfections and minor errors—thus continually finding the mistakes that create more anxiety. Victims of posttraumatic stress disorders try to avoid thinking of the stressful event (Horowitz, 1979a) and thus cannot process the event, leaving them open to intrusive thoughts about the event that, because of their overwhelming quality, lead them to avoid thinking about the event. Then there are therapists who make repeated transference interpretations in order to "resolve" the transference: The more transference interpretations they make, the further they heat up the patient–therapist relationship, and the more the transference blossoms. This last example is just a specific case of the more general situation where therapists attempt to solve problems and thereby create them. Strategic therapists are not exempt from this phenomenon, and occasionally "problem-solving therapies" can, by singling out problems, reinforce them. To the extent that strategic therapists see solutions in problems and problems in solutions, however, they often can utilize the very complaints clients bring in to effect change.

6. *Only a small change is necessary.* Because we can view problems as dependent upon a particular context that maintains them and gives them meaning, a small change in the problem can result in rapid change, if it alters the defining context. Because all aspects of the behavioral loop participate in the pattern or framing of experience, altering one part of the system will alter all parts. This is possible without insight and with minimal effort. Systems being complex, they react to a perturbation anywhere in the system in a way that can be disproportionate to the intensity of the change in the signal. For example, imagine a speaker addressing a postdinner gathering of sleepy people, gathered reluctantly to hear a political speech. If the speaker feels he can gain their attention only by being stimulating and intelligent, he could be at his work for a long time. Yet a single word would be enough to rouse everyone in the audience to their feet: "Fire!"

Small interventions can lead to large changes. Generally speaking, the challenge of strategic therapy is finding the smallest possible change, one acceptable to patients in their present world view, which will alter the context sufficiently to create the possibility for new behaviors that are consistent with the patient's current life goals.

Skeptics raise the issue of symptom substitution, but this does not generally arise. Because client's problems are not necessarily the expression of something "deeper," no new symptom need arise. If my car is misfiring, I often can adjust the timing, and my car will have lower fuel consumption, better acceleration, and so forth. There is no reason to necessarily posit a "deep" problem in my car requiring regrinding the valves, or that "merely" providing a tuneup will be a palliative that will result in some other serious malfunction occurring.

7. *Strategic therapy is brief therapy.* Problems need not be viewed as representing the outcome of "deeper" forces. In fact, the "deeper" psychological forces traditional theories posit often are dormitive principles, which repackage a description and call it an explanation. Systems theory, in contrast, allows us to focus on the problem at hand; this problem can often be seen as a function of a particular framing patients employ of their experience, which then leads patients to attempt solutions that deriving from the same frame as the problem, help to perpetuate the problem (Fisch *et al.*, 1982). Essentially, strategic therapists find patients' main difficulty is that in attempting to solve a problem, they keep doing "the same damn thing over and over" (De Shazer, 1985). This means that *any* change in what the patient is doing has the potential to create a set of new experiences that depotentiates the identified problem. Furthermore, after the initiation of a small change, strategic therapists tend to find that clients become involved in positive new life experiences that continue to promote further changes in an adaptive, positive feedback system.

Strategic therapists approach *every* session as if it were possible to create an appropriate context for change to occur. Because strategic therapists focus on the patient's actual behaviors, there is a rich field for possible interventions. It is extremely important for the therapist to begin each session, including the very first, with the expectation that it may be possible to solve the patient's problems within that session. Simply having the expectation for change creates a difference, within the therapeutic relationship, of how the problem is framed. Many clients come in to treatment with the expectation that their problem is due to some "inner badness" or that, because their previous efforts at solving the problem have failed, they are doomed to experience the problem for a long time. At the same time, paradoxically, even though patients may be pessimistic about change, research shows (Garfield, 1978) that most patients expect therapy to consist of only a few sessions, typically no more than six.

Clearly it will not be useful for the strategic therapist to simply reassure a client that change will be rapid: This fails to meet clients at their view of the world. Instead, the strategic therapist meet clients by offering a view that change is perhaps undesirable, that their pain and suffering are likely continue but *in a different form when* (not if) *the problem changes.* The therapist's attitude is that the nature of the change is unclear, and thus perhaps worrisome, but change is nonetheless inevitable and in fact is *already* happening, though the client may not have noticed yet. This is consistent with strategic therapy's roots in hypnosis. It is common, in hypnosis, to say to a patient, "I don't know if you've noticed yet how deeply you've begun to go into trance . . . how your rate of breathing is different now. . . " Here the hypnotist takes an inevitable phenomenon (the rate of respiration naturally fluctuates, so by calling attention to "a difference" in breathing the therapist takes advantage of something the patient will be experiencing), then punctuates it as a sign of something else (the beginning of trance), which ratifies and creates the phenomenon it purportedly is describing. Furthermore, use of the word *yet* allows patients the freedom to experience the new phenomenon any way they want but has a strongly implied suggestion that if they have not noticed up until now, they will in the future.

By coming in to see a therapist and by listening to a therapist's reframing, a change in the situation has already occurred, whether the client has acknowledged it or not. The strategic therapist does not structure the therapy to continue until change occurs because it has *already* occurred. Thus strategic therapists do not take long-term, open-ended approaches to therapy. Similarly, strategic therapists may not adopt a "time-limited" framework for therapy, in the sense of setting a contract with a client to work for a set number of sessions. Such a time-limited contract assumes the client cannot get better until the therapy is complete; clients may well wish to get better faster (although it is usually part and parcel of the strategic technique to paradoxically discourage this). The most common strategic treatment strategy is to set up a contract to meet until the problem is solved, or a maximum number of sessions is reached, whichever occurs sooner. This is similar to the Ericksonian hypnotherapist, who will say to a client: "I don't know whether you'll notice some change in the next few days, or it may take as long as a week or two." This is an illusion of alternatives, in which the occurrence of change is presumed, but the client is given the freedom to find *any* change he or she wants in the time he or she needs.

The hallmark of brief therapy is flexibility: Within the therapeutic system, as in any system, the most flexible member will have the most control (Keeney, 1983). Length of sessions can be varied to achieve maximum treatment impact: If an important point has been highlighted, it is useful to end the therapy session at that point, rather than let the message become diluted. Duration of therapy can also be flexible. It is not always necessary to set a contract with a specified number of sessions as a maximum. Sometimes, even a single therapy session will highlight what changes have already occurred or clarify what changes a client is clear about making.[1] It is then possible to suggest to clients that they go off and continue these changes at the pace they find appropriate and set up a follow-up appointment for some time in the future, often 4 to 6 weeks. Clients are informed they can cancel this appointment if they do not need it but should come to the appointment if they have run into difficulties from changing too much too fast or have encountered something different and unanticipated. This kind of contract can be quite valuable because, while presuming change, it gives the client the opportunity to not change or have troubles. From a systemic point of view, this depotentiates the pressure for forcing a solution that tends to maintain the problem. It is also possible to conceptualize this kind of termination from a psychodynamic viewpoint: By leaving the possibility of a return visit open, this approach bypasses resistances clients may feel about being abandoned or not being given enough. I have found that clients are less likely to return for further treatment about the presenting problem when they are given the option to return. Clients do sometimes come back with a different issue or problem, but then this is treated as requiring a whole new treatment contract. In this instance, it is important to clearly mark the previous therapy as terminated, in order to set off the work that follows.

Whatever method is employed, any strategic therapy needs a clear frame that defines the starting and stopping points. Such a frame highlights what changes have occurred, by demarcating a specified temporal interval in a client's life that then allows it to be assigned meaning. As in so much of strategic therapy, there is a kind of dialectic involved here: Because strategic therapists see life as an ongoing flow of constantly changing experience, it needs an artificial punctuation to allow a certain piece of it to become reorganized. Music must occur against a background of silence; symphonies are divided into movements, in order to give coherence to their parts. It is possible to approach clients' lives as "stories" or narratives (Strupp & Binder, 1984): Although we can never know the meaning of our actions and stories until our death (Arendt, 1978), which finally interrupts the flow of being, we can divide the novels of our lives into discrete chapters. Therapies must have ending points to give an opportunity to pretend we can stop changing and look back on what has occurred.

Clients' journeys are continuous as long as they live but must occur via a progression of discrete starts and stops. Some clients will make large changes, others small ones: Strategic therapists respect the right of clients to change as little or as much as works for them. The only option that is precluded for clients is that they cannot not change.

8. *Strategic therapists utilize whatever clients brings in order to help them make a*

---

[1]Single sessions of psychodynamic therapies can also have significant long-term effects (cf. Malan, Heath, Bacal, & Balfour, 1975; Hoyt, Rosenbaum, & Talmon, 1987; Bloom, 1981). Strategic therapists are, however, more likely than psychodynamic therapists to intentionally work within a single-session framework.

satisfactory life. The Lanktons phrase this more economically: They suggest therapists respect *all* messages from the client (Lankton & Lankton, 1983). This is
obviously related to meeting patients at their model of the world, but it goes
further and embraces whatever the client brings.

Most therapeutic schools would say that they respect their clients, but most
therapeutic schools also view certain behaviors or traits of their clients as pathological, something to be "gotten rid of." Implicitly, most therapists split their
client into the "good client"—the "healthy, cooperative, adaptively functioning
client"—and the "bad client"—the "neurotic, resistant, or symptomatic" part.
In doing so, therapists unconsciously make the same epistemological mistake
the client does. Clients generally come to us with a view that there are parts of
them that are "really" them and that they have other ego-dystonic symptomatic
parts that they disavow. As we have discussed, it is this dissociated view that, in
itself, can help create the client's problems, and to the extent the therapist goes
along with the client in this, he or she can help make the problematic behaviors
more entrenched.

Strategic therapists are much more radical in their respect for the client: *All*
the client's behaviors, including the resistant and symptomatic ones, are seen as
representing the best possible choice the client can make, given his or her
(necessarily distorted) perception of the world and the range of his or her
choices. Thus strategic therapists prefer, rather than take a symptom away, to
make it part of the solution. When strategic therapists utilize "paradoxical"
techniques, such as prescribing the symptom, they are not being manipulative,
but sincere; strategic therapists respect the symptom as providing something
useful the patient might continue to need. There are many techniques to utilize
symptoms (cf. Mazza, 1984), some of which will be described further on in this
chapter. It is worth noting here the profundity of the paradox: Acknowledging
the usefulness of the client's problems can make it easier to find alternative
choices for handling the issue the problem is currently solving.

Acknowledging the usefulness of the patient's problems is not a matter of
interpreting the "secondary gain" from a symptom but rather a question of
using the symptom to discover what a patient's needs are at this particular time.
Strategic therapists feel no need to eliminate "bad" client traits and replace them
with "good" ones. Strategic therapists try to never take anything away from a
client. Instead, strategic therapists will take whatever a client brings to them and
try to expand its utility. A widely cited (cf. Haley, 1973) classic example of this
was when Erickson encountered a schizophrenic who claimed to be Jesus Christ.
Rather than "cure" him of his delusion, Erickson instead said to him, "I assume
you've had experience as a carpenter?" and proceeded putting him to work
building a bookcase (Haley, 1973, p. 28). This was enough to allow the patient to
return to socially useful activity.

There is a certain delicacy required in positively reframing patients' problems. The therapist must not come across as flip or sarcastic; the appreciation of
the patients' problems must be real. Furthermore, to note the positive aspects of
the problem does not deny the real pain the patient may be experiencing with
the problem; generally, without empathically acknowledging the patient's pain,

positive reframings go unheeded at best or come out as insults at worst. At its best, though, the proper respect and utilization of the patient's problems leads to an alteration in the concept of resistance.

9. *Strategic therapists do not punctuate client actions with the concept of resistance.* By utilizing *everything* a client brings to them, strategic therapists tend to see all client behaviors as messages offering important information that provides corrective feedback to therapist interventions. In this light, the distinction between resistance and cooperation tends to drop out. If a client is given an assignment and comes back the next week not having done it, this is seen not as resistance but as the client's method of communicating something important. Perhaps the therapist gave an assignment that was too difficult, or perhaps was unsuccessful at meeting clients at their view of the world. Perhaps the therapist was not synchronized with the client's goals. Furthermore, if the client did perform the task, this sends a message about the patient's position in the therapeutic relationship (i.e., compliant), but there is nothing to say this patient's position is "better" than a noncompliant one; patients who let themselves be abused are often compliant with therapists.

The issue here is that patients cannot not communicate; *any* client behavior will have some significance. Furthermore, as noted meaning relies in part on how we draw distinctions and punctuate behavior. Although clients tend to be locked into assigning rather rigid meanings to events, strategic therapists have considerable flexibility. It is possible, for example, to positively connote all client behavior, framing it as cooperative (cf. De Shazer, 1984a,b). At that point, because there are no longer any distinctions being made along the cooperative/ noncooperative dimension, it is no longer meaningful to talk of resistance or compliance. This derives in part from the recursive, self-referential nature of the therapeutic system.

If a Cretan says to you, "All Cretans always lie," you cannot judge the truth value of that statement. If the Cretan is lying, he is telling the truth; if he is telling the truth, then he is lying. The meaning of the statement oscillates and shimmers. It is no longer useful to talk about the truth/falsehood value of the statement. In the same way, if the therapist structures the treatment situation so that cooperative behavior is cooperative and resistant behavior is cooperative and neutral behavior is cooperative, then it is rather like a painting of white on white: The distinction of "cooperative/resistant" loses its meaning. Instead, therapist and client can focus on the task at hand.

It is possible to frame the therapy situation this way because all people are constantly making distinctions that then create the realities we are attempting to label. Because this labeling can be done in a variety of ways, strategic therapists have the *choice* of whether or not to label client responses resistant. In keeping with the utilization approach that respects all client messages, strategic therapists choose not to view client actions as resistant in the usual meaning of the term. If you label a client resistant, he or she will be resistant, not just because the client will live up to your expectation, but because in looking for resistance you will find it. (It should be noted, though, that if a strategic therapist attempts to frame all client behaviors as cooperative, the client has the option of rejecting the therapist's labeling. In order for such a frame to be effective, the therapist must meet clients at their view of the world, using their language and ideas with a "hinge" or "pivot" still acceptable to clients that simultaneously alters the meaning ascribed to behaviors or symptoms.)

It is not necessary to remove resistance from the strategic therapist's lexicon. Indeed, if the goal is to teach clients assertive behavior, it is often useful to "find" resistance in compliant patients and praise them for it. Of course, there is then a paradox: Resistance leads the way to change.

Some systems therapists have argued that it is still necessary to deal with client resistance (Anderson & Stewart, 1983; Stewart & Anderson, 1984); others (De Shazer, 1984) have argued we should eliminate the concept of resistance entirely. I prefer to avoid such a dichotomy and see resistance as a matter of punctuation, where it is possible to view resistance as the twin sibling of change: No change occurs without resistance, and no resistance occurs without change. (Keeney, 1983; Rosenbaum, 1988). Each heralds and contains the other. Just as you cannot take a step forward without letting one of your feet go back behind the other, in the very act of backing off from a new behavior, you are anticipating and reacting to the new behavior, making it a part of you. Stopping implies starting; holding your breath implies letting it out. Strategic therapists view life as an ebb and flow of constant experience: just as you can arbitrarily start the nagging/withdrawing/nagging/withdrawing sequence anywhere in the chain, you can begin change and wait for resistance, or begin with resistance and then wait for change. If you punctuate the flow of experience with the idea of resistance, the other side of the punctuation is change. Resistance is not the opposite of change: Rather, change/resistance forms a pair, in which each member of the pair implies a linear direction. Whether it be forward or back, there will still be direction. If we want to find an opposite or complement to the linear framework of change/resistance, we would look to "continuous directionless being." This, in fact, is the framework the strategic therapist operates from: Knowing that life is a continuous flow of experience that neither changes nor stays the same until we punctuate it, the strategic therapist is then able to find a punctuation that makes a difference and introduces a new direction.

Once such a punctuation of experience is made, one thing is clear to the strategic therapist: *Something* will happen. Often, it seems that almost anything new in the symptomatic context will be enough to change the patient's experience (De Shazer, 1985). It turns out, though, that there are certain "differences that make a difference" (Bateson, 1972, 1979), and certain differences that do not make a difference. Determining what kind of difference will be effective is the task of the strategic therapist, and this leads us to the last distinguishing characteristic of strategic therapy.

10. *Strategic therapists tend to design a particular approach for each problem.* Milton Erickson stated that he made up a new theory and a new technique for each client (Lankton & Lankton, 1983). This follows directly from strategic therapists' desire to meet the patient at the patient's view of the world, in order to build on and expand that world view. This precludes devising a single global technique (free association, relaxation training, attending to thoughts, express-

ing affect, etc.) that would be suitable for all patients. Patients who are logical must have interventions that appeal to logic (but that usually incorporate "logically illogical" actions); patients who describe themselves as "sensitive" must have interventions where they are encouraged to "follow their feelings" (usually, by thinking about them). This crafting of intervention to client is what distinguishes strategic therapy from being a unitary "method" of treatment (Madanes, 1980).

Furthermore, strategic therapists see problems as patterns embedded in contexts that punctuate, describe, and maintain the problem. It is therefore essential to work with the specific context the patient brings in. We cited Erickson's asking a patient who thought he was Jesus Christ to help out with some carpentry work. This was effective, but if the patient had previously been a construction worker and developed his delusion after a conflict with his supervisor in which he had to adopt a submissive, self-sacrificing role, it is unlikely a "carpentry" intervention would work. In fact, this specific intervention would not work for most patients with that particular delusion; at a minimum, the patient would have to fit the following: (1) premorbidly had a strong work ethic, (2) work competence was not currently conflictual, and (3) had previous carpentry experience.

This may sound obvious when detailed in print, but the field of psychotherapy is sufficiently stressful so that therapists tend to look for "answers" and apply them indiscriminately. Therapists read a "cookbook," enthusiastically attempt to apply its techniques to all cases fitting the model, and find it works to varying extents. Gradually, enthusiasm wanes, and clinicians once again must confront the small details of real-life patients.

> One day in [Carl Whitaker's] office, a mother left her infant's bottle. When the next patient commented on it, Whitaker offered him the bottle. From then on, bottle feeding became an important technique . . . therapists were full of excitement, and so were the sessions. . . . For a while, it seemed that The Technique had been found. But with the passage of time, the excitement wore off. Patients and therapists became less enthusiastic, and ultimately bored. Finally milk became not a pathway, but plain milk. (Minuchin & Fishman, 1981, pp. 286–287)

The search for "formula" solutions is not simply a matter of anxious therapists seeking security blankets. Psychology as a whole has, since its inception, been confronted with the nomothetic/idiothetic problem. There is so much individual richness that the single case study, with interventions tailored for that specific individual, has tremendous appeal: On the other hand, there is a recognition that if we only have information about an individual, without finding some kind of classificatory schemata, it will be hard to organize a coherent theory and proceed in a classical scientific fashion. Notice that this is related to but not the same as "differential diagnosis." In differential diagnosis there is an attempt to classify patients according to a *typology* of some sort and match a class of treatments to a class of patients. How can we reconcile this with Erickson's objective of creating a new theory and technique for each patient?

Some strategic therapists have tried to bring a sort of nosology to the field. For example, Fisch *et al.* (1982) list types of patient positions the therapist must take into account and classify their major tactical interventions according to various schema (patient attempting to force something that can only occur spontaneously; attempting to master a feared event by postponing it; attempting to reach accord through opposition; attempting to attain compliance through voluntarism; confirming an accuser's suspicions by defending oneself). They also offer general rules of thumb that work well in a variety of situations. Jay Haley (1980, 1984) offers "leaving home" and "ordeal" therapies. De Shazer (1985) not only offers techniques for specific conditions ("read, write and burn" for ego-dystonic intrusive thoughts; structured fights for battling couples, etc.), but has also come up with the idea of "fit" for utilizing a variety of generic strategic interventions. In De Shazer's view, it is not necessary to match a technique to a specific condition; often any change in a recurrent pattern is sufficient, so that a merely adequate fit of intervention to problem will do. Rather than offering tailormade suits, he suggests clothes sized off the racks will fit adequately.

The attempt to provide some classificatory schemata and to provide generic techniques that go beyond the individual case are both laudatory as teaching tools. In my view, however, these attempts are problematical insofar as they go contrary to the basic spirit of strategic therapy. In my experience, these attempts to treat patients by reference to a kind of "strategic cookbook" often fail.

Most strategic therapists would agree that an important element of being strategic involves having a "map" of the therapy in mind, a sense of the layout of the problematical land, and a direction in which to go. Classificatory schema attempt to provide the beginnings of such maps. The problem with any nosology, however, is that it can be no more than the *outlines* of a map, one that perhaps shows the major roadways but leaves off the individual side streets. Each patient, however, lives in a house with a specific number, and which he or she has furnished in idiosyncratic ways.

In addition to the problem of the lack of detail in most nosological maps, there is a more serious problem that is inherent even in the most detailed of maps: the danger of mistaking the map for the territory (Bateson, 1979). There is a considerable gap from looking at a piece of paper with little grids, red squiggles, and street names, no matter how detailed the map may be, and translating it into the actual scenery you see in the car. As you drive along the actual territory, you discover some street signs are missing from corners; some streets have been renamed since the map was published; road work may be going on that requires detours, and straight lines often have bumps in them. Maps are fine as rules of thumb, but they do not substitute for the actual experience of navigating the land. Strategic therapy is essentially about a therapist taking responsibility for traversing a *unique* piece of land toward a *unique* goal.

There is nothing wrong with nosology and classification in and of itself. However, there is a real danger that users of nosology make an error of logical typing. A nosology specifies *classes*; a therapist, however, is with working with discrete entities. We can characterize a group accurately statistically, but the degree of fit an individual member has to the group picture can vary widely. Strategic therapists have been more than usually creative in their nosologies: They tend to depict patterns of interactions rather than reified disease entities.

However, it is quite possible for a patient's behavior to appear similar to a behavior that often fits a characteristic pattern, but in this case the pattern is not applicable.

The following case illustrates the need for adequate assessment in strategic therapy, in which not only the initial pattern is taken into account, but the individual details necessary for the "working-through" process:

L. R. came in complaining of problems of urinating in public restrooms. She desired to be able to urinate on demand. This would seem to fall into the Fisch *et al.* category of "attempting to force something that can only occur spontaneously"; the presumption is that the problem is one of overcontrol, where the very attempt to control shuts down the possibility of the desired behavior. "Be spontaneous" is the classic example of such situation. The usual tactic to apply is to jam the overcontrol aspects with some variant of instructing the patient to intentionally fail in the attempt at performance.

This tactic was used as part of the treatment package with L. R. It was not effective. On further examination, it turned out that L. R. had very mild cerebral palsy, undetectable in most interpersonal interactions, but sufficient to have left the patient with a self-image of being physically unable to adequately control herself. Intentionally failing merely reinforced her idea that there was something congenitally wrong with her. In addition, she felt resentful at her perceived disabilities: thus, the idea of intentionally retaining her urine for a time (which occasioned some minor physical sensation of pressure) left her feeling resentful at having to "suffer more pain." It eventually turned out that one of the major aspects of her symptom had to do with her embarrassment that someone in an adjoining stall would hear that she was not urinating and so be aware of her "lack of control." What turned out to be the effective intervention was to have her obtain a small squeeze bottle, go into toilet stalls and, without attempting to urinate, experiment squeezing out the fluid from the bottle to imitate the variety of urinary sounds (steady streams, dribbles, etc.). Having the control to sound any way she wanted, she then found herself progressively more able to use public restrooms. It turned out, however, that this was tied in to whether she would then have to enter the job market and also to whether she would have to go on her honeymoon, both of which had been postponed by the symptom, and both of which needed further discussion before the presenting problem was effectively resolved.

ASSESSMENT AND THE INITIAL INTERVIEW

The process of assessment in strategic therapy is not distinct from the treatment process; treatment and assessment are continuously ongoing. Treatment in all therapies may be successful within a single session (Bloom, 1981; Hoyt, Rosembaum, & Talmon, 1987), but strategic therapy takes this seriously, trying to make each session a complete treatment in and of itself. Most therapies segment the notion of "client," "client problem," "therapist," and "treatment" into discrete packages. The client is thought of as someone who has a distinctive identity that can be pointed to and described, and this identity persists outside of the treatment situation. In other words, most therapies subscribe to the idea that people have personalities: They carry their selves around with themselves.

In contrast, strategic therapy does not conceive of clients except as they exist in certain contexts. There is no "stable personality" except as it interacts with, is observed, and responded to, by other people. The very act of coming in to therapy creates a new entity, the client(s)–therapist(s)–identified problem system. The therapist is thus not in a situation where he or she must identify and evaluate a situation that exists objectively "in reality out there." Instead, the therapist is called upon to observe the interaction of the client with the therapist and to see what happens as each adjusts to the other. The traditional therapist adopts the position of a member of an audience watching a performance; the strategic therapist adopts a position of being a partner dancing with the client, constantly watching the steps the client makes, the responses of the client to the therapist's steps, and how they are moving in rhythm to the music of the presenting problem that draws them together.

Assessment is not directed toward describing an unchanging entity. Rather, assessment is geared toward participating in a constantly changing process. The only way to assess a system is to introduce a perturbation into the system and see how it responds. If our phone is broken, we do not assess it by peering at it: We examine it via a series of interactions, trying to dial out, by having people dial in, by running electrical current through it, and seeing what happens. Similarly, we assess clients by trying to "dial in" to them and asking them to call out to us.

We cannot approach patients as if they are one of those puzzles that ask us, "How many things can you find wrong in this picture?" Pictures are static, frozen: People are constantly moving and changing, even if only to remain the same. A patient is a tightrope walker on his or her symptom. From far below, the tightrope walker looks motionless, but when we get up close, we see the tightrope walker can only balance by making constant slight movements to one side and another; if he or she stands still for any length of time he or she risks falling.

Patients may be worried about falling off their symptom tightrope: They do not know where they will land. When patients come in to therapy, they have asked us to join them on the tightrope. Our job then is to walk with them and see how they adjust to us. As soon as we take a step onto the tightrope, we *inevitably* alter the tension in the rope, its motion, and stability; the patient must compensate in order to stay on the rope. Assessment in strategic therapy involves two main components: noticing the wider surrounding context that surrounds the tightrope, and observing what the patient does to maintain his or her balance on the symptom tightrope as we introduce perturbations. As far as the surrounding context goes, perhaps we will notice that the tightrope is poised only inches above firm ground; alternatively, we may notice the tightrope is stretched over quicksand, or over a long fall. Perhaps the tightrope walk involves a performance before an appreciative or critical audience; perhaps the tightrope has been stretched by the client, either as a bridge to a new location, or as a means of practicing balance. Perhaps the client is rather near the platform which terminates the tightrope; perhaps he or she is in the center. Perhaps we will ask the patient to look in a different direction. Meanwhile, we will observe how the patient responds to those of our moves that cause the tightrope to sway a bit. Perhaps the patient will balance faster: Perhaps he or she will grab onto the rope with his or her hands; perhaps he or she will attempt to grab onto us. We may twitch the rope slightly, join hands with the patient, or give a gentle push.

What this means, practically, is that the strategic therapist sees the therapy as a constant feedback situation, with client and therapist responding to each other's input from the moment the client makes the phone call. It is impossible to be an objective, outside observer of a system where you are a member of the system; we cannot hope to be a camera, simply recording data. We can, however, notice how our dance is going while we keep on dancing with our partner(s). We touch the patient, and then touch ourselves touching (Merleau-Ponty, 1964).

This is obviously a situation of considerable complexity. It would be easy to be paralyzed, and in fact the novice dancer sometimes goes onto the floor and does not know what to do. It is helpful, at such times, to know how to waltz and do a tango (the specific "techniques" described by strategic therapists). When in doubt, however, you can simply follow your partner, the client: learn his or her moves, then introduce a few of your own and see what happens.

The strategic therapist is guided by a view heuristic rules of thumb in the assessment/treatment process. First of all, the goal of the therapist is not to identify a problem and find a solution for a client. Rather, the goal is to set up a situation that allows for spontaneous goal attainment, rather like the hypnotist who directs the patient to voluntarily allow something involuntary to happen (Haley, 1973, pp. 21–22) (e.g., "prepare to let yourself be surprised"). The therapist may seed certain ideas, and then, seeing what direction the patient goes in, continue in that direction with the patient. (As in hypnosis: the therapist says, "I don't know if your arm will continue to float or will start to get heavier. . . ." and then monitors for patient movements; once the patient starts in a certain direction, the therapist expands on and develops the direction the patient takes.) De Shazer (1985) gives some suggestions for making the first interview effective. The therapist can look for something the client is already doing different and compliment him or her on that; or the therapist can suggest something new. The therapist will try to potentiate change by connecting the present up to the future, ignoring the past.

Meanwhile, it is important to focus in on the client's description of the problem and his or her past and current attempts to solve it. Because clients' problems are maintained by their attempts at solution, it is important to avoid suggesting a solution that the client or others have tried unsuccessfully, unless the previous attempted solution is modified in some way (Fisch et al., 1982). The therapist can always have clients perform more of their usual solution, or less of their solution, or modify it by performing it in a different context (a different place, a different time, etc.), or, of course, propose a completely different type of solution. The therapist is trying to avoid, at all costs, "more of the same damn thing over and over," and instead institute an environment in which *something* different is going to occur (De Shazer et al., 1986).

As the therapist assesses the focal problem, the therapist is making an inventory of the client's behavioral repertoire. The therapist is not looking for

client "strengths" and "weaknesses." Categorizing a client's repertoire of behaviors into this dichotomy creates pathology: It is more useful to look at each
behavior as having the seed of being useful in some situations and maladaptive
in others.

A couple came in, with the husband the identified patient. He complained of problems controlling his temper. His wife explained that when he became excited in conversations with their friends he would speak in a loud, stentorian voice which came across as
hostile and angry; it attracted attention, embarrassed her, and offended her sensibilities.
He would then become annoyed at her criticism of him in public but would not attack her
directly but would withdraw in sulky silences which would go on for a week. He stated
that in retrospect he could believe his wife and sympathize with her but got angry at
hearing others' "stupid opinions" although he wasn't aware he became so loud and
overbearing. I enquired whether the patient ever got hoarse or breathless after being loud
and was told no. I then explained to the patient how most people hurt their voices if they
talked over a certain volume, but that he had obviously acquired a natural ability at breath
control which allowed him to project his voice effectively. We discussed the diaphrag-
matic breathing which allowed him to maintain his volume, and converted that into
taking deep breaths when he felt the urge to become angry. At the same time, I complimented the patient on his ability to project his voice, as well as his lack of self-
consciousness, and commented it would make him a natural for theatrical performances.
This pleased the patient greatly. He was then open to the idea of practicing projecting his
voice and his breathing while doing dramatic soliloquies in their living room at home.
The wife could then be praised for her sensitivity and discrimination and was enlisted to
offer helpful critiques of her husband' home performances. The patient found he was
better able to participate in friendly discussions and acquired an interest in amateur
theatrics. The temper tantrums disappeared.

The therapist is looking for ways to reframe or repunctuate behavior while
exploring the presenting problem. The therapist is also looking for the exact
sequence of behaviors as well as the situational and interactional contexts in
which they occur. For example, in the preceding case, the husband's shouting
was defined as a problem in public places: Having him shout in private places
shifts the nature of the "problem" into something else. Furthermore, the problem shouting occurred in a context where the wife got to comment on and
critique the husband; it turned out she rarely did this otherwise, and removing
this opportunity would have upset the interpersonal balance. It was important
to find a way to allow the positive parts of the interpersonal process to be
maintained, in this case by making her a helpful, rather than a humiliated, critic.

The content of the behaviors is not so important as the context. Take the
following example and contrast it to the one immediately preceding it:

Another patient, a high-functioning professional, came in complaining of problems
controlling his temper. He stated in an analytical, controlled fashion that he would
frequently spout off while on the job, causing distress in those around him. He had done
this for many years, pretty much voluntarily, and essentially felt that it was productive to
be able to explode briefly and then go about his work refreshed. He did not often become
angry at home, however, because his wife reacted negatively. The immediate reason he

came in was that his wife considered the situation no longer tolerable. He had had an outburst of temper in a public place, his wife had become angry at him, feeling he was demeaning her; she had insisted he change his behavior or risk losing their relationship. He was also concerned that he did not have a good memory of the incident and worried his temper was getting out of control. An arrangement was made to see the couple on the subsequent session. In the meantime, since the client took pride in being able to exercise self-control, I suggested he keep a log of when he had temper outbursts at work so that he could "analyze his behavior and have even more control of it"; in the meantime, he was directed to not alter his behavior too much over the next week, so that we could study it properly.

The next week he came in with his wife, reporting that he had had no temper outbursts, as he did not want to have to go to the trouble of writing them down. He had spontaneously begun a number of stress reduction exercises and was feeling much calmer. He and his wife discussed their relationship, and how they would avoid getting into disagreements out of fear that an explosion would occur. If explosions did occur, he would get over his anger quickly, but she would seethe with cold anger for days. This precluded their resolving conflicts. An initial assignment to have intentional "small fights to let the steam off" was given.

At the next session, they had not tried having small fights, since they were still fearful of getting into a conflict they could not resolve. They had, however, decided that they were managing their relationship according to a 10-year-old, outdated agreement: that while the wife had previously been intimidated by husband's anger, she was "much tougher" now with higher self-esteem. During the session, it was clear each could appreciate and acknowledge the other's position, and have insight into their own foibles, as long as they talked directly to the therapist. When they talked to each other, they began getting defensive and angry. I complimented them on their ability to acknowledge each other and also on their courage on beginning a small fight within the session. I also complimented them on their wisdom of knowing what they were and were not ready to do in the way of assignments and suggested they not take too many risks too fast. I then suggested that they could try a "structured communication" exercise which would utilize their abilities to listen to each other; the exercise was designed to avoid fights and help them air their ideas in a cool fashion while preparing them to disagree constructively. They were to meet on a regular basis, at a regular time, flip a coin for who was to go first, and then have one of them speak for 10 minutes continuously without the other making any responses or rejoinders. Then the other would speak for 10 minutes without interruption. Then they would separate and go about their business.

At the next meeting, the husband reported he was still keeping his log with him but still had not had a temper outburst. He reported still more stress reduction methods he was using and described a variety of stressful events which would normally prod him to an outburst where he had instead gone to his office and done some effective breathing exercises. They had found the structured communication exercises useful, and when a serious topic of disagreement arose during the week they did not avoid it nor explode but to their surprise successfully negotiated it in a manner they had never previously been able to do in their marriage.

In both of the examples, the "presenting problem" appears initially the same: temper outbursts in a husband that are objected to by his wife. Different interventions were required, however, because the interactional context was quite different. In the first case, the wife felt embarrassed but did not feel demeaned or attacked; in the second case, the wife did. In the first case, the husband presented the volume of his anger as something that was unconscious and involuntary; in the second case, the husband saw it as an intentional, controlled coping mechanism that was now having unfortunate consequences. In the first case, the problem was confined to public settings, where an excess of interaction occurred; in the second case, the problem froze interaction in private settings and required some private rituals. These contextual elements are inseparable from the "main" presenting problem, which has no independent existence except in its defining context.

In order to find what avenues of change exist in a system, it is necessary first to decide what parts of the system you are going to work with. Strategic therapists vary somewhat in this regard. Because strategic therapy derives from a systemic viewpoint, some strategic therapists adopt a family therapy orientation and try, whenever possible, to meet with all people who interact together over a problem. This is most often the family but may include employers, schools, friends, neighbors, and so forth. In contrast, many strategic therapists will be more interested in working just with the complainant, that is, that person in a system who is stating that there is a problem (cf. Weakland *et al.*, 1974; Fisch *et al.*, 1982). There are advantages to both methods.

The reason for meeting only with the complainant is simple: The complainant is the person in the system most motivated for change. The complainant is thus more likely to be interested in coming to therapy and following directives, as long as any changes required of the complainant are justified as being overtly targeted toward altering the other person (the subject of the complaints). Altering the complainants's behavior introduces an element of surprise in a "stuck" system; this element of newness can be watered down if all participants discuss the problem and proposed interventions together. Furthermore, because problems are seen as a function of ongoing interactions *between* people, rather than *inside* a single person, the rationale is that changing the behavior of any member in a system is likely to result in changes in the behavior of other members of the system. Recent research has indicated (Wells & Giannetti, 1986) that doing systemic "family" therapy with a single person can be as efficacious as doing therapy with the entire family network.

Working with the entire system has the advantage of letting the therapist see the actual systemic transactions in process in the therapy, rather than rely on the complainant's report which will always *necessarily* omit or distort important information. More precise interventions may be tailor-crafted for a situation. Meeting with all the participants also grants the therapist greater control over the system's reaction to any changes in behavior initiated by one of its members; this increases the probability that it will be possible to protect a person who initiates a change from having an experience of failure, something that is generally to be avoided (unless failure is prescribed as an exercise).

The strategic therapist, ever flexible, is not bound to conform to one or the other of these models, and in fact may mix them within a single case. When mixing models, it is generally easier to start by meeting with larger groups of people and then focus down to meet with different subsets or individuals. If you do meet with one member of a system and then elect to meet with others, they may perceive an alliance between you and the original help seeker. It is necessary to take care then to join with the new members, usually by taking a "one-down" position; although strategic therapists do not believe in an "even-handed" approach and will want to make alliances with various family members and family subsystems, they want to be have the freedom to move into and out of these alliances freely, at their discretion.

Consider, for example, a family where the mother is distraught over her teenage son's failing grades. The boy's older sister is a model student who teases him about his "stupidity." Father remains aloof and unconcerned so long as the boy maintains an interest in athletics, and the boy himself couldn't care less about his school grades. The therapist may choose to meet only with the mother: perhaps she will be directed to compliment the boy on his thoughtfulness on failing his grades, since that will allow him to remain at home another year and the family can make use of his labor around the house. The therapist may choose to meet with the parents: the boy's "failures" may be redefined as "disobedience" and the parents instructed they should stop asking their son to voluntarily involve himself in school, but rather implement a series of behavioral consequences. Alternatively, the father may be asked to "distract" his wife from her son, and give her what her son never can, since he's going to grow up and leave soon, anyway. Or the therapist may meet with the whole family: the therapist may worry about the daughter's "lack of knowledge of how to enjoy life;" or the therapist might praise the son for bringing the family together; or the therapist might send the children out of the room "while we adults talk."

There are many possible interventions in the example; we cannot choose between them without knowing more specifics about the interactional context. How do we decide when to meet with whom? Prior to the first session, it is largely a matter of personal predilection and convenience. Notice, though, that as the number of people in the room goes up, the number of possible interventions goes up accordingly. Families are overrich in meanings and potential transactions. Just as strategic therapists generally like to make the smallest change possible to effect a resolution of the problem, so they often prefer to meet with the fewest people necessary. This is often more efficient and has the advantage of not burdening you and them with an overabundance of information and potential alternatives. I generally use the rule of "meeting people at their view of the world." For the first session, if there is an identified "couples" issue, I will suggest both members of the couple come in; for other issues I will meet with the complainant on his or her terms (if they want to come in alone, I will meet with them alone; if they want to bring others, and are successful at getting them to the session, I will meet with whoever comes).

By the end of the first session, a decision should usually be made on who to invite to the next session. This is determined as part of the assessment procedure, which focuses on the presenting problem but that attends to a variety of dimensions outlined next:

1. *What parties are involved in the transaction, and what is their mode of involvement?* The strategic therapist is rather like a journalist, in that he or she wants to

know who does exactly what with whom, as well as when and where they do it. The "why" is flexibly framed to aid in promoting solutions rather than maintaining problems.

In terms of who does what with whom, a person who is apparently peripheral or withdrawn may, in fact, be involved but in a different modality: A family member may never be seen yet in everyone's thoughts (i.e., "what would your grandfather think about this if he were around to see it"). Conversely, family members may spend large quantities of time in the same house but nearly never be in the same room. Someone who seems to be spending a good deal of time on the problem may not be much concerned about it. It is important to find out how much time various parties spend doing something about the problem, worrying about, or avoiding it.

The mode of interaction of the participants around a problem must also be determined. This is generally either symmetrical or complementary (Bateson, 1979, pp. 116–117). In symmetrical relationships, an increase in an action by Party A results in a corresponding increase in Party B's response. In complementary interactions, as Party A escalates Party B does less. The complementary/symmetrical quality refers not to the *content* of behavior, but to its pattern. Person A might nag, whenever Person B withdraws; this can involve either symmetrical or complementary patterns. If the sequence is symmetrical, more nagging by A will result in more withdrawal by B. If the sequence is complementary, more nagging by A will result in less withdrawal by B (or some different behavior by B, such as angry overinvolvement). Knowledge of who is involved and what pattern allows the therapist greater prediction over how interventions will affect the interaction.

A patient came in complaining she procrastinated too much. She was self-employed and each day, she said, she obsessed over how much time she was wasting. She got down on herself for putting things off until the last minute. An initial series of interventions aimed at dealing with the concerns about procrastination were only partly successful. Further enquiry showed that the patient rather enjoyed tinkering with her work to get it right: She did not become aware of "wasting time" until her husband would come home from his job and ask her what she had done during the day. She also would always meet her deadlines, but her husband, an ex-military man, expected her to adhere to a rigid schedule. He would object whenever she deviated from her usual daily schedule.

In this case, an "uninvolved" family member (i.e., the husband) formed a key part of the interaction. The patient, however, did not consider the marital interaction a problem and saw no point in having her husband come to sessions. It turned out that the patient responded well to hypnotherapy, but the symptoms did not remit when the focus was exclusively on self-directed behavior. The hypnotherapy became effective when multiple embedded metaphors were used in which there were *two* elements with different time frames (for example, one metaphor involved gardening "on schedule—mowing the lawn at set times" versus gardening "as needed—when the tulips need planting"; another metaphor involved writing music on commission for a certain occasion versus writing when inspired). The patient was able to discover a work rhythm which suited her but which was different from the one she had originally thought she "ought" to subscribe to.

2. *Patients' positions.* Patient position refers to a variety of issues: What meanings do the parties ascribe to their and others' actions? What position does the patient see him or herself occupying vis-à-vis the problem? Does the patient see himself as sick? as bad or evil? as a failure? as "self-actualizing?" as healthy, but earnestly concerned about another? Is the problem seen as a medical illness, a problem in living, a judgment from God?

What position does the patient(s) see him or herself occupying vis-à-vis the therapist? As a reluctant supplicant for the therapist's help? As an eager learner? Is the therapist a challenge to the patient's authority or competence? Is the therapist seen as an expert, or as a charlatan? The therapist must be able to understand the patient's position, because it defines the patient's view of the world, and the therapist must meet the patient at that view of the world. If a patient sees his or her problem as somatic, the strategic therapist will not waste time trying to convince the patient that it is "really" psychological but instead will talk "body talk" to the patient and frame an intervention around somatic issues. If the patient sees the problem as a punishment, the therapist will devise an atonement. If the patient sees the therapist as a competitor, the therapist will take a one-down position; if the patient needs an expert, the therapist can be expert.

In all of this, the task is not for the therapist to become a chameleon who *pretends* to adopt patient positions: Rather, the task is to find something in the patient's position the therapist can genuinely and authentically relate to and build on that bridge to the patient. For example, if the patient needs an expert, the therapist can be an expert "on problem solving" but need not pretend to be expert about the patient's life (the patient always remains the expert on that, whether he or she wants to or not). If a therapist needs to take a one-down position, there is always something to be genuinely humble about, without turning into a Uriah Heep. The task for therapists is to be big enough to acknowledge all the different parts of themselves—even the parts they do not like much—as potentially useful in certain contexts. Doing this, we model for our clients that their discounted parts, too—including their "problems"—may hold seeds of usefulness. Speaking the client's language, we attempt to extend a hand to him or her in the way he or she wants it extended. This flexibility is often confused, by critics, with manipulation. It is simply our way of showing our clients we care enough to meet them half-way.

As a subset of investigating patient positions, it is useful to determine who in the system is most concerned about solving the problem, as well as who is the most flexible member of the system. These two are rarely the same person. This is not quite the same thing as a straight assessment of who are the therapist's allies in the system, because often being concerned about a problem is different from working usefully to solve it. Nonetheless, it is useful to find out who is most likely to promote the "cause" of the therapy, if only because this often frees us to then work with other members of the system. In line with the fact that attempted solutions maintain problems, often the more concerned members are contributing to the problem, whereas the more peripheral members of a system have other resources that, uncommitted in the past, can be drawn upon in the present. The task of therapy is often figuring out how to get the flexible member of the system to aid the motivated member in a way the motivated member may not have anticipated but can still accept. It is rather like directing a bout of tag wrestling.

3. *What is the recursive sequence of behaviors in the problem, and what kinds of feedback maintain which behaviors?* This is often assessed by examining previously unsuccessful attempted solutions, seeing these as one step in a feedback cycle in which solutions and problems are intertwined. Another way of putting this is, in addition to assessing what a person's intent is (as manifested in attitudes and beliefs), we want to be sure to assess what the impact of the actions are which he or she uses to implement his or her intent. The mother who belittles her son for getting poor grades may intend to motivate him, but the impact of this may be to make schoolwork more aversive for the son, which will lead to more scoldings, and so forth. Rather than attend to good intentions, the cardinal rule for analyzing the sequence of behaviors is to just see it as a "black box" situation where the input and output are visible and subject to change, and what is "inside" the black box is irrelevant.

4. *What is the context in which the problem occurs?* As noted previously, it is not enough to specify a series of behaviors without placing them in their contextual setting. This has to do with ascertaining how frequently the problem occurs, under what circumstances, with which people, in what locations. Each of these contextual factors is a possible nodal point for change. The initiation and termination of a sequence of problem behaviors often is contextually determined: For examine, marital arguments often are initiated in automobiles and frequently are terminated if third parties enter the room.

5. *What will change in the patient's life* when *the problem is resolved?* By phrasing this as what will happen when, rather than if, the problem is solved, asking this question orients the client toward the future with a presupposition that change will occur. It helps the therapist to know what the client values, which will help the therapist frame interventions in the client's language, and also helps the therapist know what direction to head toward. Often, simply having clients think about where they are heading for is therapeutic, changing their mental set and initiating a hopeful unconscious search for pathways to their goal.

This question is *not* necessarily designed to elicit the "function" of the problem or the "secondary gain" it is providing to the system. Strategic therapists differ from systems therapists in that they are leery about talking of the function of a symptom. It is possible to frame the symptom as "serving a purpose for the system," but this is only one way among many of describing the interaction, and talking of symptomatic function runs the risk of getting you stuck in a perspective that emphasizes motivations, resistance to change, and potential problems on the horizon. For this reason, strategic therapists do not assume all symptoms serve a function. If you have a crack in a phonograph, so that the needle repeatedly goes over and over the same groove, it is possible to talk of how this "prevents" the record from playing further and reaching the next selection. Strategic therapists are more interested in jolting the player or lifting the arm so that the music may proceed. Alternatively, it is possible to listen again and again to the same section of a piece as a way of fully appreciating nuances of its aesthetic beauty. It is also possible to turn off the phonograph and turn on the radio.

This is not to say that strategic therapists do not attend to how symptoms fit into peoples' lives; strategic therapists are simply careful to consider the possibility that the symptom may not be serving a function. Sometimes a symptom may fill a role in an individual or family negotiating a stage in the family life cycle (Carter & McGoldrick, 1980), but sometimes a symptom may have been introduced by a chance fluctuation and gotten stuck as people put excessive unproductive energies into solving it. This is not to say the symptom does not have meaning to the recipients: People always ascribe meaning to their experience. The meanings people assign may, however, contribute to their difficulties: Calling something a "random glitch" is less likely to make a person feel stuck than calling it a "problem whose deeper meaning we will have to uncover." In the former case the therapist will assume, as described, that the people involved are making the best possible choices available to them. The symptom thus must be respected as accomplishing something valuable, and alternative avenues for accomplishing the relevant tasks must be created before removing the symptom. In the latter case, where there is more of a "random glitch" component, troubleshooting may proceed immediately.

Many therapists seem to have troubles with the idea that not all symptoms serve important functions in the family. It is important to realize that viewing all symptoms as functional can lead to serious errors. Imagine if you had an old car which began to stall out on you. You don't know it, but while driving along a country road, an insect flew into your carburetor and is blocking proper airflow. If you didn't know what was wrong, you might turn your engine over again and again, and in the process burn out the starter. Now the engine really has a problem starting up! If you took it to a mechanic who said, "Your car's pretty old, it's at a stage in its life-cycle where we're going to have to do an engine overhaul," you might be inclined to believe the mechanic and let yourself in for a lot of unnecessary expense. All this could have been avoided by simply removing the fly in the ointment.

What follow are two cases in which the presenting problem is similar. In the first case, the symptom did not appear to serve a functional purpose in the marital relationship; in the second case, the symptom did serve such a purpose.

A 30-year-old married man came to therapy because he had been having ego-dystonic intrusive homosexual thoughts.[2] These began shortly after a brief period of impotence in his sexual relations with his wife. The impotence appeared to have been caused by a recent physical illness and its treatment, from which he was not fully recovered. Behavioral sex therapy was successful in restoring his potency, but he continued to have some intrusive homosexual ideation, which he related to feeling that his impotency proved he wasn't a "real man." Marriage and family life were proceeding well, though his wife was beginning to get annoyed about his continuing insecurities. After eliciting his ideas about what constituted a real man, he was hypnotized. The patient enjoyed

[2]In both the following cases, homosexuality was explored as a possible positive choice, but the patient rejected this option.

fishing, and so the induction made use of his "good knowledge of how to use the reel and rod." A confusion technique was utilized which talked about movie actors, all of whom were "reel men" but not all of whom were "real men," while most men of course are not "reel men" but are "real men." I told him a true story about John Wayne visiting a Marine Corps hospital during World War II, in a ward of men who had been injured at Iwo Jima. These men had injuries, but were looking forward to recovery: Wayne appeared before them in his cowboy hat and boots, and struck a macho pose. One man, then another, then the entire hospital ward booed and hissed. These men knew how to tell who was a real man, and it wasn't something they had to talk about, think about, worry about, or prove to anybody, least of all themselves. After the hypnosis, the patient was told that as the finishing part of the sex therapy, he needed to go fish around a video store and get a reel of videotape with a "blue movie" that would be acceptable for his wife and he to watch together. The patient called back later and told how he had started laughing while watching the videotape at the "phoniness" of the actors and how much he enjoyed having his wife suggest they turn off the tape and make love for real rather than just watch it. The ego-dystonic homosexual thoughts did not return.

In another case, a 28-year-old married man came in to therapy because he had been having ego-dystonic intrusive homosexual thoughts. These began shortly after a brief period of impotence in his sexual relations with his wife. The exact precipitant of the impotence was not exactly clear; it appeared to coincide in time with his wife's becoming more withdrawn, perhaps as a reaction to illness in her family of origin and with the patient's father having a heart attack. Behavioral sex therapy was successful in restoring his potency, but he continued to have some intrusive homosexual ideation, which he related to feeling that his impotency proved he wasn't a "real man." He presented his marriage and family life as proceeding well, though his wife was beginning to get more withdrawn in reaction to his continuing insecurities. Initial interventions involved self-monitoring his symptoms; the patient was very compliant with the intervention, but it turned up no useful information nor did it suggest any interventions. The patient spontaneously offered detailed explicit memories of repeatedly hearing his parents in the "primal scene" and also discussed significant distressing dynamics in his family of origin involving accidental death of a sibling which his mother blamed on his father's negligence and used as a means to browbeat his father. Responding to the patient's apparent wishes, psychodynamic psychotherapy was instituted, which proved ineffective. The patient was extremely vague, passive, looking for guidance from the therapist and unable to respond to transference interpretations. After a while, further enquiry was made into the patient's relationship with his wife. It turned out the ego-dystonic homosexual thoughts increased inversely with the frequency of sexual intercourse with his wife. He felt angry that his wife never initiated sexual intercourse and left him to always make the first move. An intervention in which he refrained from initiating intercourse while attempting to covertly stimulate his wife sexually (undressing in her sight rather than in another room, stroking her and then wishing her good night, etc.) proved unsuccessful. It turned out patient and his wife had for some time avoided any kind of communication which could lead to disagreement. I hypothesized that the issue of whether to have children was looming and highly charged for each of them. Patient was told to simply point out babies to his wife when they went for walks together and comment on whether or not they looked cute. This led to the initiation of couples' therapy; an increase in direct marital communication led to the resolution of the ego-dystonic homosexual thoughts.

6. *Look for pivot chords.* The final part of the assessment process involves searching out where the potential "pivot chords" for change exist. In music, a

pivot chord makes it possible to modulate from one key to another. The pivot chord is ambiguous, containing notes which may appear in more than one key; the chord thus can imply several "directions" to the music. Music, like therapy, is a sequential process occurring in real time. If you approach a pivot chord from one key (say, C minor), the pivot chord will sound like it "belongs" to C minor; if the material following the pivot chord is in a close key relative, (say, C major), retrospectively the pivot chord will appear to "belong" to C major. The pivot chord facilitates the transition from one key to another.

The art of musical composition is not a matter of simply generating beautiful tunes but of linking them together in a way that makes sense. Similarly, the art of the strategic therapist is not just to come up with good "content" material (interventions, reframings, interpretations) but to link them to the client's current framework in a way that facilitates a transition to a new framework that makes sense to the client. The strategic therapist is looking to create just sufficient ambiguity and confusion regarding the meaning of a problematical behavior so that it can be used as a bridge to new behaviors.

This involves finding areas of flexibility or leverage in the system. Flexibility and leverage are two rather different things. Flexibility indicates a preexisting range of behaviors combined with an ability and willingness to shift between them. Assessing this resource involves finding out which members of the system have tried or at least thought about a variety of responses to the problem and which are committed to a particular path. Investigating for leverage, on the other hand, involves discovering precisely those values and attitudes held most dear by the client(s) that they are likely to dig in their heels on, and how to use this intransigence as a motivation for change.

For example: A young woman in her mid-20s came in to therapy complaining of irrational jealousy directed toward her husband. Sobbing, she related how whenever he went away from the home, she was tormented by thoughts that he was having an affair. He had given her absolutely no cause to mistrust him, but his reassurances to her were in vain. She felt she was not worthwhile enough to keep him interested and occupied and regretted that he spent so much time at home with her. In fact, it turned out husband had very few outside interests, and it was hard to motivate him to leave the home for recreational activities. She worried constantly, however, that her irrational fears and insecurities would alienate her husband; he would abandon her and their 1-year-old son. If given the chance to be alone, without her, he would cheat on her. She had tried a number of solutions to the problem: putting the "bad, jealous" thoughts out of her mind; reassuring herself about her husband's fidelity; calling him up to check on him at work; avoiding calling him up to give him some "space"; encouraging him to go out with male friends. This last solution worked best, clearing up her symptom for several days at a time.

This woman showed considerable flexibility in her attempts at solutions. She also showed flexibility in adjusting to her role as a new mother and learning how to take care of her infant in a way that showed good parenting. She felt very strongly, however, that (a) she was worthless, (b) being loved and loving were vital to existence, and (c) an intact nuclear family was highly prized.

There were a number of potential pivot chords. The patient's jealousy was redefined as consuming romantic love, the kind found usually in novels and movies, and only rarely in real life. I worried about the husband getting depressed if the patient stopped showing so much love for him, especially since he had so little else to occupy him. The husband's staying home became the essential pivot: It was defined as part of the problem, and the patient's worries about what would happen if the husband went out redirected to worries about what would happen if he stayed home. If he stayed home, she wouldn't be able to be constantly interesting to him; constant exposure to something satiates anybody's appetite. Attraction needed some mystery: "Absence makes the heart grow fonder." The patient might feel worthless (thus accepting rather than challenging her view of herself) but, being worthless, it was especially important that she "demonstrate her love" for her husband by "sacrificing herself" and taking an art class at the local community college (art being an area in which she had previously shown talent and interest). I told her this would make her more interesting to her spouse; also, leaving her husband alone at home with the baby while she went out and took art classes (something she hesitated to do, fearing he would use the opportunity for an affair) might be risky, but was the only way I could think of to cement the father's ties with his son.

Thus all the interventions were used to create a pivot whereby the husband being alone, without her, became a desirable or necessary state rather than a feared one. At the same time, she was given a task calculated to increase her self-esteem. Other interventions (not described here) were used to decrease the negative interactions between her husband and herself. The interventions resulted in considerable symptomatic reduction. Over time, the husband became rather bored staying at home. The couple decided to take a parenting class together, met some other couples, developed a support network and a group of friends that each of them could spend time with apart from the other.

INTERVENTIONS AND THE PROCESS OF THERAPY

I have indicated how the basic process of strategic therapy involves a continuous feedback system. The therapist does not "do" an intervention "to" a patient. Rather, the therapist joins with the patient on a tour of the patient's house. During the tour, the therapist discovers doorways that have always been there but that may have been overlooked before; on opening the doors, each turns out to have several corridors. The therapist notes the patient's choice of pathways and accompanies them until they arrive at a mutually agreed upon destination. Throughout the tour, the therapist is guided by the patient as much as (or perhaps more than) the patient is guided by the therapist. It is the therapist's responsibility to set up situations that facilitate the patient's search for new directions and choices, and the therapist does this by

> responding to the patient's responses
> to the therapist's responses
> to the patient's responses
> to the therapist's responses
> to the patient's responses
> to the therapist's responses
> to the patient's responses
> to the therapist's responses
> to the patient's responses
> to the therapist's responses
> to the patient's responses
> to the therapist's responses

until a resolution of the problem is reached.

The therapeutic relationship in strategic therapy is a cooperative one (De Shazer, 1984a, 1985). This sometimes surprises people who think of strategic therapy as "manipulative." The fact is that any therapy, to be successful, must proceed from a positive therapeutic alliance (e.g., Frieswyk *et al.*, 1986; Lansford, 1986). The psychodynamic literature has noted that the therapeutic alliance is based, in part, on the real relationship with the therapist (Greenson, 1981a–c). Strategic therapy differs from other therapies in that it enlarges the scope of how to form a therapeutic alliance. In traditional psychodynamic therapies, the real relationship is distinguished from the transference. Strategic therapists do not choose to punctuate the therapeutic relationship in such a dichotomous fashion. Any patient will of course come to therapy with a variety of attitudes; they will have mixed feelings about being in therapy, about seeing the therapist as an authority figure, a fool, a parent. The strategic therapist does not ask the question: Which of these feelings are real and which are transference? All these feelings are "real," in that we construct (i.e., punctuate and frame) their reality at will. The strategic therapist accepts all of these offered potentialities for relationship and asks: Which of these forms a basis for connecting helpfully with the patient? The task is to find out not whether the client is cooperative or noncooperative, but *how* to be cooperative with the client. Erickson used to say he could only hypnotize somebody who would cooperate, but he could virtually always find some part of the person to be cooperative with (Lankton & Lankton, 1983).

The point here is that, as in any therapy, the therapeutic relationship is the vehicle for any interventions that occur. Therapy involves a minimum of two people: it is not possible to not have a relationship. Strategic therapists, however, do not *interpret* the relationship but rather *utilize* it as a vehicle for change. Simply having another human being take the time to try to be helpful to you can be therapeutic; if a therapist needs to employ paradoxical techniques, and thus be seemingly unhelpful, it is always within the larger framework of attempting to be helpful. Strategic therapists may be tricksters, but they are human beings first.

Having acknowledged the importance of relationship, the strategic therapist is not content to *just* utilize the therapeutic relationship for a "corrective emotional experience." Within the frame of the relationship, it is necessary to find interventions that will mobilize change in the patient's actual life. These interventions must (1) fit with the patient's view of the world, so the patient will be able to understand and utilize them; (2) differ from the patient's view of the world, so as to create the opportunity for change; (3) offer a novel approach that fits with the patient's defined problem; and (4) fit within the context of the therapeutic relationship. (Patients vary in terms of what they see as the therapist's prerogative to offer suggestions and advice in various areas, and the therapist must respect this. For example, a patient is unlikely to respond to a therapist who intervenes by proposing that the client buy or sell certain of their stock investments: This would not be seen as falling within the therapist's purview.)

It may seem difficult to come up with interventions that meet these criteria. Notice, however, that the requirement is that the therapist come up with an intervention that is an adequate *fit;* the therapist need not come up with an exact *match* (De Shazer, 1985). The closer the match, the better, of course, but we expect clients to alter our interventions to suit their needs. We merely need to give them some new "hook" which provides some impetus to a new direction. As I mentioned earlier, I am not a proponent of the "cookbook" school of strategic therapy, and I rather doubt that any strategic therapist goes by "formula" interventions. There are, however, some rough guidelines and rules of thumb which can be useful, which I will list below.

1. *Expect change.* As noted repeatedly, change is not only possible but inevitable. The strategic therapist takes advantage of this by taking a "present and future" stance (De Shazer, 1985): What is the patient already doing that leads him or her in new directions?

There are multiple ways of perpetuating the expectation of change. In virtually every initial interview, the therapist will want to ask "what will your life be like *when* this problem is resolved?" The strategic therapist can look for "exceptions to the rule" by enquiring into those times the symptom does not occur (since no symptoms ever occurs continuously, 24 hours a day, without ceasing), or by enquiring about what is occurring when the symptom lessens. De Shazer (1985) has a particularly elegant technique he calls the "crystal ball technique," in which he has patients imagine themselves at a future session telling the therapist how they solved the problem. The strategic therapist can take *any* new behavior—even one seemingly unrelated to the symptom—and label it as a harbinger of change. Perhaps the therapist will ask what actions the patient intends to take *first;* or the therapist will ask what the patient intends to do *before* changing: Both phrases presume change will occur. The therapist can ask the patient to pay attention, in the time between the current and the next session, to what he or she is doing that is helpful and which they wish to continue doing. When the therapist does enquire into the past, it is to search out past successes and link them to the present.

A couple came to therapy who complained about coldness in their relationship. They avoided arguing, fearing it would turn into a big blowup. They were both afraid that if things got "hot," they'd never recover. During the session, I had them discuss a small issue they had a minor disagreement about. Sure enough, the emotional level escalated. They attempted to avoid further confrontation, but I had them continue past their usual point; the emotional level escalated further and then, as you could predict, they engaged in their predicable avoidance behavior. After letting the conversation wander offsubject for a few minutes, I asked whether things had gotten "hot": Both confirmed they had. I asked them if they felt "hot" now: Both did not. I then congratulated them on their ability to cool things off. The couple looked surprised ad pleased and were more willing to work on direct communication with each other from then on. This was a simple case of punctuating the behavior at an appropriate point. This technique of enactment of the presenting problem to achieve intensity, followed by punctuation of it at a successful point, has been described well by Minuchin and Fishman (1981).

2. *Make the smallest change possible.* The rationale behind this technique is self-evident: Patients will be more willing to make changes that do not sound too difficult. Any change, of course, has the potential to grow into a powerful force:

The patient will allow the change to grow just enough so that it works. If you plant a few wildflower seeds in a plot, from two or three seeds you soon get quite a few pretty flowers. If the flowers start taking over your yard, you can always cut them back. "Seeding ideas" is a hypnotic technique in which you sprinkle small intimations of a suggestion or image throughout the initial portion of an induction, preparing to build on these seeds later in the trance. Here, for example, is a portion of a trance induction I use to aid pregnant women anticipating childbirth.

. . . trance gives birth to comfortable new sensations you can experience with pleasure . . . for you can let your inner mind contract and expand the focus of your attention to whatever is most useful for you . . . for example, you can notice any part you want to of your breathing . . . you can notice how your chest expands, or how your diaphragm contracts . . . or how your lungs contract or your diaphragm expands . . . or how your diaphragm expands and contracts . . . expanding your awareness to the contraction of your chest or contracting your awareness to the expansion of your lungs. . . .

The use of the words *contraction* and *expansion* provides seeds for later suggestions about comfortable contractions accompanying expansion of the birth canal.

Although it is possible to devise new behaviors that are small enough to be navigable by patients, it is generally preferable to build on behaviors people are already manifesting. Behaviorists talk about behavioral shaping: Systems therapists talk about "amplifying a deviation." The principle tends to be the same: Find an already existing response, utilize, and reinforce it.

K. M., a passive, unassertive, quite depressed client complained that whenever she thought of doing things for herself or enjoying herself, she felt guilty; she was also scared to attempt any assertive behavior for fear of failure. She came in one day and told me she still couldn't imagine herself acting assertively, but she did have an image of what she'd be like if she did improve. She could see herself on a mountaintop. I asked for more detail, and she was able to describe the colors of the sky, and a yellow flag waving in the breeze. I suggested that she buy a yellow scarf and keep it out of sight in her purse; she shouldn't actually wear it "until she was ready." The next session, she had complied with the suggestion: She was markedly less depressed and had even begun enjoying a few activities.

3. *Reframing the problem.* I have talked about reframing rather extensively so will only deal briefly with it here. Generally speaking, reframing tries to find the positive aspects of what the client sees as an exclusively bad situation, but the task of the therapist is not to impose "positive thinking" on the patient, but rather, while acknowledging the problem, to reconstruct it in a way that makes it more solvable by the client. Perhaps the most common example of this is working with families complaining of the behavior of one of their children. Often, they will label the acting-out child *bad.* Now, it is not possible for therapists or parents to make children bad or good, which is something having to do with the inner soul: That is a matter for priests, theologians, and philosophers. If the

therapist reframes the child as *disobedient* rather than *bad*, it becomes easier for the parents to develop solutions.

The task for any kind of reframing, of course, is to simultaneously meet clients at their view of the world, so they feel understood and validated, while at the same time offering a new perspective. *Notice that the therapist's task here is isomorphic to the patient's.* Patients generally come in because they can only see one side of a situation: they are either healthy OR well; assertive OR passive; successful OR a failure. In reality, all people have a multitude of competing qualities present all the time. The therapist's task is to substitute a "both-and" orientation for the "either-or" orientation. Thus therapists must struggle against adopting an "either-or" attitude themselves: "pathological patient attitude OR healthy therapist attitude." The patient's world view is pathological AND healthy: The therapist's world view is healthy AND pathological. All therapies face the challenge of joining and empathizing with the patient's attitude while trying to change it: To my mind, the value of strategic reframing is that it accomplishes the shift in perspective without blaming the client, as psycho-dynamic interpretations often implicitly do (Wile, 1984) or convincing the patient they are a passive product of what they have learned in past experiences, as behaviorists sometimes imply (Wolpe, 1973).

There are many varieties of strategic reframing, ranging from positive connotation (Selvini-Palazzoli *et al.*, 1978) to "splitting the symptom" (Lankton & Lankton, 1983) (i.e., having the patient refocus attention to an unattended portion of the symptom. For example, a patient with panic attacks might be told to "continue, if you must, to experience your rapid heart rate, but notice at the same time the tremendous surge of energy you suddenly have available"). Reframing can, however, be considerably simpler. The therapist wants to initiate some element of doubt in the patient's world view without denying or confronting it. Raising your eyebrows while maintaining a sympathetic facial expression is a type of reframing.

4. *Direct techniques.* These involve virtually anything you ask a patient to do directly, and they can involve any technique from any school of psychotherapy: asking phobic patients to accompany you *in vivo* to their phobia; asking a patient to do relaxation exercises; suggesting a husband buy his wife flowers; requesting a patient to draw a picture of his problem; asking a patient to talk to her mother in the empty chair. Strategic therapists will use whatever seems useful, but there are a few categories of techniques that are especially heavily employed:

Get the patient to do something unpredictable or anything new. I've emphasized the importance of this repeatedly. You may start by having a patient do more of what he or she is already doing, or less of what he or she is already doing, but this often is not effective except insofar as it convinces them they have to try something new. When they do try something new, virtually *anything* will do for a starter; a good rule of thumb is to try something that is a 180° turn from their usual solution.

One patient (K. M.) was having trouble with her teenage children. Whenever she made requests of them to do some chore or attempted to impose some limits, they would ask her why, and (attempting to avoid being overly strict as her own mother had been), the patient would provide elaborate reasons. Her children then engaged her in long discussions as to the validity of her reasons, which then led her to become angry and erratically severe in her punishments. Clearly, this patient's children were able to predict her behavior overmuch. I suggested that she become more unpredictable by becoming more mysterious. I did not think she would be able to set limits by fiat and thought she would need to tell her children something. I suggested she use the opportunity to not only set limits but to sharpen her children's thinking skills. The patient was to memorize several pages of pithy but obscure proverbs, Sufi stories, and Zen parables. When her children asked her for reasons, she would choose the first proverb or story she could remember and tell it to the children, leaving them to figure it out. The children soon got tired of asking her for her reasons.

Restructuring the symptomatic experience via symptom prescription. This is a favorite strategic therapy tool, encompassing a variety of techniques in which there is no attempt to eliminate the symptom but where the symptom is placed in a different context that thereby alters its meanings. The simplest form of this is to prescribe the symptom, asking the patient to practice the symptom at set times "in order to get it under control" or "in order to learn more about it." Symptom prescription is sometimes regarded as a paradoxical intervention because there is no attempt to eliminate the symptom. This misses the true meaning of paradox, which, as we shall see, is always based on an interpersonal relationship. Symptom prescription is a direct technique because it is embedded in a direct use of the therapeutic relationship: The therapist suggests this to the patient, and the patient does it. (Suggesting to an oppositional patient that he or she needs to continue to have his or her symptom, in hopes that he or she will defy you by dropping the symptom, is a true paradoxical technique but it is not symptom prescription.)

Symptom prescription is a powerful technique, which I have found especially useful with nonpsychologically minded patients who have psychogenic somatic complaints. In general, it is useful where the patient(s) complain of some ego-dystonic symptom that feels out of voluntary control. Symptom prescriptions (1) alter the context of the symptom (i.e., by making the symptom occur at a particular place or at a particular time, where it has not occurred before), and (2) ask for voluntary production of a previously involuntary response (similar to the production of hypnotic trance). Symptom prescriptions can also involve *negative practice* (the behavioral term) of specific problems:

A patient came in complaining of "strange feelings in her tongue" that she had had for several years. She was upset that her physicians, on finding nothing wrong, had told her she was "hysterical." After empathizing and assuring her I believed she was quite discomforted by the symptom, I enquired exhaustively about specific details of the symptom, asking her several questions she was unable to answer. In order to learn more about the symptom, she was to sit down for 15 minutes each morning and night and attempt to bring on the symptom by pressing her tongue against her teeth, wiggling the tongue, tensing her jaw, etc. When she returned the next week there was a substantial diminution of symptoms. She realized the symptom was often associated with muscle tension in her neck and shoulders: Relaxation exercises were sufficient to cure the problem.

Notice that in this example there was no need to enquire into the *function* of the symptom.

Other examples of symptom prescription include De Shazer's (1985) "write, read, and burn" technique for ego-dystonic thoughts and a variety of structured fights for battling couples.

In a couples' communication group that I co-lead, we regularly do a didactic class where we describe positive and negative communication skills, then suggest that before the next class either member of the couple can "make up at least one fight each" in which he or she uses the negative communications "so that they can learn to recognize them," while the other member of the couple tries to guess whether the fight is real or sincere. This ordinarily interrupts the usual sequence of behavior and results in a decrease in fights.

We also discuss the value of having fights in different contexts. In a recent couples' class, one couple came up with the idea of having their fights only in bed, naked, regardless of the time of day. Another couple decided to have their fights only in the shower. Both these couples had initially seemed rigid and intractable in the early group sessions; when they returned the following week, they were teasing each other, laughing about how they had enjoyed their "fights."

Notice how in the example I have put the word *fights* in quotation marks. This is what symptom prescription does: It allows the patient to put the symptom in quotation marks and thus changes it to an "as-if" symptom.

Providing a worse alternative. This is a direct technique that can often set up a therapeutic double bind. Jay Haley (1984) has been instrumental in describing uses of this technique, which he sometimes refers to as "ordeal therapy," and which he first encountered in Erickson's work. Although there are considerable subtleties to the technique, essentially this technique makes maintaining the symptom more distasteful than giving it up. It is especially useful in cases where clients maintain they want to make a change but "just don't have the willpower" to do it. Thus, for example, a patient may be willing to contract to perform a certain task but is uncertain about carrying it out. The therapist might have the patient write out a check for a painful sum to a cause the client detests (for example, a Jewish client might make out a check to the Palestine Liberation Organization) and then contract with the patient to mail the check if the client does not perform the desired task and to rip it up if the client does perform as he or she wishes. This might sound simplistic, but it is rather impressive how effective it can be.

Personally, I do not often use this technique because the external locus of control is rather too severe for my taste. I will use the task somewhat differently; because I sincerely do wish my clients to consider the disadvantages involved in changing, if patients are insisting they want to alter a problem and are unwilling to respond at all to my worrying about their changing too fast or too much, I will sometimes pose an ordeal to help the client cool any excessive ardor to change.

I much prefer "providing a worse alternative" when the worse alternative to the symptom is at least potentially in the patient's best interest. That is, I prefer to create a situation where if the patient changes, he or she will feel better, and if he or she does not change and have to perform the assigned task, he or she will feel better. This kind of therapeutic double bind can be difficult to construct on a spur of the moment but results in dramatic improvements when designed properly.

One day all the participants in our crisis drop-in group happened to be women, and the talk centered around how these women had been taken advantage of by men. They discussed how important it was to be assertive. One woman in particular had been severely abused by the men in her life, from the time she was a child. She was currently in a physically abusive relationship. Often her husband would leave her for other women, then return without apology; she would let him back to abuse her more. Normally silent, in this session she burst out, exclaiming that it was easy to say you should be assertive, but how do you do it? Various group members tried to give her advice, but she rejected all of it, insisting she "just couldn't" stand up for herself. I told her that she could learn to stand up for herself by simply stating, out loud, "I am going to do everything in my power to not let myself be taken advantage of or abused again." She again stated she "just couldn't." I persisted, and she still "just couldn't." I then pressured and badgered her, asking her again and again to make the statement, "or you can tell me assertively to stop pressuring you and you'll do this in your own time and way." As I repeated this message time and again to her—"say you won't let yourself be abused, or tell me to stop"—she became quite upset. I persisted; finally she told me in a firm voice to stop badgering her.

The next session she came in and told the group that her abusive husband (who had left her recently) had told her he was moving back in, but she told him she wouldn't allow it—the first time in her life she had stood up to a man.

In this example, the patient was placed in a therapeutic double bind. If she made a statement she would no longer stand for being abused by men, she would start to change. If she told me to stop pressuring/abusing her, she would already be standing up for herself. This experience was sufficient to help her begin major changes in her life.

Another patient (K. M.) complained she just couldn't allow herself to enjoy anything without feeling guilty. She couldn't ask for anything for herself; she certainly couldn't ask her family for a half hour now and then to use as she wanted. Whenever she tried anything new, she told herself she was doing it wrong. She also complained that while she knew her husband was well intentioned, she just couldn't allow herself to get intimate with him, because then he would "want more and more from me." She felt controlled by others, especially by her family, and simultaneously resented feeling controlled and told herself she was bad for feeling angry. She had been in an unsuccessful insight-oriented interpretive psychotherapy for 4 years. I gave her the following task:

1. Go home tonight, plan out seven different activities between now and the next time we meet which will let you enjoy yourself or be happy for at least 5 minutes but not more than half hour each time.

2. Since the purpose of this exercise is to learn to tolerate failure, it would be best to choose at least a few things which won't work.
3. When you fail to enjoy yourself, rather than get down on yourself, you should spend 15 minutes (but no more than that) with your husband doing something to help him enjoy himself. (Don't tell him why you're spending the extra time with him).
4. If you can figure out some other way of learning to tolerate and REALLY ACCEPT your failings without getting depressed or mad, you can do that instead of #3.

The patient responded angrily, stating "this is enforced intimacy." She came back the following week and after complaining of feeling I was coercing her and threatening to abandon her if she didn't follow directions, she reported that for the first time in her life she had had an "image of freedom" (the picture of herself on a mountaintop, described previously). She reported that after the last session, she was so mad she left her house, went out, used her "angry energy" to buy a tape, dance with daughter, "act crazy"— and—to her surprise—enjoy herself. She continued the exercise over the week, and found (1) if you try too hard, you don't enjoy yourself (this from a woman who had always equated pushing herself with "being good" and not trying hard with "being bad"), (2) you have to take one day at a time, (3) she realized she had a tendency to disqualify the positive things she does, and (4) when she didn't enjoy herself and did things for her husband, it wasn't so bad after all.

The "worse alternative" in this case was spending time with her husband; however, since her husband sounded reasonably well-intentioned toward her, time-limited positive actions by her toward him would probably result in a positive feedback loop which would reinforce her ability to get close to him and then withdraw. There was a double bind, in that since she was instructed to fail sometimes, failing would become success and success "failure," and the whole either/or dichotomy of "fail or succeed" would be short circuited.

Indirect Interventions. Strategic therapy is usually associated with indirect interventions. I have not emphasized them here, because although the indirect interventions are "flashy" and distinctive, they do not define strategic therapy. Strategic therapy is distinguished, rather, by its propensity for flexibly utilizing whatever is most likely to serve the client's best interests. Generally speaking, I will use standard, direct interventions first of all, and turn to indirect interventions only when direct ones are stymied. Even direct interventions, however, are often "packaged" in an indirect fashion.

Psychotherapy often makes use of suggestion in a process of interpersonal influence (Frank, 1973). As noted at the beginning of this chapter, strategic therapists often make use of indirect suggestion in a manner similar to Ericksonian hypnosis, to minimize the likelihood that a client will feel a need to "resist" the suggestion. The use of indirect suggestion is described well in a variety of places (cf. Lankton & Lankton, 1983; Erickson et al., 1976). In general, indirect suggestions tend to be more open ended, covering a variety of possibilities that define a field of positive choices for a client. If you suggest to a client that he or she may, next week, start by discussing what things he or she did differently that he or she wants to continue doing (De Shazer, 1985), this focuses the client's attention away from hopelessness about the problem and onto what is changing, but it leaves the choices of changes up to the client.

A strategic therapist will not say "why don't you try, then, doing some relaxation exercises between now and next time?" because such a statement asks the patient to find reasons to explain why he or she *won't* try doing the exercises. Instead, the therapist might ask, "do you think you'll start learning relaxation by noticing your breathing sometime [thus stating an almost-inevitable occurrence], or will you begin with some scheduled muscle tensing and relaxing exercises?" This phrasing of a "direct" intervention (i.e., starting relaxation exercises) in an "indirect" fashion (i.e., it does not *tell* the patient "do this" but rather asks the patient how he or she wants to do it) offers an illusion of alternatives, either one of which presumes the patient will begin relaxing in his or her own way, at his or her own time. It should be noted that for this "indirect directness" to be effective, the therapist must first have assured a cooperative relationship with the client.

When the relationship with the client is less than fully cooperative, more indirect methods may be useful. Clients often are *attached* to their problems: Their problems are what they know and constitute part of their self-identity. Being too optimistic or too quick to change can be disrespectful to clients, denying their misery and the actuality of their present existence. In such situations, clients often will overtly agree with the therapist's efforts at change while holding back a part of themselves. At such times, it is often useful to communicate in metaphor (Lankton & Lankton, 1983).

Communicating in metaphors has numerous advantages. First of all, metaphors typically have multiple levels of meaning, and clients are given the freedom to choose what meanings are most suitable for them at the present time. This potentiates the client's own search for solutions, rather than imposing them from without. Second, metaphors are excellent for engaging a client's attention because they always begin by matching a client's current experience, but in a novel, somewhat puzzling format. Because the metaphor is isomorphic to the client's experience of the world, it empathically acknowledges his or her sufferings, hopes, and dreams. Once having ratified the client's experience, however, metaphor allows an opportunity for altering the experience; because the metaphor is presented in a different format, it is already a "same but different" framing of the problem that allows for experimentation with creative solutions. A metaphor thus acts as a therapeutic pivot chord. Finally, metaphors create intensity in the therapeutic process, in that they tend to encapsulate a client's situation in some vivid, concrete, immediate fashion.

There are many different kinds of metaphors. Most common, perhaps, is the use of therapeutic teaching tales, of the kind utilized by Erickson (1967, 1980). Sometimes you can reach into your "stock" of experiences and find a useful tale: Other times you can craft a tale to precisely match a patient's situation. Many beginning strategic therapists try too hard to either remember a "proper" tale from their readings or to construct a "correct" tale on the spot. Beginnings are often difficult when you focus on them too much.

My 7-year-old daughter, Anna, had a terrible time learning to swim. Anna was rather thin and didn't have much natural buoyancy. She had also picked up that learning to swim was important to me and was caught between conflicting desires: She wanted to please me but wanted to do things her way; she wanted to be brave but was in fact scared; she wanted to swim like her friends but had learned to get the attention of her swim teachers by being distressed. She had learned the fundamentals in her swim classes but was scared to take off on her own—but also could not let it go and just splash around in the water and play. I was in the pool with her once, and she would, at my urging, try to swim a few feet to me. Anna would try so hard that she would tighten her muscles, and this would make her start to sink: This would make her try harder, and she would arch her back, lifting her head out of the water, which would make her sink more, and frighten her the more. After a few attempts, I urged her to stop swimming and just play, but she was determined to swim, and time and again she would plunge in, splash, sink down, and then grab at me gasping, spluttering, scared.

A stranger in the pool with his children offered my daughter a little inflatable, brightly colored plastic float to put under her. I nearly refused. I had been taught never to teach swimming with the use of flotation aids, since supposedly you get dependent on them, and can go out too far, and slip off, and not knowing how to swim, drown. But my 2-year-old was also there and needed attention, and my 7-year-old was trying too hard, and she wanted to play on the float.

So Anna put the float under her stomach and paddled off around the pool. At first she was enthused. Gradually, she got bored with the float. She slipped off and swam a few yards to me. I asked her to go back and get the float so we could return it. She splashed and swam back to the float. She got on for a while again, got bored again, slipped off and swam to me. Suddenly she stood up, surprised. "Daddy," she said. "Look! I'm swimming."

After that she couldn't get enough of swimming . . . for a while. Eventually, when the novelty of swimming wore off, she would sometimes enjoy playing around with floats as well, basking in the sun or swimming as her fancy suited her.

Besides stories, the use of space and position is often extremely useful to metaphorically encode a situation. This is a very common technique in structural family therapy (Minuchin & Fishman, 1981), and Peggy Papp has developed an excellent method of sculpting (Papp, 1980) I find especially useful when working with couples' groups. Sculpting involves having each member of a couple position group members "playing" family members at different distances from each other and in different poses, symbolizing the degree of emotional closeness existing in various relationships. For example, the person playing an authoritarian father overinvolved with his ineffectually rebellious daughter might be instructed to stand up on a table while the surrogate daughter kneels at his feet, trying to topple him by grabbing his toes. After both members of the couple depict the situation as they see it, both can be asked to depict their view of the ideal situation they would like to have. Then the entire group can participate in trying to find a way to make the transition from the current problematical situation to the ideal outcomes, by having the people in the sculpture move around in various directions. Almost invariably, I find people come back from sculpting stating they obtained a whole new perspective on their situation, and the depiction of the relationships in visuospatial, as opposed to verbal, terms, allowed them to generate a whole new series of possible avenues for change.

Metaphors may also be used to dramatize and replay between therapist and patient an important situation in a person's life in a way that moves the therapy forward.

This case example is derived from material presented in supervision to Eric Green-leaf, an Ericksonian therapist. An extremely obsessional patient complained of inhibitions in completing projects and being successful. The patient described a memory of being 10 years old, on a baseball diamond playing second base. His team was about to win the championship if they could only get the last out. The batter hit the ball to the shortstop, who was the team coach, described as a "father figure" to the patient. The patient could see the coach cock his arm and prepare to throw the ball to the patient to win the game: The patient recalls becoming numb, paralyzed, and seeing the ball approach him in slow motion. It hit the patient, bouncing off his chest as he remained paralyzed, and his team lost.

The thing to do here is for the therapist to reach down, pick up anything that comes to hand, and throw it at the patient. If the patient catches it, the therapist can smile at him, and change the subject to other things, so as not to dilute the patient's success. If the patient drops it, the therapist can empathize with the sadness. Either way breaks through the patient's obsessional, affect-less portrayal and brings a "thinned-out" past incident into the present, where it has opportunities for alteration.

Metaphors can make the past vivid in the present. The use of transference in psychodynamic therapies is simply another form of metaphor, if a somewhat less efficient one in that it takes more time to generate. Strategic therapists can certainly use psychodynamic interpretation of the transference in cases where this is the language the patient is most likely to be able to create images of change. Any kind of use of imagery is a use of metaphor, of course. The strategic therapist can employ cognitive therapy's techniques of guided imagery to good effect.

One last type of metaphor should be mentioned—ritual. Rituals are structured enactments of a situation in a set sequence that somehow symbolizes or encapsulates some central aspect of the experience. It is often useful to prescribe rituals to patients, in that it brings symptomatic behavior under their voluntary control; furthermore, the ritual can often include acts that are partial solutions of the problem. Although the use of rituals in strategic therapy is widespread and varied, perhaps it is most common in grief work, where patients might be instructed to put a picture of the deceased on their mantelpiece and pray before it for 5 minutes nightly. Rituals that match a patient's propensities can sometimes seem strange because they are so individualized, but often they are the most effective.

I remember one case where the patient was a young man who had had multiple deaths in his family over a period of about 2 years. One death in particular, that of his sister, haunted him, in that he did not visit her much while she was in the hospital in another city during her final days. Instead, he spent much of his time playing softball.

Since then, he had devoted a good deal of his time to helping acting-out high-school students by organizing and coaching softball leagues and teams. This patient came to therapy because of intrusive thoughts that he might run his truck over and hurt somebody accidentally. The effective intervention for his problem turned out to be a grief ritual, in which he was to make periodic pilgrimmages to his sister's grave (which was several hours' drive away). Each time he visited her grave, he was to leave, as an offering, a new softball on her grave, as a penance and an offering. His symptoms, which had been of at least a year's duration, disappeared within 2 weeks and, 2 years later, had not returned.

Besides metaphors, the most common indirect interventions by strategic therapists are paradoxical ones. Paradoxical interventions are not exclusive to strategic therapy—they are common, for example, in behavioral therapies (Espie & Lindsay, 1985; Riebel, 1984) and logotherapy (Frankl, 1960)—but strategic therapy is often associated with paradox. There is a large literature on paradox (cf. Dell, 1981; Driscoll, 1985; Fisher, Anderson, & Jones, 1981; Rosenbaum, 1982), and the very meaning of the term tends to be subject to interpretation (Dell, 1986). In general, paradoxical interventions refer to those therapeutic efforts that attempt to solve a problem by trying to not solve it or even maintain it. Haley (1973, 1976) describes a variety of types of paradoxical interventions. These include encouraging resistance, encouraging a response by frustrating it, discouraging patients from changing, and encouraging relapses in order to prevent them. Selvini-Palazzoli *et al.* (1978) have made paradoxical interventions the centerpiece of their therapeutic endeavors, with a special emphasis on the value of positive connotation (i.e., finding the useful and helpful parts of *all* behaviors in a system).

As noted, symptom prescription is often thought of as a paradoxical intervention, but I would argue that for an intervention to be paradoxical, the communicated *intent* of the intervention must be to *not* remove the symptom. Interventions that ask patients to practice the symptom with the intent of helping them "get control" of it in order to subsequently "get rid" of it are not paradoxical in spirit. Similarly, if a therapist asks an oppositional patient to do something, hoping the patient will defy the therapist and do the opposite, this is a strategic use of "reverse psychology," but it is not paradoxical. You cannot "paradox a patient," for this implies a unidirectional epistemology in which the therapist "tricks" the patient into getting better; in reality, paradoxes only work well if the therapist is *sincere* in encouraging the symptom (Rosenbaum, 1982). Only in this fashion can the therapist generate a true paradox, one that turns in on itself, implying directly contradictory meanings simultaneously. For an intervention to be truly paradoxical, it must involve an inherent conflict within itself, an oscillation of mutually exclusive, equally valid meanings. This is usually obtained by having paradoxical interventions be self-referential.

> There is a famous Zen koan. A monk says to the master, "master, I cannot pacify my mind." The master responds, "Bring out that mind before me, and I shall pacify it for you." The monk despairing, cries out: "But I cannot grasp it, to hold it out before you." Says the master: "There, you see? Already it is pacified." At this point the monk is enlightened. (Reps, 1964, pp. 121–122)

A paradoxical intervention is self-referential when it comments on itself in contradictory ways. When a Cretan says, "all Cretans are liars," if the Cretan is telling the truth, he is lying, and if he is lying, he is telling the truth. This kind of paradox occurs because there is a confusion of logical types: the Cretan speaker is simultaneously one frame "above" his utterance, as an observer, and one frame "below" being observer, as the object of the observation. In a similar fashion, paradoxical interventions invoke themselves in contradictory ways. Having a patient perform an involuntary symptom voluntarily makes the patient simultaneously subject and object, controller and controlled. Furthermore, when the therapist requests the patient to have his or her symptom, the therapist is creating a paradoxical therapeutic relationship (Rosenbaum, 1982) in which the therapist is simultaneously powerful and impotent, wise person and fool, and the patient is simultaneously helpless and empowered, passive yet active. The therapeutic relationship then embodies a "both-and" epistemology in which change is maintained through stability and stability maintained through change (Keeney, 1983). When a system is sufficiently complex, it usually becomes self-referential, (Keeney, 1983), and Gödel has demonstrated mathematically that any system sufficiently complex to be self-referential is necessarily incomplete (Hofstadter, 1980). Paradoxical interventions thus tend to be seemingly closed, but by being self-referential they strangely loop around recursively in a kind of Möbius strip that, being "closed" is open; the intervention "infolds" on itself creating novel perspectives and openings on the world, thus potentiating change. By creating an experience in which the perspective on the symptom shimmers and oscillates, you create the creative ambiguity and confusion that is the hallmark of pivot chords, that allow modulation to remote keys.

A young woman came in worried about her relationship with her fiancee. She had been engaged to him for some years, but he had always backed out at the last minute from going through with several marriage plans. She loved him very much and felt loved in return but could not tolerate his relationship with his alcoholic mother. His mother was very demanding, and he would repeatedly try to placate her and satisfy her, despite the fact that whatever he did was never good enough for her and would end in her becoming enraged with him. The mother also viewed the patient as a competitor for her son and would call up and abuse the patient at unpredictable times. The patient felt disgusted at her fiancee's "puppy dog" behavior toward his mother and angry that he would spend too much of his time attending to his mother and ignoring her. She was very concerned at having him resolve this problem with his mother and attempted to "help" him by nagging him to stand up to her (thus unwittingly being demanding of the patient, as his mother was). The fiancee would then become angry at the patient for interfering.

I suggested to the patient that it was very important for her to help her fiancee resolve this problem but that she hadn't worked hard enough at it. She needed to insist that her fiancee spend more time with his mother, so that he could realize he could never satisfy her. We devised a program whereby she would encourage him to do more for his mother, and if he protested he had done all he could, to ask him skeptically whether he really believed this in his heart. I told the patient I was worried, however, that this job of helping out her fiancee would be very difficult for her, but I appreciated her nobility in pursuing the issue rather than just leaving it between him and his mother so that the patient could have peace of mind. I suggested that she continue to try to help her fiancee resolve his issues with his mother until it became clear to her what she should do next. (Clearly, this was encouraging the behavior which was causing problems between her and her fiancee—he saw her as overly intrusive, just as his mother was—but the "valence" of her meddling was changed).

The goal here was not to resolve the issue between the fiancee and his mother but rather to defuse the issue for the patient. She was overinvolved in a triangle which gave her no perspective to determine what was going to be helpful for her. This intervention allowed her to either engage with her fiancee in a different way than previously or to detach herself from his relationship with his mother while staying involved with him, or to decide he would never change and satisfy her and she was best off leaving the relationship. The intervention was paradoxical in that it did not ask her to stop being involved in the triangle, but rather positively connoted her involvement and used it as a vehicle to turning her thoughts to what decisions she needed to make for herself. Follow-up revealed that the fiancee became progressively more assertive with not only his mother but also with the patient. She is now deciding whether she likes this more assertive man.

In another case, an extremely driven, obsessional patient, an artist, complained he could "never accomplish anything" and would "just let himself drift." In one session, I talked to him about the different ways you can drift, how you can drift with the current or against it, drift in a certain direction or round and round . . . and how you could notice things around you while drifting, or just attend to the drifting . . . and how he could rely on certain things happening with regularity while he drifted, such as breathing in and out . . . but then certain things could happen in the body which you couldn't predict . . . and from there, helped the patient enter a deep hypnotic trance in which he could learn the value and pleasure of being surprised. I was then able to point out how he had accomplished entering a creative hypnotic trance by using his ability to drift and how he could prepare to be surprised at other things happening along the way sometime in the future. After coming out of the trance, the patient expressed pleasure and surprise at the achievement of hypnosis and a sense of relief and curiosity markedly at variance with his obsessional style. This allowed him to begin to make creative use of his drifting states to accomplish various artistic projects.

In yet another case, that of K. M., after several extremely productive sessions following the generation of the image of herself feeling free on a mountaintop, the patient came in anxious, depressed, and had great difficulty talking. This was a patient who often had reacted to any ideas about termination with passive aggression and accusations I was abandoning her; in addition, she was often unable to do things because she wanted to but instead was motivated to do those things she felt she "should" do and then felt angry at feeling compelled and simultaneously inadequate to do what she ought. Rather than analyze "why she was becoming resistant," I told her I was very relieved she had begun to slow down her pace of changes and learnings. She became inquisitive, and I told her that she was at the cusp of change, and if she started changing now, she could do so very rapidly, and I was worried she would then have to face all kinds of decisions, and I wasn't sure she was ready for that yet. In fact, I thought it was my job to keep her from plunging ahead and to only let her work on things she absolutely felt she had to. She then became markedly less anxious, abandoned her "tortured, helpless" demeanor and began talking in a realistic way of some of the major concerns and decisions which faced her, stating that she knew they were tough, and she knew she could put them off and didn't have to tackle them, but she really wanted to work on them now.

I meant all of what I said about not changing too fast quite sincerely, and yet simultaneously I was hopeful that saying this would give her the freedom to continue changing.

Some last words about interventions. Many times, when reading of therapies that utilize specific kinds of interventions, the reader is left with the impression that therapy is a kind of story where the client comes in with a problem, the therapist mysteriously comes up with some magical intervention, and the client goes away cured and happy. And they all live happily ever after.

The realities of therapy are, of course, quite different. Strategic therapists, like all therapists, indeed like all people are often groping about for what to do, puzzled and confused. An intervention that seems brilliant in a session may not lead to anything useful in the client's life outside the sessions; as mentioned repeatedly, it is what happens outside the sessions that really counts, and the actual therapy meetings are only springboards to potentiate changes in daily living. Once an intervention is selected and tried, often clients do not like the intervention (in which case, the therapist is confronted with how to "sell" the intervention (Fisch et al., 1982) or must come up with some new intervention. If clients do agree to work with an intervention, they often come back the next session with experiences the therapist did not expect. This, in fact, is one of the pleasures of strategic therapy: expecting the unexpected. In any event, after an intervention, there is often still much to be done. Just because strategic therapy is brief does not mean there is not a "working through."

Again, strategic therapists must respond flexibly to the feedback they receive from clients. If an intervention worked, you might ask the client to do more about it, or you might worry out loud to the client that they are changing too much too fast. It is always fine to explore what the implications of an intervention's working mean to the client's life. If the intervention did not work, you might come up with another—always taking full responsibility for the failure of the intervention. One of the more salubrious things about strategic therapy is that it *never* blames the victim (Ryan, 1972). If a client has not done an assignment, you might want to shy away from assignments, or you might want to rework your assignment to better fit the client's world view. If the client modifies the assignment, you may want to offer future assignments with choices. If you have tried something direct which has not worked, try working indirectly: If indirective does not work, be pragmatically directive. There is also nothing sinful about sitting back and taking refuge in empathic Rogerian reflections while you try to figure out what to do next (if anything—sometimes no treatment is the treatment of choice) (Frances & Clarkin, 1981; Jones, 1985). In all cases you take your lead from clients, see how they respond, with all participants altering and adapting to each other to achieve a reasonable, productive fit. Although strategic therapy's theory offers some blueprints, building the house itself always requires tinkering.

As far as outcome is concerned, the "formal" kind of strategic therapy studied in psychotherapy outcome research seems to indicate strategic therapy works about as well as other kinds of therapies (De Shazer, 1985; Gurman, Kniskern, & Pinsof, 1986), and working with the complainant seems to work as well as working with entire systems, at least in marital therapy (Wells & Giannetti, 1986). Unfortunately, psychotherapy research that attempts to isolate "pure" forms of "manualized" strategic therapy obscures the essential nature of the treatment, which always molds itself to the situation at hand.

Strategic therapy is not a solution, but tools toward solutions (Madanes, 1980). Strategic therapy is really not a "school" of therapy. It is rather a way of gaining flexibility, of developing an attitude to allow you to freely intervene with clients, using all the tools at your disposal, then respond to the feedback you receive. In this way, in its most general form, strategic therapy is integrated psychotherapy.

POSTSCRIPT: AWAKENING AND REORIENTATION

Having begun this chapter with an *in*(tro)*duction*, it seems only fitting to end it by awakening the reader from whatever trance state you may have achieved through reading, orienting you to your future work with a few "posthypnotic" suggestions.

Strategic therapy is ultimately about freedom. I want to give patients the freedom to change, and often that is best done by giving them freedom not to change. Strategic therapy teaches choice: not the choice of obsessive ruminating and intellectualized decision making but the choice of embarking on different roads when you have reached a crossroad. When you are walking in a forest and come to a path, sometimes it is useful to consult your map and pick the route that will get you to your destination. Sometimes, though, you may be walking for the sheer pleasure of it, and you may choose a path almost randomly, without thinking about it, to immerse yourself further in the experience of the woods. As therapists, we see people who often are so intent on reaching their destination that they get lost in the woods; we also see people who are so lost in the woods they have lost sight of their destination. To some we give a compass; with others, we walk along by their sides; and with yet others, we may urge them to sit down awhile and look around before moving further. The paradox of strategic therapy is that, after mastering its techniques, ultimately we employ them almost playfully, in an effort to just be with our patients as they find the changes inherent in them they brought with them with their "problems." In this way the strategic therapist is not a "doctor" but rather a midwife. The pleasures of strategic therapy are the pleasures of aiding in a birth and wondering at what emerges inevitably. The strategic therapist looks not for finalities but for changes setting off in new directions. The completion of the birth is not an end, but yet another beginning.

May you enjoy your learnings on unexpectedly pleasant walks and planned interesting journeys.

REFERENCES

Anderson, C. M., & Stewart, S. (1983). *Mastering resistance*. New York: The Guilford Press.
Arendt, H. (1978). *The life of the mind*. New York: Harcourt Brace Jovanovich.

Bateson, G. (1972). *Steps to an ecology of mind*. New York: Ballantine.

Bateson, G. (1979). *Mind and nature: A necessary unity*. New York: E. P. Dutton.

Bergman, J. (1985). *Fishing for baracuda: Pragmatics of brief systemic therapy*. New York: W. W. Norton.

Bloom, B. (1981). Focused single-session psychotherapy: Initial development and evaluation. In S. H. Budman (Ed.), *Forms of brief therapy* (pp. 167–218). New York: Guilford.

Carter, E., & McGoldrick, M. (1980). *The family life cycle*. New York: Gardner Press.

Dell, P. (1981). Some irreverent thoughts on paradox. *Family Process, 20*, 37–41.

Dell, P. (1986). Why do we still call them "paradoxes?" *Family Process, 25*(2), 223–235.

De Shazer, S. (1984a). Post-mortem: Mark Twain did die in 1910. *Family Process, 23*(1), 20–22.

De Shazer, S. (1984b). The death of resistance. *Family Process, 23*(1), 11–16.

De Shazer, S. (1985). *Keys to solution in brief therapy*. New York: W. W. Norton.

De Shazer, S., Berg, I. K., Lipchik, E., Nunnally, E. *et al.* (1986). Brief therapy: Focused Solution Development. *Family Process, 25*(2), 207–223.

Driscoll, R. (1985). Commonsense objectives in paradoxical interventions. *Psychotherapy, 22*(4), 774–778.

Efron, D. (1986). *Journeys: Expansion of the strategic-systemic therapies*. New York: Bruner/Mazel.

Ellis, A., & Harper, R. A. (1975). *A new guide to rational living*. New York: Prentice-Hall.

Espie, C., & Lindsay, W. (1985). Paradoxical intention in the treatment of chronic insomnia: Six case studies illustrating variability in therapeutic response. *Behavioral Research, 23*(6), 703–709.

Erickson, M. H. (1967). *Advanced techniques of hypnosis and therapy: Selected papers of M. H. Erickson*. J. Haley, Ed. New York: Grune & Stratton.

Erickson, M. H. (1980). *A teaching seminar with Milton H. Erickson*. J. Zeig, New York: Bruner/Mazel.

Erickson, M. H., Rossi, E., & Rossi, S. (1976). *Hypnotic realities: The induction of clinical hypnosis and forms of indirect suggestion*. New York: Irvington Publishers.

Fisch, R., Weakland, J. H., & Segal, L. (1982). *The tactics of change*. San Francisco: Jossey-Bass.

Fisher, L., Anderson, A., & Jones, J. (1981). Types of paradoxical intervention and indications/con- traindictionas for use in clinical practice. *Family Process, 20* 25–36.

Frances, A., & Clarkin, J. (1981). No treatment as the prescription of choice. *Archives of General Psychiatry, 38* (May), 542–545.

Frank, J. D. (1973). *Persuasion and healing*. New York: Shocken.

Frankl, V. (1960). Paradoxical intention: A logo-therapeutic technique. *American Journal of Psycho- therapy, 14*, 520–535.

Fraser, J. (1986). Integrating system-based therapies: Similarities, differences, and some critical question. In D. Efron, (Ed.), *Journeys: Expansion of the strategic-sytemic therapies* (pp. 125–149). New York: Bruner/Mazel.

Frieswyk, S. H., Allen, J., Colson, D., Coyne, L., Gabbard, G., Horwitz, L., & Newsom, G. (1986). Therapeutic alliance: Its place as a process and outcome variable in dynamic psychotherapy research. *Journal of Consulting & Clinical Psychology, 54*(1), 32–38.

Garfield, S. (1978). Research on client variables in psychotherapy. In S. Garfield & A. E. Bergin (Eds.), *Handbook of psychotherapy and behavior change* (2nd edition, pp. 195–197). New York: John Wiley.

Greenson, R. (1981a). The working alliance and the transference neurosis. In R. Langs (Ed.), *Classics in Psychoanalytic Technique*, (pp. 319–331). New York: Jason Aronson.

Greenson, R. (1981b). Beyond transference and interpretation. In R. Langs (Ed.), *Classics in psycho- analytic technique*, (pp. 97–103). New York: Jason Aronson.

Greenson, R. (1981c). The 'Real' relationship between the patient and the psychoanalyst. In R. Langs (Ed.), *Classics in Psychoanalytic Technique*, (pp. 87–97). New York: Jason Aronson.

Gurman, A., Kniskern, D., & Pinsof, W. (1986). Research on the process and outcome of marital and family therapy. In S. Garfield & A. E. Bergin (Eds.), *Handbook of psychotherapy and behavior change* (3rd ed., pp. 565–625). New York: John Wiley.

Haley, J. (1973). *Uncommon therapy: The psychiatric techniques of Milton H. Erickson*. New York: Norton.

Haley, J. (1976). *Problem-solving therapy*. San Francisco: Jossey-Bass.

Haley, J. (1980). *Leaving home*. New York: McGraw-Hill.

Haley, J. (1984). *Ordeal therapy*. San Francisco: Jossey-Bass.

Hofstadter, D. (1980). *Gödel, Escher, Bach: An eternal golden braid*. New York: Vintage Books.

Horowitz, M. J. (1979a). *Stress response syndromes*. New York: Jason Aronson.

Horowitz, M. J. (1979b). *States of mind*. New York: Plenum Press.

Hoyt, M., Rosenbaum, R., Talmon, M. (1987, Summer). *Treating patients in single-session psychotherapies*. Workshop presented at the American Psychological Association meeting, New York.

Jones, C. W. (1985). Strategic interventions within a no-treatment frame. *Family Process, 24,* 583–595.

Keeney, B. P. (1983). *Aesthetics of change*. New York: Guilford.

Lankton, S., & Lankton, C. H. (1983). *The answer within: A clinical framework of Ericksonian hypnotherapy*. New York: Bruner-Mazel.

Lansford, E. (1986). Weakenings and repairs of the working alliance in short-term psychotherapy. *Professional Psychology: Research and Practice, 17*(4), 364–366.

Madanes, C. (1980). *Strategic family therapy*. San Francisco: Jossey-Bass.

Malan, D. H., Heath, E. S., Bacal, H., & Balfour, F. H. G. (1975). Psychodynamic changes in untreated neurotic patients: Apparently genuine improvements. *Archives of General Psychiatry, 32,* 110–126.

Mazza, J. (1984). Symptom utilization in strategic therapy. *Family Process, 23*(4), 487–501.

Merleau-Ponty, M. (1964). *Signs* (R. McCleary, trans.). Evanston, IL: Northwestern University Press.

Minuchin, S., & Fishman, H. C. (1981). *Family therapy techniques*. Cambridge: Harvard University Press.

Papp, P. (1980). The Greek chorus and other techniques of paradoxical therapy. *Family Process, 19,* 45–57.

Peterfreund, E., & Schwartz, J. (1971). *Information, systems, and psychoanalysis. Psychological Issues.* Monograph 25/26. New York: International Universities Press.

Reps, P. (1964). *Zen flesh, Zen bones*. Garden City, NY: Doubleday.

Riebel, L. (1984). Paradoxical intervention strategies: A review of rationales. *Psychotherapy, 21,* 260–272.

Roberts, J. (1986). An evolving model: Links between the milan approach and strategic models of family therapy. In D. Efron (Ed.), *Journeys: Expansion of the strategic-systemic therapies* (pp. 150–173). New York: Bruner/Mazel.

Rosenbaum, R. (1982). Paradox as epistemological jump. *Family Process, 21*(1), 85–90.

Rosenbaum, R. (1988). Feelings toward integration. *International Journal of Eclectic Psychotherapy, 7*(1), 52–60.

Ryan, W. (1972). *Blaming the victim*. New York: Random House.

Schaefer, R. (1976). *A new language for psychoanalysis*. New Haven, CT: Yale University Press.

Selvini-Palazolli, M., Boscolo, L., Cecchin, G., & Prata, G. (1978). *Paradox and counterparadox*. New York: Jason Aronson.

Stewart, S., & Anderson, C. M. (1984). Resistance revisited: or, Tales of my death have been greatly exaggerated (Mark Twain). *Family Process, 23*(1), 17–19.

Strupp, H., & Binder, J. (1984). *Psychotherapy in a new key: A Manual for time-limited dynamic psychotherapy*. New York: Basic Books.

Watzlawick, P. (1983). *The situation is hopeless but not serious: The pursuit of unhappiness*. New York: Norton.

Watzlawick, P. (Ed.). (1984). *The invented reality: How do we know what we believe we know? (Contributions to constructivism)*. New York: W. W. Norton.

Watzlawick, P., Beavin, J., & Jackson, D. (1967). *Pragmatics of human communication: A study of interactional patterns, pathologies, and paradoxes*. New York: Norton.

Watzlawick, P., Weakland, H., & Fisch, R. (1974). *Change: Principles of problem formation and problem resolution*. New York: W. W. Norton.

Weakland, J., Fisch, R., Watzlawick, P., & Bodin, A. M. (1974). Brief therapy: Focused problem resolution. *Family Process, 13,* 141–168.

Wells, R., & Gianetti, V. J. (1986). Individual marital therapy: A critical reappraisal. *Family Process, 25* (1), 43–51.

Wile, D. (1984). Kohut, Kernberg, and accusatory interpretations. *Psychotherapy, 21*(3), 353–364.

Wolpe, J. (1973). *The practice of behavior therapy* (2nd ed.). New York: Pergamon.

17

A Systems Therapy
Problem-Centered Systems Therapy of the Family

NATHAN B. EPSTEIN, DUANE S. BISHOP,
GABOR I. KEITNER, AND IVAN W. MILLER

Family therapy has become an increasingly popular mode of treatment over the last two decades (Epstein & Bishop, 1973; Group for the Advancement of Psychiatry, 1970; Gurman & Kniskern, 1978, 1981; Haley, 1971; Olson, 1970; Zuk, 1971). Its acceptance has not been limited to psychiatry and other mental health fields, for it is increasingly viewed as an important development by family medicine (Comley, 1973; Epstein & McAuley, 1978; McFarlane, Norman, & Spitzer, 1971; McFarlane, O'Connell, & Hay, 1971; Patriarche, 1974; Stanford, 1972), by pediatrics (Finkel, personal communciation, 1974; McClelland, Staples, Weisberg, & Bergin, 1973; Tomm, 1973), and by those working with the disabled (Bishop & Epstein, 1980). Training programs and study curricula in family therapy have grown tremendously in the last 10 years (Bishop & Epstein, 1979; Liddle & Halpin, 1978). Reports of a significant amount of research have also appeared (DeWitt, 1978; Glick & Haley, 1971; Gurman & Kniskern, 1978; Guttman, Spector, Sigal, Rakoff, & Epstein, 1971; Olson, 1970; Santa-Barbara, Woodward, Levin, Streiner, Goodman, & Epstein, 1977, 1979; Wells, Dilkes, & Trivelli, 1972; Woodward, Santa-Barbara, Levin, & Epstein, 1978; Woodward, Santa-Barbara, Levin, & Epstein, 1978; Woodward, Santa-Barbara, Levin, Goodman, Streiner, Muzzin, & Epstein, 1974). Several authors have pointed to the need for clear descriptions of conceptual orientations and the specifics of the therapy process (Epstein & Bishop, 1973; Liddle & Halpin, 1978).

However, approaches to working with family problems are still basically limited to clinical judgment and intuition. Literature reviews expose the variety of theoretical models underlying clinical work in this area, and there is no generally accepted framework within which to perform family assessment and treatment. This variety is no justification for an undisciplined approach and it is

NATHAN B. EPSTEIN, DUANE S. BISHOP, GABOR I. KEITNER, AND IVAN W. MILLER • Department of Psychiatry and Human Behavior, Brown University, Providence, Rhode Island 02912.

important for those treating families to be clear and consistent about the conceptual frameworks they use. We feel that professionals working with families require both (1) a model that forms the basis for their understanding of family functioning, and (2) a model that guides their approach to treatment.

We have described two such models that in combination, can form the basis for family work. The McMaster Model of Family Functioning (Epstein, Bishop, & Levin, 1978) provides a conceptual framework for assessing and diagnosing family functioning. The Problem-Centered Systems Therapy of the Family model (Epstein & Bishop, 1981) provides an operationalized guide to the assessment and treatment of families.

Previous publication of our work (Epstein & Bishop, 1973, 1981; Epstein, Bishop, & Baldwin, 1981) resulted in numerous comments and inquiries from interested professionals. Such responses indicated a desire for more detailed explication of the Problem-Centered Systems Therapy of the Family.

It is impossible to cover in detail every aspect of a system of therapy within the scope of one chapter. Psychotherapy of any type is a highly complex process, full of limitless nuances determined by multiple factors operating at any one time and changing rapidly in response to continually changing issues. To consider that it can be satisfactorily reported is almost foolhardy. Bearing this in mind, in this chapter we will attempt to respond to the numerous comments and questions raised.

In what follows we will present some historical background, a brief introduction to the family functioning model, and then focus on treatment. In the process, we will detail the clinical use of both the family functioning and treatment models.

BACKGROUND

The senior author was first trained as a general adult and child psychiatrist and then went on to receive training in psychoanalysis. In those days, workers in child psychiatry began to highlight the role of the mother in the behavior of the child and also, to a considerably lesser extent, to take some note of the effect of other family members on the identified patient. Work with children and their mothers, plus exposure to Nathan Ackerman and Abram Kardiner during psychoanalytic training, led the senior author to an awareness of the need for a total systems approach in order to understand and help patients. Earlier research experience with a multidisciplinary medical research group studying the application of hormones to human patients had already resulted in his becoming aware of the powerful forces wrought by biological agents on human behavior.

Kardiner, a pioneer in transcultural psychiatry and a brilliantly effective teacher, demonstrated the effect of culture, values, religion, economics, history, social patterns, and practices, and so on on behavior. His major works (Kardiner, 1939; Kardiner, Linton, Du Bois, & West, 1945) remain classics in the field.

Ackerman at that time (1951–1955) was developing his ideas on working with the family group in psychotherapy (e.g., Ackerman, 1958)—a radical notion during that period for which he received much abuse from his more conservative analytic colleagues. Although Ackerman had not yet developed clear formulations of family theories or family therapy technique (Ackerman, 1966), it seemed that he was moving toward a more effective way of understanding and treating patients by having the significant actors in the patient's life in the therapy situation at the same time, thereby easing the job of "teasing out" the family interactions that led to the behavior being treated.

Struck by the exciting potential and common sense inherent in this approach, Epstein began to experiment with methods of involving family members of patients in the course of therapy. Various approaches were used, such as seeing the mother together with the child patient in play therapy; having both parents in for occasional sessions either with or without the child or adolescent patient present; having the mothers participate in activity group therapy with children and seeing those mothers in a separate weekly group without the children; seeing two spouses together when only one of them was the presenting patient; and bringing in different members of the individual patient's family at various times during the course of that individual's analytic therapy. As time went on, the approach being used most frequently was that where all members were seen together for conjoint family therapy regardless of the presenting problem.

During these early years, the conceptual model and therapy approach used were intrapsychic psychoanalytic, somewhat modified to fit the new situations. The actual family interactional patterns postulated as responsible for the creation of the intrapsychic and behavioral pathologies in the identified patient were being observed, stimulated, inferred, and interpreted. The analytic concepts most frequently used in interpreting the behavior observed in family sessions were those of role projection, displacement, incorporation and projection of part objects, oedipal strivings, sibling rivalry, denial, and affective repression. As described elsewhere (Epstein, 1963), this primarily analytic approach changed gradually to one with more focusing on the interactional aspects of the intrafamilial behavior. There was much stress on releasing the affect underlying the inferred important family interactions and the associated intrapsychic conflicts and fantasies. The primary objective remained that of easing the intrapsychic conflicts of the identified patient, which were inferred to result in the pathological symptoms and/or behavior for which treatment was undertaken. In the late 1950s, research was started on "nonclinical" families. This was reported in the *Silent Majority* (Westley & Epstein, 1969). It was only then, when we found that the family as a "system" was more powerful than intrapsychic factors in determining the behavior of individual family members that our therapy approach began to change to a systems-oriented approach. Since this occurred, around 1963–1964, our approach has been continually evolving. The early change from a primarily psychoanalytic-interactional mode to a systems mode, where the family system itself is looked at as the factor to be evaluated as centrally involved in the difficulty in the behavior being examined, was most difficult. Fifteen years of training and orientation had to be strongly modified, and a new approach based on controversial research findings had to be developed. The tendency to slip automatically into a primarily psychoanalytic approach to the therapy was great and occurred frequently. With careful self-monitoring and experience this now happens very rarely, and only when it is based upon a conscious decision for purposes of generating another viewpoint that might further understanding and therapeutic progress. As stated, our therapeutic approach has been continually modified as the results from our research, clinical work, and teaching indicated the need for same.

A conceptual framework, the Family Categories Schema (Epstein, Rakoff, & Sigal, 1968), originally developed in the course of the study of 110 "nonclinical" families (Westley & Epstein, 1969) mentioned previously, formed the basis of thinking for the current model. The model that follows is the result of the many significant revisions and developments of the original concepts since they were first generated.

Theory: Underlying Concepts[1]

The McMaster Model of Family Functioning

The McMaster Model of Family Functioning has evolved over a period of 30 years. Ideas gained from reading the family literature have been incorporated into the model in various ways. The development of the model has involved the development of a concept, then testing of the concept in clinical work, in research, and in teaching. Problems discovered in these applications have led to reformulations of the model. These were then tested out, new problems appeared, and further reformulations occurred. The result of this pattern of development has been that the model is pragmatic. Ideas that work have been kept. Ideas that did not work in therapy, could not be measured reliably, or could not be communicated in teaching were discarded or modified.

The model has been used extensively in a variety of psychiatric and family practice clinics (Comley, 1973; Epstein & Westley, 1959; Guttman *et al.*, 1971; Guttman, Spector, Sigal, Epstein, & Rakoff, 1972; Postner, Guttman, Sigal, Epstein, & Rakoff, 1971; Rakoff, Sigal, Spector, & Guttman, 1967; Sigal, Rakoff, & Epstein, 1967; Westley & Epstein, 1960) and by therapists who treated families as part of a large family therapy outcome study (Guttman *et al.*, 1971; Santa-Barbara *et al.*, 1977, 1979; Woodward *et al.*, 1974, 1978a,b). The framework has also been used in a number of family therapy training programs and found to be readily teachable (Bishop & Epstein, 1979).

The McMaster model does not cover all aspects of family functioning but identifies a number of dimensions that we have found important in dealing with

[1]The development of these concepts, the research, and training programs were supported by a number of grants from the Firestone Foundation and the Firan Foundation. Lawrence M. Baldwin, our former senior research associate, made special contributions for which we are particularly grateful. Our patient families, our trainees, and special colleagues, Sol Levin, Dorothy Horn, and J. Rubenstein, all provided special experiences, support, and ideas necessary for the development of our approach.

clinically presenting families. A family can be evaluated on the effectiveness of its functioning with respect to each dimension. On each dimension, a family may range from most ineffective to most effective functioning.

Because the development of the model has been oriented toward its applicability in the clinical setting, theoretical elegance has not been a major concern. Ideas from a variety of sources have been incorporated when they were useful. Spiegel (1971) presents a theoretical elaboration of many ideas we use. Many others have discussed some of the same concepts, but we do not wish to dwell here on the similarities and differences in usage between ourselves and other writers in the field.

The model is based on a systems approach in which the family is seen as an "open system" consisting of systems within systems (individual, marital, dyad) and relating to other systems (extended family, schools, industry, religions). The unique aspect of the dynamic family group cannot be simply reduced to the characteristics of the individual or interactions between pairs of members. Rather, there are explicit and imlicit rules, plus action by members, that govern and monitor each other's behavior. Therapy must be directed at changing the system and hopefully the behavior of the individual identified patient. The concepts of communication theory, learning theory, transaction approach, and biology are drawn on, although the infrastructure remains the systems model.

The crucial assumptions of systems theory that underlie the model to be presented can be summarized as follows:

1. The parts of the family are interrelated.
2. One part of the family cannot be understood in isolation from the rest of the system.
3. Family functioning cannot be fully understood by simply understanding each of the parts.
4. A family's structure and organization are important factors determining the behavior of family members.
5. Transactional patterns of the family system shape the behavior of family members.

The systems approach to the family is obviously an important feature of our model. Another feature we should note is that of values. Because cultural, ethical, and other similar values play such an important role in influencing human behavior, they must be sensitively appreciated and handled with care by practicing clinicians. Our approach to families is rooted in the Judaeo–Christian value system that emphasizes the optimal development of each human being. Other systems may emphasize other values and may be equally valid. We try not to impose our values in conducting therapy but recognize that we do make value judgments and believe that behavioral scientists working in the field should be prepared to state the value base underlying their approach (Epstein, 1958).

Before proceeding, it is important to emphasize our previously stated assumption that "the primary function of today's family unit appears to be that of a laboratory for the social, psychological, and biological development and maintenance of family members" (Epstein, Levin, & Bishop, 1976, p. 1411). In the course of fulfilling this role, families deal with a variety of other issues and problems. These we group into three areas: the basic task area, the developmental task area, and the hazardous task area.

The basic task area includes issues that are instrumental and fundamental in nature. Examples are the provision of food, money, transportation, and shelter. The developmental task area encompasses those family issues that arise as part of the natural processes of individual and family growth and development over time. We differentiate two sets: those associated with the individual developmental stages that each family member goes through (e.g., infancy, childhood, adolescence, middle and old age crises); and those associated with family stages (e.g., the beginning of the marriage, the first pregnancy, and the birth of the first child). Developmental concepts and family functioning have been referred to by a number of authors (Berman & Lief, 1975; Brody, 1974; Group for the Advancement of Psychiatry, 1970; Hadley, Jacob, Milliones, Caplan, & Spitz, 1974; Solomon, 1973). The hazardous task area includes the crises that arise in association with critical experiences such as illness, accidents, loss of income, job changes, and moves. There is substantial literature dealing with these topics (Comley, 1973; Hill, 1965; Langsley & Kaplan, 1968; Minuchin & Barcai, 1969; Parad & Caplan, 1965; Rapoport, 1965). The task areas are important because, in our experience, clinical presentation is often associated with the family's being unable to deal effectively with some of the tasks and issues subsumed under these three domains.

To understand the family structure, organization, and transactional pattern dysfunctions associated with family difficulties, we focus on the following six dimensions: problem solving, communication, roles, affective responsiveness, affective involvement, and behavior control. Some groups studying family functioning conceptualize much of family behavior as occurring within a single dimension such as communication (e.g., Bateson, Jackson, Haley, & Weakland, 1956; Watzlawick, Beavin, & Jackson, 1967; Weakland, Fisch, Watzlawick, & Bodin, 1974) or role behaviors (Parsons, 1951; Parsons & Bales, 1955; Spiegel, 1971). They seem to imply that these "single dimensions" subsume all aspects of family functioning. The McMaster model does not focus on any one dimension as the foundation for conceptualizing family behavior. We argue that many dimensions need to be assessed for a fuller understanding of such a complex entity as the family. Although we attempt to clearly define and delineate the dimensions, we recognize the potential overlap and/or possible interaction that may occur between them. Further clarification will undoubtedly result from our continuing research. The dimensions of family functioning will be discussed in more detail later and elaborated in the context of our treatment model.

PROBLEM-CENTERED SYSTEMS THERAPY OF THE FAMILY

This model grew out of research and clinical work in the Departments of Psychiatry at McGill and McMaster Universities in Canada (Bishop & Epstein,

1979; Comley, 1973; Epstein & Westley, 1959; Epstein & McAuley, 1978; Guttman *et al.*, 1971, 1972; McFarlane, Norman, & Spitzer, 1971; McFarlane, O'Connell, & Hay, 1971; Postner *et al.*, 1971; Rakoff *et al.*, 1967; Sigal *et al.*, 1967;
Westley & Epstein, 1960, 1969). The senior author and a colleague had previously worked together at McGill but had not observed each other's work with
families for some years. While reviewing videotapes of each doing family therapy, clear differences were observed with respect to the minor moves and interventions they both made. This was not the case for the major steps they followed. Surprisingly, these showed striking consistency. Both therapists
followed the same sequence of major steps, which we labeled the *macrostages* of
therapy.

The effect of this observation was to substantially alter our thinking about
family treatment. Perhaps we had been focusing on the wrong level in trying to
teach therapy skills. Many psychotherapists value highly the subtle interventions, strategies, and interpretations—the "art" of therapy. However, our observation of these two advanced therapists demonstrated significant differences
in these areas and, yet, a striking similarity at a more general level of conducting
therapy. We began to think that the subtle interventions, and so forth were
simply the tools therapists use to build the therapy structure. Our work since
then has reinforced the view that the major structural components or stages of
therapy are the essential building blocks of treatment. An added benefit is that
these macrostages can be clearly operationalized, and they are, therefore, more
easily followed by therapists of a wide range of abilities. This led us to further
delineate and analyze the differences between the major and minor therapy
moves and the utility of these concepts in the teaching and research of family
therapy.

We use the term *macrostages* to define the major stages of treatment. They
are the large sequential blocks of the treatment process such as assessment,
contracting, treatment, and closure. Each incorporates a number of substages,
which will be discussed later. Therapists make use of a variety of strategies and
interventions in the course of leading a family through these macrostages. Here,
strategy refers to the options and courses of action that may be taken to successfully complete a macro stage.

We differentiate the macrostages and the strategies required to negotiate
them from the micromoves, the specific intervention skills, such as those outlined by Cleghorn and Levin (1973) and by Tomm and Wright (1979). These
micromoves are the numerous interventions made by a therapist while carrying
out the macrostages and include, for example, techniques for labeling, focusing,
and clarifying.

Neither the macrostages nor the micromoves should be confused with
"style," which is based more on the personal qualities of the therapist. Different
individuals can intervene (focus) in very different ways. The differences are
style, the intervention (micromove) is focusing, and both are directed at negotiating a course of treatment, the major steps of which are the macrostages.

Returning to our earlier discussion, we would emphasize that the macrostages of therapy are the most important level of focus at this point in the

development of research in family therapy. We are aware that intervention skills (the micromoves) are important and will touch on general strategies when we feel they are important for an adequate and efficient completion of a given stage. We refer readers to the works of Cleghorn and Levin (1973) and Tomm and Wright (1979) for a detailed discussion of the many execution skill possibilities. In our experience, therapists vary in both their repertoire and number of such skills, and we have no clear empirical data to indicate specifically which ones are required to negotiate most effectively given stages of the model. We feel, rather, that the wider the range of skills available to therapists, the more effectively and efficiently they will carry out treatment. The macrostages are, therefore, the focus of what follows; we feel strongly that they play a major role in effective treatment and, therefore, require special emphasis.

We are interested in studying and delineating the basic family functioning and treatment concepts, which, if consistently applied, will allow therapists to be reasonably effective with the majority of their cases. These concepts should be readily teachable to nonexperts, be transferable to different settings, and be applicable to a variety of clinical family problems. The ability to operationally define these concepts facilitates research on therapy process and outcome, as it allows the therapeutic process to be broken down into simple, discrete components that can then be analyzed and measured.

We believe that the problem-centered model meets these objectives. We are also aware that it has been criticized as being too simplistic. Some comments are, therefore, in order. First, the model was developed with research needs in mind and, as noted, this requires clear and precise description. Clarity of definition often leads to the erroneous opinion that substantive truth is missing or that the underlying concepts are too simplistic. At the same time, complexity, density, and even incomprehensibility are often equated with wisdom and truth. Second, we hypothesize that adherence to the steps and sequences defined in the model will yield effective results, and we have initiated studies to test that hypothesis. Third, we are obviously aware that expert therapists bring a wealth of experience and skill to their treatment, but we believe that this model provides an important basic framework, particularly when dealing with difficult and complex cases. While following the macrostages as outlined, expert therapists can use the full range of their skills to enrich the treatment with their advanced techniques. However, for beginning therapists, the model provides the basis for a structured treatment approach on which to develop more focal skills. By using this model, the beginning therapist will be reasonably effective in the treatment of uncomplicated family problems. From a cursory, initial reading, the model may seem "simple," but the complexity of its concepts and its many nuances are soon recognized when it is applied to actual treatment. Before starting a detailed description of the Problem-Centered Family Systems Therapy model, there are a few important general issues that need to be addressed.

The focus of therapy is on the specific problems of the family. These include not only those problems presented by the family on coming to therapy, but also those identified during the assessment stage.

The model stresses the active collaboration of the family members with the therapist at each stage. The family must agree to and work for this collaboration throughout the therapy process, or else there is no therapy. The therapeutic contract is based upon this total mutual commitment to work at the therapy. The therapist's ideal role function in this model is that of a catalyst, clarifier, and facilitator. The family members should do, and actually do, most of the therapy work. They are involved openly and directly in identifying, clarifying, and resolving the difficulties and problems of the family. The therapist carefully explains his actions to the family every step of the way and makes sure they clearly understand and agree to what he/she is doing. This open approach throws the responsibility for its own actions to the family and ensures that the family understands, accepts, and is prepared for each step of the therapeutic process. This approach fosters a very positive collaborative response on the part of the family to the treatment (Hoehn-Saric, Frank, Imber, Nash, Stone, & Battle, 1964; Orne & Wender, 1968).

The therapist's stance during therapy facilitates the achievement of such major objectives of therapy as family openness, clarity of communication, and the development of active problem-solving abilities on the part of the family members. In the process, family members become aware of their strengths as well as their shortcomings and develop effective problem-solving methods that can be generalized for use in resolving future difficulties. They are trained to become their own family therapists and problem solvers, thereby diminishing the need for the therapist.

This therapy model is tailored to a treatment encounter involving from 6 to 12 sessions stretched over a period of time, varying from weeks to months to years, depending on the issues of each case. Length of the individual sessions may also vary considerably. The early assessment sessions may be longer (sometimes up to $2\frac{1}{2}$ hours), depending upon the needs of the case, the setting, and the stamina of family and therapist. The later task-setting treatment sessions may be as short as 15 to 20 minutes. Beginning therapists obviously will need more time to complete a satisfactory assessment. They should not feel daunted by this and should not feel under pressure to "begin treatment." Except in an emergency, families usually respond positively to such thorough assessment. They respect and feel reassured by the therapist's obvious desire to know and to understand thoroughly the family before offering a prescription for and/or beginning treatment. Beginners, and even advanced therapists in complicated cases, should not feel they have to include the number of assessment sessions in the 6 to 12 treatment sessions we advocate.

In the assessment and very early treatment sessions, the family may be seen weekly. If all goes well, the sessions may then be spread out to every 2 weeks, then to once a month and, in some cases, gradually increased to once every 3 to 6 months or so. During these intervals, the family works on its own. Families should be encouraged to contact the therapist during these interim periods. We have found that most rarely abuse this privilege.

Our stress on limiting the number of treatment sessions is due to a number of factors. Our experience has been that imposing such limits on therapy stimulates therapists and families to more active involvement in the therapeutic work, and this facilitates change. They keep the objectives of therapy more clearly to the forefront of their work together. It has been our experience that when no limits are set, families and therapists often develop a mutually satisfying relationship that they are reluctant to relinquish. Such therapy can, and often does, drag on for long periods to the seemingly mutual enjoyment of all concerned but usually without any demonstrable relationship between length of therapy and effectiveness of results. In family therapy, as in other forms of psychotherapies, there has been as yet no evidence that long-term therapy is more effective than time-limited treatment (Gurman & Kniskern, 1978).

Frequently, holding the family members to a limited number of sessions communicates to them that the therapist is confident of their ability to work at effecting change. This approach tends to emphasize the strengths rather than the weakness of the family and often leads to a quick reduction of the doubt and anxious tension often experienced when they first come for treatment. Family comments on termination of treatment, such as "the fact that you felt you could treat us in so few sessions was really a relief which helped us to regroup and get on with it" support this view. We believe that, whenever it is felt that treatment should continue beyond 12 sessions, a reevaluation of the treatment situation should take place and, if possible, a consultation should be sought. Obviously, there are times when the therapy has been going well and requires more sessions because of the complexity of the issues being dealt with or the fact that important new problems have arisen that have to be resolved. In our experience, these situations are much rarer than the cases where the therapy has gotten off track and become bogged down for various reasons. This may be due to inexperience of the therapist, but even experienced and skillful therapists can get caught in a pathological family system. Putting a time limit on the number of sessions, with a request for consultation and discussion built into such limits, is a very useful mechanism for all concerned.

Our concern for the cost-effectiveness of treatment is an important factor involved in our advocacy of limiting the number of therapy sessions. Long-term multiple sessions are very expensive financially as well as an exorbitant use of limited skilled resources.

Lastly, it should be clear that even upon termination, the family members are encouraged to call upon the therapist at any time they may wish in the future. In our experience, this is rarely abused and is a very helpful way of maintaining contact over the years. This approach allows us to act as real "family doctors" for the families we work with.

The macrostages are assessment, contracting, treatment, and closure (Table 1). Each stage contains a sequence of substages, the first of which is always orientation. A major problem in clinical work is that practitioners often take too much for granted and suppose that patients know what to expect and what we are doing. The effect of this is to dehumanize patients, not because we as professionals are unsympathetic, but because we unjustifiably assume a knowledge and understanding on the part of the patients about the way we work. From the moment the family members come in, we repeatedly orient them to what we are doing and seek their permission and agreement before proceeding

TABLE 1. Stages and Steps in Problem-
Centered Systems Therapy of the Family

Assessment
1. Orientation
2. Data gathering
3. Problem description
4. Clarification and agreement on a problem list

Contracting
1. Orientation
2. Outlining options
3. Negotiating expectations
4. Contract signing

Treatment
1. Orientation
2. Clarifying priorities
3. Setting tasks
4. Task evaluation

Closure
1. Orientation
2. Summary of treatment
3. Long-term goals
4. Follow-up (optional)

from one step to another. This is done out of our respect for the families we work with and our belief in their right to know exactly what is going on at all times. Furthermore, we believe that therapy can be more effective when the families are fully aware of and in agreement with what is being done. We do not believe in conducting therapy when these conditions are not present.

The orientation to the assessment stage is quite detailed and sets the tone and direction of therapy. All later orientations are much briefer and are used to indicate a change in the focus and task. We do not use orientation to allow for an easier and later interpretation regarding the violation of explicit expectations or rules. However, the family's agreement with the summary at the end of each stage does allow us to confront later resistance by reiterating the family agreement previously obtained up to that point.

After a general orientation, each substage needs to be approached systematically, with the therapist guiding the process. At the conclusion of each step, the therapist and family also need to review and reach agreement on what has been accomplished before moving on to the next stage. As we review each stage, the goals and methods for assessing achievement will be discussed.

Assessment Stage

The first major stage is assessment, consisting of four steps: (1) orientation, (2) data gathering, (3) problem description, and (4) clarifying and agreeing on a problem list. During the assessment stage, we are concerned with orienting the family to the beginning of the treatment process, identifying and detailing the structure, organization, and transactional patterns of the family, and carefully elucidating all the problems that currently exist. The current problems consist of the presenting problem, as well as those that are identified during the course of a careful and complete assessment. Before proceeding with "therapy," we believe that it is mandatory that we understand the family system and its problems and strengths as fully as possible. The diagnostic workup must be thorough and complete before the treatment is prescribed, much less embarked upon.

The fact that this statement must be frequently repeated and even defended is a sad comment on the current practice of family therapy. We believe that the usual procedure—(followed by many if not most practitioners)—of running off in all directions to do "therapeutic battle" at the beginning of therapy before doing a comprehensive assessment is not only unscientific and bad clinical practice but is most unethical. It is unethical in our opinion because of the important potential life commitments involved in the undertaking of treatment by a family. The changes frequently resulting from family therapy—positive as well as negative—involve radically different family orientations, interactions with each other and people outside the family, behavior, life-style, and so forth. Elements such as marital separation or divorce, children leaving home, power shifts, and the like within the family should never be taken lightly even if welcomed by all family members. Only following a thorough, comprehensive assessment can these possibilities even be considered with some degree of objectivity. That family members should obviously be helped to be aware of these possibilities by the therapist in the course of the assessment and later in the contracting phase should certainly be a minimal ethical expectation. For a family to be manipulated into a situation as complex as family therapy without such awareness and the opportunity to make an informed decision based upon as much data as possible should never be an acceptable possibility. Knowing the potential outcome, many families might exercise their right to refuse therapy despite the therapist's contrary opinion.

We consider not conducting a full assessment to be unscientific and bad clinical practice because we cannot conceive of beginning treatment before we are aware of what all the problems are. The surgical analogy would be to make an incision in the general area of the pain—and to "poke around" with the possibility of finding the true source(s) of the problem(s).

A most surprising but welcome clinical finding resulting from our thorough approach to assessment has been the degree to which it facilitates the therapy process and leads to more satisfactory outcomes. We find that in many cases the thorough assessment stage actually seems to achieve 90% of the healing process and leaves little to be done after it is completed in order to achieve a satisfactory outcome. This pleasant and serendipitous finding seems to be due to several factors. When the assessment stage is properly executed, it brings about an extremely satisfactory and fruitful "engagement" process with the family that seems to induce the family members into very active collaborative functioning throughout treatment. The assessment procedure filters out the poorly motivated and strongly reinforces the positive motivation for treatment where it is present—even in highly latent form.

In uncomplicated cases, the family problems become so clearly defined by a good assessment procedure that the well-motivated families quickly become aware—often spontaneously with minimal, if any, input by the therapist—of the steps that need to be taken to achieve satisfactory problem resolution and on their own initiative go on to develop and achieve the actions necessary.

In "simple" uncomplicated cases, beginning therapists can achieve a satisfactory assessment following the model. On the other hand—the model enables sophisticated and experienced therapists to assure themselves of a well-defined, thorough, and comprehensive evaluation.

The therapist should take as many sessions as necessary to complete a full assessment. The number of assessment sessions required will vary with both the therapist's expertise and the nature of the family problems. Beginning therapists can be expected to take longer in the assessment stage, whereas advanced therapists may also take longer with more complex problems and families.

If further time is needed to complete the assessment stage when a session comes to an end, we summarize our findings to that point and clarify that we require more information before a decision is reached regarding diagnosis and treatment. Assessment should, however, be active, and we seldom space the sessions more than a week apart at this stage. On the other hand, most families appreciate that relatively longer-standing problems can wait for completion of the assessment.

When confronted with a family emergency or acute crisis, a different and much more active intervention is called for. Appropriately dealing with immediate issues delays the full assessment in such cases, but, once the crisis has been settled, it is important to return to and complete the full assessment stage before proceeding on to other stages of the model.

When seeing a family for the first time, we prefer to have present all the family members living at home. We also include others living in the home and may subsequently include significant extended family and outsiders who are actively involved with the family. This allows us to obtain a full range of views, resulting in a clear, comprehensive assessment of the situation, an indication of potential allies and supports, and direct observation of parent–child and sibling interactions, and enables us to clarify the general future course of action for everyone. We either set a separate session for the parents or have the children wait outside when assessing the parents' sexual relationship.

Again, there are some exceptions. In cases of significant emergency, we vigorously attempt to have everyone present but will not refuse a beginning initial assessment solely on the grounds of all members not being present. Reasonable medical illness and the inability of an acutely psychotic individual to participate without major disruption are other exceptions.

When a significant member, such as a spouse or the identified patient, fails to show for an appointment, the situation obviates against open and collaborative assessment and must, therefore, be dealt with directly by confronting the difficulty before beginning. We also insist that members who are a focus of discussion attend, so that if issues involving them arise they will be present for discussion.

When no emergency exists and a significant member has not shown up, we will sometimes cancel the session, pointing out that it makes no sense to begin the process without the presence of such an important member. We let the family members know that should they really want our help it is their job to bring the absent member and that we would be glad to give them another appointment.

All exceptions require careful consideration. However, our experience is that the therapist's confidence, clarity, sensitive understanding and intervention usually result in the desired members' being present for the first assessment.

The model also allows for a therapist knowledgeable in several conceptual models to translate the data being gathered into any one of these models if it is so desired. Although we generally utilize a systems-oriented, largely behavioral, and cognitive approach in our work, occasionally we may process the data gathered within a more psychodynamic, psychoanalytic model to give ourselves another viewpoint of the problems being investigated. This does not mean that we will necessarily share this formulation with the family. We simply find it may occasionally improve our understanding of the case and thereby facilitate the treatment procedure while following our model. An example of this is a case currently in treatment under supervision of one of us. The family presented with the wife suffering from a most severe obsessive-compulsive disorder. When this family was assessed following our model, it was found that there was severe pathology in each of the family dimensions. The family agreed to and understood the complete details of the malfunctioning as well as the positive findings elucidated in the course of assessment. The latter included the couple's love for each other, the husband's devotion, loyalty, and concern, and the wife's genuine conscious desire for relief and restoration of the couple's relationship to the mutually satisfactory level attained prior to the onset of her illness. The couple and therapist focused on tasks in the task-setting stage of therapy that if carried out would help them resolve the problems generated by the symptomatic behavior. A psychodynamic interpretation of this patient's condition led to the formulation that the patient's symptoms were the expression of an underlying sexual conflict and served to help her avoid the feared sexual contact with her husband. Although these concepts undoubtedly added another dimension to the usual behavioral, phenomenological, and cognitive approach utilized within our model and enriched our understanding of the case, their utilization in the form of interpretation might be quite redundant and unhelpful. Indeed, this couple had been treated for several years prior to coming to our clinic by a therapist who utilized the psychoanalytic approach to no avail. Although our approach may ultimately yield no more satisfactory results than the previous attempts—at the time of this writing, the couple seemed to be making changes in their functioning never achieved with the previous therapeutic approaches.

Many family therapists use a potpourri of conceptual models in their conduct of family therapy—much of it undisciplined and at times "wild." Others such as Will and Wrate (1985) developed an approach composed of a number of conceptual models in a well-thought-out, disciplined manner. We differ from the latter groups in our belief that such a theoretical melange is unnecessarily complex, mostly redundant, and clinically often quite unhelpful, and at times harmful when literally applied in the actual therapy situation. We argue that utilization of other models to improve one's understanding of complex cases and/or to facilitate movement in a "blocked" therapy situation is quite justifiable—but that complexity and redundancy without purpose other than gratifying our need for intellectual and theoretical compulsiveness is uncalled for. In our experience, theoretical parsimony and elegance go hand in hand with efficacy.

Orientation

We orient the family by clarifying what each member expects will happen during the session, why they think they are here, how they think the session was arranged, and what they hope will come out of it. This often provides useful information and helps to avoid later resistance.
    Example:

T: I'd like to find out from each of you what you thought was going to take place here today? Okay, I'd also like to know why you think all the family is here? And, I'd like to know what you'd like to see come out of this session: What do you particularly want to see addressed or have an answer to?

We condense and feed back their ideas and then briefly outline our ideas, including why we understand the family is there, what we already know about them in general, what we plan to do, and what we hope to achieve. At this time, we obtain their permission to proceed. We also explain our rationale for seeing them as a family.
    Example (after summarizing the family's understanding and expectations):

T: Fine, now I have your ideas, let me explain mine. I asked you all to come in because I need to have a clear idea of how you function as a family. This gives me a much clearer understanding of the entire picture and so helps me to work out with you how things can be more helpful for John and all of you. I know you have concerns about John's getting upset and being hard to manage. That obviously affects all of you and not just John. Part of the reason it is important for me to meet with all of you and understand how you function is that I know that the way a family functions and operates strongly influences what happens to each family member. If that's not the case, then serious events affecting one individual member will also affect the family and the way it operates. So, for both of those reasons I need to have a clear picture of how you function as a family before deciding on possible treatment. I'm going to jump around a bit to find out about your family and ask a number of questions in a range of areas. Some may seem quite unrelated to John's problem, but they're important for me to know about. I'll clarify as I go along to make sure that I have a correct impression of how you operate as a family. At this point, I don't know where we're going to go. At the end of this session, however, I will summarize where we seem to be at that point. Do you have any questions? . . . Is that okay, then? . . . Can we go ahead with my finding out more about your family?

Data Gathering: Presenting Problem(s)

During this step, data is gathered about (1) the presenting problem(s), (2) overall family functioning, (3) additional investigations, and (4) other problems.

The therapist begins by asking the family to describe the problem(s) that brought them to treatment. Sufficient time is spent in gathering data so that the therapist develops an accurate picture of the nature and history of each problem. In doing so, the therapist explores the factual details, the affective components of the problem, the historical perspective, the precipitating events, and who is mainly involved with the problem and how.

An example will help. John's teacher's calling about his problems, what the teacher said, and the mother's observation of John's withdrawal and increased disobedience would be factual details. Mother's reaction of frustration and later helplessness, father's being furious at John and at mother for not disciplining him, and John's feeling guilty and sad would be effective components. Information that the problem began 6 months ago, got better for a short while, and then deteriorated further shows historical components. Father's having changed his job about that time is an example of a precipitating event, and John's just entering adolescence is a developmental issue.

In detailing the presenting problem, we also utilize appropriate dimensions of the McMaster model (Epstein et al., 1978). For example, in the the previously mentioned presenting problem, we would also explore how the family has attempted to solve the difficulty, how they communicated about it, and the behavior control issues (see later).

In doing such an exploration of the presenting problem, other issues may arise and be defined as difficulties. (In addition to the presentation of John "as the problem," this stage of evaluation might also uncover that mother feels father is not supporting her in dealing with any of the children, the father does not feel that she understands his situation, and that John recognizes conflict in Mom and Dad, tells no one, and takes off.)

We then feed back to the family our understanding of the presenting problem and make sure that everyone feels we have a clear picture about it. We do this for each problem by feeding back condensations of our understanding. Haley has also supported the need to obtain a clear picture of the presenting problem (Haley, 1976).

Example (after a detailed exploration of the presenting problem):

T: At this point I'd like to make sure that I'm seeing things correctly. We seem to agree that (1) John has been harder to manage, particularly for you, Mom. John, you and your sister both notice Mom and Dad disagreeing, but this upsets you more than your sister, and you take off, which gets you into even more trouble. (2) You, Mother, feel your husband has not been supporting you—not just with John but also in dealing with the other children, and (3) Dad, you've been down because of changes at work and don't feel your wife is understanding of that. The effect is you feel you're failing not just in the work area but also as a husband and father. All of this has recently developed within the past 6 months and was not the case previously and Dad's job change seems to be the biggest stress associated with it all. Do I have it right to that point?

Data Gathering: Overall Family Functioning

This next step moves from an assessment of the presenting problem to an exploration of overall family functioning. We first orient the family to this change in focus:
Example:

T: Okay, now I'd like to switch to some general ideas of how you operate as a family. It that all right?

Using the McMaster model, the family is assessed on the six dimensions of problem solving, communication, roles, affective responsiveness, affective involvement, and behavior control. This assessment focuses on detailing strengths and difficulties in each dimension and allows us to determine aspects of overall family functioning that influence the emotional and/or physical health of family members.

This assessment is based on family member reports. However, the therapist confirms the impressions gained in this manner by observation of behavior in the session and by confronting and clarifying contradictions between stated information and observed behavior and between information offered by different family members. The therapist's impressions are condensed and fed back until the family agrees that an honest appreciation of the family's functioning in that area has been obtained. The therapist should be careful to gather firm evidence to support any hypotheses before putting them forward to the family as opinion. If the practitioner has a strong hypothesis (clinical hunch) but can gather no confirmatory evidence, it should be presented to the family as just that, a hunch or an impression, and they should be asked for their opinion as to the validity of the impression. This approach prevents the therapist from taking off into flights of fantasy without evidence, yet allows for the testing of clinical hunches while exercising clinical intuition. It also engenders confidence and respect on the part of the family for the therapist's objectivity, impartiality, and respect for data. Further, it reinforces the role of the family members as participants in the treatment process. If there is substantial disagreement, but the therapist has sufficiently clear data to make an accurate judgment, the therapist makes a statement such as, "Okay, you (we) disagree in this area, so let's agree it is at least problematic in that regard and move on to another area I wish to explore."

The important point is that this stage focuses on assessing overall family functioning and helps to avoid developing formulations based only on data related to the presenting problem, data that by their nature are more likely to be negative. The assessment is approached tactfully, directly, and honestly. We explain carefully what we are doing, and all issues are discussed openly. As we examine each dimension, we feed back to the family members our understanding of both their assets and shortcomings in that particular area. We emphasize strengths, because this is helpful and supportive, as well as being central to any therapeutic planning that may follow.

The clinical use of each dimension has been extensively detailed in a previous publication (Epstein, Bishop, & Baldwin, 1981, pp. 455–467) and will not be repeated here. Readers are urged to refer to the previous presentation. The dimensions are summarized herein in Table 2.

The McMaster model provides a useful conceptual framework for understanding the functioning of clinically presenting families and for assessing their effectiveness on each dimension. We cannot overemphasize the need to do such a careful exploration as part of the assessment process. Assessment of families on each of these dimensions is clinically useful in two ways. First, it allows the therapist to assess areas of strength in contrast to the more negative picture gained by only looking at the presenting problem. These areas of strength can be utilized in the therapy. Second, exploration of these dimensions often turns up significant family problems other than those identified when only the presenting problem is considered. The fuller assessment allows the therapist to be more aware of problems that will be operative during the course of treatment.

The next step of data gathering is to consider the need for additional investigations.

Data Gathering: Additional Investigations

Use of the "systems approach" in family therapy extends the factors considered in the assessment and diagnostic process. As the Group for Advancement of Psychiatry (1970) pointed out, the family's behavior can be influenced by factors at numerous levels, such as the physical universe, the biological systems involved, the intrapsychic status of the individuals concerned, small groups, in this instance, the family, the extended social system, and the values existing at that time and place. The diagnostic workup, therefore, comprises, in addition to what has previously been described, the necessary individual psychological and biological studies as well as those studies of the family's broader social system such as the extended family, school, place of work, patterns of social recreation, and the like. Such additional investigations are basic to comprehensive work. Failure to make this point explicit has often led to the erroneous impression that a systems approach does not involve data obtained from such investigations.

The data gathered in the family workup to this point determines the further specific investigations to be carried out. They might include any or all of the following procedures. In the case of children, these procedures include developmental history, pediatric examinations including all necessary laboratory and X-ray studies, biopsychosocial assessment of child, intelligence, and other psychological investigations. For the adults, there could be psychosocial history and

TABLE 2. Summary of Dimension Concepts

Dimensions	Key concepts

Problem solving	—Two types of problems: Instrumental and affective
	—Seven stages to the process:
	  1. Identification of the problem
	  2. Communication of the problem to the appropriate person(s)
	  3. Development of action alternatives
	  4. Decision of one alternative
	  5. Action
	  6. Monitoring the action
	  7. Evaluation of success
	
	Postulated
	—Most effective: When all seven stages are carried out
	—Least effective: When cannot identify problem (stop before stage 1)

Communication	—Instrumental and affective areas
	—Two independent dimensions:
	  1. Clear versus masked
	  2. Direct versus indirect
	—Above two dimensions yield four patterns of communication:
	  1. Clear and direct
	  2. Clear and indirect
	  3. Masked and direct
	  4. Masked and indirect
	
	Postulated
	—Most effective: Clear and direct
	—Least effective: Masked and indirect

Roles	—Two family function types: Necessary and other
	—Two areas of family functions: Instrumental and affective
	—Necessary family function groupings:
	A. *Instrumental*
	  1. Provision of resources
	B. *Affective*
	  1. Nurturance and support
	  2. Adult sexual gratification
	C. *Mixed*
	  1. Life skills development
	  2. Systems maintenance and management
	—Other family functions: Adaptive and maladaptive
	—Role functioning is assessed by considering how the family allocates responsibilities and handles accountability for them.

(continued)

TABLE 2. (Continued)

Dimensions	Key concepts
	Postulated
	—Most effective: When all necessary family functions have clear allocation to reasonable individual(s) and accountability built in
	—Least effective: When necessary family functions are not addressed and/or allocation and accountability not maintained.
Affective responsiveness	—Two groupings: Welfare emotions and Emergency emotions
	Postulated
	—Most effective: When full range of responses are appropriate in amount and quality to stimulus
	—Least effective: When very narrow range (one to two affects only) and/or amount and quality is distorted, given the context.
Affective involvement	—A range of involvement with six styles identified:
	1. Absence of involvement
	2. Involvement devoid of feelings
	3. Narcissistic involvement
	4. Empathic involvement
	5. Overinvolvement
	6. Symbiotic involvement
	Postulated
	—Most effective: Empathic involvement
	—Least effective: Symbiotic and absence of involvement
Behavior control	—Applies to three situations:
	1. Dangerous situations
	2. Meeting and expressing psychobiological needs and drives (eating, drinking, sleeping, eliminating, sex, and aggression)
	3. Interpersonal socializing behavior inside and outside the family
	—Standard and latitude of acceptable behavior determined by four styles:
	1. Rigid
	2. Flexible
	3. Laissez-faire
	4. Chaotic
	—To maintain the style, various techniques are used and implemented under role functions (systems maintenance and management)
	Postulated
	—Most effective: Flexible behavior control
	—Least effective: Chaotic behavior control

formulation, psychiatric examination, medical history and physical examination, all the necessary laboratory and radiological studies, and psychological assessments as appropriate. Neurological investigations are becoming even more important as investigative technologies such as CAT, MRI, and PET scanners are becoming increasingly sophisticated and available. Neuropsychological workups have also become increasingly helpful and utilized.

Data Gathering: Other Problems

Finally, in concluding the data-gathering step, we ask if there are any other significant problems or difficulties that we have not touched upon. If there are, these are explored in appropriate detail.

Problem Description

The purpose of this step is to develop a list of problems. First, the family members are asked to indicate the problems they would identify now that a detailed assessment has been completed. The therapist then adds any additional difficulties he has noted. The list should highlight the major issues but be comprehensive.

Problem Clarification

The final step in the assessment process is to obtain partial or complete agreement regarding problems listed by the family and/or therapist in the problem description step. The family usually agrees to the list if the therapist has been active in clarifying and obtaining agreement during evaluation of the presenting problem and dimensions of family functioning and in the feedback of the results of other investigations.

Two types of disagreements can arise. First, family members may disagree among themselves, in which case the therapist can attempt to negotiate a resolution, reopen the area for further exploration and clarification, or obtain a temporary "agreement to disagree." If the problem differences are relatively minor, the therapeutic process can go on and, usually, the differences will resolve themselves in the course of the work. An example of this type of situation might be where one parent may feel the child is lazy and performing very badly at school, whereas the other parent feels the child is showing behavior normally appropriate for his/her age. This usually resolves itself as the work goes on and the family members become more collaborative and understanding of each other. However, if the differences regarding the child's behavior extend more deeply into basic and wider disagreements as to values related to child rearing and goals for the children, these could lead to an impasse further along in the therapy process.

The second type of disagreement that can occur is between the family and the therapist regarding the problems added to the list by the latter. Here again, if the therapist considers the differences relatively minor in importance as far as the central therapeutic issues are concerned, he or she may decide to come to an "agree-to-disagree" solution for the moment and return to them later in the therapy process. If the therapy has gone well, these disagreements usually dissolve almost automatically in the course of dealing with the more important issues and rarely have to be dealt with again. An example of this type of disagreement is that of a family where the father drinks moderately heavily and there is disagreement between the family and therapist on the degree of this drinking and its effect on the family. If this is not the central issue and the problem drinking is not too severe, the therapy can go on if the therapist shelves the disagreement. When the therapy goes well, the question of the father's drinking invariably comes up and is usually resolved by the family without any disagreement and with the father's participation. Rarely do the initial differences of opinion of this type have to be formally brought forward.

If the case were one in which the father's alcoholism was severe and a marked factor in the family problems such as violence, disruption, personal difficulties, and the like, disagreement between the family and the therapist on the presence and importance of this issue would be basic and would preclude the continuation of the therapy process beyond this point. Were the therapist to "agree to disagree" in this case, he or she would merely be colluding with the existing pathological family system, and this would obviate any successful therapy. The disagreement would have to be resolved at this point by the family's accepting the problem as is, or they would have to withdraw from the therapy process at this time with the option of resuming the procedure should they change their mind.

At times, in cases of basic disagreement, the areas may be reexplored, or the family may be asked to think about them for some time at home and return later for more discussion. With continued disagreement, the family might be offered the possibility of consultation with another therapist rather than termination at that point.

The assessment stage ends when mutual agreement is reached on a problem list. We cannot emphasize strongly enough the importance of basing such a listing on a full, thorough, and comprehensive history before embarking on therapeutic interventions. Treatment should not begin without a full knowledge of the problems and strengths existing in the family.

Contracting Stage

The second macrostage is contracting. Its goal is to prepare a written contract that delineates the mutual expectations, goals, and commitments regarding therapy. The steps in this stage are (1) orientation, (2) outlining options, (3) negotiating expectations, and (4) contract signing.

Orientation

The first step is to orient the family to the tasks in this stage and obtain their agreement to proceed.

Example:

T: If those are the problems, let's move on to discuss what you might or might not do about them. Is that okay with you?

Options. We then outline the treatment options that are open to the family, which will vary according to the situation.
   Example:

T: You have a number of options. You may choose to not do anything about the problems we've listed and make no changes. I'm sure you will hope that things will improve somehow, but they may also stay the same or get worse as a consequence of that choice. The second option is to try and work on changing the difficulties on your own now that we've clarified them. Third, you may decide that you want a different kind of treatment not involving all of you. The difficulty there is that you've all agreed that family issues have a part to play so that option would be a bit like trying to balance the books with only half the figures. But it is an option you have. A fourth option is that we agree to work together and deal with the problems as a family. Which option seems best to you?

For each option, it is the therapist's responsibility to clarify what his or her function, if any, might be (some of the options would require no input from the therapist), and to explore the possible consequences of each alternative. Obviously, if somebody is significantly depressed and suicidal, the options and consequences are quite different than if the problem is minor in nature.
   If the family chooses treatment, we then proceed to the next step. If any of the other options are chosen, they are handled appropriately.

Negotiating Expectations

Family members are asked to negotiate among themselves what they will want from each other (i.e., how they want each to change) if they are to feel they have been successful in treatment. The family is given the major responsibility for defining their expectations, whereas the therapist's responsibility is in clarifying and helping family members to express their expectations in concrete behavioral terms to allow for clearly identifying and assessing progress.
   The therapist monitors the process so that unrealistic goals such as wishing "to never again fight" are moderated into more reasonable statements like, "to be able to disagree and get angry but resolve the problem without a physical fight." Examples of expectations are shown in Figure 1, a sample treatment contract.
   The therapist may make suggestions that might be included in their negotiations and also indicates his or her own expectations, including the commitment that all of the family will attend each session. The family is also given the approximate number of sessions that are anticipated with the proviso that this can easily be changed should the situation call for it.

Family: ___Smith___   Date: ___11/27/78___

Problems	Family Expectations and Goal
1. John's behavior at home and school.	1. No negative reports from school and positive reports at home.
2. Father not supporting mother with children.	2. Mother will report that father and she satisfactorily share dealing with children.
3. Father does not feel wife understands his situation.	3. Father reports he feels involved and that his wife and he can comfortably discuss his work problems.

THERAPIST EXPECTATIONS

1. All family members will attend.
2. The family will call in advance if unable to attend.
3. The family will work hard.

SIGNATURES

Family _____

_____

_____

Therapist _____

FIGURE 1. A sample family treatment contract.

We insist that all members of the family be present for the data-gathering and contracting stages. As a general rule, we prefer that all members participate in the total treatment process. Obviously, this is not always possible for various reasons, such as illness and absolutely necessary absences of some members, and so on. There are also some situations where it is clinically advisable to see only some of the members and to exclude others. This would include sessions when the focus is on the sexual life of the parental couple. The therapeutic values and ethics and the therapist's judgment must be relied upon at other times when a decision is to be made regarding exclusion of some of the members. It is our experience that, except when the parental sexual relationship is being discussed, the need to exclude members occurs very rarely. Despite the concern of some, it is rare that members of the family (at whatever age) are hurt significantly by exposure to the family therapy process.

There are many reasons for including all members in the therapy. Because the basic aim of the therapy is to modify the total system of the family, all the members are involved whether they like it or not. Even members not directly involved may be extremely helpful to the therapy process in the informal roles of co-therapists or auxiliary therapists. (Indeed, this is one of the basic strengths of family therapy. It trains family members to be therapists and more effective problem solvers within their own family.) The presence and participation of all members allows the therapist to better evaluate the change process in the system as a whole.

Contract Signing

We then establish a written contract (see Figure 1) that lists the problems and specifies for each what has been agreed to as a satisfactory outcome. In addition, the negotiated conditions of treatment are included. The contract is signed by the therapist and the family members. It is emphasized that most of the work will be done by the family, but at the same time it is made clear that we, too, will work hard. We do not tolerate a dilatory approach, either by ourselves or by our patients!

Treatment Stage

The third macrostage is treatment, consisting of four steps: (1) orientation, (2) clarifying priorities, (3) setting tasks, and (4) task evaluation.

Orientation

Again, the first step is to orient the family to the new stage and to obtain their permission to proceed. We do this with a statement such as, "Well, now that we have agreed to work together, how would you like to begin?"

Clarification of Priorities

This step involves ordering the problem list according to the family's priorities. We establish which problems they wish to tackle first, second, and so on, in order. Though we prefer to follow the order established by the family, we would have the therapist actively intervene to change the priority list if the family ignored urgent problems demanding immediate action (anorexia, suicide potential, severe alcoholism, etc.). Allowing the family to set the priority list reinforces the general emphasis for our approach, that is, giving as much of the responsibility for the therapeutic work as possible to the family. We repeatedly make it clear that we do not consider the family to be passive partners in the therapeutic process.

Setting Tasks

Taking their first priority, the therapist asks the family to negotiate and set a task, which if carried out during the next week would represent a move in the direction of meeting their expectations. This negotiation includes identifying individual responsibilities with regard to the task. If the family is unable to do this, the therapist suggests a task and checks to see if it is agreeable to the family.

In negotiating and assigning tasks, the following general principles need to be considered:

1. The task should have maximum potential for success.

2. The task should be reasonable with regard to age, sex, and sociocultural variables.
3. Tasks should be oriented primarily toward increasing positive behaviors rather than decreasing negative ones. Families often ask someone to stop a behavior rather than asking him/her to do something. We prefer to request positive actions.
4. A task should be behavioral and concrete enough so that it can be clearly understood and easily evaluated.
5. A task should be meaningful and important to everyone involved.
6. Family members should feel that they can accomplish the task and they should individually commit themselves to carry out their part.
7. Emotionally oriented tasks should emphasize positive, not negative, feeling. Fighting, arguing, and open display of hostility should be strongly discouraged.
8. Tasks should fit reasonably into the family's schedule and activities.
9. Overloading should be avoided. A maximum of two tasks per session is usually reasonable.
10. Assignments to family members should be balanced so that the major responsibility for completing a task does not reside with just one or two members.
11. Vindictiveness and digging up the past should be avoided, with the focus placed on constructive dealings with current situations.

These principles are made explicit to the family in the form of instructions or suggestions when necessary. For example, if one spouse wants the other spouse to "stop nagging" (violation of principle 3), we would respond with a statement such as, "I'm sure you do and can understand that, but it's harder to ask someone to stop doing something than to start to do something. So what would you like your husband to do in the next week that would give you the sense that he is trying and that would begin to help in solving the problem?"

Examples:

Using our previous case of John and his family, we can indicate an example of negotiated tasks that follow the previously mentioned principles.

A 16-year-old son agrees to come in by an agreed-upon time; the father agrees to take the son to a ballgame later in the week if he does well and to deal with the son if he is late; the mother agrees to back the father and send the son to him as well as agreeing to spend more time with the 15-year-old daughter, who agrees to keep her room tidy.

Examples of other family tasks are the following:

Father will take mother out once; mother agrees to go even if she does not want to; the older son agrees to baby-sit, and the younger brother agrees to behave. A couple agrees to set aside 15 minutes after supper to talk about "good things," and the children agree to clear the table and do the dishes.

Once tasks have been assigned, it is important and valuable to designate a family member to monitor and report on performance at the next therapy session. Designating a monitor increases the involvement of the family, increases expectations regarding their sense of responsibility and accountability, and rais-es individual self-esteem. The role of the monitor may be rotated among members or may vary with the tasks (e.g., one member reports on one task and someone else on another). The role of the monitor should be given to members who are most objective, not actively involved in the area being dealt with, and most likely to keep the family at the task. We have not experienced any particular difficulties with this role.

Task Evaluation

During this step we assess whether or not the task was accomplished. Information is obtained from the monitor and other appropriate family members as necessary. If the task was accomplished, we provide positive reinforcement, highlighting the positive aspects of the family's performance, including what particular individuals did which made things go so well.

Example:

T: Well, how did the tasks go? . . . Okay, so _____ got done but _____ didn't. Is that right? We'll come back to the difficult one in a minute, but first what made the other go so well? Can you tell me what each of you did to help that go well? What did others do that made it easier for you to do your part? That's very good, and I'm sure you're pleased. Okay, let's return to the area you had difficulty with.

We would then explore with questions such as: What was the problem? Did nothing get done, or did you do part of it? Were you aware of thinking about it? What could others do that would make it possible? Do you think it's possible to do it? Do you agree that if the task were carried out it would make things better?

If there is a major block, the therapist should cycle back to the original assessment discussions and clarify that there was agreement regarding the problem and then renegotiate a related task. Perhaps the task was too difficult for this stage of treatment, and the family and therapist should generate a simpler task having to do with the same problem. In general, after checking on the successfully accomplished tasks, the family and therapist then move on to negotiate the next task.

If all goes well, the process of task setting and evaluation continues, at times negotiating new priorities, at times recontracting, until all contract expectations have been fulfilled.

If a family fails to complete its tasks and/or demonstrates no improvement over a period of three successive sessions, we share our feelings with the family that there is need for serious stocktaking. We indicate that, perhaps without being aware of it or without informing the therapist, they have changed their chosen option from the stated one of family therapy to the option of no treatment. We then give them an opportunity to formalize the change if so desired. If the family members insist they still want family treatment, we point to the fact that they do not seem to be working at their tasks and that perhaps there is something wrong with the treatment process or the therapist's handling of the case, and a consultation is therefore indicated. Should the family reject the suggestion for consultation, we then recommend termination of therapy because we have adequate evidence of failure, and there is no point in denying it while continuing to spin our wheels in a charade of the treatment process.

Acute situational disturbances in previously well-functioning families do well with this approach. However, at this stage of our studies we can make no definitive statements about which therapist skills, family problems, or degrees of dimension ineffectiveness are most predictive of success or failure in our treatment approach. Hopefully, we will be able to gather accurate answers as our research continues into the future. At present, we have only soft clinical impressions as partial answers to the questions. We feel problem severity is as yet an unreliable predictor of outcome in any given case. We are continually surprised by positive outcomes in cases that at intake appeared hopeless.

We feel that the success of outcome in most cases directly reflects the degree of rigor and thoroughness that the therapist maintains in family sessions. This includes following the principle of keeping the family actively involved in working with the therapist at each step of all the stages. The therapist must learn to function as a thorough assessor, evaluator and diagnostician, clarifier, investigator, catalyst, facilitator, and, at times, a confronter. The major responsibility for treatment is given to the family while the therapist remains intensely involved in the treatment process. The therapist must not need to feel so omnipotent that he or she cannot delegate the responsibility for working on its own problems to the family and cannot terminate therapy when there is ample evidence the family is not working adequately to resolve its problems. The family should be aware at all times that the therapist expects full commitment to change. We do not believe in "seducing" the family into a state of positive motivation. Families can always return for another trial of therapy at some future time should their motivation to change increase. We have had many positive experiences terminating some families on this basis and then having them return spontaneously at a later time ready to work hard at change they are more prepared to handle. There is no ill will generated in such terminations, and they are left with the assurance that they can contact us any time they change their mind. This is further evidence that we respect their opinions, values, goals, and objectives whereas, at the same time, making it clear we respect our craft to the point of not wanting to participate in "sham" therapy or merely going through the motions of a therapeutic process that continues interminably without evidence of successful change. We believe that by developing these skills and approach, therapists can look forward to quite successful outcomes.

Closure Stage

The final stage is closure, consisting of four steps: (1) orientation, (2) summary of treatment, (3) long-term goals, and (4) follow-up (optional).

Orientation

As an orientation to treatment termination, we point out that the family expectations, as set forth in the contract, have been met and that perhaps we should stop now.

If the family wants more therapy, we are willing to explore the issues or problems they wish to deal with and consider continuing. Although treatment might occasionally continue, most of the time families should be encouraged to resolve the new issues they want to work on by themselves. They should be encouraged to get in touch with the therapist any time they so desire. At such a time, the therapist could decide whether to see them again for another session or not, depending on the situation.

Summary of Treatment

The family members are asked to summarize what has happened during treatment and what they have learned. We then confirm or elaborate on their perceptions, adding any points that may have been overlooked.

Long-Term Goals

At this point, we ask the family to discuss and set some long-term goals. We also ask them to identify how they will recognize if things are going well or badly, and what they will do if the latter occurs. We then ask them to identify those issues that they anticipate might either come up or become problematic in the future. The family is reinforced regarding their ability to cope with such problems, whereas at the same time the option of returning to obtain help is clarified.

Follow-Up

Therapy ends at this point, although an optional follow-up appointment may be arranged. When a follow-up is arranged, it is scheduled far enough into the future to allow the family a full opportunity to deal with issues as they arise. It is also stressed that the follow-up visit is for monitoring and is not a treatment session.

Conclusion

We hope we have presented our approach in adequate detail to at least whet the appetite of other therapists as yet unfamiliar with it and thereby encourage them to investigate this approach further and to include it in their therapeutic armamentarium.

References

Ackerman, N. W. (1958). *The psychodynamics of family life*, New York: Basic Books.
Ackerman, N. W. (1966). *Treating the troubled family*, New York: Basic Books.
Bateson, D., Jackson, D. D., Haley, J., & Weakland, J. (1956). Towards a theory of schizophrenia. *Behavioral Science, 1*, 251–264.

Berman, E. M., & Lief, H. I. (1975). Marital therapy from a psychiatric perspective: An overview. *American Journal of Psychiatry, 132,* 583–592.

Bishop, D. S., & Epstein, N. B. (1979). *Research on teaching methods.* Paper presented at the International Forum for Trainers and Family Therapists, Tavistock Clinic, London, England.

Bishop, D. S., & Epstein, N. B. (1980). Family problems and disabilities. In D. S. Bishop (Ed.), *Behavioral problems and the disabled* (pp. 337–364). Baltimore: Williams & Wilkins.

Brody, E. M. (1974). Aging and family personality: A developmental view. *Family Process, 13,* 23–37.

Cleghorn, J., & Levin, S. (1973). Training family therapists by setting learning objectives. *American Journal of Orthopsychiatry, 43,* 439–446.

Comley, A. (1973). Family therapy and the family physician. *Canadian Family Physician, 19,* 78–81.

DeWitt, K. N. (1978). The effectiveness of family therapy: A review of outcome research. *Archives of General Psychiatry, 35,* 549–561.

Epstein, N. B. (1958). Concepts of normality or evaluation of emotional health. *Behavioral Science, 3,* 335–343.

Epstein, N. B. (1963). Pratiques nouvelles dans le traitement de l'enfant et de la famille. *Service Social,* 12(1&2), 159–164.

Epstein, N. B., & Bishop, D. S. (1973). State of the Art—1973. *Canadian Psychiatric Association Journal, 18,* 175–183.

Epstein, N. B., & Bishop, D. S. (1981). Problem-centered systems therapy of the family. *Journal of Marital and Family Therapy, 7,* 23–31.

Epstein, N. B., & McAuley, R. G. (1978). A family systems approach to patients' emotional problems in family practice. In J. H. Medalie (Ed.), *Family medicine: principles and applications,* (pp. 223–229). Baltimore: Williams & Wilkins.

Epstein, N. B., & Westley, W. A. (1959). Patterns of intra-familial communication. *Psychiatric Research Reports 11,* American Psychiatric Association, 1–9.

Epstein, N. B., Bishop, D. S., & Levin, S. (1978). The McMaster Model of Family Functioning. *Journal of Marriage and Family Counseling, 4,* 19–31.

Epstein, N. B., Levin, S., & Bishop, D. S. (1976). The family as a social unit. *Canadian Family Physician, 22,* 1411–1413.

Epstein, N. B., Rakoff, V., & Sigal, J. J. (1968). *The family category schema.* Unpublished manuscript. Jewish General Hospital. Department of Psychiatry. Montreal.

Epstein, N. B., Bishop, D. S., & Baldwin, L. M. (1981). Problem-Centered Systems Therapy of the Family. In A. Gurman & D. Kniskern (Eds.), *Handbook of family therapy* (pp. 444–482). New York: Brunner/Mazel, 1981.

Glick, I. D., & Haley, J. (1971). *Family therapy and research: An annotated bibliography of articles and books published 1950–1970.* New York: Grune & Stratton.

Group for the Advancement of Psychiatry. (1970). *The field of family therapy, Report 78,* Volume 7.

Gurman, A. S., & Kniskern, D. P. (1978). Research on marital and family therapy: Progress, perspective and prospect. In S. L. Garfield & A. E. Bergin (Eds.), *Handbook of psychotherapy and behavior Change: An empirical analysis* (2nd ed.) (pp. 817–901). New York: Wiley.

Gurman, A. S. & Kniskern, D. P. (Eds.) (1981). *Handbook of family therapy,* New York: Brunner/Mazel.

Guttman, H. A., Spector, R. M., Sigal, J. J., Rakoff, V., & Epstein, N. B. (1971). Reliability of coding affective communication in family therapy sessions: Problems of measurement and interpretation. *Journal of Consulting and Clinical Psychology, 37,* 397–402.

Guttman, H. A., Spector, R. M., Sigal, J. J., Epstein, N. B., & Rakoff, V. (1972). Coding of affective expressions in conjoint family therapy. *American Journal of Psychotherapy, 26,* 185–194.

Hadley, T. R., Jacob, T., Milliones, J., Caplan, J., & Spitz, D. (1974). The relationship between family developmental crisis and the appearance of symptoms in a family member. *Family Process, 13,* 207–214.

Haley, J. (1971). A review of the family therapy field. In J. Haley (Ed.), *Changing families: A family therapy reader* (pp. 1–12). New York: Grune & Stratton.

Haley, J. (1976). *Problem-Solving Therapy,* San Francisco: Jossey-Bass.

Hill, R. (1965). Generic features of families under stress. In H. N. Parad (Ed.), *Crisis intervention: Selected readings* (pp. 32–52). New York: Family Services Association of America.

Hoehn-Saric, R., Frank, J. D., Imber, S. D., Nash, E. H., Stone, A. R., & Battle, C. C. (1964).

Systematic preparation of patients for psychotherapy. Effects on therapy behavior and outcome. *Journal of Psychiatric Research, 2,* 267–281.

Kardiner, A. (1939). *The individual and his society.* New York: Columbia University Press.

Kardiner, A., Linton, R., DuBois, C., & West, J. (1945). *The psychological frontiers of society.* New York: Columbia University Press.

Langsley, D. G., & Kaplan D. M. (1968). *The treatment of families in crisis.* New York: Grune & Stratton.

Liddle, H. A., & Halpin, R. J. (1978). Family therapy training and supervision literature: A comparative review. *Journal of Marriage and Family Counseling. 4,* 77–98.

McClelland, C. Q., Staples, W. I., Weisberg, I., & Bergin, M. E. (1973). The practitioner's role in behavioral pediatrics. *Journal of Pediatrics, 82,* 325–331.

McFarlane, A. H., Norman, G. R., & Spitzer, W. O. (1971). Family medicine: The dilemma of defining the discipline. *Canadian Medical Association Journal, 105,* 397–401.

McFarlane, A. H, O'Connell, B., & Hay, J. (1971). Demand for care model: Its use in program planning for primary physician education. *Journal of Medical Education, 46,* 436–442.

Minuchin, S., & Barcai, A. (1969). Therapeutically induced family crisis. In J. H. Masserman (Ed.), *Science and psychoanalysis, Vol. XIV, Childhood and Adolescence* (pp. 199–205). New York: Grune & Stratton.

Olson, D. H. (1970). Marital and family therapy: Integrative review and critique. *Journal of Marriage and the Family, 32,* 501–538.

Orne, M. T., & Wender, P. H. (1968). Anticipatory socialization for psychotherapy: Method and rationale. *American Journal of Psychiatry, 124,* 88–98.

Parad, H. J., & Caplan, G. (1965). A framework for studying families in crisis. In H. J. Parad (Ed.), *Crisis intervention: Selected readings* (pp. 53–72). New York: Family Service Association of America.

Parsons, T. (1951). *The social system.* Glencoe, IL: Free Press.

Parsons, T., & Bales, R. P. (1955). *Family socialization and interaction process.* Glencoe, IL: Free Press.

Patriarche, M. E. (1974). Finding time for counseling. *Canadian Family Physician, 20,* 91–93.

Postner, R. S., Guttman, H. A., Sigal, J. J., Epstein, N. B., & Rakoff, V. (1971). Process and outcome in conjoint family therapy. *Family Process, 10,* 451–473.

Rakoff, V., Sigal, J. J., Spector, R., & Guttman, H. A. (1967). *Communications in families.* Paper presented on investigation aided by grants from Foundations Fund for Research in Psychiatry, Laidlaw Foundation.

Rapoport, L. (1965). The state of crisis: Some theoretical considerations, In H. J. Parad (Ed.), *Crisis intervention: Selected readings* (pp. 22–31). New York: Family Service Association of America.

Santa-Barbara, J., Woodward, C. A., Levin, S., Streiner, D., Goodman, J., & Epstein, N. B. (1977). Interrelationships among outcome measures in the McMaster Family Therapy outcome study. *Goal Attainment Review, 3,* 47–58.

Santa-Barbara, J., Woodward, C. A., Levin, S., Goodman, J., Streiner, D., & Epstein, N. B. (1979). The McMaster Family Therapy outcome study: An Overview of methods & results. *International Journal of Family Therapy, 1,* 304–323.

Sigan, J. J., Rakoff, V., & Epstein, N. B. (1967). Indicators of therapeutic outcome in conjoint family therapy. *Family Process, 6,* 215–226.

Solomon, M. A. (1973). A developmental, conceptual premise for family therapy. *Family Process, 12,* 179–188.

Spiegel, J. (1971). *Transactions.* New York: Science House.

Stanford, B. J. (1972). Counseling—A prime area for family doctors. *American Family Physician, 5,* 183–185.

Tomm, K. M. (1973). A family approach to emotional problems of children. *Canadian Family Physician, 19,* 51–54.

Tomm, K. M., & Wright, L. M. (1979). Training in family therapy: Perceptual, conceptual, and executive skills, *Family Process, 18,* 227–250.

Watlzlawick, P., Beavin, J. H., & Jackson, D. D. (1967). *Pragmatics of human communication.* New York: W. W. Norton & Company.

Weakland, J., Fisch, R., Waltzlawick, P., & Brodin, A. M. (1974). Brief therapy: Focused problem resolutions. *Family Process, 13*, 141–168.

Wells, R. A., Dilkes, T. C., & Trivelli, N. (1972). The results of family therapy: A critical review of the literature. *Family Process, 11*, 89–107.

Westley, W. A., & Epstein, N. B. (1960). Report on the psychosocial organization of the family and mental health. In D. Willner (Ed.), *Decisions, values and groups* (Vol. 1) (pp. 278–303). New York: Pergamon.

Westley, W. A., & Epstein, N. B. (1969). *The silent majority.* San Francisco: Jossey-Bass.

Will, D., & Wrate, R. (1985). *Integrated family therapy: A problem-centered psycho-dynamic approach,* London: Tavistock.

Woodward, C. A., Santa-Barbara, J., Levin, S., Goodman, J., Streiner, D., Muzzin, L., & Epstein, N. B. (1974). *Outcome research in family therapy: On the growing edginess of family therapists.* Paper presented at the Nathan W. Ackerman Memorial Conference, Margarita Island.

Woodward, C. A., Santa-Barbara, J., Levin, S., & Epstein, N. B. (1978a). The role of goal attainment scaling in the evaluating of family therapy outcome. *American Journal of Orthopsychiatry, 3*, 464–476.

Woodward, C. A., Santa-Barbara, J., Levin, S., & Epstein, N. B. (1978b). Aspects of consumer satisfaction with brief family therapy. *Family Process, 17*, 399–407.

Zuk, G. H. (1971). Family therapy during 1964–1970. *Psychotherapy: Theory, Research and Practice, 8*, 90–97.

18

Short-Term Marital Therapy

R. Taylor Segraves

Considerable evidence documents that the quality of intimate interpersonal relationships is related to one's subjective sense of well-being and that the presence of intimate relationships may aid in the ability to withstand life stress (Segraves, 1982). It is also clear that marital disruption is a severe stress for most individuals (Bloom *et al.*, 1977) and is associated with a higher incidence of suicide (Weissman, 1974), homicide (Carter & Click, 1976), alcohol abuse (Bachrach, 1975a,b,c), accidental death (Gove, 1973), and the use of mental health services. On most indexes of psychopathology, the divorced and separated score higher than their married, never married, or widowed counterparts (Segraves, 1980). Other research has suggested that the "protective" function of marriage is related to the quality of the marital relationship and that the unhappily married may resemble the recently divorced in terms of their psychological turmoil (Renne, 1971). Various hypotheses have been put forth to explain the consistent findings of strong associations between marital status and psychiatric morbidity. Current evidence suggests that a large part of this association is due to the protective influence of intimate interpersonal relationships, social networks, and kinship networks that occur in marriage (Segraves, 1982).

Given the high divorce rate in the United States and the disruptive influences of marital discord and separation on the individuals involved, it appears that there is a clear need to provide effective interventions for couples experiencing serious discord. The frequent lack of third-party reimbursement for the provision of marital therapy mandates the development of brief therapies. Unfortunately, most graduate programs in the mental health field provide minimal training in the provision of marital therapy (Martin & Lief, 1973; Prochaska & Prochaska, 1978). This lack of training in marital therapy may partially reflect the absence of an adequate conceptual model for marital interventions.

Marital therapy has been described as a therapy without a theory (Manus, 1966), although it can best be described as consisting of numerous partial theories, which either focus on observable behavior or upon inferences about internal cognitive emotional events within the marital partners (Segraves, 1978).

R. Taylor Segraves • Case Western Reserve University and Metrohealth Systems, 3395 Scranton Road, Cleveland, Ohio 44109.

Three major theoretical systems—general system theory, behavioral marital therapy, and psychoanalytic theory—have influenced the practice of marital therapy. Each of these systems offers the clinician a set of explanatory concepts and a suggested format for interventions. The major theoretical schisms appear to be between those schools that focus on the direct modification of observable behavior (e.g., behavioral, general systems) and those that focus on putative internal psychological events (e.g., psychodynamic). The degree of possible overlap between the various theoretical approaches is obscured by the absence of common terminology and by polemical disputes between representatives of the various schools (e.g., Gurman & Knudson, 1978; Jacobson & Weiss, 1978). In the recent past, a similar situation existed within the field of individual psychotherapy, and the scientific literature contained similar polemical arguments (Breger & McCaugh, 1965; Eysenck & Rachmam, 1965). However, numerous individual psychotherapists have shown a willingness to attempt to bridge concepts from differing schools of thought in order to attempt to build a unified approach to psychotherapy, which encompasses both observable behavior and inner psychological events (e.g., Hunt & Dyrud, 1968; Segraves, 1986; Wachtel, 1977). The author feels strongly that a similar blending of therapeutic approaches is required in the field of marital therapy. In the marital context, the therapist needs to consider both past and present determinants of discord, individual and interactional contributions, and the interplay of maladaptive behavior patterns with internal representational systems to be maximally effective. In addition, the therapist must be able to flexibly intervene at both the observable interactional level as well as at the inner psychological level.

The purpose of this chapter is to describe a theoretically integrative approach to the short-term treatment of marital discord. This approach can be described as a sequentially integrative cognitive behavioral approach to the treatment of chronic marital discord and is based on the assumption that the goal of therapy is twofold: (1) to disrupt the repetitive maladaptive behavior patterns, and (2) to dislodge the internal schemata maintaining such patterns. This chapter will proceed by first describing the basic assumptions upon which the therapy is based and then to selection criteria, therapeutic objectives, assessment, and a description of the therapeutic process itself.

Basic Assumptions

A key concept in understanding the author's approach to short-term marital therapy is the viewpoint that marital difficulties are not substantially different from other types of interpersonal conflicts for which individuals seek psychotherapy. In this context, the goals of marital therapy are similar to the goals of individual psychotherapy. For example, in many forms of interpersonal individual psychotherapy, the therapist attempts to identify dysfunctional attitudes, cognitions, and behavior patterns that interfere with the patient's interpersonal adjustment with significant individuals in his or her life and to teach the patient alternative strategies of interpersonal interaction. In psychoanalytically oriented psychotherapy, the therapist interprets the irrational attitudes, cognitions, and behavior patterns that the patient displays toward the therapist in the "transference reaction." The implicit assumption of this form of psychotherapy is that correction of these cognitive-emotional distortions (resolution of the transference neurosis) will enable patients to recognize their propensity to interpersonal distortions and thus transfer this new learning to interpersonal contexts outside of the therapeutic situation. In marital therapy, the therapist has the unique opportunity to observe individual interactional difficulties in a meaningful relationship that freely evolved in the natural environment. The observational base is somewhat more complex in marital therapy in that the maladaptive behavior patterns often exist in both spouses and that certain maladaptive interactional patterns appear to have a life of their own.

It appears reasonable to assume that one's pleasure in a marital relationship is partially dependent on the spouse's behavior toward oneself. It is also reasonable to assume that one's behavior toward a spouse is a major determinant of that spouse's behavior to oneself. It also appears reasonable to assume that one's past experiences will influence one's perception of the spouse and thus one's behavior toward that spouse. Within this viewpoint, marital conflict offers the therapist an opportunity to observe the interaction between inner representational worlds and observable behavioral patterns. By necessity, the therapist is forced to attend to the past history and individual psychopathology of each spouse as well as to the evolved dysfunctional interactional pattern in the marriage. Thus the marital therapist is forced to consider data encompassed by both psychodynamic and behavioral schools of thought.

The author's approach to the conceptualization of chronic marital discord is based upon a number of assumptions held explicitly or implicitly by many integrative psychotherapists, family therapists, and cognitive social psychologists. The first assumption is that dysfunctional interpersonal schemata for the perception of intimate members of the opposite sex are of primary importance in both the genesis and maintenance of chronic marital discord. In other words, individuals have predispositions to organize perceptions of intimate others in characteristic ways, and these internal representations of significant others are instrumental in determining one's behavior toward others. This assumption is clearly analogous to the concepts of schema, interpersonal template, and personal construct system introduced by social psychologists such as Kelly (1955), Stotland and Canon (1972), and Carson (1969). This concept is also similar to the psychoanalytic concept of transference. Numerous psychoanalytic therapists have hypothesized that maladaptive behavior patterns are related to transference distortions (Kaplan, 1976; Offendrantz & Tobin, 1975). Transference distortions can be redefined in the language of cognitive social psychology as learned expectations from significant others and the carryover of this to new relationships (Segraves & Smith, 1976). Many psychoanalytically oriented marital therapists have observed that the significant transference reactions in marital discord manifest themselves between spouses rather than to the therapist (Gurman, 1978; Meissner, 1978; Nadelson, 1978; Sager, 1967). In other words, many experienced psychodynamically oriented marital therapists have observed that dysfunctional and inaccurate perceptions of the mate's character and intentions underlie severe marital discord. Analytic therapists have tended to assume that such distorted expectations can only be corrected by interpretation. For this reason, the author prefers the term *schemata*. This concept derived from cognitive social psychology assumes that faulty inner representational systems can be corrected by disconfirmatory life experiences in a variety of contexts. As mentioned in the preceding paragraph, the interactional problems encountered in marital therapy are not substantially different from those encountered in individual psychotherapy or group therapy. It is assumed that individuals have patterns of disturbed interpersonal behavior that manifest themselves in various contexts and theoretically can be modified in various contexts. In most forms of individual psychotherapy, one hopes that the learning within the therapeutic context will then transfer to relationships in the world outside of the therpist's office. The advantage of marital therapy is that the new learning occurs within a significant relationship in the patient's life. Indeed, certain patients appear to have quite successful professional and social relationships and to have their disturbed interactional patterns restricted to ongoing intimate relationships such as marriage or intensive psychotherapy.

The second major assumption of the author's model is that individuals have inner representational models for significant others and tend to behave toward others in such a way as to invite behaviors that are congruent with that schemata. This hypothesis clearly implies that patients partially create their own interpersonal universes by the effects of their behavior on significant others. Leary (1957) described how certain eliciting interpersonal behavior has a high probability of being self-sustaining because of its effects of eliciting confirmatory behavior from others. He gave an example of a 30-year-old man who entered group therapy complaining of depression, social isolation, and that no one cared for him. Within eight sessions, this patient had reproduced his microcosm by provoking the other group members into critical, unsympathetic behavior toward him. Other social psychologists have made similar observations and have proposed similar mechanisms (Carson, 1969; Stotland & Cannon, 1972). Theorists as dissimilar as Bandura (1977) and Wachtel (1977) have spoken about how certain interpersonal behavior can be self-sustaining by its tendency to encourage self-confirmatory reactions from others. Such observations have also been noted by analytically oriented therapists, such as Offenkrantz and Tobin (1975) who spoke of the self-fulfilling interpersonal prophecies of the neurotic, and Kaplan (1976) who remarked on the tendency of patients to "repeatedly provoke the analyst to react in a manner similar to past object relations." Other analytic therapists such as Selwyn Brody, have noted how spouses elicit self-confirmatory behavior from one another:

> While the wife feels unloved and has never felt consistently loved, she compensates by romantic day-dreaming of an ideal lover. The more the husband feels rejected, the more recalcitrant he is about modifying careless—even repulsive personal habits which readily justify some of his wife's behavior. In effect, while contemptuously blaming him, she successfully provokes him to remain as he is. (Brody, 1961, pp. 100–101)

The third major assumption is that in cases of chronic marital discord, the discord itself plays a crucial role in maintaining the individual psychopathology of each of the spouses. Thus there is a reciprocal linkage between inner representational reality and observable behavior such that the recurring maladaptive interactional patterns are largely responsible for maintaining individual psychopathology in each of the spouses. The actual behavior of the spouse is confirmatory to the spouse's distorted view of interpersonal reality and thus contributes to its permanence. The therapeutic corollary of this assumption is that repetitive observation of spouse behavior that is discrepant with the inner representational model for that spouse will result in a change in the representational model. This assumption is clearly compatible with the cognitive psychology assumption that faulty cognitions can be disproven by discongruent life experiences. It is similar to the family therapy concept of acting in (Ackerman, 1966) and the concepts of integrative psychotherapists such as Wachtel (1977), Birk and Brinkley-Birk (1974), and Marmor (1971) that the development of new patterns of behavior that are incongruent with the usual defensive structure will lead to intrapsychic change.

This last assumption forms the basis of the brief cognitive/behavioral model of marital therapy to be described. If one assumes that the maladaptive behavior patterns observed in marital discord are the result of one or both spouses attempting to influence the other to act in accord with the inner representational model for the opposite sex, it then follows that the primary goal of therapy is both to dislodge the confirmatory behavior patterns and to modify the fixated misperceptions. Thus the initial thrust of therapy is to reduce the congruence between inner representational systems and the actual behavior of marital partners. One can restate the goal of therapy in a different language system by saying that the goal of therapy is to arrange a cognitive/behavioral disproof of transference distortions. If significant pathology is present in both spouses; the disproof of the transference distortion may need to be bilateral.

The theoretical assumptions previously discussed are illustrated in Figure 1. This schematic illustrates the reciprocal interaction between inner representational events and maladaptive behavior as well as the multiple levels of possible intervention.

SELECTION CRITERIA

The selection criteria for this approach are relatively straightforward. This approach was designed for the treatment of marital discord in which characterological issues in one or both spouses are presumed to be etiologically significant. Couples with an identifiable recent precipitant for their discord (e.g., death of child) are excluded from this model as far simpler approaches may suffice. Newlyweds are similarly excluded as their turmoil may represent a normal phase in their evolving a satisfactory marriage contract. In general, the discord must be chronic (at least 6 months in duration) for this model to be employed.

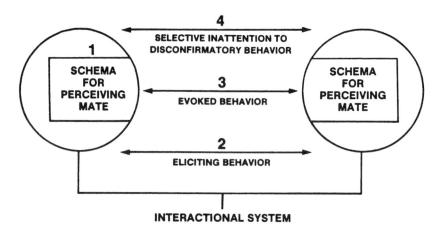

FIGURE 1. Schematic of theoretical assumption. Interpersonal discord is conceptualized as maladaptive person–environment interaction that can be disrupted in various ways. The therapist can attempt direct change of the schema (interpretation, cognitive relabeling, discrimination training), modification of eliciting behavior, or modification of the evoked behavior. Modification of the interactional system would include reciprocity training and communication training.

This arbitrary distinction is made to exclude transitory disturbances that do not involve character pathology.

Another inclusion criteria is commitment to the relationship. In cases of severe marital turmoil, threats of divorce are common, and commitment to the relationship may not be readily verbalized. For this reason, some basic behavioral requirements are used: (1) both spouses are living in the same household; (2) there are no currently active extramarital affairs—if so, this affair must be terminated completely until the termination of therapy; and (3) there are no currently active steps toward separation or divorce—if so, these actions must cease until the conclusion of therapy.

The most difficult inclusion criteria to evaluate are the couple's ability to tolerate uncertainty, rapid changes in behavior and perceptions, and intense emotion. The author's model involves a rapid and unrelenting attempt to disrupt long-standing behavior patterns and usual ways of perceiving the mate. In some patients, the pace of this therapy may be more than they can tolerate. The fleeting perception of the spouse as a potentially safe companion and the experience of adult bonding may be extremely disruptive emotionally. In my experience, this situation will manifest itself early in therapy by failure to follow suggestions or premature termination in therapy.

Structure of Therapy

The therapeutic model is structured for 15 to 20 hour-long sessions, typically occurring at weekly intervals. The time limit is set for a 20-session maximum as the goal of therapy is to foster healthy interdependence between the spouses, rather than dependence on the therapist. These guidelines are not absolute. On rare occasions, the session length may be extended to 90 minutes. This typically occurs with extremely intelligent couples with restricted expression of affect. With such couples, the therapist may need a longer observation period to decipher the specific maladaptive patterns in operation. On very rare occasions, the 20-session maximum may be waived if the couple appears to be making genuine progress but at a slower pace than most couples.

Except in unusual circumstances, all sessions are conjoint. There are several reasons for this approach: (1) the therapist is interested in continually monitoring the couple's interactional pattern, (2) individual historical data are important to this treatment approach only to the extent that they affect the current interactional difficulty, (3) the therapist wants to foster greater communication between the spouses, and (4) this is an attempt to avoid the problems of "secrets" shared by one spouse with the therapist. Similar to all rules of psychotherapy, the conjoint-only rule is also broken on occasions. If the attempt to obtain information concerning the couple's history is problematic and the therapist feels that one spouse is withholding information, individual sessions may be scheduled. The other situation in which individual sessions might be utilized is when one spouse strongly suggests such, and the other spouse does not object. Certain patients apparently feel safer sharing particularly painful memories (i.e., childhood molestation) first with the therapist and then the spouse. At the conclusion of individual sessions, the therapist will usually request that this newly divulged information be introduced into the conjoint session. This is especially true if one spouse is seriously considering an extramarital affair or divorce. If the "guilty" spouse refuses to divulge this information to the spouse, the therapist makes a decision as to whether or not maintaining the secret will interfere with the work in couple therapy. If so, the clinician may elect to tell the couple that she or he cannot in good conscience proceed with therapy. In actuality, such situations are rarely encountered as the "guilty" spouse is usually thankful to have a safe context in which to bring up the forbidden subject. If the situation involves a past affair of which the spouse is truly unaware, the therapist may elect not to press for a confession with the spouse. In such situations, the therapist suspects that the probable harm may outweigh any probable benefits.

This therapeutic approach has been employed both with a dual-sexed co-therapy team and with a single therapist of either sex. For practical reasons, the single therapist model is almost universally employed. The dual therapy model is occasionally used for training new therapists, but financial considerations limit its use. Another difficulty with the dual therapy model is the importance of the relationship between the co-therapists. In the author's experience, marital therapy has a unique propensity to evoke strong emotions in the therapists and to evoke a tendency to choose sides. Unless the co-therapists have a good working relationship, there is tremendous potential for destructive influence from co-therapists rivalry or disagreement.

The disadvantage of the single therapist approach is that one sex may feel that the therapist does not really comprehend the position and problems of the opposite sex. This can usually be circumvented if the therapist is quite active in verbalizing an understanding of each spouse's perspective.

GOALS OF THERAPY

The primary goal of therapy is to reduce interpersonal discord and to modify dysfunctional schemata regarding intimate relationships with the opposite sex such that the couple can have the experience of a safe, mutually pleasurable, pair-bonding experiencing. In couples in which a mutually pleasurable pair-bonding experience is unrealistic, a minimal goal of therapy is for the couple to experience periods of nontumultuous interaction and a realistic perception of the other spouse's character. Even if the couple decides to dissolve the relationship, it is crucial that the separation be from real individuals rather than from distorted perceptions of the mate. In other words, individuals experiencing discord frequently have fixated and limited perceptions of their foe's personality and intentions. The goal of therapy is to broaden that perception to a more realistic perception. For example, a wife in a dysfunctional marriage may state with conviction that her husband "has no feelings." In many cases, a more realistic description of the husband might be that of a man who is unskilled in the verbal expression and acknowledgment of affective states and who questions the importance of such behavior. With assistance, such a man can often be helped to realize the importance of such behavior for his spouse and assisted in the learning of such behavior. Although such an individual may never achieve the same skill in verbal expression of emotions as someone raised in a household that fostered such behavior, he can be taught at least rudimentary skills. In turn, his spouse can be taught to appreciate her husband's different way of handling and expressing emotions. She can also be helped to increase her recognition of his expression of emotion, which may be terse, indirect, or stated in a monotone. If this couple recognized their differences without antipathy and decided that their interpersonal priorities might be more easily achieved with alternative partners, the therapeutic goals of this model would be satisfied.

A secondary goal of therapy is to educate both members of the couple as to their unique predispositions to fall into disruptive interactional patterns and ways to circumvent such patterns in the future. For example, the woman who stated that her husband has no feelings can be taught to recognize her tendency under duress to perceive her husband as unfeeling. She can be taught to recognize his expressions of emotion and to reinforce his attempts at emotional expression. She can be taught to recognize how her angry outbursts at her husband for not expressing his feelings contribute to his difficulty and reticence to attempt such behavior. In other words, she can be taught how her behavior unwittingly decreases the behavior in her husband that she overtly desires. In other words, she is made fully aware of how she is partially responsible for the behavior of her husband toward her. The husband can be shown how his lack of emotional expressiveness contributes to his wife's anger and be specifically instructed to increase such behavior. It is unlikely that brief therapy will be successful in eliminating long-standing behavior patterns. Thus, each spouse is informed that under times of stress in the future, that here is a high likelihood of reverting to previous patterns. In couples in which divorce or separation appears likely, each member of the couple will be rehearsed in his or her unique contribution to interpersonal discord such that he or she may recognize and be able to self-correct such behavior in future relationships.

Certain individuals in troubled marriages enter therapy with the expressed goal of saving the marriage. In such situations, the therapist expresses hope that the relationship will persist but that the overt goal is not to save the marriage at all costs. The therapeutic goal is to reduce discord and to allow the couple to realistically appraise each other as partners and to independently decide the future of their relationship.

It should be clear by this point that the goal of this therapy is to modify the marital relationship. Individual psychopathology, relationships with families of origin, and other issues are addressed only to the extent that they are relevant to this goal.

The model of mental health underlying the treatment goals of this model is the assumption that successful pair bonding with an intimate other serves a protective function versus psychiatric impairment. It is assumed that psychiatric impairment is the result of biological vulnerability interacting with environmental stress and that interpersonal connectedness serves a protective function against such impairment. Although extended social and kinship networks also serve protective functions, it is assumed that pair-bonding with an intimate other is a major source of such stability.

ASSESSMENT

The demarcation between assessment and treatment sessions is seldom clear. In many couples, assessment will coexist with initial treatment interventions until the therapist has a clear formulation of the problem. In emotionally distant couples, formulation of the difficulty may require observation of the couple's response to initial therapeutic maneuvers.

The goals of assessment are (1) to observe the couple's interactional behavior, (2) to form provisional hypotheses concerning the behavior's maintaining the interactional problem, (3) to form provisional hypotheses concerning the cognitive contributions to the interactional difficulty, (4) to obtain provisional information concerning the best ways to interrupt the dysfunctional interactional pattern and the couples' capacity for change, and (5) to gather information regarding each spouse's capacity for change, and any special assistance required by each spouse. The therapist begins by asking the couple to describe their difficulty, its duration and onset, and their opinions regarding its etiology. As the therapist elicits information concerning the marital difficulty as experienced by the couple, he or she listens on multiple levels. The actual verbal description of the conflict may be of less importance than direct observation of the couple's interactional style. For example, the therapist observes who speaks first and dominates the conversation, at the same time noting the quiet spouse's reaction as the first spouse speaks (i.e., attentive listening, bored inattention, facial grimaces indicating disagreement, etc.). The practitioner also observes each spouse's characteristic response to hearing unpleasant things being said about him or her (i.e., passive withdrawal, verbal obfuscation, open warfare, indirect putdowns, etc.). At this point, the therapist begins to form hypotheses concerning the forces maintaining the marital discord. For example, it may be observed that one spouse voices his or her wishes in an angry authoritative style and that the other spouse repeatedly agrees with the first spouse verbally while expressing disagreement by voice tone or gesture. such an interactional style can generate an interactional impasse with each spouse silently concluding that effective interaction with the other spouse is impossible. In this example, the eliciting behavior to be changed is the first spouse's authoritative manner of expressing a desire for behavior change from his or her mate. The confirming behavior to be modified is the second spouse's passive noncompliance. Another interactional problem targeted for change is each spouse's unwillingness to confront the issue of his or her inability to resolve differences by open discourse and negotiation.

At the same time that the therapist is identifying dysfunctional interactional patterns specific to this couple, she or he searches for information concerning the perceptual distortions maintaining and being maintained by the interactional sequence. For example, the therapist may wonder why this husband continued to order his wife to do certain things when it is clear that his interactional style is seldom effective with her. It is reasonable to assume that this man does not feel that his wife would respond to simple requests from an equal partner. Further information concerning this hypothesis consists of the husband's statement that his wife is similar to his mother who dominated and ruined his father. Additional information is provided when the husband in a frustrated rage states, "She's impossible. She's defiant, controlling, and cold." Thus a provisional hypothesis that the husband sees his wife as dangerously powerful and controlling is obtained from (1) inferences from interactional data, (2) descriptions of past interactions with members of the opposite sex, and (3) the husband's actual verbal descriptions of his spouse. This assessment approach is analogous to the psychoanalytic assessment described by Menniger (1958) and Malan (1976) when behavior is assessed in the current therapeutic context (i.e., transference), the distant past, and in current relationships outside of therapy. The crucial difference in the marital therapy context is that the transference and current relationship both involve the spouse. Feelings evoked in the therapist (countertransference) are of less significance in the marital therapy content as most of the emotional intensity is directed toward the spouse. The authoritative husband is unaware of how his behavior evokes confirmatory behavior from his spouse while she meets his demands with passive noncompliance, reinforcing his view of her as uncontrollable and defiant.

The therapist also wonders why this otherwise competent woman reacts to her authoritative husband with passive noncompliance rather than open disagreement. Noting that she holds an executive position in a medium-sized business, the therapist postulates that her interactional deficit may be restricted to her intimate relationships with men. He suspects that this woman has a fear of confrontation with her husband and may be afraid of his anger. He learns that her father had an explosive temper and had struck her on numerous occasions when she had disagreed with him. Subsequently, he hears her say that much of their marital life could be peaceful if only her husband learned to control his temper. She continually describes her husband as explosively angry at times when the therapist perceives her husband as irritated or frustrated. When asked directly if her husband has ever struck her, she answers that he has not yet but has come close on numerous occasions. When pressed for examples, she recalls her husband pounding the refrigerator door and looking as if he wanted to hit her when he learned of her past affair with a friend of his. She states that she has seldom gotten her way in the marriage because of her husband's temper. At this point, it is reasonable to conclude that she views her husband as a powerful man with an explosive temper and that her estimation of his explosiveness is exaggerated. It is also reasonable to conclude that this cognition relates to her style of passive defiance and that her failure to directly disagree with her husband reinforces her perceptual distortion of him. She is unaware of how her passive noncompliance contributes to her husband's resorting to authoritative demands and to his frustration (and thus, her fear of his anger).

At this point, the therapist has a set of hypotheses concerning the perceptual distortions in each spouse, how these perceptual distortions interact, and how these distortions are related to the observable interaction. He or she has various therapeutic options available and can begin to test the marital system to find its weak points. For example, he or she could attempt to get the husband to try a different way of obtaining what he wants from his wife; he or she could attempt to get the husband to confront his wife's passive noncompliance, or he or she could attempt to get the wife to openly disagree with her husband. Alternatively, he or she could begin to challenge their perceptions of one another. If all of these trial forays fail, he or she could resort to a variation of reciprocity counseling to help the couple to, at least, have the experience of negotiation and compromise on some point, or he or she could use a variation of communication training to help the couple achieve a better understanding of each other as complex human beings. In the actual clinical situation, assessment merges with intervention as the therapist begins testing the marital system for its point of least resistance.

Although the therapist is focusing his or her major attention to their marital problems, he or she is also assessing each spouse's capacity for change and any special support they may require as individuals. For example, if he or she notes that one spouse is especially sensitive to the idea of marital therapy and regards the need to seek professional guidance as a personal failure, the therapist may search for small ways to bolster this spouse's self-esteem. For example, an older businessman regarded seeking help for a younger male professional as a major blow to his self-esteem. In this situation, the therapist's repeated genuine interest in the businessman's accomplishments was sufficient to enable the man to benefit from the therapist's interventions. In another case, a female attorney was especially sensitive to criticism. Thus the therapist continually monitored her emotional reactions (primarily through nonverbal cues) and was extremely careful to phrase his interventions in a manner that would not be perceived as criticism.

Treatment

The phases of treatment can be arbitrarily described as: (1) engagement, (2) nonspecific initial interventions, (3) the cognitive therapy phase, and (4) termination. The goals of the engagement phase of therapy are to establish a working alliance with the couple and to restore hope. It is critical that each spouse feels that his or her problem has been heard and is respected by the therapist. During the early sessions, the therapist strives to give each spouse roughly equal time to present his or her side of the story without undue interruption. After each spouse present his or her viewpoint, the therapist paraphrases what was heard and asks if this is an accurate representation of what was said. If the previously silent spouse attempts to interrupt at this point and to point out the gross distortions of reality by the mate, the therapist politely but firmly instructs the second spouse to be silent ("You had your turn to give your view of the situation. Now I want to devote my full attention to understanding your spouse's view of the problem"); with respect to her insistence that the other spouse is distorting reality, the therapist may say "There is no reality here. There are only your separate perceptions of reality." To make certain that each spouse feels that his or her position has been heard and at the same time maintain neutrality in the dispute, the therapist may begin his paraphrasing of each spouse's position with the statement, "According to your perception . . ." At this stage, the therapist is also particularly careful to be certain that any statements that might be construed as attributing blame are bilateral. For example, if he or she comments that the wife appears to perceive many of her husband's comments as criticisms, he or she would also comment that the husband's style of communication is often unclear and easily misinterpreted. The therapist strives to lower defensiveness ("It's extremely difficult for most couples to resolve these kinds of problems") and to restore hope.

The major thing that the therapist can do to restore hope may be to take control of the interaction and to prevent further escalations of accusations and counteraccusations. Many couples enter therapy, arguing even as they introduce themselves to the therapist. The emotional intensity of such intervention is rarely approached in individual psychotherapy. For example, it is not unusual for the couple to drift into a heated exchange within 10 minutes of first meeting the therapist. In the confusion, the therapist may not even be able to decipher the specific issue being argued. In such situations, the therapist has to be extremely active to take control and prevent escalations and thus prevent further demoralization. As most couples who enter marital therapy are somewhat demoralized by their failure to resolve their difficulties, the therapist may wish to initially make some comment about the problem to be resolved. "One of the major things that I've noted so far is how often the two of you misunderstand each other. We need to note how often the two of you misundertand each other. We need to start working on communication skills." This type of action-oriented feedback can be reassuring to many couples.

NONSPECIFIC INITIAL INTERVENTIONS

The treatment approach of the author has been described as a sequential integrative approach (Johnson, 1986). In the early phases of therapy, the therapist uses procedures developed by behavior therapists in order to gain control of the interaction and to set the stage for cognitive learning. in subsequent phases, the therapist may focus on modifying the dysfunctional behavior specific to the couple. For the reader's convenience, the stages in this sequential intervention model are outlined in Table 1. It is important to emphasize that these stages do not represent a rigid protocol but consist of a general battle plan that is modified to fit each couple's unique difficulty. In certain couples in which the therapist can rapidly target the dysfunctional behaviors to be changed, the interaction stage of therapy may be quite short-lived. Unfortunately, in most couples, the therapist is immediately faced with a baffling complexity of data. Arguments escalate, issues are not resolved, behavior is variously interpreted, and speech is often tangential or obscure. In such situations, the therapist needs to gain control of the interaction before he or she can pinpoint the dysfunctional interactional pattern specific to that couple. Procedures borrowed from communication training and reciprocity counseling programs are ideally suited for this purpose.

Communication training and reciprocity counseling are reviewed in the chapters in this text on brief behavioral marital therapy. Procedures from these approaches are selectively employed in this treatment approach as a nonspecific way for the therapist to gain control of the couple's interaction. In other words, these procedures are used for the express purpose of reestablishing an equi-

TABLE 1. Stages of Therapy

Stage	Technique	Rationale
Interaction	Reciprocity counseling, communication training	Nonspecific modification of current interactional pattern
Eliciting behavior	Label, identify, probable consequence, teach alternative behavior	Modify behavior that elicits confirmatory behavior from spouse
Evoked behavior	Label, identify probable consequence, teach alternative response	Modify confirmatory behavior
Inner-representational	Discrimination training, repetitive emphasis of discrepancy between spouse's behavior and interpretation of that behavior	Disproof of faulty perception

librium or state of relative calm. Once this state is reached, the therapist can better assess the couple's specific difficulties and begin cognitive therapy. The choice of behavioral procedures is individualized for each couple and will vary considerably from couple to couple.

Numerous marital therapists have noted that faculty communication patterns appear to help stabilize dysfunctional interaction (e.g., Satir, 1976; Weiss, Hops, & Patterson, 1973; Gottman, Notarius, Gonso, & Markham, 1976). As the therapist observes the couple's interaction, he or she may readily identify such patterns. Common examples of dysfluent communication include presumptive attribution, incorrect usage of first person plural pronouns, and topic shifting. The therapist can coach the couple into alternative communication patterns as he or she listens to their verbal interchanges. For example, an attempt to achieve change in an interactional pattern can be effectively sabotaged by one or both spouses assuming that they know what the other spouse is really thinking. This type of communication pattern can lead to considerable confusion as to who feels what and can immobilize the interaction pattern. For example, the most difficult couple encountered by this therapist was a married couple in which both spouses were skilled psychodynamic psychotherapists. The wife continually interpreted her husband's hostility as being related to his past relationship with his mother, and the husband interpreted his wife's difficulty with control as being related to her relationship with her father. The only way out of this impasse was for the therapist to say, "You're both right, but it's essentially irrelevant to our solution of your current dispute. What do you want from each other now?" The pattern of presumptive attribution had to be broken for any change to occur. In subsequent interactions, the therapist had to repeatedly block instances of presumptive attribution and to insist that each spouse only speak of his or her own feelings. The accuracy or inaccuracy of their intuited perceptions of one another was not the issue; this style of interaction immobilized the interactional system. A similar type of problem occurs when genuine differences are obscured by one or both spouses speaking for the two of them. For example, a minister and his wife were in therapy, and the therapy was initially deadlocked by the minister continually being the couple's spokesperson. On one occasion, he stated, "Our sex life isn't too great, but we as born again Christians aren't too concerned about that." In actuality, his born-again Christian wife was extremely concerned about their sex life. This situation was handled by the therapist tactfully inquiring from the minister's wife some of the details of their sex life and her feelings about that. Her minister husband seemed genuinely surprised by her comments, and this new information led to the possibility of their open discussion of their sex life. The therapist never directly confronted the minister about the fact that the minister frequently used his assumptions about religious principles to control his spouse. Instead, the therapist coached the wife into expressing her independent feelings and assisted the minister in realizing that his wife frequently had differing opinions from him. Thereafter, the therapist repeatedly but tactfully insisted that the minister not speak for his wife. In other couples, any potential resolution of issues appears to be blocked by frequent topic shifting. Just as the wife begins to feel that a dispute concerning child rearing is about to be resolved, the husband begins discussing his wife's lack of sexual responsivity. In this case, the therapist has to quickly intervene (i.e., "I'm glad that you brought that up. Your sexual interaction is extremely important. But let's solve one problem at a time. For now, we'll discuss your children.") In this case, the therapist defuses the husband's attempted topic shift. If the husband persists in his tactic of topic shifting, the therapist will label such behavior and repeatedly block the husband's attempt to use this tactic to stall resolution of issues.

Modification of expression of anger is critical in the early stages of therapy as escalating battles are counterproductive and demoralizing to the therapist as well as to the couple. A technique that is often useful is to translate terminal blaming statements (which invite retaliation) into requests for change (Hurvitz, 1975). For example, if a wife states that her husband has no feelings, this will most likely elicit a counterattack or denial, both of which stabilize the angry interactional pattern. In such a situation, the therapist might attempt to retranslate this terminal statement into a request for change: "You seem to be saying that you desire greater sharing of feelings between you and your husband. I agree that this is important for your marriage. How can the three of us work together to achieve that?" Subsequently, the therapist will point out that requests for change are more likely to be successful than condemnation of the mate's personality. He or she will then model and have the couple role play alternative style of communication. Similarly, it is important to train the couple to shift from derogatory character descriptions to specific complaints. For example, the statement, "My husband is a selfish son-of-a-bitch," will evoke a different response than "I get angry when he doesn't help out around the house." Another common disruptive pattern are what have been labeled "zings" or indirect putdowns. For example, a husband who is displeased with his wife's sexual responsiveness, rather than confront the issue directly, may suddenly describe how good in bed a previous lover was. Clearly, such a comment will engender defensiveness in the spouse rather than a desire to change her sexual behavior. The principle behind most of these interventions is to have each spouse clearly identify the area of personal displeasure without casting aspersions on the spouse's character. These interventions are employed in the course of interaction as the couple discuss their difficulties. One spouse will use a dysfluent communication pattern, and the therapist will immediately intervene, provoking and/or modeling a different style of communicating. Subsequently, he or she will have the spouse role play the new pattern of communicating.

COGNITIVE THERAPY PHASE

Once a period of relative tranquility has been established in the couple's interactional pattern and the partners are able to discuss their differences without escalations or recriminations, obsessive battling over minor disputes, or incessant verbal diversions and obfuscations, the therapist is ready to begin the cognitive therapy phase. The goals of this phase are twofold: (1) to disrupt the

Table 2. Specific Cognitive Interventions

1. Identify the distorted or incomplete perception of the spouse.
2. Identify eliciting behavior and its probable consequences; teach alternative behaviors.
3. Identify confirmatory behavior; teach alternative responses.
4. Emphasize counterinstances to the fixated perception.
5. Emphasize minimally perceived parts of the spouse's character.
6. Require accurate paraphrasing of the spouse's comments; confront distortions.
7. Use immediate observational disconfirmation when available.
8. Discriminate repeatedly between the spouse's observable behavior and the schema for perceiving the spouse.

behavior patterns that maintain the distorted perceptions of one another's character, and (2) to directly challenge these dysfunctional interpersonal schemata. The major components of this cognitive phase of therapy include (1) disrupting the usual confirmatory elicited and eliciting behaviors, (2) emphasizing counterinstances between the perceived spouse and that spouse's actual behavior, and (3) helping each spouse to begin to experience the multidimensional complexity of the other spouse's personality. For the reader's convenience, the specific steps in this approach are listed in Table 2.

By this point in therapy, the therapist has formed hypotheses concerning the dysfunctional interpersonal schemata involved in the marital discord and how each spouse elicits confirmatory behavior from the other. Thus, the husband who describes his wife as emotionally dependent and insatiable emotionally has been observed to be unusually emotionally reserved and to not give the verbal and nonverbal reassurances common in our culture. For example, the therapist notes that this man rarely compliments his wife and seldom nonverbally acknowledges agreement with her comments. The wife, devoid of any of the usual signs of her loveability, may constantly seek reassurances of her husband's love. This otherwise competent professional woman seems continually to be seeking her husband's approval for trivial matters. Thus the wife's behavior confirms her husband's view of her as dependent and emotionally demanding.

At this point, a verbal interpretation of the husband's tendency to perceive his wife as weak and dependent would be useless as her observed behavior is indeed consistent with that description. What the husband does not realize is how his withholding behavior tends to elicit his wife's seeming insatiable need for reassurance. Without intervention, this couple can easily become stuck in this interactional pattern. Marital therapists of the general systems theory approach have brilliantly described how because of the reactive nature of interpersonal behavior (circular casuality) that one can punctuate this interactional sequence in various ways (Haley, 1963; Lederer & Jackson, 1968). In this instance, we focus on the husband's eliciting behavior of emotional distance. Thus the therapist begins scanning their interaction for aspects of the wife's behavior which the husband silently approves. The therapist knows of the husband's concern with social appearances and that his wife had recently arranged a quite successful dinner party for his business associates. Of course, the husband had never complimented his wife concerning this. The therapist begins inquiring about the party, who was there, how his wife related to his friends, how she appeared, and what his business associates thought of her and the evening. What slowly evolves is a description of a vivacious, strikingly attractive woman whom everyone regarded as quite charming. The therapist then makes the implicit comment explicit, "Gosh, you must be really proud of her." As expected by the therapist, the husband quickly backtracks, pointing out how a few guests arrived before everything was ready and they ran short of brandy before the evening was over, and so forth. At this point, his wife becomes irritated and starts to criticize the husband again as being a cold fish who never appreciates anything. The therapist politely, but firmly, instructs the wife to be silent while he questions the husband's reluctance to be complimentary. Eventually, he drags a thinly disguised compliment from the husband. Again, the wife becomes angry and tries to interrupt, but the therapist again cuts her off saying, "We have to start somewhere. If you demand it all at once, you won't get anything. He's not used to complimenting people. Give him a change."

In a series of similar steps in subsequent sessions, the therapist coaxes the husband into giving his wife genuine compliments while at the same time keeping his wife's anger in bay. He points out to the husband that his series of compliments have not unleashed a massively dependent lioness. In fact, her demand for attention and approval has decreased since her husband has begun to compliment her. He then tries to help the husband realize how his behavior of never giving his wife approval is partially responsible for his wife's apparent insatiable need for approval. To briefly summarize, the therapist first makes the implicit approval explicit by first speaking for the husband. Subsequently, the therapist coaches the husband to spontaneously express approval as well as disapproval of his wife's behavior.

The therapist then focuses on the wife's part of the self-perpetuating cycle. She views her husband as cold and withholding. She is noted to constantly fish for compliments from her husband in a girllike coquettish manner that is repeatedly unsuccessful. She is also noted to ignore or dismiss most of her husband's statements of admiration or approval of her. At other times, she becomes angry that he seldom expresses total approval of her actions. In effect, this woman, although overtly stating her need for admiration and approval from her husband, effectively extinguishes such behavior on his part by not noticing such behavior or being angry that such efforts on his part do not meet her exacting standards. Thus the therapist begins pointing out in each session all of the statements by her husband that imply explicit or at least strongly implicit approval of his wife's behavior and/or actions. The therapist then suggests that she acknowledge her husband's statements of approval either verbally or nonverbally and subsequently points out to her how her "fishing" for approval in manner similar to an adolescent rather than a grown woman has never been effective. In fact, it can be observed to decrease the probability of her husband's responding in the way she states that she wants. It is also pointed out how her anger at small compliments from her husband also decreases the likelihood of future compliments. In effect, the therapist teaches this woman how to shape her husband's behavior by positive reinforcement and to abandon unsuccessful behavioral change techniques. He explicitly states that her own behavior is in part responsible for her failure to get what she says that she wants from her husband.

The therapist then attempts to convince the couple that the wife's perception of the husband as withholding and the husband's perception of the wife as demanding, although accurate, are also partially an artifact of their style of interaction. He emphasizes that their perceptions of one another, although qualitatively accurate are quantitatively distorted (i.e., the husband subjectively exaggerates the extent of his wife's emotional neediness). He also emphasizes how they are perceiving limited aspects of one another's personality. For example, the wife is not noticing the caring actions of her husband, and the husband is not noting the competent aspects of his wife's personality. In subsequent sessions, the therapist repeatedly comments on behaviors of each spouse that do not fit the stereotyped perception. For example, he will assist the husband in noting the things that his wife does on her own without asking for or even desiring his reassurance.

Later in the therapy, the therapist may inquire of each spouse past situations in which similar feelings were evoked. For example, the husband may have a predisposition to see women as needy because of his relationship with his first wife or mother. The wife may remember her father as distant and withholding. The purpose of this diversion into past determinants of current behavior is not individual psychodynamic insight about the origins of one's behavior. The purpose is to have the spouse realize that his or her mate's behavior is not totally determined by feelings in the present. In many couples, such realization can damper the intensity of the disappointment in a spouse's behavior. For example, if the wife realizes that her husband has difficulty expressing admiration and affection for her because he perceived his mother as overly demanding, she then has the realization that his "withholding" behavior is not directed solely at her.

In another couple, significant discord recurred around how to raise their only child. The husband described his wife as impossible, stubborn, and willful—"I can't get her to do anything that I want. Everything has to be her way." In actual fact, his wife appeared uneasy compromising and was frequently defiant of her husband's wishes. However, her husband's behavior appeared to play a large role in her defiance. Earlier communication training has decreased the husband's tendency to express his wishes as moral imperatives—"All women should" or orders "It's your responsibility, just do it and be quiet." However, his requests to his wife were often criticisms mixed with requests for change, "Charlie's wife does that without complaining. I don't see what's wrong with you." On other occasions, his mixed messages were a bit more sophisticated. He would seemingly innocently drift into a conversation about some couple they both knew, a conflict they had, and imply without stating so explicitly that the resolution of the conflict had occurred because the friend's wife had agreed to compromise. Five minutes later, he would ask his wife to do something analogous to what his friend's wife had allegedly done. When his wife would refuse, this man could be seen silently nodding to himself that this indeed proved his case.

This man pleaded complete innocence when the therapist pointed out what seemed to be an obvious connection. His wife's usual response was passive noncompliance ("That's right, Dear," stated in a voice tone suggesting noncompliance), counterattack ("Well, you never do anything for me"), or topic shifting ("Sally's husband helps out more with child rearing than most"). The husband's behavior elicited the responses from his wife that confirmed his view of her as unyielding and controlling. In turn, his wife viewed him as cold and authoritative. What she did not perceive was how her defiance of her husband contributed to the maintenance of his authoritative style. The initial intervention was twofold: to change the elicited behavior and the evoked confirmatory behavior. The therapist modeled for the husband alternative ways of asking his wife to do things. Considerable effort was expended to find a behavioral strategy that was acceptable to the wife (not seen as dictatorial) and also to the husband (not experienced as begging). At the same time that the therapist helped the husband try out alternative ways of relating to his wife, the therapist repetitively emphasized to the wife that her genuine willingness to cooperate and compromise or minor issues was crucial to the success of the therapy.

Once the therapist was successful in partially modifying the husband's behavior, he focused more attention to the wife's role. She felt that her father has continually dominated her mother and that this had led to her mother's "emotional breakdown" from which her mother never recovered. Thus, this woman understandably had a fear of being dominated by her husband, while at the same time unwittingly evoked such behavior from her husband. The therapist challenged her perception of her husband, repeatedly emphasizing instances in which her husband had gone out of his way to foster her independent goals. At the same time, the therapist helped this woman to realize that there was a large middle ground between total submission and total defiance. As her husband practices alternative ways of asking his wife to do things, the therapist intervenes before she can reply. He asks her to state her range of feelings about what her husband is requesting. In this way, he finds out to what extent she genuinely agrees or disagrees with her husband's request and assists her in making small compromises, at the same time emphasizing that this does not represent dangerous submission to her husband's tyranny. In other words, the therapist helps shape his wife's behavior and at the same time reassures her that this behavioral change is safe.

In this particular case, as the therapist is gently assisting the wife in small comprises, he notes that her husband has tears in his eyes. He asks the husband what is happening. The husband starts crying openly and says, "I never knew it was so difficult for her. I just thought that she was stubborn. It made me feel so helpless." The therapist closely monitors the wife's reaction to this incident. At first, she appears puzzled, then she looks as if she is about to cry. At this point, the therapist gently inquires what she is feeling and what she heard her husband say. He then points out the discrepancy between what her husband is saying and her previous description of her husband. At this point, the therapist is attempting to help the wife have an experience of her husband as a safe partner. This subjective experience may be a more powerful counterinstance to her perception of her spouse than anything the therapist can do or say. The artistry of this form of therapy is the therapist's ability to monitor the emotional readiness of each partner to have a different emotional experience of the other. Both partners have to be ready before an experience such as that previously described can occur.

In most cases of chronic marital discord, one or both spouses will have a perceptual distortion of the other's personality that is partially accurate but represents a quite limited perception of the mate's character. For example, the spouse described as totally helpless can usually be observed to be competent in some area, and the spouse described as having no feeling usually has some cracks in his armor that the other spouse overlooks. The therapist plans an assault on the fixated perception of the spouse. As mentioned previously, part of this assault involves pointing out exceptions to the restricted description of the spouse. Another technique is to gradually shift the description of the spouse by subtle relabeling of the spouse's behavior. For example, if a wife states that her husband has no feelings, the therapist can nod in agreement while stating ("He's a bit gruff" or "He's a bit out of touch with his feelings"). Later, the therapist can then ask the spouse how she might be able to help her husband express his feelings.

In other cases, the therapist may have to directly confront the distortion. For example, in one couple, the wife was convinced that her husband really did not care about her as a person. She felt that he only valued her for the functions she served—hostess, housekeeper, and companion for social gatherings. Her husband was a driven, highly competitive man who had difficulty expressing feelings of endearment. In a gruff manner, her husband responded to her accusation by a long monologue that included comments on the importance of the well-functioning marital unit to career advancement, and so forth. In the midst of the confused monologue, he states unambiguously that his marriage comes first, although he does not want his marriage to interfere with his career. The therapist asked the wife what she heard her husband say. She replied that he said that he did not want her to interfere with his career. The therapist replies that he indeed heard that but that he also heard something quite different. He then asks the husband to repeat his statement and for his wife to repeat verbatim what her husband says. He makes absolutely certain that she does not omit the part when he says that his marriage to her is more important than his career. He then asks his wife to explain how this statement fits with her opinion of her husband. When she tries to explain away what her husband has said, the therapist asks her bluntly if she thinks that her husband is lying. The therapist states unequivocally that he believes the husband and marshalls evidence to support that viewpoint (meetings the husband missed to be with his wife, etc.).

Termination

The couple is ready for termination when the following criteria have been met: (1) destructive discord has ended, (2) the repetitive eliciting and confirmatory behavioral cycles have been eliminated, (3) the couple has begun to perceive one another as multidimensional complex beings, (4) the couple is aware of their unique propensity to get caught in a repetitive destructive cycle and have demonstrated an ability to extricate themselves from it without the therapist's assistance, and (5) the couple have had the experience of a safe and pleasurable bonding. As termination becomes close, the therapist requests that both spouses describe what they have learned about themselves and their interaction and specifically to state the problem areas and how to extricate themselves from old patterns. Approximately one half way through the therapy, the therapist has purposely begun being progressively less active so that the couple has had the experience of successful problem resolution with minimal assistance. The other part of termination, similar to individual psychotherapy, consists of the couple expressing their fears of being on their own and saying their goodbyes to the therapist. Follow-up sessions are not routinely scheduled as the therapist does not want to foster dependence on therapy.

CONCLUSION

In this chapter, I have attempted to outline a brief therapy model for chronic marital discord. Although procedures are borrowed from differing therapeutic schools, the unifying principle is the use of behavioral and cognitive procedures to provoke a change in the perception of the spouse.

REFERENCES

Ackerman, N. W. (1966). *Treating the troubled family*. New York: Basic Books.
Bachrach, L. L. (1975a). *Marital status and mental disorder: An analytic review* (DHEW Publication No. 75-217). Washington, DC: U.S. Government Printing Office.
Bachrach, L. L. (1975b). *Marital status and age of male admissions with diagnosed alcohol disorders to state and county hospitals in 1972* (Statistical Note 12). Washington, DC: U.S. Government Printing Office.
Bachrach, L. L. (1975c). Mental health, marital status and mental disorders: An analytic review (DHEW Publication No. ADM 75-217). Washington, DC: U.S. Government Printing Office.
Bandura, A. (1977). *Social learning theory*. Englewood Cliffs, NJ: Prentice-Hall.
Birk, L., & Brinkley-Birk, A. W. (1974). Psychoanalysis and behavior therapy. *American Journal of Psychiatry, 131*, 499–510.
Bloom, B. L., Hodges, W. F., Caldwell, R. A., Systra, L., & Cedrone, A. R. (1977). Marital separation: A community study. *Journal of Divorce, 1*, 7–19.
Breger, L., & McCaugh, J. L. (1965). Critique and reformulation of learning theory approach to psychotherapy and neurosis. *Psychological Bulletin, 63*, 338–358.
Brody, S. (1961). Simultaneous psychotherapy of married couples: Preliminary observations. *Psychoanalytic Review, 48*, 94–107.
Carson, R. C. (1969). *Interaction concepts of personality*. Chicago: Aldine.
Carter, H., & Glick, P. C. (1976). *Marriage and divorce: A social and economic study*. Cambridge, MA: Harvard University Press.
Eysenck, H. J., & Rachman, S. (1965). *The causes and cures of neurosis*. London: Routledge & Kegan Paul.

Gottman, J., Notarius, C., Gonso, J., & Markman, H. (1976). *A couple's guide to communication.* Champaign, IL: Research Press.

Gove, W. R. (1973). Sex, marital status, and morality. *American Journal of Sociology, 79,* 45–67.

Gurman, A. S. (1978). Contemporary marital therapies: A critique and comparative analysis of psychoanalytic, behavioral and system theory approaches. In T. J. Paolino & B. S. McGrady (Eds.), *Marriage and marital therapy* (pp. 445–566). New York: Brunner/Mazel.

Gurman, A. S. & Knudson, R. M. (1978). Behavioral marriage therapy I: A psychodynamic systems analysis and critique. *Family Process, 17,* 121–138.

Haley, J. (1978). Marriage therapy. (1963). *Archives of General Psychiatry, 8,* 213–234.

Hunt, H. F., & Dyrud, J. E. (1968). Commentary: Perspective in behavior therapy. *Research in Psychotherapy, 3,* 149–152.

Hurvitz, N. (1975). Interaction hypotheses in marriage counseling. In A. S. Gurman & D. G. Rice (Eds.), *Couples in conflict* (pp. 225–240). New York: Jason Aronson.

Jacobson, N. S., & Weiss, R. L. (1978). Behavioral marriage therapy III. Critique: The contents of Gurman *et al.* may be hazardous to your health. *Family Process, 17,* 149–164.

Johnson, S. (1986). *Integration in marital therapy.* Paper read at the annual meeting of the Society for the Exploration of Psychotherapy Integration, Toronto.

Kaplan, S. M. (1976). The analyst, the transference, and the representational world. *Comprehensive Psychiatry, 17,* 47–54.

Kelly, G. A. (1955). *The psychology of personal constructs.* New York: Norton.

Leary, T. (1957). *Interpersonal diagnosis of personality.* New York: Ronald Press.

Lederer, W. J., & Jackson, D. D. (1968). *The mirages of marriage.* New York: W. W. Norton.

Malan, D. N. (1976). *The frontier of brief psychotherapy.* New York: Plenum Press.

Manus, G. L. (1966). Marriage counseling: A technique in search of a theory. *Journal of Marriage and the Family, 28,* 449–453.

Marmor, J. (1971). Dynamic psychotherapy and behavior therapy: Are they irreconcilable? *Archives of General Psychiatry, 24,* 22–28.

Martin, P. A., & Lief, H. I. (1973). Resistance to innovation in psychiatric training as exemplified by marital therapy. In G. Usdin (Ed.), *Psychiatry education and image* (pp. 123–140). New York: Brunner/Mazel.

Meissner, W. W. (1978). The conceptualization of marriage and family dynamics from a psycho-analytic perspective. In T. J. Paolino & B. S. McGrady (Eds.), *Marriage and marital therapy* (pp. 25–88). New York: Brunner/Mazel.

Menniger, K. (1985). *Theory of psychoanalytic technique.* New York: Basic Books.

Nadelson, C. C. (1978). Marriage therapy from a psychoanalytic perspective. In T. J. Paolino & B. S. McGrady (Eds.), *Marriage and marital therapy* (pp. 89–164). New York: Brunner/Mazel.

Offenkrantz, W., & Tobin, A. (1975). Psychoanalytic psychotherapy. In D. X. Freedman & J. E. Drud (Eds.), *American handbook of psychiatry* (Volume 5, pp. 183–205). New York: Basic Books.

Prochaska, J., & Prochaska, J. (1978). Twentieth century trends in marriage and marital therapy. In T. J. Paolino & B. S. McGrady (Eds.), *Marriage and marital therapy.* New York: Brunner/Mazel.

Renne, K. S. (1971). Health and marital experience in a urban population. *Journal of Marriage and the Family, 33,* 338–350.

Sager, C. J. (1967). Transference in conjoint treatment of married couples. *Archives of General Psychiatry, 16,* 185–193.

Satir, V. (1967). *Conjoint marital therapy.* Palo Alto: Science and Behavior Books.

Segraves, R. T. (1978). Conjoint marital therapy: A cognitive behavioral model. *Archives of General Psychiatry, 35,* 450–455.

Segraves, R. T. (1980). Marriage and mental health. *Journal of Sex and Marital Therapy, 6,* 187–198.

Segraves, R. T. (1982). *Marital therapy: A combined psychodynamic behavioral approach.* New York: Plenum Press.

Segraves, R. T. (1986). Implications of the behavioral sex therapy for psychoanalytic theory and practice: Intrapsychic sequelae of symptom removal in the patient and spouse. *Journal of the American Academy of Psychoanalysis, 14,* 485–493.

Segraves, R. T., & Smith, R. C. (1976). Concurrent psychotherapy and behavioral therapy. *Archives of General Psychiatry, 33,* 756–763.

Stuart, R. B. (1972). Operant-interpersonal treatment for marital discord. In C. J. Sager & H. S. Kaplan (Eds.), *Progress in group and family therapy* (pp. 125–132). New York: Brunner/Mazel.

Wachtel, P. L. (1977). *Psychoanalysis and behavior therapy*. New York: Basic Books.

Weiss, R. L., Birchler, G. L., & Vincent, J. D. (1974). Contractual models for negotiation training in marital dyads. *Journal of Marriage and the Family, 36,* 321–330.

Weiss, R. L., Hops, H., & Patterson, G. R. (1973). A framework for conceptualizing marital conflict, a technology for altering it, some data for evaluating it. In A. Hammerlynck, L. C., Handy, & E. J. Mash (Eds.), *Behavior change, methodology and practice,* Champaign, IL: Research Press.

Weissman, M. M. (1974). The epidemiology of suicide attempts, 1960 to 1971. *Archives of General Psychiatry, 30,* 737–746.

19

Brief Psychotherapy for the Sexual Dysfunctions

J. Gayle Beck

> If your life at night is good, you think you have Everything; but, if in that
> quarter things go wrong, You will consider your best and truest interests
> Most hateful
> —Euripides, *Medea*

Sex therapy, as we know it today, is a relatively new therapeutic approach within the history of psychology, psychiatry, and related disciplines. The earliest appearance of problem-focused techniques for sexual disorders occurred in the late 1950s, with Wolpe's successful application of classical conditioning procedures to anxiety-based sexual dysfunction (Wolpe, 1958) and Semans' 1956 article describing the "stop–start" method for premature ejaculation. Since this time, a number of approaches to time-limited sex therapy have been developed, in particular Masters and Johnson's (1970) conjoint sex therapy, Kaplan's (1974) integration of analytic and behavioral approaches, Lazarus' (1971) multimodal behavior therapy, and LoPiccolo's (1978) direct treatment of low sexual arousal. Each of these therapeutic models shares the basic assumption that sexual behavior can be treated directly, without long-term exploration of underlying psychological dynamics, and in most cases, utilizes skill acquisition and anxiety reduction techniques to accomplish this goal.

Had this chapter appeared 10 years earlier, the next sentence would have stated that these approaches have produced startlingly high success rates and appear able to be adapted by clinicians varying in experience and orientation (e.g., Masters & Johnson, 1970; Kinder & Blakeney, 1977). In the intervening decade, it has become apparent that the simplistic use of sex therapy techniques cannot adequately address the complexity of many cases of sexual dysfunction, particularly given the changing nature of sexual problems presenting to clinics. This chapter will present current approaches to time-limited sex therapy, with emphasis on the role of pretreatment assessment and definition of problem-focused goals. The various types of sexual dysfunctions will be outlined, along

---

J. Gayle Beck • Department of Psychology, University of Houston, Houston, Texas 77204-5341.

with approaches to assessment. Presentation of specific therapeutic approaches will include treatment parameters and determination and evaluation of therapeutic goals. Clinical issues such as resistance, difficulties arising at termination, and the integration of sex and marital therapy approaches also will be included. Despite growing recognition that the practice of sex therapy can be fraught with subtle difficulties, brief therapeutic approaches remain the primary mode of intervention for the sexual dysfunction. The advances of the past 20 years have, in many respects, produced a body of knowledge that simultaneously reflects our sophistication and our ignorance about human sexual behavior.

UNDERLYING THEORETICAL ASSUMPTIONS

The foundation of sex therapy rests upon the assumption that the sexual response can be affected by cognitive, behavioral, and emotional factors, each of which may increase or decrease sexual arousal depending on an individual's sexual history and current relationship. Precluding the existence of an organic etiology, sexual dysfunction is conceptualized as learned behavior, resulting from an array of factors that can be assessed and addressed directly in treatment. Although similarities exist between approaches to sex therapy and behavioral interventions with respect to this assumption, the theoretical underpinnings of sex therapy are considerably more diverse and include tenets of systems theory (e.g., Jackman, 1976), social psychological theories of attraction and love (e.g., Tennov, 1979), and gestalt therapy (e.g., Perls, 1960). In many respects, the development of sex therapy has relied on empirical evaluation of specific interventions, creating an eclectic, data-based approach to psychotherapy that escapes easy theoretical categorization. Thus the inclusion of ongoing evaluation could be seen as a second underlying assumption of sex therapy, as patient progress is monitored throughout treatment with the aim of refining treatment formulation and expanding knowledge of factors influencing outcome.

Another central assumption of sex therapy relies upon conceptualization of the sexual response. Beginning with the landmark studies of Masters and Johnson (1966, 1970), treatment approaches have focused on dysfunctions occurring at specific points in the "sexual response cycle." Specifically, Masters and Johnson (1966) categorized the sexual response as occurring in four discrete phases: excitement, plateau, orgasm, and resolution. Physiological responses of each phase have been delineated by these authors, with the greatest attention devoted to disorders occurring during the excitement and orgasm phases. Although the notion of discrete phases of sexual responding has been questioned, both conceptually (Robinson, 1976) and empirically (Rosen & Beck, 1988), this nomenclature has remained influential in formulations of sex therapy. More recent nosologies have elaborated on this basic scheme and have included facets of sexual behavior such as sexual desire (Kaplan, 1979), coital pain, and sexual satisfaction (Schover, Friedman, Weiler, Heiman, & LoPiccolo, 1982). Refinements such as these have expanded the conceptualization of the sexual response, allowed for precise description of multiple dysfunctions in the same patient, and permitted the inclusion of sexual disorders involving subjective components of sexual arousal.

In conceptualizing sex therapy, one should not assume that this type of psychotherapy is designed exclusively for couples or individuals who have a regular sexual partner. Although certain approaches to treatment, such as the Masters and Johnson model, are designed for couples, a variety of other techniques and treatment formats have proven useful with individual patients. Given that most individuals who seek sex therapy are involved in a steady relationship, the majority of this chapter will focus on couple-oriented assessment and treatment, with treatment approaches for individuals without partners highlighted where relevant. In treating a couple with sexual dysfunction, it is assumed that the problem resides with the couple rather than one of the partners. This assumption helps to reduce the guilt and blame that may be compounding the presenting problem and assures that both partners share responsibility in working to resolve the sexual dysfunction.

TYPES OF MALE AND FEMALE SEXUAL DYSFUNCTIONS

In considering the available forms of sex therapies, it is first necessary to review the male and female sexual dysfunctions, particularly given the importance of tailoring treatment strategies to the presenting disorder. In some respects, the term *sexual dysfunction* implies that a clear distinction can be made between "normal" and "impaired" sexual functioning. The doubtful validity of this assumption is most sharply illustrated in a report by Frank, Anderson, and Rubenstein (1978). These authors demonstrated that couples who considered themselves free of sexual problems reported some of the same sexual behaviors as couples presenting for treatment (e.g., erectile failure, difficulties in reaching orgasm). Thus, definition of a sexual dysfunction *always* requires patient labeling of a particular aspect of sexual functioning as problematic. To neglect this feature of diagnosis is an almost certain predictor of a poor therapeutic outcome (Everaerd, 1983; Fordney-Settlage, 1975).

Inhibited Sexual Excitement

Disorders of low arousal in the early stages of sexual responding have been termed *inhibited sexual excitement* in females and *erectile dysfunction* in males. Both forms of this disorder are characterized by a failure to achieve or sustain sexual arousal: vaginal vasocongestion and lubrication in females and penile tumescence in males. As with all of the sexual disorders, inhibited sexual excitement can be primary, meaning that the patient reports no history of adequate sexual functioning, or secondary, meaning that a period of adequate responding preceded the dysfunction. Some sex therapists have found that the additional classification of dysfunctions as situation-specific or generalized is useful in conceptualizing individual cases (Friedman & Hogan, 1985; Wincze, 1981).

The differential diagnosis of male erectile dysfunction as psychogenic or organic has received considerable attention, particularly given the availability of surgical treatment for known cases of organic erectile failure (e.g., Bennett, 1982; Sotile, 1979). A number of neurologic, vascular, and hormonal abnormalities may impair the tumescence response (see Kolodny, Masters, & Johnson, 1979, for a review) that would suggest medical intervention, with the possible addition of sex therapy to address psychological, marital, or sexual technique problems. Use of nocturnal penile tumescence (NPT) recording (Karacan, 1970) has become the primary method for establishing a differential diagnosis. This procedure relies on laboratory sleep evaluation, with assessment of nocturnal tumescence and penile rigidity using the penile strain gauge, to be discussed later. More recent data indicate that classification based on NPT alone is inadequate (Wasserman, Pollak, Spielman, & Weitzman, 1980) and may result in falsely labeling a patient with an abnormal NPT as *organic*, when in fact his nocturnal erectile response is the result of measurement artifact (Procci, Moss, Boyd, & Barron, 1983; Schiavi & Fisher, 1982), alcoholism (Mandell & Miller, 1983), depression, or another factor. Thus thorough assessment of psychological and organic causes of erectile failure is necessary in each case.

Isolated cases of inhibited sexual excitement are considerably less common in women and often are presented in conjunction with orgasmic dysfunction. Although much of the empirical research on sexual dysfunction in women has relied on patients presenting with complaints of both low arousal and impairment of the orgasmic response (e.g., Heiman, 1976; Rosen & Beck, 1988), inhibited sexual excitement also can present clinically as a report of pain during coitus (dyspareunia), owing to lack of vaginal lubrication. It is particularly important to assess situational factors in these cases, specifically sexual interaction styles, the partner's level of sexual skill, communication patterns, and the overall quality of the relationship. To date, little information has emerged on the role of organic factors in inhibited sexual excitement in women, although it is recognized that the onset of menopause can decrease vaginal lubrication and impair the arousal response (Myers & Morokoff, 1986).

Inhibited Sexual Orgasm

Difficulties in achieving orgasm are termed *orgasmic dysfunction* in women and *retarded ejaculation* in males. The prevalence of women reporting an inability to reach orgasm during intercourse appears high (Hite, 1976), although these data indicate that most women experience orgasm during noncoital interactions and masturbation. Thus the definition of female orgasmic dysfunction depends on a patient's sexual history, awareness of sexual techniques, religious and moral beliefs, and, if applicable, relationship with her partner. Orgasmic dysfunction can be primary, indicating that the woman has never experienced orgasm through any means, or secondary, which includes the woman who was able to reach orgasm previously but is currently rarely orgasmic, as well as the woman who can attain orgasm only in response to a restricted type of stimulation. Orgasmic dysfunction is often accompanied by low sexual arousal, and occasionally, excessive anxiety concerning sexual interaction.

Retarded ejaculation in males is considerably less prevalent than orgasmic difficulty in females. In this condition, the man has little difficulty in achieving and sustaining an erection but can ejaculate intravaginally only with considerable stimulation. Because of the infrequency with which these cases occur clinically, little is known about relevant maintaining factors and etiology (Dow, 1981; Munjack & Kanno, 1979). Although certain medications can produce delays in ejaculation, often the patient who presents with retarded ejaculation previously has contacted a physician and ruled out an organic cause for this problem.

Premature Ejaculation

A more common form of male orgasmic dysfunction is premature ejaculation. The ejaculatory reflex is controlled sympathetically by the lumbar portion of the spinal cord and once triggered cannot be voluntarily stopped. Occasionally, a patient presenting with this disorder actually is reporting a normal latency to ejaculation (average time from intromission to ejaculation of about 2 minutes, Masters & Johnson, 1970), with unrealistic expectations for his own performance derived from the media. Generally, however, patients with ejaculatory control problems report a greatly heightened awareness of their own degree of arousal (Spiess, Geer, & O'Donohue, 1984) and extremely rapid onset of ejaculation once sexual contact begins. Men with this problem tend to be younger than those presenting with erectile dysfunction and often report a low frequency of sexual partner contact (Spiess et al., 1984). Whether this reduced pattern of sexual activity is a cause or an effect of premature ejaculation is difficult to establish (Kedia, 1983; Kinsey, Pomeroy, & Martin, 1948), although treatment of this disorder remains one of the most efficacious forms of sex therapies to date.

Inhibited Sexual Desire

Inclusion of sexual desire disorders is a relatively new addition to classification schemes for the sexual dysfunctions. Inhibited sexual desire is particularly difficult to define, given a lack of normative information on "usual" levels of sexual interest and the uncertain relationship between desire and sexual behavior. Generally, inhibited desire problems are presented by a couple, with one member stating that his or her partner rarely initiates sex and often is unresponsive to overtures. This has led Zilbergeld and Ellison (1980) to suggest that sexual desire problems be viewed as a "desire discrepancy" within a particular couple, to avoid labeling of one partner as "sick." Low sexual desire is not a unidimensional phenomenon, as one may note a decrease in sexual interest with one partner (e.g., the spouse) with no impairment in other sexual relationships. Currently, little empirical data exist on men and women with inhibited sexual desire, although three major etiological factors have been proposed: hormonal problems (Bancroft, 1984), family of origin theories (Kaplan, 1979), and problems in the dynamics of the sexual relationship (Friedman & Hogan, 1985). The lack of a specific behavioral or physiological referent that defines low levels of sexual desire necessitates reliance on subjective criteria in diagnosing inhibited sexual desire.

Vaginismus

Vaginismus is a female dysfunction in which spastic contractions of the circumvaginal musculature occur, such that the penis (or sometimes any other object) cannot be admitted to the vagina without difficulty and pain. Vaginismus is distinguished from dyspareunia (pain during coitus resulting from an organic etiology; Sarrel, 1977). By definition, no physical lesion exists in vaginismus; it results from a fear of penetration and may be situation specific. That is, the woman may be able to tolerate penetration during a gynecological pelvic exam but not during sexual contact with her partner. LoPiccolo and Stock (1987) note that vaginismus often is presented by women who have a history of incestuous molestation in childhood or adolescence, and it frequently is accompanied by inhibited sexual excitement and lack of orgasm.

Sexual Aversion

Recently sexual aversion has been differentiated from other forms of sexual dysfunction, particularly inhibited sexual desire, due to differences in clinical profiles and treatment formulation. Sexual aversion is characterized by repugnance or disgust at sexual activity and initially may appear as difficulties with low arousal or inhibited interest (Caird & Wincze, 1977). Clinical practice suggests the role of extreme religious beliefs, conflicts in sexual partner preference, and general psychopathology in cases presenting with sexual aversion.

General Considerations in Selecting Patients for Sex Therapy

A number of related considerations are germane in determining if an individual is an appropriate candidate for sex therapy. After screening for physical factors that may account for the dysfunction, it is useful to assess the existence of other primary psychiatric disorders because the presence of psychopathology is a predictor of poor treatment response (Chapman, 1982; Reynolds, 1977; Wright, Perreault, & Mathieu, 1977). If other disorders are present, particularly depression or an anxiety disorder such as agoraphobia, successful sex therapy can often follow therapeutic intervention for the primary problem (e.g., Beck, 1985). Although age and social class do not appear to be associated with treatment outcome (Ansari, 1976; Hawton & Catalan, 1986), the prospective patient's orientation toward treatment can determine treatment progress (Chapman, 1982). Factors such as a belief that sex therapy will be potentially useful, motivation to carry out homework tasks, and ability to afford treatment can shape the process of sex therapy, much as with any type of psychotherapy.

Previous sexual experience may also influence the course of sex therapy, although in no way should this be regarded as an exclusionary factor in evaluating a potential patient. Hawton and Catalan (1986) report that positive therapeutic outcome was not related to whether the male partner was sexually experienced before the current relationship began, although women with vaginismus who had not had intercourse prior to the current relationship tended to have a better outcome than those who had. In this study, therapist and patient ratings of the overall quality of the relationship predicted outcome, with higher ratings of satisfaction and committment at pretreatment predicting more favorable outcomes. Similar findings have been reported by a number of other authors (Abramowitz & Sewell, 1980; Hartman & Daly, 1983; Lansky & Davenport, 1975; Levay & Kagle, 1983), suggesting that assessment of relationship functioning is an important component in evaluating whether sex or marital therapy is an appropriate first step in treatment.

Another consideration in formulating cases presenting for sex therapy is whether the dysfunction is primary or secondary, that is, whether the patient has ever experienced an interval of satisfactory sexual functioning prior to seeking therapeutic help. For women, primary dysfunctions appear relatively responsive to sex therapy (Kilmann, 1978; Kinder & Blakeney, 1977), whereas secondary dysfunctions frequently require more careful treatment formulation, often with the addition of interventions aimed at the couple's interaction pattern (e.g., Everaerd & Dekker, 1981). For men, data on this issue are mixed, although the duration of the dysfunction appears to predict treatment response, with dysfunctions of longer duration showing greater resistance to change (Cooper, 1981). For males, acute onset of the dysfunction appears to predict favorable treatment response, relative to an insidious onset (Cooper, 1981).

PRETREATMENT EVALUATION PROCEDURES

An integral ingredient of successful sex therapy is a thorough assessment of the patient's functioning prior to intervention. This often involves several methods of evaluation, including the interview, questionnaires, monitoring of sexual behavior using weekly self-report recording, and occasionally, psychophysiological and medical evaluation. Optimally the selection of questionnaires and behavioral records can be tailored to allow repeat administration throughout the course of treatment, to index patient progress.

Interview Format

The clinical interview is still the most valuable tool for diagnostic assessment and initial evaluation of a sex therapy candidate. Although the structure of the interview can vary, it is important to collect information necessary for understanding the frame of reference in which the sexual dysfunction occurs in order to provide a basis for treatment formulation. If a couple presents for sex therapy, some time should be spent with each individual alone, as well as interviewing the dyad. In cases where male and female co-therapists are working together, many clinicians chose same-sex therapist–patient pairs for the individual portions of the interview, to provide a more comfortable environment for the (often awkward) initial discussion of the problem. It is important for the clinician to help the patient to discuss sexual material in as open and candid fashion as possible. Thus, interviewers who rely on open-ended questions and use straightforward language, rather than sexual slang, frequently are more successful at eliciting details relevant to the individual's dysfunction, attitudes about sexuality, early education about sex, feelings toward his or her partner, and other sensitive issues. Lobitz and Lobitz (1978) have reviewed factors that influence the initial clinical interview, to assist in organizing this information for treatment formulation.

In considering the choice of topics for the initial interview, one may ask where to begin. LoPiccolo and Heiman (1978) have provided an extensive outline of topics to serve as a guide in interviewing. Included are questions concerning family background, religious influences, medical history and current physical status, early sexual experience, puberty and adolescence, current attitudes towards sex, perceptions of the general and sexual relationship, and the nature of the sexual difficulty. These authors caution against beginning an interview by inquiring about sexual dysfunction because therapeutic rapport has not yet been established fully and useful information may be neglected or understated. Thus conceptualization of the interview as a "funnel" may be useful (Hawkins, 1979) with the initial introduction of nonthreatening questions (e.g., "how did the two of you first meet?"), followed by open-ended questions concerning the sexual problem (e.g., "could each of you describe the problem that brought you here?"), which can be specified through greater inquiry (e.g., "I'd like a more detailed picture of what happens when you relate sexually . . . for example, who initiates sex? what types of foreplay do you usually engage in?"). The more detailed and specific the information gathered during the initial interview, the lower the chance of misdiagnosing the sexual problem or overlooking a contraindication to sex therapy, such as an ongoing extramarital affair.

Questionnaires

The use of questionnaires is a cost-effective means of obtaining information, although the manner in which these instruments are presented initially to patients is an important consideration. Some prospective sex therapy candidates react strongly to extensive questionnaire batteries, particularly those who already resent being in therapy. There are various opinions about how to handle such resistance (e.g., Friedman & Hogan, 1985; Nowinski & LoPiccolo, 1979), with some indicating that questionnaires are necessary for a complete pretreatment evaluation and others suggesting that the clinician should exercise his/her judgment in cases where such a request may lead individuals to decline treatment.

A number of instruments exist for the assessment of sexual function and related areas (Corcoran & Fischer, 1987). Selection of specific instruments depends largely on time constraints and any limitations imposed by the patient's reading ability. Many of these inventories have been validated empirically, with normative data available for some. Little is known concerning the clinical utility of most of the questionnaires to be mentioned here (Conte, 1986), suggesting that some trial and error may be involved in selecting questionnaires for a comprehensive battery. A typical array of questionnaires might include the Sexual Interaction Inventory (LoPiccolo & Steger, 1974), which assesses dyadic sexual interaction patterns, the Derogatis Sexual Functioning Inventory (Derogatis, 1978), which assesses sexual functioning in 10 areas, including sexual fantasies, attitudes, and general sexual satisfaction, the Locke–Wallace Marital Adjustment Test (Locke & Wallace, 1959), the Beck Depression Inventory (Beck, 1967), and the SCL-90R (Derogatis, Rickels, & Rock, 1976), which measures general psychological disturbance. Taken together, these questionnaires can be time consuming, and often patients are requested to complete the battery at home, with instructions that individuals not reveal their responses to one another.

Behavioral Records

While Masters and Johnson (1966) pioneered the use of direct behavioral observations as a method for assessing sexual behavior, the obvious disadvantages of this approach have yielded to the use of self-report behavioral records of sexual behavior. Several models exist that vary in the degree to which they are standardized or tailored to the individual. Barlow (1977) has described a format where patients are asked to record all instances of sexual interaction with a partner, masturbation and accompanying fantasies, and fantasies occurring in the absence of sexual behavior. Obler (1973) have described a similar approach to behavioral recording, in which couples are given forms to indicate successful and unsuccessful sexual interactions, defined within the context of sex therapy.

The Weekly Sexual Activity Checklist (Caird & Wincze, 1977) is a more standardized approach to behavioral recording. In this format, patients are asked to check any of 10 sexual behaviors that they have engaged in and to indicate if these activities created anxiety and/or sexual arousal at the time of occurrence (see Figure 1). Completed forms are given to the therapist at weekly sessions, providing an ongoing index of therapeutic progress. Each of these behavioral recording formats provides specific information on the frequency and quality of sexual interactions, alone and with a partner, and each has been used clinically. Although no psychometric data exist for these approaches to monitoring sexual activity, their use has proven valuable both for pretreatment assessment and for examining changes across time.

Psychophysiological and Medical Assessment

The inclusion of laboratory psychophysiological evaluation is a relatively new addition in pretreatment assessment for male sexual dysfunction. In part, based on the growing recognition that a high percentage (50% to 60%) of men with erectile dysfunction may have an organic basis for this disorder (e.g., Fisher, Schiavi, Edwards, Davis, Reitman, & Fine, 1979), the use of NPT assessment has become somewhat routine in cases where a neurological, vascular, or

For week ending _____

WEEKLY SEXUAL ACTIVITY CHECK LIST

Sexual Activity	Check if the activity occurred	If it occurred check if it caused you any anxiety	If it occurred, check if it caused you any arousal
Being seen in the nude	_____	_____	_____
Orgasm (yours)	_____	_____	_____
Seeing partner nude	_____	_____	_____
Having genitals caressed	_____	_____	_____
Caressing partner's genitals	_____	_____	_____
Intercourse	_____	_____	_____
Kissing, embracing, caressing (no genital contact)	_____	_____	_____
deep kissing with tongue contact	_____	_____	_____
Orgasm (partner's)	_____	_____	_____
Caressing breasts (or having breasts caressed)	_____	_____	_____

Note. You should not include on this check list any sexual activity engaged in during the home practice sessions.

Figure 1. Weekly sexual activity check list. (Reprinted from W. Caird & J. P. Wincz (1977), *Sex Therapy*. Hagerstown, MD: Harper & Row Publishers. Reprinted with permission.)

hormonal etiology is suspected. Although organic factors may be equally prevalent in cases of female dysfunction (Hatch, 1981), psychophysiological procedures have not achieved methodological sophistication or widespread use with women.

The NPT procedure is based on Ohlmeyer, Brilmayer, and Hullstrung's observation in 1944 of regular and consistent patterns of penile tumescence occurring during rapid eye movement (REM) sleep in normal males. The procedure involves a 3-night laboratory sleep assessment, including direct monitoring of erectile capacity using a strain gauge to detect changes in penile circumference (see Figure 2). Recently measurement of penile rigidity during erection has been recommended (Karacan, 1978), because some forms of vascular disease may result in partial occlusion of the corpora bodies, impairing complete vasocongestion during tumescence (e.g., Wagner, 1981; Wein, Fishkin, Carpiniello,

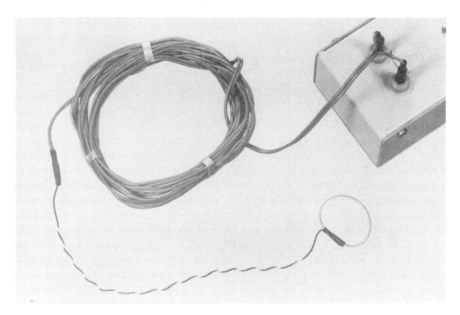

FIGURE 2. Mercury-in-rubber strain gauge used in the NPT procedure for assessment of penile circumference (gauge is shown attached to a resistance bridge, which is interfaced to the polygraph). (Reprinted from R. C. Rosen & J. G. Beck (1986). Models and measures of sexual response: Psychophysiological assessment of male and female arousal. In D. Byrne & K. Kelley (Eds.), *Alternative approaches to the study of sexual behavior* (pp. 43–86). Hillsdale, NJ: Erlbaum.)

& Malloy, 1981). Because psychological and situational influences are minimized during sleep, it is assumed that a diminished or absent NPT is the result of organic factors, whereas a demonstration of normal capacity during NPT suggests a psychological etiology. Recent data, reviewed here, indicate that this assumption may be misleading and that a variety of factors can influence NPT recording. Additionally, portable home monitoring units for NPT have been developed, including NPT "stamps" (Barry, Blank, & Bioleau, 1980) and plastic strip methods (Schwartz, 1983). These methods are not recommended as substitutes for laboratory evaluation, despite their ease and simplicity of use, given the inability to determine whether normal sleep patterns occurred and the lack of quantification of the frequency and magnitude of NPT (Melman, Kaplan, & Redfield, 1984; Rosen & Beck, 1988; Wasserman *et al.*, 1980).

The use of psychophysiological assessment can be a useful adjunct in pretreatment evaluation for sex therapy, particularly if an organic cause is suspected for a male patient. Exclusive reliance on NPT for differential diagnosis is not possible at present, despite early claims about the accuracy of this procedure (e.g., Karacan, 1970). In each case where a potential organic etiology exists, referral for a medical evaluation is recommended. For males, this includes a physical exam by a urologist and where possible, hormonal analyses, including total testosterone, free testosterone, estradiol, and prolactin. For women, a gynecological exam is necessary to correctly diagnose cases of dyspareunia and vaginismus. Information from physical evaluation can augment the medical history taken during the interview.

SEX THERAPY: GOALS, TREATMENT STRATEGIES, AND THERAPEUTIC PROCESS

The foundation for many techniques utilized in sex therapy was designed by Masters and Johnson in their 1970 treatment program for couples. Since initial presentation, many of these approaches have been modified and adapted to a broader range of patients and service delivery styles. Following pretreatment assessment, the first step in sex therapy is determination of treatment goals. Often the type, frequency, and spacing of therapy sessions can be decided, based on the patient's desired outcome and availability of a sexual partner for inclusion in treatment. Next, specific treatment strategies and techniques are selected, based on the presenting problem(s). The integration of assessment instruments that can be administered repeatedly throughout the course of therapy is an integral component in formulating therapy and usually involves an extension of instruments used during the pretreatment assessment phase. A number of therapeutic process considerations are relevant, including patient resistance, the use of homework, therapeutic adjuncts such as reading assignments, and integration of marital and sex therapy. Termination and follow-up are the final component of sex therapy, which may involve booster sessions or periodic assessment to determine the stability of therapeutic change.

Determination of Therapeutic Goals

It is the rare patient who comes to therapy without an agenda, whether explicit or unarticulated, for what he or she would like to happen during treatment. Often patients will discuss specific goals during the initial interview, allowing the therapist an opportunity to determine if the individual has unrealistic expectations of the therapeutic process or is anticipating that therapy will change "only" his or her partner. More systematic determination of goals occurs following the initial assessment and should be conducted conjointly, to prevent differences between partners from arising midtreatment. This is particularly important for cases of inhibited sexual desire and sexual aversion, where the problem may have been defined as one individual's "illness" or where one partner is not invested in the change process. The specification of therapeutic goals most often involves an interplay between patient and therapist, with the latter assisting in formulating measurable objectives and integrating the use of weekly records and other instruments for assessing progress.

Selection of goals generally extends beyond the presenting problem itself and often includes dimensions such as increasing the amount of sexual satisfaction experienced by both partners, improving sexual communication, diminishing the level of anxiety concerning sexual interaction, and increasing pleasurable sexual activities that are not oriented specifically toward intercourse. The inclusion of related goals can help the couple to decrease anxious concern over the presenting problem, whereas also introducing the notion that sex therapy is designed to foster gradual relearning of sexual interaction patterns that are more arousing and satisfying for both. Changes in behavior and general orientation toward sex as identified by the patients themselves should be included in determining goals for therapy, particularly given the wide range of patterns that are considered typical and the difficulty in empirically differentiating functional from dysfunctional sexual behavior. In the context of specifying goals, it can be helpful for the therapist to explain the rationale and assumptions behind sex therapy, in order to dispell any mistaken preconceptions about therapy and to heighten motivation.

The Format of Treatment

A number of decisions concerning the format of therapy arise following specification of therapeutic goals. These include the approximate number and spacing of sessions, whether an individual therapist or male–female therapy team are best suited for the patient, whether individual or group sessions are appropriate, and whether marital therapy is necessary, either as a therapeutic adjunct or prior to beginning sex therapy. Sex therapy, as conceptualized here, is a time-limited process, ranging from 8 to 25 sessions depending on the complexity of the presenting problem, the therapeutic goals, and the clinician. The use of a time-limited format can provide structure for therapeutic tasks as well as emphasizing to patients the importance of consistent adherence with homework assignments. Although some authors have noted that increasing time in treatment and utilizing an open-ended format can prove helpful when faced with difficulties in achieving desired outcomes (e.g., Kaplan, 1974; Levay & Kagle, 1977), this can also result in "interminable" sex therapy, where therapeutic deadlocks are not acknowledged and efforts persist beyond their useful limit (Levay & Kagle, 1983).

Although Masters and Johnson's original treatment format involved an intensive 2-week visit to their clinic in St. Louis, most sex therapy is conducted using weekly sessions, ranging from 1 to 2 hours depending on whether group or individual sessions are employed. In one of the few empirical investigations of treatment format, Heiman and LoPiccolo (1983) reported little differential effectiveness of daily versus weekly treatment sessions. Similar findings have been reported in Europe and England (Marks, 1981); in these reports, the data suggest that weekly sessions may be slightly superior to daily treatment for cases of female secondary orgasmic dysfunction and male erectile failure. It is possible that the longer time course offered by weekly sessions allows for greater resolution of relationship problems.

Similarly, the Masters and Johnson tradition prescribes the use of male and female co-therapists, with the stated rationale that co-therapy teams provide the opportunity for each member of the couple to identify with a therapeutic model, who can demonstrate effective communication. However two studies have shown equal effectiveness for single therapist treatment and dual-sex co-therapists treatment (Arentewicz & Schmidt, 1983; LoPiccolo, Heiman, Hogan, & Roberts, 1985). This suggests that given a skilled, knowledgable, and sophisticated therapist, the practice of sex therapy can be conducted in a more cost-effective fashion, relative to the use of co-therapist teams.

A related concern is the choice of group or individual treatment sessions, a decision that can be shaped by the availability of a sexual partner, willingness of a patient to enter into group therapy, and related factors. In particular, group sessions as a useful treatment format for women with orgasmic dysfunction were first popularized by Wallace and Barbach (1974). Although group treatment can be varied on a number of dimensions, such the inclusion of sexual partners, number of therapy sessions, and choice of specific treatment techniques, the empirical literature suggests that group sessions can provide a supportive therapeutic environment for patients without severe psychopathology, relationship distress, or presence of other psychological problems (LoPiccolo & Stock, 1986). Barbach (1974, 1975) and others (e.g., Ersner-Hershfield & Kopel, 1979; Golden, Price, Heinrich, & Lobitz, 1978; Schneidman & McGuire, 1976) have reported that group treatment generally produces increases in sexual satisfaction, ability to reach orgasm with masturbation (and occasionally during coitus), increased sexual communication, and greater happiness with the relationship in women with primary and secondary orgasmic dysfunctions.

In considering the use of group treatment for female orgasmic dysfunction, Schneidman and McGuire (1976) have noted that inclusion of male partners was necessary midtreatment to alleviate anxieties concerning changing patterns of sexual interaction and reduce resistance in homework compliance. Ersner-Hershfield and Kopel (1979) examined this observation systematically, comparing two groups that did not include partners with a third group where partners were invited to attend two sessions. The majority of women in all three groups became orgasmic with self-stimulation during treatment, although generalization of orgasm to partner stimulation or coitus was rare, irrespective of whether partners were included in therapy. This lack of generalization has been reported by other authors (e.g., Kuriansky & Sharpe, 1976; Leiblum & Ersner-Hirshfield, 1977) and does not appear to be related to treatment format.

A final consideration in selecting a treatment format is the inclusion of marital or couples counseling. Although sex therapy includes some elements of marital therapy, such as communication training, discussion of life-style patterns that preclude attention to sexuality, emphasis on increasing the quantity and frequency of pleasurable, nonsexual activities, it is not a substitute for marital counseling. When severe marital discord exists, sex therapy should be postponed until the couple has received help with their nonsexual relationship. Occasionally, marital and sex therapy can be integrated, particularly if the nature of the couple's distress involves a focused problem, such as changes in usual patterns of dependence and independence (e.g., a wife returning to work following childbirth). Generally, this type of integration requires clinical skill with both forms of treatment and can extend the time limit of therapy by 10 to 12 sessions.

Strategies for Intervention

In the past two decades, a number of specific techniques have been developed for sexual dysfunctions. Despite the existence of a treatment technology for sexual dysfunction, there is a danger in indiscriminate, simplistic application of these strategies. Thus the following is intended as a descriptive introduction to available treatment approaches, rather than a training guide. Interested readers are referred to Masters and Johnson (1970), Caird and Wincze (1977), and LoPiccolo and LoPiccolo (1978) for further information.

Intervention for Low Sexual Excitement Dysfunctions

Techniques designed to increase sexual arousal constitute the foundation of sex therapy and tend to be used with most other forms of sexual dysfunctions. These approaches are derived from Masters and Johnson's 1970 conceptualization of etiological factors in sexual dysfunction, which includes lack of adequate information about the sexual response, negative attitudes toward sexuality, past sexual experiences that have been unarousing and frustrating, and anxiety concerning the adequacy of current sexual performance. One of the first therapeutic instructions that couples receive is a ban on intercourse, with the rationale that continuation of negative sexual interactions will tend to compound feelings of failure and will counteract treatment gains in related areas. Although there is little dispute concerning the utility of this prohibition (see Madsen & Ullmann, 1967, and Lipsius, 1987, for dissenting viewpoints), no empirical data exist to confirm its therapeutic value. However, a ban on intercourse does not preclude other forms of sexual contact and often encourages the couple to expand their sexual repetoire.

Nongenital pleasuring and sensate focus exercises have been used to help individuals identify types of stimulations that are pleasurable and exciting. The couple is instructed to begin by giving nongenital massage to one another, alternating the roles of giver and receiver. Practice with improving sexual communication styles is integrated with nongenital pleasuring, as couples are coached in ways to express their likes and dislikes clearly. The emphasis throughout these exercises is on pleasure, with a concomitant deemphasis on whether one or both partners experience sexual arousal and orgasm. Sensate focus exercises follow this same format, with the inclusion of genital pleasuring; these exercises minimize the importance of achieving an erection (for males) or experiencing vaginal lubrication (for females). The goal of this series of graduated pleasuring exercises is to eliminate the performance demands of intercourse that perpetuate low arousal states and to help the couple develop new patterns of relating sexually. Generally, by the time that the couple has established a comfortable pattern of genital pleasuring, changes have been noted in the presenting problem and individuals are eager to resume intercourse. It is unwise to rush this process, particularly if it appears guided by a belief that noncoital activity is not "genuine" sex, for this may recreate a demand for performance and diminish arousal.

As an addition to sensate focus, many therapists provide accurate information concerning the sexual response. For example, many men with erectile dysfunction feel hopeless and stop sexual activity if they lose their erection during foreplay. Description of the sexual response, including the fact that sexual excitement typically waxes and wanes during the process of arousal, can help to allay fears concerning a lack of "normal" functioning and encourage the individual to focus his or her attention on sensations of pleasure and arousal, rather than his or her physical responsivity. In cases where strong negative attitudes exist concerning sexuality, the introduction of self-help texts can assist the therapist in presenting sexual activity in a more positive light. Zilbergeld's book, entitled *Male Sexuality*, and Barbach's volume, *For Yourself*, are excellent examples of the type of reading that can serve as therapeutic adjuncts.

Inclusion of techniques designed to enhance sexual fantasies also is a component of treatment strategies for low sexual excitement. This can include identification of fantasy themes that each partner finds arousing, prescribing fantasy breaks throughout the day to enhance the use of imagination in facilitating arousal, helping the couple share fantasies together, and possibly, acting out a particular fantasy. The role of fantasy in increasing sexual arousal is clear, and explicit therapeutic focus on fantasy allows the couple to experiment with sexual activity in a playful, nonjudgmental fashion. The use of reading material, such as Friday's *My Secret Garden: Women's Sexual Fantasies* and *Men in Love*, can help patients to elaborate fantasy material and often normalizes any concerns about specific images (e.g., fantasies about coercive sexual contact).

In cases where excessive anxiety is present, systematic desensitization has been used successfully (e.g., Caird & Wincze, 1977; Husted, 1975; Obler, 1973). This technique involves construction of a hierarchy of sexual activities, ranging from least to most anxiety provoking, and teaching the patient progressive muscle relaxation. Presentation of hierarchy items proceeds either imaginally or using videotapes, paired with relaxation, until the individual can visualize the most anxiety-provoking activity in a relaxed state. Desensitization has been used with individuals as well as groups and appears to produce positive benefit (e.g., Andersen, 1983).

Intervention for Orgasmic Dysfunctions

In addition to the strategies outlined to enhance sexual arousal, several specific techniques have been used in the treatment of orgasmic dysfunction. For women, these include directed masturbation and Kegel exercises. The masturbation program developed by LoPiccolo and Lobitz (1972) is based on a sexual skills model and includes education, genital self-exploration, and masturbation, both with and without the partner present. A self-help book, *Becoming Orgasmic* (Heiman & LoPiccolo, 1988) can assist the woman in progressing through this series of programmed exercises and helps her share the process with her partner. Variations on this approach have been presented by others (e.g., Annon, 1973; Barbach, 1975; Kline-Graber & Graber, 1975), but each of these approaches maintains the goal of enhancing body awareness and increasing the women's ability to achieve orgasm through structured practice with various forms of clitoral stimulation. In later phases of the program, the partner is asked to participate, in order to learn which body areas are sensitive to erotic stimulation and to receive feedback from the woman during pleasuring exercises. Controlled studies support the use of directed masturbation in the treatment of orgasmic dysfunction, with 65% to 100% of patients reporting orgasm during masturbation at the termination of treatment (e.g., Andersen, 1983; McMullen & Rosen, 1979; Riley & Riley, 1978).

Masturbation exercises are regarded as potentially therapeutic for women with primary and secondary orgasmic dysfunction for several reasons. First, relative to coitus, masturbation is regarded as the most probable method of producing orgasm (Kinsey, Pomeroy, Martin, & Gebhard, 1953) as well as producing the most intense orgasms. Second, during self-stimulation, the woman can learn to redirect her attention to her own physical responses and sexual sensations. Third, masturbation is potentially less anxiety producing and more sexually arousing because pressures from partner evaluation are removed and the intensity of the stimulation is under the woman's control.

Finally, it has been suggested that orgasm leads to increased vascularity of the vagina, labia, and clitoris (Bardwick, 1971), resulting in greater orgasmic potential. This observation also supports the use of Kegel exercises in the treatment of orgasmic dysfunction. Kegel (1952) originally reported that patients who strengthened the pubococcygeus (PC) muscle reported an increase in the frequency and intensity of orgasm. In treating women with orgasmic dysfunction, PC exercises are recommended daily to assist in strengthening the musculature surrounding the introitus (see Table 1). Although clinical reports support their

TABLE 1. At-Home Practice for Kegel Exercises

Slow Kegels—Tighten the P.C. muscle and hold it as you do when you stop the flow of urine for a slow count of 3. Then relax the muscle.

Quick Kegels—Tighten and relax the P.C. muscle as rapidly as you can. At first it will feel like a flutter. You will gradually gain more control.

Pull in/push out—Pull of the entire pelvic area as though trying to suck up water into the genitals. Then push out or bear down as if trying to push the imaginary water out. (This exercise will use a number of stomach or abdominal muscles as well as the P.C. muscle.)

Repetitions—At first do 10 of these exercises (one set), 3 times a day (3 exercises × 10 times × 3 times a day = 90 total exercises to start). Each week add 5 more times to each exercise. Example: Week 2: 3 sets × 15 times × 3 times a day; Week 3: 3 sets × 20 times × 3 times a day; Week 4: 3 sets × 25 times × 3 times a day. Keep doing 3 sets a day.

You can help yourself remember to do the exercises by associating them with some activity you do every day: talking on the phone, watching television, waiting in line, or lying in bed. Think of activities that don't require much moving around.

Don't worry if your muscles seem to get tired easily at first; that's normal for exercising any new muscle group. Rest between sets for a few seconds and start again. Remember to keep breathing naturally.

Women can place one or two fingers into the vagina and men one finger on each side of the base of the penis in order to feel the movement and strength of the muscle. You may also watch the movement by looking at your genitals in a hand mirror. Doing these things with your Kegels will help you learn them more rapidly.

---

value (e.g., Graber & Kline-Graber, 1979), other empirical investigations have failed to demonstrate a consistent relationship between PC muscle strength and orgasmic potential (Chambless, Stern, Sultan, Williams, Goldstein, Hazzard-Lineberger, Lifshitz, & Kelly, 1982; Chambless, Sultan, Stern, O'Neill, Garrison, & Jackson, 1984; Messé & Geer, 1985). In considering available treatment strategies for orgasmic dysfunction, it is important to recognize that these approaches do not necessarily ensure the transfer of orgasmic potential to sexual interactions with a partner. In fact, of those women who successfully acquire orgasmic ability with masturbation, only 9% to 55% transfer this ability to coital interactions (de Bruijn, 1982). However, sexual satisfaction does not appear to depend exclusively on orgasm during intercourse (Jayne, 1981). Generally, therapeutic focus on sexual technique and education concerning the anatomy and physiology of the female sexual response appears important in the treatment of orgasmic dysfunction in women.

Treatment of premature ejaculation in males is one of the more effective forms of sex therapy developed to date. Two similar techniques have been used extensively with men presenting with rapid, uncontrolled ejaculation: the squeeze technique (Semans, 1956) and the pause procedure (Masters & Johnson, 1970). Both rely on stimulation of the penis until high levels of sexual arousal but not threshold to ejaculation (ejaculatory inevitability) are reached. With the squeeze technique, pressure is applied beneath the coronal ridge at this point, reducing arousal and permitting resumption of sexual stimulation. The pause procedure similarly stops sexual activity at the point where high arousal is achieved, with the couple allowing arousal to diminish prior to reengaging in sex play. These procedures work well in group and individual treatment formats, and can be used with men who are not currently involved in a sexual relationship, with relatively good transfer of ejaculatory control to sex with a partner. Success rates of 90% to 98% have been reported at termination of treatment, although the long-term maintenance of these gains is more difficult to determine (Kilmann & Auerbach, 1979). Currently, there is little understanding of the mechanism through which these techniques operate. It is speculated that the ejaculatory threshold is raised through enhancing the man's accurate awareness of his arousal response.

Retarded ejaculation has received little attention in the therapeutic literature, perhaps owing to the rare nature of this dysfunction. Assuming the absence of an organic factor in the etiology of inhibited ejaculation, reduction of performance anxiety and increasing physical stimulation through sensate focus exercises are the primary treatment strategies used with this problem. LoPiccolo (1977) has suggested the adaptation of strategies used for anorgasmia in the treatment of retarded ejaculation. These include Kegel exercises, the use of electric vibrators to heighten stimulation, and role plays of exaggerated orgasm.

Intervention for Inhibited Sexual Desire

Despite the fact that considerable attention has been focused upon disorders of sexual desire (Leiblum & Rosen, 1988), the development of effective treatment for this disorder has lagged behind intervention for other sexual dysfunctions. It is recognized that standard sex therapy often fails to increase sexual desire (Kaplan, 1979), suggesting that separate therapeutic strategies are necessary for enhancing sexual interest. The most complete treatment program has been described by Friedman and Hogan (1985). This treatment model relies on a thorough assessment of the presenting problem, with individually tailored homework assignments revolving around four treatment elements. These include heightening experiential and sensory awareness of a range of emotional states, including sexual desire, expanding insight concerning factors that cause and maintain low desire, cognitive restructuring of thoughts that interfere with sexual functioning, particularly attributions concerning the sexual partner, and behavioral techniques as already outlined for enhancing arousal.

The experiential phase of treatment is designed to help patients differentiate various emotional states and to develop greater awareness of cues that evoke anxiety, anger, disgust, and other negative feelings. Friedman and Hogan include body awareness training and other interventions derived from the gestalt tradition during this phase of therapy, with the goal of enabling patients to recognize emotional influences in their verbal and nonverbal interactions. This phase of treatment often is integrated with the insight phase, where the therapist explores potential reasons for the desire discrepancy with the couple. This can include examination of family of origin issues, religious and attitudinal responses, and other material derived from the pretherapy assessment. Insight exercises can help to diffuse anger within the couple and prepare them for cognitive and behavioral interventions. Cognitive restructuring follows the systematic rational restructuring model of Goldfried (Goldfried & Davison, 1976) and focuses upon identifying self-statements that mediate negative and positive emotional responses. Friedman and Hogan include exercises derived from transactional analysis to facilitate patients' recognition that their feelings are under their control and to bridge the gap between cognition and emotion. Finally, behavioral techniques are used, including nongenital pleasuring, sensate focus, bibliotherapy, use of erotic films, and training in initiation and refusal of sexual activity. These clinical procedures appear effective for individual cases. To date, one outcome study, using a preliminary version of this treatment approach, has shown positive results (Schover & LoPiccolo, 1982).

Intervention for Vaginismus

Treatment of vaginismus involves several strategies designed to help the woman learn to relax her vaginal musculature and to experience penetration as pleasurable rather than painful. The first step in treatment involves teaching the woman relaxation, often using sensual message, progressive muscle relaxation, deep breathing, and imagery (Leiblum, Pervin, & Campbell, 1980). Once this has been achieved, the second step is to reduce her sensitivity to vaginal penetration. Dilators of increasing thickness may be used (often initially inserted in a gynecologist's office) or alternatively, the couple may practice insertion at home, using fingers instead of dilators. Often several repetitions of each step are required in order for the woman to feel relaxed and comfortable with vaginal penetration. The final step in treatment involves penile insertion, which generally occurs weeks (or months) following initiation of treatment. Structured treatment of vaginismus, when followed carefully, is highly effective, with an estimated 99% success rate (Kolodny, 1981). This high success rate may mask the importance of a past history of sexual trauma or couple systems issues in the etiology of vaginismus. Failure to address these concerns often results in unwillingness to undertake a program of relaxation and dilation.

Intervention for Other Sexual Dysfunctions

By definition, dyspareunia results from a physical etiology and should not be treated with sex therapy approaches. However, it is not uncommon for dyspareunia to be misdiagnosed as vaginismus, thus highlighting the importance of a medical evaluation prior to formulating treatment. Similarly, successful treatment of sexual aversion depends on identification of contributing factors at pretreatment. In cases where a conflict in sexual-partner-preference exists, the clinician is cautioned to explore several alternative treatment approaches, including helping the individual to adjust to a homosexual orientation, particularly given the ethical issues and clinical difficulty in changing partner preference.

The Process of Sex Therapy

In addition to specific intervention strategies, a number of therapeutic process concerns are relevant in the practice of sex therapy. The use of homework exercises is integral to treatment, particularly given the skills-training model that underlines their use. Anecdotal reports suggest that compliance with at-home exercises is a critical component to successful treatment (e.g., Lansky & Davenport, 1975) and point to noncompliance as an indicator of severe marital distress, precluding the couple from active resolution of sexual difficulties. Little systematic data exist to suggest particular homework exercises or formats that might be maximally effective. However, there is little question about the utility of at-home practice in treating sexual dysfunctions.

A related concern involves the use of self-help books, either alone or as an adjunct to traditional sex therapy. Several excellent books of this type currently exist (already mentioned), as well as more specialized texts, for older patients (e.g., Schover, *Prime Time: Sexual Health for Men over Fifty*) and couples (Barbach, *For Each Other*). The availability of these self-help programs allows a reduction in actual therapist contact and increased cost-effectiveness of sex therapy. Recent studies indicate that a minimal therapist contact format, when used in conjunction with a self-help program, can be as effective in treating female orgasmic dysfunction as a more extended course of therapy (Dodge, Glasgow, & O'Neill, 1982; Morokoff & LoPiccolo, 1986; Whitehead, Mathews, & Ramage, 1987). These studies carefully prescreened participants for the absence of other psychological disorders and couples systems issues, suggesting that self-help programs alone or with minimal therapeutic assistance may be useful with a small percentage of cases presenting for sex therapy.

As with other forms of brief psychotherapies, patient resistance can occur during sex therapy, often protracting the course of treatment. Munjack and Oziel (1978) have presented a typology of five sources of resistance that can be encountered during sex therapy, with suggestions for therapeutic management of each. The first source of resistance is related to the patient's misunderstanding of therapeutic instructions and can be handled with clarification. The second source of resistance is attributable to a deficit of skills, such as a lack of anatomical knowledge, and generally is avoided by careful pretreatment assessment. The third source of resistance, according to Munjack and Oziel, is due to lack of motivation or low expectations of success. Demonstrable evidence of change, as indicated by weekly records, can assist in heightening motivation, although this source of resistance can be difficult to distinguish from the fourth type of resistance, stemming from guilt or an excessive dependency upon the therapist's approval. In the latter case, examination of patterns of resistance with the patient can be helpful in clarifying emotional barriers to positive change and often indicates that at-home exercises be assigned at a more gradual pace, with emphasis on strengthening the patient's coping skills. The final source of resistance is due to secondary gains, including monetary benefits or attention for dysfunctional behavior. As far as possible, the therapist is advised to shift reinforcements to reward progress in therapy and to help the patient develop a belief in his or her own ability to handle future problems.

Resistance also can arise near the time of termination, taking the form of a brief relapse of sexual difficulties or a direct expression of apprehension concerning the cessation of treatment. In response to this, it is not uncommon for sessions to be scheduled at 2- to 3-week intervals near the end of treatment, to help patients develop greater confidence in their sexual problem-solving skills. Additionally one can remind patients of the continuing availability of therapy, if necessary, in the future. Generally, termination of brief sex therapy is not characterized by the type of difficulties that can arise in long-term therapy. Booster sessions are used only rarely, particularly given the availability of self-help books and emphasis throughout treatment on the integration of new skills into ongoing sexual interactions.

The following case study illustrates the treatment of a woman with secondary orgasmic dysfunction, involving some of the treatment strategies already outlined. In considering this case, it is important to note the role of cultural influences and couples systems issues in treatment.

CASE STUDY: MARY ANN AND NAV

Mary Ann and Nav, both 30 years old, had been dating for 1 year and living together for 2 months at the time they sought sex therapy. Mary Ann reported that during the past

6 months, she had experienced low arousal, a lack of orgasm during sexual interactions, and occasionally, painful intercourse with Nav. This couple had discontinued any attempts at sexual activity in the preceding month, although Nav had continued to masturbate when alone. Prior to the onset of this problem, Mary Ann had been able to achieve high levels of sexual arousal, including orgasm, both alone and with Nav. Mary Ann had recently begun a new job as an independent writer for a small consulting firm, and Nav was employed as an engineer in a *Fortune 500* company. They were engaged and planned to marry within the year.

Background: Mary Ann

Mary Ann had been born and raised in a small rural town in west Texas. Her parents were described as "traditional," as evidenced by their emphasis on marriage and child rearing as appropriate career goals for their daughters. Mary Ann was the elder of two children; her younger sister had married a man that Mary Ann referred to as "a little boy" and was fulfilling parental expectations. In contrast, Mary Ann had completed a master's degree in business administration and, prior to her current job, had been employed as a consultant in a high-pressure company. Her parents had divorced when she was 18, and each had remarried within 3 years. Her current relationship with her father was strained, and she stated that she did not get along well with her stepmother. Mary Ann was close to her mother and stepfather and enjoyed her frequent visits with them.

During her childhood, affection and caring were not shown often at home, and Mary Ann stated that she could not imagine that her parents' sex lives were satisfying. Although her mother was described as warm and giving, she never discussed sexuality with Mary Ann during childhood or adolescence, except for a brief explanation of female anatomy when Mary Ann began to menstruate. Her father was quite involved with his job during these years and spent little time with his family. Mary Ann perceived that her mother held much of the power in the family, although she always deferred to her husband on matters of child rearing. Their divorce followed many years of strained communication and arguments and occurred during the year that Mary Ann was a freshman in college. During high school Mary Ann dated infrequently, stating that she dreaded bringing a boy home to meet her parents, for fear that they would immediately begin to pressure her to marry. She began to date more frequently in college and had her first sexual experience when she was 20, which she described as "pleasant enough." She first masturbated to orgasm when she was 25, after a boyfriend explained male and female anatomy to her. She was unaware of any sexual fantasies that were arousing for her. Mary Ann had dated two boys seriously before meeting Nav and had been sexually active in both of these relationships.

Background: Nav

Nav was born in India and had moved to the United States at age 22 to pursue graduate studies. He described his family as "strict and successful" and stated that both of his parents had emphasized the importance of formal education throughout his childhood. He had two younger sisters who were still living in India. Despite the distance, Nav visited his family at least once a year. Nav stated that he was close to both parents and enjoyed the accumulated business wisdom that his father shared with him.

Nav had attended a boy's military school, beginning at age 5 and had lived on-campus throughout most of his childhood and adolescence. Sex education had occurred in the context of his peer group, and Nav had never discussed sexuality with either of his parents. He described his parents' relationship as close and caring but emphasized that they rarely touched one another in front of their children. He imagined that their sexual relationship was mutually satisfying but admitted that this was speculation, given the absence of communication concerning sex in the household. He had first masturbated at age 16, which was accompanied by guilt and anxiety at the prospect of being discovered, and had intercourse for the first time at age 19. Upon moving to this country, Nav was startled by the availability of sexually explicit books and films and initially had made every effort to expand his knowledge about sexuality through reading. Before meeting Mary Ann, Nav had maintained a sexual relationship with a girl whom he described as "knowing even less about sex" than himself. His sexual fantasies were exclusively heterosexual and included intercourse, oral, and anal sex. He stated that he had never experienced difficulty in achieving or maintaining an erection or rapid ejaculation.

Presenting Problem

During the initial interview, both Mary Ann and Nav described a pattern of sexual interaction that had becoming extremely uncomfortable prior to the complete cessation of sexual contact. They had been extremely attracted to one another upon meeting during a business transaction and had begun to date shortly thereafter. Sexual activity was initiated by Nav and was arousing and satisfying for both at first. Mary Ann was orgasmic with manual stimulation during intercourse, and each stated that sex was spontaneous, highly enjoyable, and "natural." After several months, Mary Ann found it difficult to achieve orgasm with Nav, which she did not reveal to him, and had attempted to remedy this problem herself by increasing her frequency of solitary masturbation to orgasm. This approach did not generalize to her sexual interactions with Nav, and she became more anxious as she found herself less aroused by his touch.

Their decision to live together had been precipitated by Mary Ann's job change, which had reduced her income and allowed her to spend considerably more time writing at home. Nav expressed satisfaction with this new arrangement, as he appreciated the flexibility that this offered Mary Ann with respect to both housekeeping and working. Mary Ann stated that she enjoyed her new work colleagues but felt displaced without a regular schedule. Their free time was spent at home, as Nav usually was exhausted at the end of the workday.

Mary Ann's goals for treatment were to enjoy sex more, to achieve orgasm during sexual interactions, and to be able to communicate more effectively. Nav's goals for treatment included increasing the amount of leisure activities they shared together, including social contacts with other couples, and to feel less inhibited during sex. Neither indicated significant medical, health, or other psychological problems. At the time of intake, they were relying on oral contraceptives for birth control, although Mary Ann stated that she had not been consistent in her use of these in the month preceding therapy. Both were judged to be above average in intelligence and appeared to have good communication skills. The exception to this was their ability to resolve conflict, as Nav frequently would withdraw from an impending argument by leaving the room. Mary Ann often yielded to his wishes on matters where they disagreed, in fear of this approach–avoidance pattern.

Table 2. Assessment Information Pre- and Posttherapy

	Intake	Post
Male Locke–Wallace score	110	120
Female Locke–Wallace score	98	123
Male Overall Sexual Satisfaction (DSFI)	6	10
Female Overall Sexual Satisfaction (DSFI)	2	9
Male SII Scaled score (Overall)	70	56
Female SII Scaled score (Overall)	83	59
Male BDI	2	0
Female BDI	9	1
Male estimate of intercourse frequency (weekly)	0	4
Female estimate of intercourse frequency (weekly)	0	4

Formulation

Based on pretherapy assessment (see Table 2), several factors appeared relevant in the etiology and maintenance of Mary Ann's secondary orgasmic dysfunction. These included:

- *Performance anxiety.* Both individuals expressed considerable apprehension concerning the quality of their own sexual performance, particularly Nav, who stated that he was particularly concerned about his ability to please Mary Ann.
- *Inadequate knowledge about sexual functioning.* Nav's previous sexual contacts had been characterized as "fumbling," suggesting that he knew little about male and female sexual function and was unsure of what constituted typical sexual behavior.
- *Couples issues relating to dependence/independence.* In light of the recent changes in their relationship, a number of unresolved conflicts appeared to exist concerning the extent of independence that each was comfortable with. A lack of methods for resolving these differences was noted.
- *Sexual communication skills.* Mary Ann appeared reticent to discuss the specifics of her sexual interactions with Nav. This included communication concerning sexual technique, frequency of intercourse, and expression of likes and dislikes.
- *Differences in expectations for their relationship.* During the individual portion of the interview, Mary Ann and Nav had expressed markedly discrepant expectations for their overall relationship. Mary Ann stated that ideally, she wished for her marriage to be characterized by equity, whereas Nav stated that he enjoyed a more traditional relationship, with his role being "breadwinner and protector." These expectations were recognized by both individuals as stemming from their own families of origin.

Treatment

In light of the factors identified as potentially maintaining this couple's problem, treatment was designed to integrate sex therapy techniques with interventions targeting the unspoken differences in their expectations for their relationship. Treatment sessions initially were held at weekly intervals and included strategies designed to address each of these areas, with homework assignments given at the end of the session. Near completion of treatment, sessions were scheduled biweekly. Given this couple's degree of psychological sophistication and expressed motivation, a single-therapist format appeared to be the most cost-effective choice.

The first intervention given to Mary Ann and Nav was individual self-exploration of pleasurable bodily sensations and a ban on intercourse. They were asked to read *For Yourself* and *Male Sexuality*, in order to expand their knowledge of female and male sexual anatomy, with discussion of details of the female sexual response pattern during the treatment session. Methods for communicating likes and dislikes were discussed during the session, with each partner sharing fears that direct communication would evoke their conflict avoidance pattern. For example, Mary Ann revealed to Nav that she felt extremely vulnerable to his unexpressed anger and withdrawal and feared destroying the relationship by expressing herself directly about sensitive issues. Nav indicated that he felt a responsibility to react logically during stressful interactions and when he felt unable to do so, would leave in order to collect himself. Role plays were used during the sessions, with each partner adopting the other's role, to clarify unspoken beliefs that influenced conflict resolution. Although both partners were able to enact these roles with humor, they appeared to gain insight into the rigid patterns that had evolved between them. These interventions were used for three treatment sessions.

Several weeks after initiating this approach, Mary Ann reported that she had begun to become aroused during nongenital pleasuring and had learned to give Nav feedback in a fashion that appeared to be well received. In addition, for the first time, they began to experiment with exchanging household responsibilities, such as preparing grocery lists and balancing the checkbook, and were actively struggling with maintaining flexibility in this role exchange. Therapy sessions included discussion of how much each partner desired this type of fluidity in their relationship. Nav indicated that he was unaccustomed to this type of relationship, particularly because Mary Ann previously had maintained responsibility for many of these tasks. This was the first time that each had shared their expectations for their relationship with one another, and several arguments resulted during the sessions. Although Nav tended to withdraw at first, with therapeutic emphasis on communication skills and the desirability of conflict resolution, they gradually began to discuss how they could compromise and still feel satisfied with the relationship. One outcome of this intervention was an overall relaxation of the demands that they placed on one another for performance of household duties, as well as a more balanced distribution of responsibility. Four sessions were spent examining these issues, during which time this couple continued nongenital pleasuring exercises.

Once some of these couple systems issues were aired and explored, the genital pleasuring exercises became the focus of treatment, as the introduction of direct genital stimulation evoked considerable performance anxiety for both Mary Ann and Nav. Instructing this couple that orgasm was not the goal at this point in treatment, as well as introducing the notion that homework exercises could be done in a variety of situations (e.g., in the shower) helped to ease tension and added an air of novelty to their sexual contacts. Mary Ann began to expand her sexual fantasies through reading, and gradually she and Nav began to "swap fantasies." Additionally, Nav surprised Mary Ann by renting an erotic movie for home viewing, which enabled them to mutually experience sexual arousal without the necessity for intercourse (which was still prohibited). The frequency of their sexual contacts had increased to three to four times per week by this point in treatment, although both were uncomfortable with the notion of masturbating in each other's presence. Given the goals outlined during the pretreatment assessment, this did not appear necessary despite its inclusion in many masturbatory training programs. Sexual contact was initiated by Mary Ann as often as by Nav; two sessions were devoted to genital pleasuring and fantasy elaboration.

During the tenth session, Mary Ann revealed that she had initiated intercourse and had been orgasmic with manual stimulation. She reported that she felt no anxiety and had not experienced pain or a lack of arousal at any point. Nav had experienced some transient anxiety at first, but this had dissipated rapidly. Part of the session was spent discussing the positive changes that each had made that allowed satisfying intercourse to occur. Additionally, the issue of how the couple spent their leisure time was raised, as Nav had targeted this as one of his pretreatment goals. With little therapeutic intervention, each was able to suggest activities and changes in work schedules that would permit greater social contact, with clear communication concerning sensitive issues, such as Mary Ann's need for uninterrupted time on the weekend for writing, given a regular Monday deadline.

Treatment sessions were spaced at 2-week intervals for the remaining two sessions, with both Nav and Mary Ann expressing continued satisfaction with the frequency and quality of sexual contact. Mary Ann remained orgasmic with manual stimulation and the couple appeared to adjust their schedules to permit leisure time together. Termination did not bring about a return of problems, although Nav expressed some apprehension about his ability to "remember" the changes that had occurred during treatment (see Table 2). A follow-up appointment was scheduled 4 weeks after termination; at this appointment Mary Ann and Nav announced their wedding date and informed the therapist that they were moving to another state, because Nav had received a promotion. Despite the stress that these life events had created, this couple had maintained the patterns of sexual and nonsexual communication that had resulted following 12 weeks of treatment.

Summary

Although this case may not be typical of most individuals presenting for sex therapy, given both partners' level of education and motivation for treatment, the integration of interventions for both sexual and couples systems problems appeared necessary for successful resolution of Mary Ann's secondary orgasmic dysfunction. The absence of other psychological problems contributed to a positive outcome, particularly given our current knowledge of factors associated with success and failure in sex therapy. Pretreatment assessment identified areas where therapeutic gains would generalize, from sexual to nonsexual interactions, and yielded a thorough picture of etiological and maintaining factors in this couple's problem.

CONCLUSION

In many respects, the practice of sex therapy has gained a startling degree of sophistication during the past 20 years. Although questions remain concerning effective treatment of specific dysfunctions such as retarded ejaculation, as well as a lack of specification of the active ingredients of the total sex therapy package, there is little dispute that this form of brief psychotherapy can be effective. Over time, the nature of sex therapy cases presenting to clinics and individual practitioners has become more complex, requiring greater clinical acumen with therapeutic strategies and highlighting the necessity of pretreatment assessment. Fortunately our empirical knowledge base has kept abreast with these changes and has greatly expanded our understanding of one of the more complex and private forms of human behavior.

References

Abramowitz, S. I., & Sewell, H. H. (1980). Marital adjustment and sex therapy outcome. *Journal of Sex Research, 16,* 325–337.

Andersen, B. L. (1983). Primary orgasmic dysfunction. Diagnostic considerations and review of treatment. *Psychological Bulletin, 93,* 105–136.

Annon, J. S. (1973). The therapeutic use of masturbation in the treatment of sexual disorders. In R. D. Rubin, J. P. Brady, & J. D. Henderson (Eds.), *Advances in behavior therapy.* New York: Academic Press.

Ansari, J. M. A. (1976). Impotence: Prognosis (a controlled study). *The British Journal of Psychiatry, 128,* 194–198.

Arentewicz, G., & Schmidt, G. (1983). *The treatment of sexual disorders.* New York: Basic Books.

Bancroft, J. (1984). Hormones and human sexual behavior. *Journal of Sex and Marital Therapy, 10,* 3–22.

Barbach, L. (1974). Group treatment of preorgasmic women. *Journal of Sex and Marital Therapy, 1,* 139–145.

Barbach, L. (1975). *For yourself: The fulfillment of female sexuality.* Garden City, NY: Doubleday.

Bardwick, J. (1971). *Psychology of women: A study of bio-cultural conflicts.* New York: Harper & Row.

Barlow, D. H. (1977). Assessment of sexual behavior. In A. Ciminero, K. Calhoun, & H. E. Adams (Eds.), *Handbook of behavioral assessment* (pp. 461–508). New York: Wiley.

Barry, J. M., Blank, B., & Bioleau, M. (1980). Nocturnal penile tumescence monitoring with stamps. *Urology, 15,* 171–172.

Beck, A. T. (1967). *Depression: Clinical, experimental, and theoretical aspects.* New York: Harper & Row.

Beck, J. G. (1985). Secondary orgasmic dysfunction: Modifying sexual and marital scripts. In M. Hersen & C. G. Last (Eds.), *Behavior therapy casebook* (pp. 185–199). New York: Springer Publishers.

Bennett, A. (1982). *Management of male impotence.* Baltimore: Williams & Wilkins.

Caird, W., & Wincze, J. P. (1977). *Sex therapy.* New York: Harper & Row.

Chambless, D. L., Stern, T., Sultan, F. E., Williams, A. J., Goldstein, A. J., Hazzard-Lineberger, M., Lifshitz, J., & Kelly, L. (1982). The pubococcygeus and female orgasm: A correlational study with normal subjects. *Archives of Sexual Behavior, 11,* 479–490.

Chambless, D. L., Sultan, F. E., Stern, T. E., O'Neill, C., Garrison, S., & Jackson, A. (1984). Effects of pubococcygeal exercise on coital orgasm in women. *Journal of Consulting and Clinical Psychology, 52,* 114–118.

Chapman, R. (1982). Criteria for diagnosing when to do sex therapy in primary relationship. *Psychotherapy: Theory, Research, and Practice, 19,* 359–367.

Conte, H. R. (1986). Multivariate assessment of sexual dysfunction. *Journal of Consulting and Clinical Psychology, 54,* 149–157.

Cooper, A. J. (1981). Short-term treatment in sexual dysfunction: A review. *Comprehensive Psychiatry, 22,* 206–217.

Corcoran, K., & Fischer, J. (1987). *Measures for clinical practice.* New York: Free Press.

de Bruijn, G. (1982). From masturbation to orgasm with a partner: How some women bridge the gap—and why others don't. *Journal of Sex and Marital Therapy, 8,* 151–167.

Derogatis, L. R. (1978). *Derogatis Sexual Functioning Inventory* (Rev. ed.) Baltimore MD: Clinical Psychometrics Research.

Derogatis, L. R., Rickels, K., & Rock, A. (1976). The SCL-90 and the MMPI: A step in the validation of a new self-report scale. *British Journal of Psychiatry, 128,* 280–289.

Dodge, L. J. T., Glasgow, R. E., & O'Neill, H. K. (1982). Bibliotherapy in the treatment of female orgasmic dysfunction. *Journal of Consulting and Clinical Psychology, 50,* 442–443.

Dow, S. (1981). Retarded ejaculation. *Journal of Sex and Marital Therapy, 7,* 49–53.

Ersner-Hershfield, R., & Kopel, S. (1979). Group treatment of preorgasmic women: Evaluation of partner involvement and spacing of sessions. *Journal of Consulting and Clinical Psychology, 47,* 750–759.

Everaerd, W. T. A. M. (1983). Failures in treating sexual dysfunctions. In E. B. Foa & P. M. G. Emmelkamp (Eds.), *Failures in behavior therapy* (pp. 392–405). New York: Wiley.

Everaerd, W., & Dekker, J. (1981). A comparison of sex therapy and communication therapy: Couples complaining of orgasmic dysfunction. *Journal of Sex and Marital Therapy, 7,* 278–289.

Fisher, C., Schiavi, R. C., Edwards, A., Davis, D. M., Reitman, M., & Fine, J. (1979). Evaluation of nocturnal penile tumescence in the differential diagnosis of sexual impotence. *Archives of General Psychiatry, 36,* 431–437.

Fordney-Settlage, D. S. (1975). Heterosexual dysfunction: Evaluation of treatment procedures. *Archives of Sexual Behavior, 4,* 367–387.

Frank, E., Anderson, C., & Rubenstein, D. (1978). Frequency of sexual dysfunction in "normal" couples. *New England Journal of Medicine, 299,* 111–115.

Friedman, J. M., & Hogan, D. R. (1985). Sexual dysfunction: Low sexual desire. In D. H. Barlow (Ed.), *Clinical handbook of psychological disorders* (pp. 417–461). New York: Guilford Press.

Golden, J. S., Price, S., Heinrich, A. G., & Lobitz, W. C. (1978). Group vs. couple treatment of sexual dysfunctions. *Archives of Sexual Behavior, 7,* 593–602.

Goldfried, M. R., & Davison, G. C. (1976). *Clinical behavior therapy.* New York: Holt, Rinehart & Winston.

Graber, B., & Kline-Graber, G. (1979). Female orgasm: Role of pubococcygeus muscle. *Journal of Clinical Psychiatry, 40,* 33–39.

Hatch, J. P. (1981). Psychophysiological aspects of sexual dysfunction. *Archives of Sexual Behavior, 10,* 49–64.

Hartman, L. M., & Daly, E. M. (1983). Relationship factors in the treatment of sexual dysfunction. *Behaviour Research and Therapy, 2,* 153–160.

Hawkins, R. P. (1979). The functions of assessment. Implications for selection and development of devices for assessing repertoires in clinical educational, and other settings. *Journal of Applied Behavior Analysis, 12,* 501–516.

Hawton, K., & Catalan, J. (1986). Prognostic factors in sex therapy. *Behavior Research and Therapy, 24,* 377–385.

Heiman, J. R. (1976). Issues in the use of psychophysiology to assess female sexual dysfunction. *Journal of Sex and Marital Therapy, 2,* 197–204.

Heiman, J. R., & LoPiccolo, J. (1983). Clinical outcome of sex therapy: Effects of daily vs. weekly treatment. *Archives of General Psychiatry, 40,* 443–449.

Heiman, J. R., & LoPiccolo, J. (1988). *Becoming orgasmic.* New York: Prentice-Hall.

Hite, S. (1976). *The Hite report.* New York: Macmillan.

Husted, J. R. (1975). Desensitization procedures in dealing with female sexual dysfunction. In J. LoPiccolo & L. LoPiccolo (Eds.), *Handbook of sex therapy* (pp. 195–208). New York: Plenum Press.

Jackman, L. S. (1976). Sexual dysfunction and the family system. In P. J. Guerin (Ed.), *Family therapy* (pp. 298–308). New York: Gardner Press.

Jayne, C. (1981). A two-dimensional model of female sexual response. *Journal of Sex and Marital Therapy, 7,* 3–30.

Karacan, I. (1970). Clinical value of nocturnal erection in the prognosis and diagnosis of impotence. *Medical Aspects of Human Sexuality, 4,* 27–34.

Karacan, I. (1978). Advances in the psychophysiological evaluation of male erectile impotence. In J. LoPiccolo & L. LoPiccolo (Eds.), *Handbook of sex therapy* (pp. 137–145). New York: Plenum Press.

Kaplan, H. S. (1974). *The new sex therapy.* New York: Brunner/Mazel.

Kaplan, H. S. (1979). *Disorders of desire.* New York: Brunner/Mazel.

Kedia, K. (1983). Ejaculation and emission: Normal physiology, dysfunction, and therapy. In R. J. Krane, M. B. Siroky, & I. Goldstein (Eds.), *Male sexual dysfunction* (pp. 37–54). Boston: Little, Brown.

Kegel, A. (1952). Sexual functions of the pubococcygeus muscle. *Western Journal of Surgery, 60*, 521–524.

Kilmann, P. R. (1978). The treatment of primary and secondary orgasmic dysfunction: A methodological review of the literature since 1970. *Journal of Sex and Marital Therapy, 1*, 155–176.

Kilmann, P. R., & Auerbach, R. (1979). Treatments of premature ejaculation and psychogenic impotence: A critical review of the literature. *Archives of Sexual Behavior, 8*, 81–100.

Kinder, B. N., & Blakeney, P. (1977). Treatment of sexual dysfunction: A review of outcome studies. *Journal of Clinical Psychology, 33*, 523–530.

Kinsey, A. C., Pomeroy, W. B., & Martin, C. E. (1948). *Sexual behavior in the human male.* Philadelphia: Saunders.

Kinsey, A. C., Pomeroy, W. B., Martin, C. E., & Gebhard, P. H. (1953. *Sexual behavior in the human female.* Philadelphia: Saunders.

Kline-Graber, G., & Graber, B. (1975). *Woman's orgasm.* New York: Popular Library.

Kolodny, R. C. (1981). Evaluating sex therapy: Process and outcome at the Masters & Johnson Institute. *Journal of Sex Research, 17*, 301–318.

Kolodny, R. C., Masters, W. H., & Johnson, V. E. (1979). *Textbook of sexual medicine.* Boston: Little, Brown.

Kuriansky, J., & Sharpe, I. (1976). Guidelines for evaluating sex therapy. *Journal of Sex and Marital Therapy, 2*, 303–308.

Lansky, M. R., & Davenport, A. E. (1975). Difficulties in brief conjoint treatment of sexual dysfunction. *American Journal of Psychiatry, 132*, 177–179.

Lazarus, A. A. (1971). *Behavior therapy and beyond.* New York: McGraw-Hill.

Leiblum, S., & Ersner-Hershfield, R. (1977). Sexual enhancement groups for dysfunctional women: An evaluation. *Journal of Sex and Marital Therapy, 3*, 139–152.

Leiblum, S., & Rosen, R. C. (Eds.). (1988). *Disorders of sexual desire.* New York: Guilford Press.

Leiblum, S. R., Pervin, L. A., & Campbell, E. H. (1980). The treatment of vaginismus: Success and failure. In S. R. Leiblum & L. A. Pervin (Eds.), *Principles and practice of sex therapy* (pp. 167–194). New York: Guilford Press.

Levay, A. N., & Kagle, A. (1983). Interminable sex therapy: A report on ten cases of therapeutic gridlock. *Journal of Marital and Family Therapy, 9*, 1–9.

Levay, A. N., & Kagle, A. (1977). A study of treatment needs following sex therapy. *American Journal of Psychiatry, 34*, 970–973.

Lipsius, S. H. (1987). Prescribing sensate focus without proscribing intercourse. *Journal of Sex and Marital Therapy, 13*, 106–111.

Lobitz, W. C., & Lobitz, G. K. (1978). Clinical assessment in the treatment of sexual dysfunctions. In J. LoPiccolo & L. LoPiccolo (Eds.), *Handbook of sex therapy* (pp. 85–102). New York: Plenum Press.

Locke, H. J., & Wallace, K. M. (1959). Short marital-adjustment and prediction tests: Their reliability and validity. *Marriage and Family Living, 21*, 251–255.

LoPiccolo, J. (1978). Direct treatment of sexual dysfunction in the couple. In J. Money & H. Musaph (Eds.), *Handbook of sexology* (pp. 1227–1244). New York: Elsevier/North Holland.

LoPiccolo, J. (1978). Direct treatment of sexual dysfunction. In J. LoPiccolo & L. LoPiccolo (Eds.), *Handbook of sex therapy* (pp. 1–17). New York: Plenum Press.

LoPiccolo, L., & Heiman, J. R. (1978). Sexual assessment and history interview. In J. LoPiccolo & L. LoPiccolo (Eds.), *Handbook of sex therapy* (pp. 103–112). New York: Plenum Press.

LoPiccolo, J., & Lobitz, W. C. (1972). The role of masturbation in the treatment of orgasmic dysfunction. *Archives of Sexual Behavior, 2*, 163–171.

LoPiccolo, J., & LoPiccolo, L. (Eds.). (1978). *Handbook of sex therapy.* New York: Plenum Press.

LoPiccolo, J., & Steger, J. C. (1974). The Sexual Interaction Inventory: A new instrument for assessment of sexual dysfunction. *Archives of Sexual Behavior, 3*, 585–595.

LoPiccolo, J., & Stock, W. (1987). Sexual counseling in gynecological practice. In Z. Rosenwaks, F. Benjamin, & M. Stone (Eds.), *Basic Gynecology* (pp. 339–371). New York: Macmillan.

LoPiccolo, J., Heiman, J. R., Hogan, D. R., & Roberts, C. W. (1985). Effectiveness of single therapists versus cotherapy teams in sex therapy. *Journal of Consulting and Clinical Psychology, 53,* 287–294.

Madsen, C. H., & Ullmann, L. (1967). Case histories and short communications. *Behaviour Research and Therapy, 5,* 67–68.

Mandell, W., & Miller, C. M. (1983). Male sexual dysfunction related to alcohol consumption: A pilot study. *Alcoholism: Clinical and Experimental Research, 7,* 65–69.

Marks, I. M. (1981). Review of behavioral psychotherapy: II. Sexual disorders. *American Journal of Psychiatry, 138,* 750–756.

Masters, W. H., & Johnson, V. E. (1966). *Human sexual response.* Boston: Little, Brown.

Masters, W. H., & Johnson, V. E. (1970). *Human sexual inadequacy.* Boston: Little, Brown.

McMullen, S., & Rosen, R. C. (1979). Self-administered masturbation training in the treatment of primary orgasmic dysfunction. *Journal of Consulting and Clinical Psychology, 47,* 912–918.

Melman, A., Kaplan, D., & Redfield, J. (1984). Evaluation of the first 70 patients in the center for male sexual dysfunction of Beth Israel Medical Center. *Journal of Urology, 131,* 53–55.

Messé, M. R., & Geer, J. H. (1985). Voluntary vaginal musculature contractions as an enhancer of sexual arousal. *Archives of Sexual Behavior, 14,* 13–28.

Morokoff, P. J., & LoPiccolo, J. (1986). A comparative evaluation of minimal therapist contact and 15-session treatment for female orgasmic dysfunction. *Journal of Consulting and Clinical Psychology, 54,* 294–300.

Munjack, D. J., & Kanno, P. H. (1979). Retarded ejaculation: A review. *Archives of Sexual Behavior, 8,* 139–150.

Munjack, D. J., & Oziel, L. J. (1978). Resistance in the behavioral treatment of sexual dysfunctions. *Journal of Sex & Marital Therapy, 4,* 122–138.

Myers, L. S. & Morokoff, P. J. (1986). Physiological and subjective sexual arousal in pre- and postmenopausal women taking replacement therapy. *Psychophysiology, 23,* 283–292.

Nowinski, J. K., & LoPiccolo, J. (1979). Assessing sexual behavior in couples. *Journal of Sex and Marital Therapy, 5,* 225–243.

Obler, M. (1973). Systematic desensitization in sexual disorder. *Journal of Behavior Therapy and Experimental Psychiatry, 4,* 93–101.

Ohlmeyer, P., Brilmayer, H., & Hullstrung, H. (1944). Periodische vorgange im schlaf. *Pfleugers Archive Gestaut Physiologie, 249,* 50–55.

Perls, F. S. (1960). *Gestault therapy verbatim.* Moab, UT: Real People Press.

Procci, W. R., Moss, H. G., Boyd, J. L., & Barron, D. A. (1983). Consecutive night reliability of portable nocturnal penile tumescence monitor. *Archives of Sexual Behavior, 12,* 307–316.

Reynolds, B. S. (1977). Psychological treatment models and outcome results for erectile dysfunction: A critical review. *Psychological Bulletin, 84,* 1218–1238.

Riley, A. J., & Riley, E. J. (1978). A controlled study to evaluate directed masturbation in the management of primary orgasmic failure in women. *British Journal of Psychiatry, 133,* 404–409.

Robinson, P. (1976). *The modernization of sex.* New York: Harper & Row.

Rosen, R. C., & Beck, J. G. (1986). Models and measures of sexual response: Psychophysiological assessment of male and female arousal. In D. Byne & K. Kelley (Eds.), *Alternative approaches to the study of sexual behavior* (pp. 43–86). Hillsdale, NJ: Erlbaum.

Rosen, R. C., & Beck, J. G. (1988). *Patterns and processes of sexual responding.* New York: Guilford Press.

Sarrel, P. (1977). Biological aspects of sexual function. In R. Gemme & C. C. Wheeler (Eds.). *Progress in sexology* (pp. 227–244). New York: Plenum Press.

Schiavi, R., & Fisher, S. (1982). Measurement of nocturnal erections. In J. Bancroft (Ed.), *Diseases of sex and sexuality: Clinics in endocrinology and metabolism* (pp. 769–784). Philadelphia: Saunders.

Schneidman, B., & McGuire, L. (1976). Group therapy for nonorgasmic women: Two age levels. *Archives of Sexual Behavior, 5,* 239–248.

Schover, L. (1984). *Prime time: sexual health for men over fifty.* New York: Holt, Rinehart and Winston.

Schover, L., & LoPiccolo, J. (1982). Treatment effectiveness for dysfunctions of sexual desire. *Journal of Sex and Marital Therapy, 8,* 179–197.

Schover, L. R., Friedman, J. M., Weiler, S. J., Heiman, J. R., & LoPiccolo, J. (1982). Multiaxial problem-oriented system for sexual dysfunctions: An alternative to DSM-III. *Archives of General Psychiatry, 39,* 617–619.

Schwartz, D. T. (1983). Role of confrontation in performance and interpretation of nocturnal penile tumescence studies. *Urology, 22,* 240–242.

Semans, J. H. (1956). Premature ejaculation: A new approach. *Southern Medical Journal, 49,* 353–357.

Sotile, W. (1979). The penile prosthesis. *Journal of Sex and Marital Therapy, 5,* 90–102.

Spiess, W. F., Geer, J. H., & O'Donohue, W. T. (1984). Premature ejaculation: Investigation of factors in ejaculatory latency. *Journal of Abnormal Psychology, 93,* 242–245.

Tennov, D. (1979). *Love and limerence.* New York: Stein and Day.

Wagner, G. (1981). Methods for differential diagnosis of psychogenic and organic erectile failure. In G. Wagner & R. Green (Eds.), *Impotence* (pp. 89–130). New York: Plenum Press.

Wallace, O. H., & Barbach, L. G. (1974). Preorgasmic group treatment. *Journal of Sex and Marital Therapy, 1,* 146–154.

Wasserman, M. D., Pollak, C. P., Spielman, A. J., & Weitzman, G. D. (1980). Theoretical and technical problems in the measurement of nocturnal penile tumescence for the differential diagnosis of impotence. *Psychosomatic Medicine, 42,* 575–585.

Wein, A. J., Fishkin, R., Carpiniello, V. L., & Malloy, T. R. (1981). Expansion without significant rigidity during nocturnal penile tumescence testing: A potential source of misinterpretation. *The Journal of Urology, 126,* 343–344.

Whitehead, A., Mathews, A., & Ramage, M. (1987). The treatment of sexually unresponsive women: A comparative evaluation. *Behavior Research and Therapy, 25,* 195–205.

Wincze, J. P. (1981). Sexual dysfunction (Distress and dissatisfaction). In S. M. Turner, K. S. Calhoun, & H. E. Adams (Eds.), *Handbook of clinical behavior therapy* (pp. 290–317). New York: Wiley.

Wolpe, J. (1958). *Psychotherapy by reciprocal inhibition.* Stanford: Stanford University Press.

Wright, J., Perreault, R., & Mathieu, M. (1977). The treatment of sexual dysfunction. *Archives of General Psychiatry, 34,* 881–890.

Zilbergeld, B. (1978). *Male sexuality.* Toronto: Bantam Books.

Zilbergeld, B., & Ellison, C. R. (1980). Desire discrepancies and arousal problems in sex therapy. In S. R. Lieblum & L. A. Pervin (Eds.), *Principles and practice of sex therapy* (pp. 65–101). New York: Guilford Press.

20

One Person Family Therapy

Jose Szapocznik, William M. Kurtines,
Angel Perez-Vidal, Olga E. Hervis,
and Franklin H. Foote

Background

This chapter introduces practitioners to the strategies and techniques of One Person Family Therapy (OPFT). It is aimed at family therapists and counselors who want to make immediate, practical use of structural and strategic family therapy techniques but who either prefer or need to work with only one person rather than a whole family in most therapy sessions. Anyone wishing to become truly expert in OPFT should become thoroughly familiar with the theory behind it. A more complete account is available in Szapocznik, Perez-Vidal, Hervis, Foote, and Spencer (1983); Szapocznik and Kurtines (1989); and Szapocznik, Kurtines, Hervis, and Spencer (1984). Briefer accounts are in Szapocznik, Kurtines, Foote, Perez-Vidal, and Hervis (1983, 1986) and Foote, Szapocznik, Kurtines, Hervis, and Perez-Vidal (1985). The structural family precursors of the work are described in Minuchin (1974, 1976) and Minuchin and Fishman (1981). Precursors of the strategic components of OPFT are described in Haley (1976) and Madanes (1981).

The strategies and techniques presented here were developed, refined, and then tested using rigorous research procedures at the Spanish Family Guidance Center at the University of Miami. They were found to be highly effective as implemented in a research project funded by the National Institute of Drug Abuse, entitled Brief Strategic Family Therapy (Szapocznik, Perez-Vidal, Hervis, Foote, & Spencer, 1984).

Jose Szapocznik, William M. Kurtines, Angel Perez-Vidal, Olga E. Hervis, and Franklin H. Foote • Spanish Family Guidance Center, Department of Psychiatry, University of Miami School of Medicine, Miami, Florida 33136. The work reported in this chapter has been adapted from a monograph, *One Person Family Therapy*, by J. Szapocznik, F. H. Foote, A. Perez-Vidal, O. E. Hervis, and W. M. Kurtines, published by the University of Miami Spanish Family Guidance Center, 1985.

One Person Family Therapy

A mother calls for help with her adolescent son, Frank, who is involved with drugs and in trouble at school. Her family is in turmoil. Emotions like anger, guilt, pity, hopelessness, and despair are rampant, and communication lines have collapsed. The mother calls out of desperation, identifying the son as the source of the family's problems. The therapist, however, recognizes that, although the problem adolescent is the only one displaying the symptom of drug abuse, the entire family contributes to maintaining the drug abuse. Thus, although the drug-abusing adolescent is the identified patient (IP), the therapist knows that the entire family is dysfunctional.

Logically, because the entire family is dysfunctional, the therapist wishes to see the entire family together in therapy. However, this is not always possible. This may be because the IP is physically separated from his family, the family is unusually strong in their belief that the IP is the only one who needs to be cured, the IP insists on being seen alone, or for some other reason. This chapter addresses the issue of how to deal with this situation: A client appears to need the benefit of family therapy but circumstances make seeing the whole family during most therapy sessions impractical or undesirable. In this chapter, we will describe the techniques we have developed for conducting OPFT. The approach is based on the same basic concepts of systems, structure, and strategy described in Chapter 5 of this volume, but is designed to accomplish the goals of family therapy while working primarily with only one family member.

A therapist using OPFT techniques tries to achieve the same two goals as *conjoint* family therapy (i.e., family therapy with the entire family present). First, the therapist works to reduce the symptoms exhibited by the IP. Second, the therapist works to change the way family members act toward each other so that they will not do or say things that might, unwittingly, contribute to maintaining or promoting the IP's symptoms. To make the changes necessary to achieve these goals, the therapist will use the joining, diagnosing, and restructuring techniques that are described in Chapter 5 (this volume), but they will be modified for use with one person, whom we will call the "OP" (i.e., "one person" in therapy). The OP, we would point out, is usually also the IP (i.e., the person the family member has identified as the patient), but we have changed the term from IP to OP in order to highlight that the reason we work with this person alone is *not* because this person is the only one in need but rather because working with this person is a strategic maneuver through which we will gain access to the entire family process, and through this OP, we will seek to change the family's maladaptive patterns of interaction. There are several characteristics of OPFT that make it brief and effective. Knowing what these characteristics are and keeping them in mind will make the reader a more effective family therapist.

Time Limitation

One of these characteristics is that it is a brief therapy: 12 to 15 therapy sessions lasting about 1 to 1½ hours once a week are usually all that is necessary.

Therapy, therefore, should take less than 4 months. For this time limit to be effective, however, it must be made explicit between the therapist and the family. Families rarely have any difficulty with limiting therapy. Therapists, however, who are not used to brief therapy find it extremely uncomfortable to make such a commitment. At the start of therapy, the client and his or her family should make a verbal or written contract with the therapist that should include the 12- to 15-session limitation. Without such a clear, strong agreement before therapy begins, limiting the length of therapy becomes very difficult. When such an agreement is made, it gives the message that "we are here to work and we intend to do it quickly."

Strategic

Another characteristic of OPFT is that it blends two of the major approaches to family therapy: strategic family therapy and structural family therapy. From strategic family therapy comes the idea of maintaining a problem focus when doing therapy. This means that the therapist must always work on reducing the problems that bring the client into therapy (e.g., the adolescent drug abuse, problems in school) and changing the underlying contributors to these problems (e.g., the things the family does unknowingly to maintain or promote the drug abuse and problem behaviors). Time is not wasted on other matters that do not directly affect the presenting problems. It is important to note, however, that the problem behaviors should not be defined too narrowly. In most cases of adolescent drug abuse, for example, there are other problem behaviors such as skipping school, fighting, being overly rebellious, and so on that cannot be ignored. Thus the problem focus usually refers to a set or problems and those family interactions that maintain them.

A special word of caution may be needed here. OPFT therapists need to change those family interactions that contribute or maintain drug abuse and other problem behavior. No time is spent in attempting to discover the "original" cause of these behaviors. OPFT is present and future oriented, never past oriented. The entire focus is on those causes of behavior that exist in the present and, in particular, family interactions.

Another element of being strategic in therapy is that, as much as possible, the therapist makes deliberate plans, both for the general therapy strategy and for each specific session. This usually means that the therapist has some specific goals for each therapy session and some specific ideas about how to achieve them. Thus some time must be set aside to plan each therapy session. Of course, the therapist must be flexible enough to make use of any opportunities or handle any crisis that may arise during a therapy session. The point is that things are not usually allowed to "just happen" during therapy; as much as possible the direction of the treatment is carefully planned. As will be seen later, the main focus in structural therapy is on the way in which family members act and interact with each other. The main interest in the therapy is to change patterns of interaction. In strategic structural family therapy, careful planning of strategies is used to change the way in which family members interact.

Another element of being strategic is being practical. The goal of therapy is to effectively and permanently reduce the identified patient's problems and constructively change the things the family does to maintain them. Anything that will most effectively achieve these goals is encouraged. For example, the therapist may want to use gestalt techniques or those from some other therapy approach, such as rational emotive therapy, behavior therapy, and so on. What is important is to be sure to use any of these "borrowed" techniques to achieve the goals of OPFT—reduction of problem behavior and constructive change in the way the family behaves toward the identified patient.

There is yet another aspect to this practical quality of the strategic family approach that is particularly important with adolescent drug abusers. Many therapists feel that drug abuse is such an overwhelming problem that they must always immediately attack it head on (e.g., forbid all drug use). An OPFT therapist would certainly agree that drug abuse is a very severe problem. However, an OPFT therapist would never agree that there is only one strategy for dealing with the problem. In some cases confronting the drug abuse might be the one most effective strategy. However, in other cases other approaches might be much more effective. In some of our cases, drug abuse was not even mentioned during therapy. Other problems were worked on—and in the course of solving these other problems the drug abuse disappeared. Of course, the therapist kept the overall goal of achieving a reduction in drug abuse in mind, even while working on other problems. The point is that whatever combination of strategy and technique is used, it must be chosen for the specific people and situation so that it will be maximally effective for that particular client.

Structure

The other major concept about therapy that is blended into OPFT is called structural family theory: The concept of structure is basic to OPFT and requires a careful explanation. The concept is based on the idea of an interaction, as in the following illustration. When two people meet, let's call them Jack and Jill, Jill responds to Jack then Jack, in turn, responds to Jill. These events of one person responding to another—either through actions or conversation—is referred to as an interaction. People pick up habits, ways they like to behave, as they go through life. Two or more people who see each other often (e.g., members of a family) form habits around the way they interact with each other. For example, Jack always pays for Jill. Jill always picks on Jack. Jack and Jill fight whenever they have to discuss the problem behavior of their son. These habitual ways of interacting or patterns of interactions are referred to as structures. When these structures first develop, they often are helpful in achieving the family members' goals. Sometimes, however, these structures become so ingrained that they are used in situations where they are no longer effective. If this happens, it means that the structure (habitual way of interacting) is no longer operating in a useful and appropriate fashion and, rather than being helpful and functional, it now has become maladaptive. A common example of a maladaptive structure that was once functional is that of a parent who treats a 15- or 16-year-old adolescent like a 7- or 8-year-old child. Limitations, punishments, and lectures that may have worked with a child, no longer work with the adolescent. The parent–child dyad is not working well, and we would say that the habitual way that this dyad interacts (i.e., this structure) has become maladaptive. The main concern of an OPFT therapist working through the one person seen in therapy is to assess family interactions/structures in order to find those that are maladaptive in order to change them.

Combining the structural approach with the strategic approach discussed earlier means that our OPFT therapist will attempt to change those family interactional patterns or structures that maintain or contribute to the IP's drug abuse and other problem behavior. Maladaptive structures that do not contribute to the IP's problem behavior perhaps should not be disturbed in a brief therapy such as OPFT. Care must be taken in deciding which maladaptive structures do and do not contribute to these problems, however. For example, whereas a marital disagreement about the wife's role outside the home might appear to be very unrelated to the issue of an adolescent's drug abuse, in a given case, the therapist could decide that it was, in fact, related and devote considerable time to resolving it.

Complementarity

Before discussing specific strategies and techniques of OPFT, one other important concept needs to be presented. This concept is called *complementarity* and is the concept that allows us to adapt family therapy to the one person situation. According to this concept, for a family to work as a unit (even if it appears to do a bad job of it), the behavior of each family member must "fit in" with the behavior of each and every one of the other family members. Thus within the family, for each action there, is a set of complementary actions. The behaviors of members of a family are like the cogs and wheels that make up the inner workings of a clock. For the clock to keep on ticking, all wheels must turn in just a certain way. When the OP seen in therapy tells the therapist that his father becomes angry at anything he says, the therapist needs to ascertain what that person said to elicit an angry response. Often what the OP tells the therapist will not be accurate because it is seen through the eyes, ears, projections, displacements, and all other senses and defenses that make up the interpretations of the OP. The therapist needs to evaluate it in terms of the complementary behaviors that exist in the family.

Thus, if an OP talks about a sibling's behavior, with knowledge of family interactions, we construct a fuller picture of what goes on. For example, if Mary complains that an older brother call her "Druggie," "bum," and "stupid," the practitioner must assume that there is a reason why this brother berates her. Perhaps you learn that Mary's reaction to her brother's attack is one of rage and hysteria. She proves to be a perfect foil to her brother's insults and because she reacts in an immature way, she gives him the ammunition he needs to continue to put her down. His behavior complements Mary's behavior, and Mary's behavior complements that of the brother. Mary continues to use drugs perhaps as a means to withdraw from his harassment or perhaps because it is the only way she has found to get his attention. There are other possibilities of course, but the point is that the behavior of Mary and her brother are interlocked.

The parents do little to chastise their son for his attitude toward his sister because he is fulfilling a function for them. He is venting the family's anger and frustration. He is saying things they, for some reason, cannot bring themselves to say. As long as they do nothing and he continuous to perform this task for them, the interaction between him and Mary will remain. So, in a way, the parent's behavior is complementary to their son's. He has taken over their parental role, and the hierarchy in the family has shifted and become diffused. This example shows how the behavior of some family members mutually reinforces and contributes to the behavior of other family members. This is the concept of complementarity that is central to all the work done in OPFT.

Now that the general notions of time limitation, strategies, structure, and complementarity have been presented, the strategies and techniques of OPFT can be discussed. As many examples will be utilized from the case of Frank, we will use masculine pronouns in referring to the OP, although in actual practice, of course, the OP may be masculine or feminine in gender.

OPFT STRATEGIES AND TECHNIQUES

Following the structural approach to family therapy (Minuchin, 1974, 1976; Minuchin & Fishman, 1981), OPFT techniques can be separated into two major types: joining and restructuring. In simplistic terms, joining can be thought of as the therapist's blending with the family to become a part of it, whereas restructuring involves changing the family. These two sets of techniques are discussed separately later, although in actual practice, joining, and restructuring occur simultaneously and their techniques are often intermixed.

Joining

As in conjoint structural family therapy, the initial task is to join the family. In OPFT, because the entire family is not available for most or all treatment sessions, the therapist must enter the family, as well as direct change, through the OP. The first step in accomplishing this is to establish a therapeutic alliance with the OP. That is, the therapist must create a close working relationship of trust and goodwill with the OP. The therapist must demonstrate to the OP that he or she is sensitive to the OP's needs and values and sufficiently skilled to help solve the OP's problems. The therapist, in the context of this therapeutic alliance, diagnoses and monitors the family through the OP's perceptions about the family's typical patterns of interactions. Later, during restructuring, the therapist will direct changes in the maladaptive family interactions by directing and encouraging change in the part the OP plays in these interactions.

In the case of Frank, the therapist began the joining process in the first session by establishing a therapeutic alliance. Frank presented himself for the first session dressed in a black jacket and gave the impression of a tough, "streetwise" adolescent who took pride in flaunting his drug experiences. He was initially cautious and cool to the therapist but later in the session began to enthusiastically recount his experiences while having run away from home. This situation provided the opportunity for the therapist to establish rapport and create a therapeutic alliance. The therapist, sensing Frank's great pride in his adventures in drug dealing and his success in the adult world, listened intently and allowed him to savor his bold adventure. (This is an example of what is called *maintenance*, i.e., supporting a behavior for the sake of establishing rapport, even if we do not agree with the behavior.) Frank was allowed to experience the opposite of his initial self-blame and negativism about what he had done. By listening attentively, the therapist and patient shared a critical experience and established a therapeutic alliance that provided a foundation from which to begin to assess the family structure and the position of Frank within it.

Diagnosis

Enactment Analog

In conjoint family therapy when the whole family is present and carrying out their typical interactional patterns in the presence of the therapist, the therapist's assessment of these interactions can be done directly. Enactment is considerably different in OPFT where just one person is present and only an enactment analog is possible. The enactment analog used in OPFT refers to constructing the family's characteristic interactional patterns through description and role play in lieu of actual direct observation.

Because we all tend to see what others do rather than our own behavior, when a typical OP like Frank is asked to describe his family, what he usually presents is the behavior of others rather than his own. The therapist assumes from systems theory that for the system to maintain itself, the OP must behave in a fashion that complements the reported behavior of others, that is, the OP has introjected the kinds of behaviors that mesh with the behavior of others in the family. Enactment analogs provide the opportunity to reconstruct the kinds of interactions that may occur in the family by making use of the concept of complementarity.

The concept of complementarity holds that the family interactional patterns are defined as comprising two complementary parts: (1) the OP's own behavior in the family context, and (2) the rest of the family's behavior. Because Frank tends to perceive the other family members' behaviors but not his own in the enactment analog, he is requested to represent what he is aware of, that is, the other family members' behaviors. The therapist learns what other family members are perceived as doing from the OP and then assumes that the OP's behavior must be the complement of their behaviors. Bringing together the family's represented behaviors and the OP's assumed behaviors provides a full picture of the family's systemic, self-reinforcing, and repetitive patterns of interactions. This process is illustrated in the diagram contained in Figure 1.

The therapist typically begins the enactment analog by asking an OP such as Frank to describe or act out interactions between himself and other family mem-

1. OP represents other family members' behaviors.

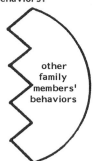

2. Therapist assumes that family is a system and thus OP's behaviors must be the complement of what s/he has represented as behaviors of others.

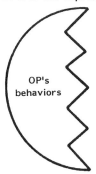

3. Therapist constructs a symbolic representation of the family system/inter-actional patterns by bringing together the two complements (adds 1 & 2 above).

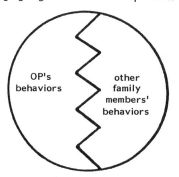

FIGURE 1. Venn diagrams of family interactions.

bers. Usually the OP will say that "Dad did this to me," "Mom yelled at me," and so on. That is, the person tends to perceive that everyone is "dumping" on him. In the case of Frank, when the therapist inquired about his perception of the problem in the family, Frank responded by complaining that he felt humiliated by his family. His mother treated him like a child, and his father was always down on him. He indicated that he had run away from home because he could not stand it anymore. "I felt asphyxiated. I couldn't breathe. I escaped and I didn't even look back." The task of the therapist is to get as much information as possible and then fill in the missing information from an understanding of complementarity. What did Frank do or say that got him in the predicaments he describes? The process is somewhat like putting together a jigsaw puzzle that has some missing pieces. The OP provides some of the pieces but the therapist must then construct the missing pieces that will fit with those provided by the OP. These missing pieces are the complements to the interactions as described by the OP. For example, if mother treats Frank as a child and father dumps on Frank, what did Frank do that may have precipitated those behaviors from his father? Once the therapist has all the pieces, both the ones that had to be constructed and the ones provided by the OP, it is possible to put together the entire puzzle and have a clear picture of the family's structure. Beyond asking for descriptions of what happens in the family, the therapist can also make use of role playing to produce the enactment analog.

Role Play

In role play, the OP enacts some of the interactions and situations that occur within the family thereby revealing the patterns of interaction. The OP pretends to be some other member of the family and acts as this person would in a given situation. For example, if the OP is role playing a strict and punitive father or controlling mother, the therapist can observe the OP's concept of such parents. In the case of Frank, his relationship with an older Anglo girlfriend (whom both of Frank's parents disliked) provided the opportunity for role playing. The therapist asked Frank to play the role of his mother and father in these interactions. This process revealed that Frank allowed himself to be placed in two conflicting roles: that of an innocent baby by his mother ("My poor little one, that terrible woman is misleading you") and that of a no-good bum by his father ("You are no son of mine to go with a woman like that!"). Frank, in portraying his parents, reveals how his behavior complements theirs and vice versa. Through this enactment process, he may also develop empathy and understanding for other members of the family, facilitating the change process.

During role playing, the therapist often helps the OP recall incidents and relieve them with almost the same emotional intensity as when they originally occurred. Or, the practitioner may help the OP devise situations that did not happen but could occur, as a way of exploring how a particular person in the family would handle a situation. Often OPs learn how they themselves may act in an imaginary situation.

At other times the therapist and OP engage in role play together. Here the therapist has a good opportunity to present various facets of family interactions, thus allowing the OP to see himself from several dimensions. This technique also enables the therapist to probe into areas the OP may possibly not delve into by himself. Thus, the therapist must be very active: like an actor when engaging in role play, like a director in encouraging the OP to assume the roles of family members, and sometimes, serving as a choreographer in physically rearranging seating patterns, and the like.

In addition to role playing, the gestalt empty chair technique is also useful in learning about family structure. Because this technique is used most often in restructuring, however, it will be discussed in that section.

Restructuring

Most therapists who do individual therapy try to change something inside their clients. Many therapists try to change their client's attitudes, thoughts, or personality. This type of change inside the person's mind we call *intrapersonal* change. Structural family therapists, on the other hand, try to change the family's structure (habitual ways family members interact with each other). That is, they try to change the way one person behaves toward another person. This type of change we call *interpersonal change.*

In OPFT, the therapist sees only one person in most therapy sessions but tries to make changes in the entire family's structure. In order to accomplish this, the therapist must make both intra- and interpersonal changes. The strategy is to first make the intrapersonal changes in the OP seen in therapy, then use that person as an ally to make interpersonal changes in the family. Sometimes the therapist will make all the necessary intrapersonal changes, then make all the interpersonal changes. Usually, however, it is more effective to select one facet of one problem (i.e., one thing that contributes to, for example, the adolescent's skipping school), do all the necessary intrapersonal and interpersonal work on that one facet, and then move on to another facet. In the case of Frank, the therapist first worked on Frank's problem of his father's always "dumping" on him, then moved on to his mother treating him like a child. This type of progression, dealing with one thing at a time, usually seems to work best and is not very different from the rule given by efficiency experts that states that one select a task and complete it before going on the next task.

We will organize restructuring techniques in this section into intrapersonal and interpersonal for purposes of explaining them. This distinction, although convenient, is somewhat artificial because many techniques can be used either intrapersonally or interpersonally.

Restructuring: Intrapersonal

During intrapersonal restructuring, the therapist changes things within the OP that will allow changes in the family structure. The therapist may work on changing or organizing attitudes, beliefs and/or feelings, as long as it is remembered that the strategic character of OPFT requires that the goal is to change only those things that must be changed in order to modify those components of family structure that are directly responsible for the undesirable symptoms. Normally the therapist will have to do three things: (1) help the OP discover or decide what he wants and needs, (2) understand what his complementary roles are in the family, and (3) realize how he contributes to the family interactions.

Some techniques that can be used to achieve the necessary intrapersonal restructuring are described next.

Making Direct Suggestions. Structural therapists have no qualms about making direct suggestions to clients: In particular, tasks are given that will directly modify interactions. General advice or value judgments are not allowed, however. Carefully considered suggestions based on the individual situation of each family, on the other hand, can be very useful, and, as an objective, outside observer, the therapist often will be able to see things that a client cannot see. In some cases a direct suggestion concerning a goal to achieve or a role relationship to change can be constructive.

Diagraming the Family. Drawing a diagram of the interaction patterns including the power hierarchy in the family can clarify some of the role relationships that are hard for the OP to understand. Mapping the family's structure—as described in Chapter 5 (this volume)—can be a useful tool in facilitating restructuring.

Gestalt Empty Chair Technique. In this technique, the OP sits facing an empty chair, imagines that some family member or other specific person is sitting in the other chair, and talks to that person in therapy. Also, the OP can imagine himself as sitting in the empty chair while he pretends he is someone else (e.g., his mother, father, or sibling). In this way, he can come to understand his role in the family. In many cases, OPs are verbalizing something they would like to say but for some reason are afraid to say. This technique is effective as a rehearsal for a later encounter with that person. For example, Frank might want to be able to tell his sister that he really likes her and wants to be her friend, but since early childhood he has felt threatened by her. He is afraid to reveal his feelings to her. When the therapist assigns this task to him, to confront his sister at home, it will be easier to carry out this difficult assignment after having practiced it during the session.

Role playing can also be used in a way similar to the gestalt empty chair technique. Sometimes having a real person play the other part adds to the realism of the play acting. On the other hand, sometimes having just an empty chair is less threatening or allows the OP greater freedom of expression. In the case of Frank, the therapist used role playing to help Frank understand his parents' behavior toward him as well as his habitual response. His parents alternately babied and denigrated him, and Frank allowed himself to be dragged to these behavioral extremes.

Reframing. In all families, the members have a certain impression of each other. This tends to color the way they regard and deal with each other. In dysfunctional families the negative aspect of some individual is highlighted, and the positive quality of others is also exaggerated. In reframing, the therapist tries to help the OP or other family members to see each other and their situation in a new light, a different way of viewing the underlying meaning of behavior and communication.

One example may be of a father such as Frank's who, in talking about his son, says, "Frank wastes his time hanging around with a bunch a useless bums." The therapist can reframe this remark with, "I would be happier to see Frank go to school or get a job? I want that for him." Frank can then see the positive aspect of the father's complaints and his underlying concern for his son. This gives the remark a new "frame" so that Frank can view it from a different perspective.

Increasing Stress and Provoking Crises. These are related techniques that are used to help motivate or mobilize a person or family to change. It is very difficult to change people if they do not believe that anything is wrong. Raising an individual's stress level or provoking a crisis makes that person acutely aware of the need for change. This technique is often needed if the family tends to deny or avoid problems. In addition, if a person is about to make a decision, experiencing stress around the decision makes it a more important decision for that person and, therefore, tends to make it a more permanent, irrevocable decision. In actual practice, there are a variety of ways to apply these techniques. In general, the therapist can emphasize or exaggerate some aspect of an issue or can needle some family members or temporarily side with one family member against other family members.

Splitting the OP's Executive Observant EGO. In this technique, after the OP has described an event, the therapist asks the OP to objectively observe himself in the scene. Thus, the OP first presents a scenario and then both the OP and the therapist remove themselves from the scenario and watch it together as if they were outsiders. The OP has two roles: One role is that of engaging in interaction and conflict with the members of his family while the other role is of an observer sitting next to the therapist, objectively watching the conflict with the therapist as if it were a movie on television. As both the therapist and the OP "watch" the imagined interaction presented by the OP, the therapist points out how the OP, for example, contributed to the interaction that caused him to be singled out as the family scapegoat. The function of the therapist is to reveal to the OP his complementary role in the family structure.

The OP, with the therapist's aid, learns how he has participated in accepting the role he is in. In that way, the OP can take responsibility for problem behavior that is a reaction to how someone in the family is relating to him and can learn to reframe his self-perception from "I am a problem person" to "I am behaving in such a way that it is placing me in a role that creates problems for me."

In Frank's case, this technique allowed Frank to "observe" the interactional sequence in which he was alternatively babied and denigrated. The therapist asked Frank to imagine seeing himself in the family context while the interaction was ongoing. Thus Frank was asked to observe along with the therapist an imagined family interaction. The part of Frank that observed the interaction is Frank's executive observant ego while the individual imagined participating in the interaction is the Frank who played the identified patient (IP) role that meshed with the rest of the family system. As Frank observed the imagined family interaction, he was taught by the therapist how he contributed to that interaction and how he contributed to being labeled the IP by quietly and passively accepting this label and role.

Restructuring: Interpersonal

When the OP has established a therapeutic alliance with the therapist, is beginning to understand his complementary role in the family, and is ready to relinquish his role, it is time to begin restructuring the family. In family therapy, when the entire family is present, restructuring takes place directly through the therapist's interventions that change family interactions as they occur during a therapy session. In OPFT, the therapist creates changes in family interactions by changing those OP behaviors that help to maintain the maladaptive interactions. The OP, as an emissary from the therapist, goes home to bring about changes in the family. As this happens, the therapist will make full use of the principle of complementarity. The therapist must plan carefully to make the most effective use of the family members' complementary role relationships with the OP. The family structure is changed when the OP changes the way he behaves and the other family members adjust to his changes. There are a number of useful restructuring techniques, and we will describe them next.

Task Setting. This is an essential ingredient of structural family therapy through which the therapist manipulates and reshapes the family. The therapist actually assigns tasks as homework but first plans the task in collaboration with the OP. After a task has been planned, the therapist usually must carefully rehearse it with the OP. Oftentimes the therapist will be trying to alter ways the family has interacted for many years, and the other family members, therefore, will be very resistant to change. The only way to overcome this resistance is for the OP to be very confident of what he is doing. Rehearsal is the best way to achieve this confidence; role playing and the gestalt empty chair technique can be very helpful for this purpose.

Tasks should focus on interactions between family members rather than on what the individual can do by himself. In the beginning sessions, the therapist should make the tasks easy to accomplish so they become a successful experience. A difficult or failed task may prove to be too discouraging and may even cause the OP and/or family to withdraw from therapy.

The therapist has to fit the task to the family. A task that can be successfully carried out by one family or OP may prove to be impossible for another. It would be fruitless for the therapist to suggest that a "macho" father, who feels that work in the kitchen is a demeaning activity, prepare dinner the next week. The therapist may suggest, however, that such a father go fishing with his son or some other task more in keeping with the father's personal style. It should be noted that tasks serve a diagnostic purpose as well. From the way they are done or not done, the therapist can gather an impression as to the flexibility or rigidity of the family.

Reversals. This maneuver is aimed at changing a rigid pattern of behavior by suggesting to the OP that he do something that is the opposite of, or very different from, his usual inclination. If the OP rarely communicates with his sister, the therapist may suggest during the session that he talk to her about a recent experience. Where such a relationship has a history of estrangement, this act can provide a breakthrough and an opening for a new behavior. Reversals are useful in creating the opportunity for new interactional patterns to emerge. In Frank's case, for example, the therapist coached Frank to stand up to his father when his father began to denigrate him. The way in which system change takes place is that when Frank changes his behavior, in effect, he has interrupted the flow of the family interactions that cast him into the IP role. This is a clear example of how OPFT differs from many other psychotherapies that focus on intrapersonal change. It does not stop at reaching awareness. Instead, it uses awareness as a tool for redirecting the interpersonal behavior of the OP, thereby bringing about change in the family.

In conjoint family therapy, the therapist could have caused this interruption of the maladaptive family interactions during family sessions in which the therapist would be present to support the change. In OPFT, however, the therapist must rely heavily on the OP's ability to change his own behavior and to maintain the change in the face of strong family pressure to return to the family's old, habitual pattern of interactions. Hence, in using reversals in OPFT, the therapist must rehearse with the OP his change in behavior. It is particularly important to role play various alternative outcomes that could ensue from the OP's change. The purpose of the rehearsal is to allow the therapist to overcome any resistance in the OP, to give the OP an experience of mastery, and to attempt to prevent possible family sabotage of the OP's new behaviors.

Detriangulation. Often when two family members have a conflict that they do not know how to resolve, one or both of them will involve a third party. This is called *triangulation* and usually is very destructive. For example, a husband and wife may have a disagreement. The wife may, without thinking about it, avoid talking it over with her husband but instead tell their son what a terrible person the father is, trying to draw the son to her side and away from the father. The therapist would have to break up or "detriangulate" the interaction, not only because the son is suffering by being deprived of the father but more importantly, because the wife is avoiding finding a solution to her conflict with her husband. If the son were the OP, the therapist might try to have him get closer to the father (e.g., going to ball games together, fixing up a car together) and may have the son just leave the scene whenever the wife tries to berate her husband. In this fashion, the son achieves a rapprochement with his father and avoids becoming a part of the conflict.

FURTHER CLINICAL ISSUES IN OPFT

It will be apparent that to achieve the goals of OPFT, the therapist must strategically restructure both intrapersonally with the OP and interpersonally in the family, using the OP as a therapeutic ally. When restructuring intraper-sonally, the therapist prepares the OP so that he can help to make the necessary changes in the family structure. Generally this means helping the OP to decide what he wants and needs, understand his complementary roles in the family, and identify how he contributes to family interactions.

Based on this intrapersonal restructuring, the therapist then focuses on changing interactions through interpersonal restructuring. The therapist works with the OP to change those parts of the family's structure (habitual ways of interacting) that maintains or contribute to the OP's problem behaviors. In order to accomplish these changes, the therapist strategically chooses to change those interactions that have two characteristics: (1) they are maladaptive, and (2) they are ones in which the OP plays an important role. The therapist chooses mal-adaptive interactions because there is no reason to change those interactions that are functioning properly. This follows from the idea of staying problem focused. The therapist chooses interactions in which the OP plays an important role because generally the OP is the only family member with whom there is ex-tended contact in OPFT.

If the OP changes his behavior in interactions in which he plays an impor-tant role, the concept of complementarity says that the others involved in the interaction must also change in order to accommodate the new behavior. In other words, if the OP's behavior changes, the behavior of the other people involved must also change in order to mesh and coordinate with the change. This complementary change cannot occur if the OP is not already involved in an interaction. The therapist might, of course, try to have the OP enter into an ongoing interaction between two other people, but this, however, is *very strongly discouraged*. It is only likely to result in a destructive triangulation that will do far more harm than good. The only way the therapist can make changes in interac-tions in which the OP is not involved is if the rest of the family is available to come in for some therapy sessions.

In the best of all worlds, when the OP changes, the family will accommo-date itself to the change, thereby reinforcing the new behavior. However, in the real world, the response to the OP's changed behavior is family pressure to return to its previous patterns of interactions. The confrontation between the OP trying to create change and the family's trying to prevent it will tend to produce a family crisis. At this point, families are often accessible to the therapist, and a crisis can be an ideal moment for the therapist to request and typically obtain a family session.

A family session or two also provides an opportunity—albeit a limited one—for the therapist to intervene directly in family interaction patterns in which the OP does not participate (e.g., in the case of Frank, the therapist may intervene in the marital relationship directly during a conjoint session). How-ever, in one or two family sessions, it may not be possible to bring about major structural changes in these other family dysfunctional patterns. Rather, it is only possible to change those aspects of these other dysfunctional interactions as they affect the OP. Thus in the case of Frank, the therapist might help Frank's parents decide what rules they will follow with Frank at home because this aspect of the marital relation (i.e., their ability to establish clear rules together) directly impacts on Frank's behavior.

When to Have Whole Family Sessions

A therapist can request the whole family, or major parts of it, to come in to the therapy sessions whenever it is considered helpful, but there are three situations in which such requests are likely to be both advantageous and complied with: the first therapy session, after a crisis has occurred in the family, and at the time of formal termination of therapy.

The First Session

If it is possible to arrange, it is very helpful to have the whole family present at the first or at least at one of the early therapy sessions. This gives the therapist the opportunity to join the family directly, establishing the therapist's leadership and obtaining the family's cooperation more easily. It also gives the therapist a firmer basis on which to construct a picture of family structure during enactment analogs. From the family's point of view, family members are often curious about the therapist. In addition, they often wish to tell the therapist just how terrible they feel the identified patient is. Family members love to share their complaints, and an alert therapist can often pick up some important structural information while listening to this complaining. There is opportunity to observe how the family behaves together in real life: Who speaks first, who speaks longest, what the fundamental complaint is, and how the identified patient and other family members react can all be important clues to the power hierarchy and structure of the family. This first session, then, gives the therapist a chance to observe the family's spontaneous interactions and gather important structural information while listening to the family's complaints.

After a Crisis

During the course of therapy, situations may arise that lead to a crisis. Crises are, in fact, quite likely to occur during interpersonal restructuring. In an ideal world, the family would accommodate to the OP's changed behavior, as predicted by the postulate of complementarity. In the real world, however, the family often resists the changed behavior of the OP. The family does not like to change and fights to maintain the old ways.

This can prove to be a very crucial time because, as the OP changes and the rigid family structures are threatened, there is a strong tendency to return to the original, habitual family patterns. As a result, a crisis usually ensues. At this time, a family session must be scheduled for several reasons. The most important is to support the OP and his new way of behaving. Another reason is to observe and directly assess the new family dynamics. A third reason is to keep the family in treatment because at times of crises, many families choose to withdraw in order to return to the pretreatment state. Unhappy as it may have been, the pretreatment status provided a structure and a manner of relating that was familiar to the family. It was a comfortable structure devised by the family. Now, with changes in the OP, the family is in turmoil and uncomfortable.

Therapy Termination

After completing therapy, the therapist should follow up with the family for several months to ensure that changes are maintained. With some families, a telephone call every month or two will be sufficient. With others it may be necessary to schedule one or two family sessions in order to provide the family with a chance to function on its own and to test its new structures, while still having the security of the therapist's continued interest and availability. During this time, the therapist can slowly reduce his or her position in the family.

CHOOSING THE ONE PERSON

In the vast majority of the situations, the drug-abusing adolescent who is the IP is the one person seen in OPFT. In other situations, there may be some latitude for choosing who will be the OP. In order to choose someone other than the IP, there are four factors to consider. These factors are (1) the rigidity of the identified patienthood, (2) centrality in family interactions, (3) power in the family, and (4) availability.

Rigidity of the IP refers to the strength of the family's belief that all their problems are caused by the IP rather than a willingness to accept the possibility that others share responsibility to some extent. In most cases the family thinks that if the IP was well, the family would not be troubled, and there would be no need for therapy. This type of thinking exemplifies a rigid identified patienthood and would suggest that the IP may need to be the OP seen for most therapy sessions because the family will accept no alternatives.

Centrality in family interactions refers to how many of the interactions in the family are funneled or routed through a particular individual. How many of the family concerns center around this person? If most of the interactions and communications are routed through this person, then such an individual is involved in a large number of interactions and for that reason has a certain amount of power in the family as well as having good potential to be the OP selected from the family to be seen for therapy.

The concept of power is closely tied into the concept of centrality because a person in the central position in the family exercises a great deal of control and power, especially if that person is also the main topic of concern of the family's interaction. This is typically an IP who derives power from his unfortunate position in what has been called "the tyranny of illness."

Often when an individual's symptoms are life-threatening or constitute a suicidal risk, when the individual is heavily into drug abuse or exhibits homicidal tendencies, this person should definitely be selected as the OP. This enables the therapist to monitor such an at-risk individual more closely.

Finally, availability is a significant factor in selecting the OP. The ease with which the therapist and OP can establish a positive working relationship is of great importance, especially in time-limited therapy. Another aspect of availability is that the OP needs to be physically available, able to keep appointments, and able to follow through on the various intervention strategies proposed by the therapist. Our experience suggests that the IP is typically the most successful choice for OPFT because of the rigidity of the identified patienthood and the centrality of the IP. Therefore, unless there is a strong reason to choose someone else, we suggest the IP as the one person to be seen in most therapy sessions.

ACKNOWLEDGMENT. This work was funded by Grant #DA03224 of The National Institute on Drug Abuse to Jose Szapocznik, principal investigator.

REFERENCES

Foote, F., Szapocznik, J., Kurtines, W., Hervis, O. & Perez-Vidal, A. (1985). One person family therapy: A modality of brief strategic family therapy. In R. S. Ashery (Ed.), *Progress in the development of cost-effective treatment for drug abusers* (pp. 51–65). National Institute on Drug Abuse Research Monograph 58. Washington, DC: U.S. Government Printing Office.

Haley, J. (1976). *Problem-solving therapy.* San Francisco; Jossey-Bass.

Madanes, C. (1981). *Strategic family therapy.* San Francisco: Jossey-Bass.

Minuchin, S. (1974). *Families and family therapy.* Cambridge: Harvard University Press.

Minuchin, S. (1976). Structural family therapy. In G. Caplan (Ed.), *American handbook of psychiatry* (Vol II, pp. 178–192). New York: Basic Books.

Minuchin, S. & Fishman, H. C. (1981). *Family therapy techniques.* Cambridge: Harvard University Press.

Szapocznik, J., & Kurtines, W. (1989). *Beyond family therapy: Breakthroughs in the treatment of drug abusing youth.* New York: Springer.

Szapocznik, J., Kurtines, W., Foote, F., Perez-Vidal, A., & Hervis, O. (1983). Conjoint versus one person family therapy: Some evidence for the effectiveness of conducting family therapy through one person. *Journal of Consulting and Clinical Psychology, 51,* 889–899.

Szapocznik, J., Perez-Vidal, A., Hervis, O., Foote, F., & Spencer, F. (1983). *Brief strategic family therapy: Final report* (NIDA Grant No. R 18 DA 03224). Miami: University of Miami Spanish Family Guidance Center.

Szapocznik, J., Kurtines, W., Hervis, O., & Spencer, F. (1984). One person family therapy. In B. Lubin & W. S. O'Connor (Eds.), *Ecological approaches to clinical and community psychology* (pp. 335–355). New York: Wiley.

Szapocznik, J., Kurtines, W., Foote, F., Perez-Vidal, A. & Hervis, O. (1986). Conjoint versus one person family therapy: Further evidence for the effectiveness of conducting family therapy through one person. *Journal of Consulting and Clinical Psychology, 54,* 395–397.

V

Brief Group Approaches

One of the underlying assumptions of this *Handbook* is that brief therapy provides a methodology for structuring psychotherapeutic services in a more efficient and cost-effective manner. Group therapy has always maintained this advantage because the therapeutic forces harnessed through group processes can benefit a number of persons simultaneously. Group approaches have traditionally been effective with populations where reality testing and confrontation are critical to successful outcome. The popularity and general effectiveness of group therapy with addictive disorders and schizophrenics are examples. The combination of group therapy techniques with the structured focus and time limitations of brief therapy offers the possibility for a wide distribution of therapeutic assistance to a variety of client populations.

The chapters in this section discuss a diverse body of approaches and techniques, some applied to specific client populations, others applicable to group intervention in general. Garvin's opening chapter (21) spells out the overarching principles common to all short-term group interventions, as well as many of the specific issues arising in selection, formation, and management of such groups. In Garvin's work, as well as in the succeeding chapters, therapeutic forces in groups such as catharsis, reality testing, consensual validation of experience, and the corrective nature of feedback are detailed.

The chapters represent a plurality of theories. The social skill training chapter by Sheldon Rose (22) provides a structured, behaviorally oriented approach to enhancing social competence that can be applied to a variety of patient populations. Although the use of social skill training is discussed in Kanas's chapter concerning groups for schizophrenics, the specific utility of using feedback and group confrontation for decreasing the severity and frequency of hallucinations and delusional thinking is also demonstrated. Naar's chapter (25) on psychodrama has a gestalt therapy flavor, discusses the concept of unfinished business, and details the use of techniques such as alter ego, role reversal, and the use of imagery and imagination. Although crisis intervention was discussed in the *Handbook* in an earlier chapter, the brief crisis chapter by Imber and Evanczuk (24) demonstrates some of the advantages of groups in working with people in crisis. These include the opportunity for group members to overcome isolation and the value of having multiple perspectives and exposure to solutions.

The techniques and strategies of group intervention presented in the chapters of this section do not drastically differ from the basic methodology common to all forms of group therapy. The difference lies in their appreciation of structure, use of time, and their general bias toward action. The point here is that the material in this group section, as well as other chapters, does not so much represent a radical departure from traditional approaches as much as an emphasis upon refining of technique and conducting therapy as if time really mattered. The operative assumption is that a good proportion of the work begins after termination. The obvious advantage of groups consists in the possibility for creating a miniature laboratory that in many ways can simulate and reenact past and current conflicts as well as provide an opportunity for the learning and rehearsal of new attitudes and skills. The added advantage of brief therapy is that there is a clear and prearranged understanding that the group is not a substitute for coping with and managing conflicts and problems but rather a training ground for living effectively with present and future challenges.

21

Short-Term Group Therapy

Charles D. Garvin

Definition of Short-Term Group Therapy

Although the terms *short-term treatment* as well as *short-term group therapy* are widely used, there is a good deal of ambiguity as to the meaning of these terms. As one expert on the subject states (Klein, 1985):

> Typically, reported sessions vary from a single meeting to as many as 50 or more, and range in overall time up to and even beyond one year. For individual short-term treatment, the mean number of sessions appears to be about 25, while for short-term group therapy the range is similar but there is a trend toward fewer sessions with a mean of about 12 to 15 sessions, apart from marathon groups. Most short-term group treatment sessions, whether in inpatient or outpatient settings, last 1 to 1½ hours on a weekly basis and utilize a variety of theoretical orientations; for example, psycho-analytic, cognitive, interpersonal, and behavioral. (p. 310)

Although we recognize that some groups that are included in this category may be conducted for as many as 50 sessions, we find that this length of time mitigates many of the forces that are brought into play by member's awareness of time limits. The limit of nearly a year may clearly be understood as a limit, but our experience is that this termination time is seen, at least at first, as so far distant that the force of operating under time pressures is lessened. We, there-fore, do not classify all time-limited groups as brief but only those of less than about 25 sessions, and this number is used as an upper limit by many writers (Butcher & Koss, 1978, p. 730). The actual number, therefore, may be as few as one, although, as we shall note later, additional considerations apply to single-session groups.

A variable that clearly affects choices regarding the number of sessions is their frequency. Meetings of short-term groups may be held daily, several times a week, weekly, or even less often. Thus a decision to have a group meet for 20 sessions will have a different impact when these sessions are held daily over a 1-month period as compared to weekly over 5 months. Members may continue to

Charles D. Garvin • School of Social Work, University of Michigan, Ann Arbor, Michigan 48109.

work on problems between sessions (or in contrast repress their memories of what happened during the session), and factors such as these will influence the decision as to how often the group will meet. Nevertheless, we reiterate our definition of short-term groups as based on the number of sessions and not their frequency.

The term *therapy* also can have many different meanings. We use it to apply to all interpersonal helping efforts employed by mental health therapists directed at aiding individuals to cope better with their social situations. *Group therapy* as we employ the term, involves the actions of a professional to enhance the way members of a therapy group help each other in this respect. Thus practitioners of group therapy must be skillful in utilizing group processes to help individuals attain their treatment goals.

Contemporary short-term group psychotherapy draws upon a number of approaches such as those developed for individual short-term, long-term group, and behavioral therapies as well as for individual enhancement as seen in sensitivity and related groups. As we shall see, these approaches have come together in an entity that, although having borrowed widely now has unique elements of its own.

THEORETICAL BASIS

Any justification for short-term group psychotherapy should note the fact that much psychotherapy, whether it is intended to or not, is of brief duration (Garfield, 1978). This holds true for group as well as individual therapies. The conclusion that must be drawn, we believe, is not to find better ways of retaining people in therapy but rather better ways of helping them through short-term contracts for service.

A number of considerations apply equally to brief individual and group therapy. One is that if the objective of extensive personality reconstruction as a result of psychotherapy is abandoned, then it become necessary to establish highly specific individual goals. These can include relief of disabling symptoms, reestablishment of a previous emotional equilibrium, or an understanding of the current situation and how the individual might cope with it (Butcher & Koss, 1978, p. 731).

Another mark of short-term therapy is its focus and present centeredness (Butcher & Koss, 1978, p. 731). The ability of the client to accomplish his or her goals is highly dependent on having the goal related to a specific problem area, having that problem area remain "center stage" during all sessions, and relating these deliberations to the client's current situation and behavior as much as possible.

The client's ability to choose a goal and focus in this manner is very dependent on the active intervention of the therapist that, according to Butcher and Koss (1978), means "talking more, directing more conversation when necessary, actively exploring areas of interest, offering support and guidance, and formulating plans of action for the patient to follow" (p. 736). These types of interventions require the therapists to engage in rapid, early assessment of the clients and their situations, to possess a broad repertoire of interventions, and to create and maintain a positive relationship with the client within a short time period.

When group therapists employ these principles, the factors that account for change through the therapy they conduct, in addition to those found in any short-term treatment, are likely to be the following:

1. From a systemic point of view, most problems of individuals are seen as stemming from the interactions among individuals in a system and between that system and other systems. These problems are often identified and brought to the attention of mental health practitioners when the stability of the interactions within and among systems breaks down. The individual is likely to feel motivated to remain in treatment until some new stability (often referred to as "equilibrium") is restored. Because the group is also a social system, it can come to parallel, for the individual, the kinds of transactions she or he experiences elsewhere. The individual can, therefore, learn how to change her or his effect on the group and transfer this to other situations, and this can occur in the short run.

2. Because short-term therapies tend to focus on specific behaviors, this will also be true for group therapy. The group, however, is also a place where these behaviors can be practiced and strengthened, thus adding to the potency of the short-term therapeutic process.

3. Research has demonstrated that an appropriate degree of emotional arousal is associated with therapeutic change (Butcher & Koss, 1978, p. 745). The feedback the individual receives in the group situation can heighten such arousal and thus increase the potency of the group as a vehicle for short-term therapy.

PURPOSES

Short-term group therapy can be employed for virtually the same purposes as short-term individual therapy. The selection of clients for short-term group rather than individual therapy, therefore, often rests with other factors than the purposes of the treatment. These factors, which will be discussed in more detail later, include individual preferences, the availability of enough members who are suitable for the group, and agency proclivities.

Thus short-term groups have been successfully developed for people of all ages. In a handbook that presents 21 case reports of short-term group psychotherapies, the examples include groups for every age in the life span (Rosenbaum, 1983). One chapter describes the author's adaptation of activity group therapy for a time-limited group of preadolescent boys. Another chapter reports on a group for female adolescent victims of sexual abuse. The chapters on short-term groups for adults include one on "a self-control therapy group" for depressed women and another on short-term group psychotherapy for newly blind men. Still other chapters present groups devised for older members such as a "staying-well" group at a senior citizen center and a reminiscence group for the institutionalized elderly.

Short-term groups have also been devised for people with problems of all types and related to all fields of human services. Groups in child welfare settings have been used to help children adapt to foster care and deal with adoption. They have also been employed to help adoptive and foster parents. In family service settings, they have assisted people to face divorce or to learn to communicate better in their marriages; in outpatient mental health settings, they have been offered to adults who have difficulty forming relationships or who are deficient in social skills; in medical settings, they have involved women with mastectomies, families of cancer patients, and patients receiving kidney dialysis; in schools, they have enabled students to handle the demands of the educational setting. Short-term groups have also been successfully conducted in prisons and other correctional settings as well as with alcoholics.

A more abstract categorization of the purposes of short-term groups is provided by Klein (1985) as follows:

> These typically include: (1) the amelioration of distress (i.e., the reduction of symptomatic discomfort); (2) prompt reestablishment of the patient's previous emotional equilibrium; (3) promoting efficient use of the patient's resources (e.g., increasing the patient's sense of control or mastery, emphasizing adaptation, or providing cognitive restructuring, aiding behavioral change, self-help, and social effectiveness); (4) developing the patient's understanding of his current disturbance and increasing coping skills for the future. (p. 312)

TYPES

As explained, therapists with short-term groups have drawn upon a variety of treatment approaches in their work, although these have commonalties because of the processes stemming from the context of the treatment as a short-term group. Nevertheless, the therapist has a number of choices among approaches, and these have an impact on the nature of the group experience.

A major choice is whether the group will be conducted in a structured manner in which there is a specific agenda for sessions or in an unstructured manner in which the group's process is determined as interactions occur in the group. Obviously few groups are conducted in entirely one mode or the other, but one typically is predominant. Because these two modes represent major differences in approach, we shall describe them as well as their appropriate uses in detail later when we consider the "middle phases" in the group.

Other therapist decisions that will be analyzed in less detail are (1) the therapist may focus upon member affect, cognition, or instrumental behavior; (2) the group may be a closed or an open group in that either all members join at the same time, or members join at different times, and each member has his or her own short-term contract; and (3) the therapist may primarily utilize verbal activities or may employ, instead, nonverbal ones such as games, art, or music to achieve therapeutic effects.

Some writers who categorize types of short-term group psychotherapies combine what we call purposes and types. Poey (1985), for example, states:

> There are four types of brief groups that are commonly run. The first is the crisis group which is designed to focus heavily on solving reality problems for its members. . . A second approach is the marathon group which employs accelerated interaction techniques in the space of a weekend. . . Third, and perhaps the most common form of brief group, is the brief open-ended inpatient group with predominantly schizophrenic patients. . . And fourth, brief topic-focused groups offer a treatment modality that is designed to focus on a specific theme such as assertiveness or self-esteem. These psychoeducational groups usually rely heavily on a structured format with a didactic leader who gives the group experiential exercises relevant to the topic. (pp. 332–333)

PLANNING FOR THE GROUP

Now that we have presented background material regarding short-term group psychotherapy, we shall move on to present concrete information on the procedures therapists employ to establish and facilitate such groups. These will be described in terms of those used to plan for the group prior to its first sessions, to select members, to compose the group, to help the group through the process of formation, to assist the group to attain its goals during its "middle phases," and to help the group to terminate. The kind of planning the therapist does before the group comes into existence includes the determination of the purpose of the group, the length and number of sessions, and the means of securing a pool of potential members.

Determination of Purpose

We believe that many of the decisions a therapist must make regarding how to secure members for the group, compose the group, and facilitate it through its various stages are made in view of the group's purposes. In addition, in short-term groups, clarity of purpose will help members to move quickly to identify and work on goals, and this is essential when time constraints are also present. Careful attention is essential, therefore, to the determination of these purposes. Therapists will generate group purposes that are consistent with the agency's purposes. In addition, they will often engage in a needs assessment by surveying colleagues or even clients to elicit information on the kinds of group purposes that would meet client needs.

For example, a therapist sought to create a short-term group in a community mental health center. Some of the agency service priorities at that time were to help families cope with the mental illness of family members, parents with the behavior of their adolescents, and the unemployed with the readjustments required by that status. Questionnaires were circulated to families of patients recently released from mental institutions, families of youth in the local high school, and to people when they applied for unemployment compensation.

A sufficient number of returns were secured from each of these sets of people. The unemployed, however, indicated very strongly that they will join a group whose purposes include helping them decide how to seek employment and how to deal with the sense of shame they have when facing other family members. Although the agency planned eventually to serve all three needs through short-term groups, the worker was immediately assigned to contact the unemployed who had responded to the questionnaire to begin the process of screening them for the group; an announcement was also placed in the local paper urging other unemployed people to contact the agency if they wished this type of service. The purposes of the group were announced as helping the unemployed find ways of seeking unemployment and dealing with the reactions of others to their unemployed status.

Length and Number of Sessions

The amount of time allotted to each meeting is dependent upon the structure of the session, the size of the group, and the capacity of the members. Groups with structured approaches such as social skills groups may well have agendas that require 1½ to 2 hours. This time span allows the therapist time to explain a skill, present a model of the behaviors that make up the skill, tailor the skill to the needs of individual members, and allow them to practice the skill, receive feedback, and secure "homework" assignments.

A less structured approach such as one centered upon group members examining their interactions with each other in the "here and now" and seeing the relationship of these to their presenting problems is likely to utilize a shorter session, often between 1¼ to 1½ hours in length. These sessions will become quite intense at times, and members may be overtaxed by too long a session unless they are carefully selected and prepared as should be done for "marathon" sessions that last for a full day or even a weekend.

The size and composition of the group also affect the length of time that should be allotted for each group sessions. Smaller groups, such as those of 5 to 8 members may be able to give a required amount of time to each member to present issues in an hour, whereas a larger group of 8 to 12 members might need more time to do the same thing. More homogeneous groups may provide for vicarious learning so that each member does not need "separate" time, whereas in heterogeneous groups this type of learning may be more difficult to attain.

The capacity of members is related to their age and their physical and mental status. Young children, low functioning psychotic individuals, and the developmentally disabled may not be able to sustain interest in a session that lasts more than 45 minutes. People who are functioning well and are seeking an experience that sensitizes them to their social interactions may be able to handle an all-day session.

The frequency of sessions and the overall number of sessions to be held are related issues. Groups in which members may only be available for a short period of time can meet daily so that members receive the maximum benefit from the group situation before they must leave. This is currently true of groups in mental hospitals inasmuch as current ideas of mental health care require the patient to be returned to the community quickly. Other residential settings, such as those for substance abusers, may also utilize a daily format in order to challenge the strong denial that is found in this population.

Skill-oriented groups will typically meet weekly or even biweekly for 8 to 12 sessions as this is the time required to learn a specific skill or a closely related set of skills. This meeting frequency allows the members to practice the skills in their roles outside of the group. Groups that seek, albeit on a short-term basis, to help members to focus on patterns of behavior and even to obtain some insight into personality tendencies will be likely to approach the upper limits on the number of sessions that still constitute short-term therapy.

SELECTION AND PREPARATION OF CLIENTS

Once therapists have selected a group purpose and through referrals, advertising, or agency intake have obtained a pool of potential members, they will make a final selection and prepare these members for their participation in the group. Close attention to these procedures will make it more likely that the group will be able to achieve its purposes within the time limits.

Selection Procedures

As Klein (1985) states, there is little, if any, research evidence regarding who will benefit from short-term group psychotherapy so that therapist and writers have to rely on clinical and anecdotal reports. Because of this, one of the first of the criteria we use is client preference. This should be an informed decision, however, so that clients should be told of the benefits of group therapy, provided with examples, and when possible be given an opportunity to observe a group.

There are a number of kinds of client problems that are very appropriate for clients to work on in groups. These are the problems that are defined in interpersonal terms such as a lack of social skills or difficulties in relationships. Groups can be helpful because they provide a place where the client can experiment with new social behaviors while receiving feedback from others. The client can also learn a variety of ways of coping with interpersonal situations because each member can provide suggestions from his or her own experience.

Klein (1985), in his review of the literature on who should be included in or excluded from short-term group psychotherapy, primarily cites literature about who should or should not be included in either long-term group therapy or short-term individual therapy. There is little on short-term groups as such. The literature, moreover, on choosing clients for group psychotherapy appears to be written from a verbal, psychodynamic perspective.

Thus some of the reasons for excluding clients are that they may heavily deny, somaticize, or externalize; be poorly motivated; not be psychologically minded; be acutely psychotic or chemically dependent; be sociopathic; or fear emotional contagion or intimacy. The problem we have with such a list is that alternative ways of working with groups other than a verbal, insight-oriented mode have been developed that address each of the mentioned reasons for exclusion. We agree, therefore, with Klein (1985) when he states:

> These "ideal" selection criteria might well be regarded by therapists in a typical outpatient clinic as frivolously luxuriant and, for the most part, irrelevant with regard to the vast majority of patients referred for group therapy. In my opinion, more seriously disturbed, chronically ill, or less well motivated patients also can benefit from a short-term therapy group. However, if such patients are selected, then the goals of the group, its structural features, and the role and techniques of the therapist need to be tailored accordingly. (p. 316)

An example of this point is provided by a demonstration of the effectiveness of short-term group for mothers receiving Aid to Families of Dependent Children grants (Navarre, Glasser, & Costabile, 1974). The purpose of the group was to help the mothers to handle problems interfering with their children's schooling. The group met for only six sessions because the mothers' motivation for group therapy as well as their ability to handle transportation, baby-sitting, and other barriers to attendance was limited. A parent-education combined with a problem-solving approach was utilized, and this, together with the time limits, undoubtedly contributed to the success of the group.

As we have stated, other reasons for recommending short-term group psychotherapy are the same as those for individual therapy. These include the bounded nature of the presenting problem and achievable expectations about treatment and change.

Assessment

Therapists will typically schedule interviews with potential group members for assessments that will aid them in making decisions as to whether the individuals are appropriate for the group and provide information that will help them plan for the group as well as ways of being helpful to each member. The types of information required for the latter purposes will vary based on the group approach the therapist intends to use. We, consequently, can only discuss the assessment process in general.

As we indicated, a primary consideration is the client's desire for a group experience. The therapist can assess this, in addition to placing the question directly, by discussing previous experiences in groups with the clients, whether they found them helpful, what their emotional reactions were to the group, and what roles they held in the group such as leader, low-level participant, scapegoat, and so forth.

As we indicated, although some form of short-term group may be devised for most types of clients, a particular group form may not be appropriate for a specific client. The range of possibilities is too great to catalogue here, but at least one caution should be noted. At times a structured group is advertised, such as an assertiveness training group, and some people may apply who really want a more classical psychotherapy group; others who apply may also suffer from some form of severe mental illness such that they will receive little benefit from the group while interfering with the group's value to others. The therapist must be skillful enough to identify these circumstances.

Part of the assessment process should also consist of helping the potential members to state their problems or focal concerns with considerable specificity. This will help the therapist to refine the group's purpose. This also has a direct relevance to the short-term nature of the group in that if group members are asked to discuss their reasons for coming to the group during early sessions, they will already have clarified this for themselves and, consequently, can more quickly do so in the group. This will help the group to move more quickly to the next stage of the process.

The therapist should be warned, however, that members may change their minds about the problems/concerns they wish to work on in the group when they are confronted with the realities of the other members and the impacts of the actual group interactions. This is not intrinsically good or bad; therapists, however, are in a better position to evaluate this matter if they know the pre-group concerns of the members.

For similar reasons, therapists will also ask potential members to express what they hope to accomplish in the group, and this will, in fact, be a first step toward articulating goals. The same cautions apply, also, in that members may reconsider their goals under the stimulus of actual group events. At times, as a reaction to goals stated by other members, they may formulate more or less ambitious ones than they presented to the therapist prior to the group.

Yalom (1985) presents a theoretical framework for assessing clients with reference to group therapy. This is based on the straightforward idea that "patients are likely to terminate membership in a therapy group, and are thereby poor candidates, when the punishments or disadvantages of group membership outweigh the rewards or the anticipated rewards" (p. 248). He discusses in detail the following ways in which group members are rewarded for group participation. We suggest that therapists bear them in mind as assessment considerations.

Members are satisfied with their groups (attracted to their groups and likely to continue membership in them) if:

1. They view the group as meeting their personal needs—that is, their goals in therapy.
2. They derive satisfaction from their relationships with the other group members.
3. They derive satisfaction from their participation in the group task.
4. They derive satisfaction from group membership vis-à-vis the outside world.

Preparation for Group

There is considerable evidence that preparing members for group therapy will contribute to the ease with which they begin to work on their issues in the group, and this is certainly of great value in a short-term experience (Garvin, 1987a; Meadow, n.d.; Poey, 1985; Yalom, 1985). Yalom (1985) begins this process by identifying and correcting the misconceptions clients have about group therapy. He also discusses with patients the "interpersonal theory of psychiatry" that focuses on relationships as central to leading a productive life and on how the group therapy experience can be a "laboratory" in which the individual works on relationships.

Yalom also explains that the best results can be secured if the member is honest in expressing feelings, particularly those toward other group members and therapists. We agree with Yalom regarding stressing openness in the initial interview while recognizing that this should be framed in terms of the amount that will be expected in this particular group. He also explains that no one will be *forced* to reveal anything. A good deal of information is also supplied on how the members are likely to react to the tensions created by group formation; we do not find that this is as important in short-term groups as in the long-term ones for which Yalom is preparing members.

Preparation of members should also include an explanation of group norms such as confidentiality, attendance, and punctuality. This type of information can often be presented in the form of written handouts.

Some authorities also suggest a "structured preparatory group workshop" before the actual group begins (Budman, Clifford, Bader, & Bader, 1981; Budman & Bennett, 1983). They propose a 3-hour session in which clients see what it is like to be in a group. This offers the clients an additional basis for making a decision on joining a group while giving additional assessment information to the therapists.

GROUP COMPOSITION

The composition of the group can have a great influence upon subsequent events. Because people differ from one another in countless respects, it is impossible to predict with certainty how a set of people who are brought together because they share some limited number of characteristics will subsequently behave. Nevertheless, there is enough research and practice experience to make some predictions as to the result of composing groups in particular ways. The therapist, therefore, can note the characteristics of people in a group and can be prepared to respond to likely responses.

Even if the therapist's intent is to compose a group in a particular manner, he or she may not have a sufficient pool of clients to do this. The question then becomes not how to compose a group to fulfill a specified purpose, but, given a group with a certain composition, what purposes might it achieve. In any case, when the group is time limited, it behooves the therapist to use any device to aid the group to accomplish its purpose within its time limits and composing the group clearly is one such.

One compositional decision is the degree of heterogeneity or homogeneity to seek. Because people do vary in so many ways, the therapist should choose a limited set of characteristics to use in selecting people. This set consists of what Bertcher and Maple (1985) term *descriptive* and *behavioral* attributes. The former consist of such demographic characteristics as age, sex, and race, whereas the latter consists of such behaviors as aggressiveness, talkativeness, friendliness, or acting bizarrely.

We agree with Yalom (1985) that group cohesiveness (that is, the attraction the group holds for the members) is one of the group conditions that most accounts for the effects of the group upon its members. In a short-term group, moreover, the therapist does not have very much time to create a cohesive group. Inasmuch as group cohesiveness is promoted when members perceive each other as possessing similar qualities, the therapist will seek out potential members who are similar. The exception will occur when the therapist chooses a group approach that requires heterogeneity such as when both men and women are included in a social skills group in which the program will include role plays involving both sexes.

Some have expressed concern that if members are too alike in behavioral attributes, they will be likely to reinforce each other's problematic behaviors rather than seek to change them. We again agree with Yalom that the diversity that exists among people often prevents too much homogeneity in any case; in addition, there are ways therapists can confront that sort of reinforcement.

We are more concerned that if a member differs too much from others in both behavioral and descriptive attributes, she or he is likely to become isolated in the group or even to be scapegoated by other members. We, consequently, have used the device of creating a chart in which each member is rated on each of the variables that the therapist deems salient for the type of group being created (for details of this procedure, see Garvin, 1987a, p. 65). This chart makes it possible for one to "eyeball" the potential composition of the group and to quickly identify potential "deviants." This can then be dealt with either by adding others with similar characteristics or by finding another service for the member in question.

An example of this procedure can be seen in a short-term group created for the purpose of helping adolescents without social skills to acquire them. The characteristics the therapist rated for purposes of this group's composition were sex, age, degree of social skill, sexual sophistication, academic performance, and level of verbal activity in groups. One youth was not referred to the group because she was younger, more sexually active, a poorer academic achiever, and more withdrawn than any of the other potential members.

Among the most important issues to consider in composition are the sex and the ethnicity of the members. The therapist should avoid composing a group in which the member represents, in these respects, a small minority (such as one or two). Such a member is likely to receive little support from others on issues very central to his or her identity and is also likely to carry the burden of having to represent "all women" or "all blacks," to name a few possibilities. At times, in contrast, the therapist will compose a group in which *all* members are of the same ethnicity or sex. Such groups are used to help members enhance their consciousness about identity related issues (Edwards, Edwards, Daines, & Eddy, 1978).

Another important point regarding black–white proportions in groups was made by Davis (1984) who wrote:

> Blacks, it appears, prefer groups that are 50 percent Black and 50 percent white— numerical equality. Whites, on the other hand, appear to prefer groups that are approximately 20 percent black and 80 percent white, societal ratios of Blacks and whites.

Needless to say, the preferences of both groups cannot be simultaneously met. This difference in preference for racial balance has the potential to lead to member dissatisfaction, discomfort, and withdrawal. (p. 102)

Davis, nevertheless, was not advocating for any particular racial composition but rather he hoped to sensitize the therapist to issues that would have to be faced if a particular kind of composition is used. Another example of the importance of racial composition is provided by Chu and Sue (1984) who stated:

In a group of very verbose, articulate, and aggressive non-Asians, the Asian member may be hesitant to speak up. In a confrontation, which inevitably happens at some point in a long-term group, the Asian may not know what to say, not being used to such interaction. (p. 30)

These authors recommend, therefore, that Asian-Americans be grouped together, at least at the beginning of a group experience. They believe this will enhance communication and empathy as well as the emergence of indigenous leadership.

Another important consideration is gender composition. Martin and Shanahan (1983), in their excellent review of this topic, point out the following:

1. Even without interpersonal interaction (e.g., verbal exchanges) females are negatively "evaluated" in all-male groups and in groups in which they are tokens.
2. The quantity and content of verbal interaction in groups varies with sex composition of the group and by gender of the participant. For example, women talk less and are talked to less in mixed groups than in all-female groups; men in all-male groups tend to concentrate on competition and status topics while females in all-female groups focus on personal, home, and family topics. Both males and females are most likely to exhibit the greatest quantity of leader-like statements in same sex groups.
3. Females are perceived of less positively than males, even when equally influential.
4. "Solo" or "token" females in otherwise male groups tend to fare poorly.
5. The findings regarding women in all-female groups are inconsistent. Variations seem to be related to whether the study focused upon attraction to group, "growth" of members, intermember influence, motivation for participation, or group effectiveness. (pp. 19–32)

To deal with these gender issues, Martin and Shanahan suggest that the therapist affirm the right of women to assume influential roles in the group and to receive "rewards" for competence. They also note that, whereas women have much to gain in all-women groups, men derive much benefit from being in a "mixed" group because they are less likely to be competitive and more likely to be "personal" under that condition.

Nevertheless, men may still be more talkative and competitive with each other in the "mixed" situation, and the therapist will have to confront this. In all-male groups, in contrast, the facilitator must help the members to accept the degree of intimacy and self-disclosure that the group requires.

GROUP FORMATION

All therapy groups encounter similar issues in their first meetings, and this is referred to as group formation. These ideas include deciding upon or clarifying individual goals and group purposes that will help members attain their goals; establishing group norms and rules; and collecting information that will help members decide how they will act to reach goals (some of this information may be in the nature of individual assessments).

The decisions members arrive at with their therapists on these issues constitute their "contracts" that are sometimes in written forms. Other formation issues that go beyond contracting are initiating relationships among the members and between the members and the therapist and resolving mixed feelings members may have about the group in a positive direction. Although all of these concerns arise in any group, they must be dealt with in short-term ones in ways that make their time frames feasible, and we now turn to a discussion of this.

As we have indicated, the process of helping members decide on the problem(s) they wish to work on in the group as well as the goals that, if attained, will help to ameliorate the problem(s) begins during the pregroup screening interview(s); yet when members meet each other, they may alter these decisions. This process as well as other aspects of contracting is essential to the future success of the group. As Poey (1985) states:

> These contracts will delineate the basic boundaries within which the group will focus its attention in depth. This is perhaps the single most challenging facet of brief group therapy because it requires that both the leaders and members struggle early on to conceptualize and circumscribe each member's symptoms into focal problems. (p. 336)

Despite our belief that this degree of specificity is important, it may be less attainable in highly structured groups that meet for few sessions. Poey (1985) recommends that if the group will have less than 12 sessions, the individual goals be expressed in the group's purpose, and he gives developing assertiveness or intimacy as examples (p. 337).

Another approach is taken by some therapists who work with groups with frequently changing membership such as inpatient groups. They may ask members to formulate goals at every session that are so specific that they can be achieved in that session (Yalom, 1983). Examples of such goals are to initiate a conversation with another member, ask for feedback on a concrete issue, express a particular emotion that the member has difficulty showing, and so forth.

Even when members do not, as a reaction to other members, alter their goals during this formation and contracting period, they should make them more specific, and they should be taught through modeling and examples how to do this. This entails a good deal of interaction as they question, give feedback, and offer suggestions to each other. This interaction can be used by the therapist to illustrate how members can be of help to one another throughout the life of the group.

Group purposes and member goals are interwoven and should be discussed in ways that closely relate the two. As indicated, the therapist will have determined a group purpose prior to creating the group, and clients have joined on this basis. As they more fully specify their individual goals, however, the original statement of purpose may be modified somewhat. An example of this was a group in which developing assertiveness was the stated purpose. Many women who joined the group indicated in its first session that sexism in their life situations hindered their development of assertiveness, and they contracted to learn how to identify the effects of sexism as another but related group purpose.

In order to expedite the group's work, the therapist will have to quickly secure the members' agreement to a set of norms and rules. As in any therapy group, these should include an agreement on confidentiality, attendance, and promptness, as well as on fees and time and length of session. If new members can be added, the procedures for doing so should be explained.

Other norms that can be more subtle are those regarding self-disclosure, openness to feedback, and members' helping one another. Although these concepts can be easily explained to members, it is another thing to make them actually occur. Therapists can design exercises to teach these concepts experientially such as using "rounds" in which members express their thoughts or feelings about some aspect of the here-and-now situation and are then invited to comment on each other's statements. Many examples of openness or lack of openness and of how members respond to one another are elicited by these types of simple devices, and these examples can be used for establishing these types of group norms.

Because the goals of short-term groups are focused on specific aspects of functioning, therapists are not required to engage in complex assessments of members. Any assessment that takes place is limited to what is necessary to achieve the goal. This means that the problematic behavior must be examined in terms of how, when, and where it occurs. The skills the member already has in coping with the situation as well as skill deficits are noted. The strengths and limitations present in the situation are also examined so that they might be dealt with in constructive ways. The degree of understanding the member has of his or her behavior or situation also is relevant when the approach of the therapist is to enhance awareness and to utilize problem-solving processes.

An example of this was a discussion that took place with a member in a group of young adults that focused on intimacy issues. The member indicated that he had close male friends but felt very uncomfortable when his girlfriend said that she wanted to get closer to him. The other members explored with him what he thought she meant by "closer" and how he felt about that. They also found out how he reacted when his girlfriend raised this issue. He indicated that he felt more comfortable talking with her about their plans for the future than about disagreements they had about immediate decisions. He thought she was very supportive, but he received many criticisms from his mother whom he thought resented any relationships he had with women. He understood that these kinds of demands from his mother were related to his apprehensiveness about close relationships with women. As the reader can see, all these pieces of information will be useful to the therapist and the other members as they seek to help this member.

The therapist must also accelerate the process whereby members develop trusting relationships with each other and with him or her in order to achieve the optimal results of a short-term group. This occurs fairly readily if the norms favoring open expression of views and emotions and mutual helping are accepted and reinforced. The therapist should be observant of members who appear to be rejecting these norms or of the group itself so that the source of this negativism can be confronted.

Another way of enhancing such relationships is to turn as much as possible of the direction of the group over to the members. In structured groups such as those focused on social skills training, members can be drawn upon to monitor the steps by which each individual acquires the social skill such as being behaviorally specific, asking for suggestions on alternative ways of handling a situation, and so forth. In less structured groups, members can be called upon to suggest ways of relating a member's concern to the here-and-now situation as well as to direct each other's attention to many other processes.

Finally, the therapist should be sensitive to the ambivalence members of groups frequently experience about the group during formation. They are likely to have positive feelings associated with the hope that they will benefit from the group; negative ones stem from fears of the responses of others, including whether they will be liked and accepted. In short-term groups, therapists should try whenever possible to accentuate the positive and to be reassuring about fears. Unfortunately, there is not as much time as in long-term groups to work with these feelings as a way for members to learn to cope better with other "beginnings."

MIDDLE PHASES

The process of formation, with some variation based on the group's purposes, the member's behaviors, and the overall time frame of the group should be well on the way to completion by about the third meeting in "closed" groups. In groups with changing memberships, on the other hand, there may be a number of times that formation issues resurface. Formation, nevertheless, is essentially completed when most if not all members demonstrate their commitment to the group and its purposes, have determined individual goals, show their understanding of group norms, and are open to ways of working to achieve their goals.

This is not meant to imply that all has been "smooth sailing." Many writers have described what Garland, Jones, and Kolodny (1965) call a power-and-control phase. We find this sometimes occurs late in the formation period of short-term groups but may also occur during the middle phase and is at least in part a reaction to authority issues. Poey (1985) puts the therapist's role with regard to these issues well:

> The leaders' major activity is to reinforce adherence to therapeutic modalities and to interpret resistances. The group usually reacts to these authoritative postures with fight and flight reactions, defensiveness, scapegoating, and, we hope, eventually a

resolution to cohere as a group whose members are willing to trust each other enough
to risk working out the problems that brought them to the group. (p. 341)

There are many strategies therapists use to help members of short-term
groups during the middle phase that transcend the particular treatment approach that has been adopted. We shall discuss these first, followed by discussions of strategies that are particular to work that is less structured and to work
that is more so.

General Strategies

The ways that therapists help all short-term groups accomplish their tasks
in the middle phases can be grouped under the headings of working with
structures, processes, and climate. In accomplishing this, certain worker styles
are preferable. Each of these topics will now be considered.

Structures

We agree with Klein (1985) that structurally the role of the therapist is to
"view the group as an open system and to regard the major function of the
leadership as the management of boundaries, both internal and external" (p.
320). One set of boundaries is external, and in this respect the therapist mediates
between the group and the agency as well as systems outside of the agency.

Thus in a group referred to earlier, whose purpose was to help welfare
mothers support the education of their children, the therapist invited speakers
in from the local school. She also asked a resource person from the welfare
department to inform the mothers about ways of securing things their children
might need just to attend school.

The therapist's role with respect to internal boundaries, according to Klein,
"involves monitoring the relationship between the task of the group and its
structures, to insure that the form of the group is appropriate to its function" (p.
320). This includes many group conditions that we have discussed elsewhere
(Garvin, 1987a) such as subgroupings, communication patterns, division of labor, and roles. Therapists can affect these patterns by the types of activities they
introduce, by directions to members, by differentially reinforcing members
when they enact some patterns and not others, and by drawing members'
attention to their patterns so that a problem-solving process could be directed at
changing them.

An example of this occurred in a group whose purpose was to help members deal with intimacy issues. The men and women in the group formed two
distinct subgroups, and individuals in each group seldom addressed those who
were not in their "clique." The worker drew the members' attention to this
phenomenon. A subsequent discussion took place on the reasons for the pattern. Members admitted fears regarding interactions with the other sex and
examined ways of coping with such fears. This led to a series of "experiments"

in which members consciously tried out asking for feedback from members of the other sex.

Processes

Two processes that therapists frequently utilize in short-term groups are task assignment/implementation and problem-solving. The former draws from task-centered theory (Reid, Chapter 3 this volume) and has been described in detail as to its application in groups by Garvin (1985). The basic idea behind task-centered work is that clients, once they have chosen the problem they wish to work on and the goals they seek to achieve, can attain these goals through devising and carrying out tasks. These tasks are typically undertaken outside of the group.

Although the task-centered approach was originally devised for one-to-one helping, it can be utilized in groups in ways that enhance its utility. This occurs because members help each other to devise tasks through the similarities that often exist in their circumstances. For the same reason, they also can provide suggestions to each other as to how to carry out tasks. Furthermore, the group constitutes a laboratory in which members can practice carrying out tasks and receive immediate feedback from each other.

Task assignments are very similar to the "homework" assignments that many therapists utilize to provide for the active influence of the group between sessions. A difference is that task assignments are always mutually developed among members and between the member in question and the therapist. Homework can be a unilateral prescription.

In the group referred to devoted to helping members with intimacy issues, one member indicated that she had not spoken to her boyfriend for a week because she thought he had made fun of her. On questioning, it appeared that she was not really sure what his reaction was at the time. Because the group was utilizing a task-centered approach, the issue was discussed as to an appropriate task. The one that she agreed to was to call her boyfriend and compare his and her perceptions of the troublesome interaction. The therapist suggested that she role play her approach to this in the group. She did so and became aware of ways in which she undercut such discussions.

In view of the here-and-now reality-oriented focus of many short-term groups, problem solving is a frequently used process. Thus, it often is necessary for the therapist to teach the group a problem-solving procedure and to reinforce this learning each time problem-solving is used. The following are the steps that we have taught to groups (Garvin, 1987a, pp. 134–135):

1. The problem is specified in detail.
2. The group members determine whether a group problem-solving process should occur.
3. Goals to be attained through problem-solving are specified.
4. Information is sought to help the group members generate possible solutions as well as to evaluate such solutions.

5. One alternative is chosen.
6. How the chosen alternative will be carried out is planned.

Climate

In order to facilitate the work of the short-term group, the therapist must maintain a climate in which members speak freely and are willing to take risks. One way to accomplish this is to create a situation in which members care what happens to each other and communicate this feeling to one another. One opportunity to develop this is provided when a member arrives late or misses a session. If others ignore this behavior, the therapist will ask him or her what he or she plans on doing about it. Members may state that they do not know what to do, and the therapist can confront this by asking, "Don't you care?" This question usually leads to a discussion of caring in groups and how it can be shown.

This is only one example of how this issue can be raised. The therapist who understands the value of a caring atmosphere will be able to perceive when this topic underlies an incident in the life of the group and will help the group to attend to it and deal with it in constructive ways.

Style

Some therapists undoubtedly are more effective than others with short-term groups. We think that one of the reasons for this is that their style coincides with the factors that promote the success of such groups. One of these is that the therapist is very active. This means that in view of time constraints, she or he frequently raises questions, makes suggestions, offers interpretations, and prescribes exercises. This has sometimes been referred to in a critical way as "manipulative." Dies (1985), in a thoughtful discussion of this in an essay entitled "Leadership in Short-Term Group Therapy: Manipulation or Facilitation" argues against this characterization. As a result of gathering data from clinicians, he concluded the following:

> Our information study demonstrates that process commentary, reflection, interpretation, introduction of structured exercises, and so forth were often regarded as helpful and not necessarily manipulative and controlling. (p. 449)

He makes another important contribution when he notes:

> A key issue appears to be the subjective experience of freedom or personal control felt by group members. The leader who can best incorporate more directive intervention strategies is probably the one who is positively oriented and personally and technically open. The same tactics practiced by a distant, indifferent, or confronting clinician would undoubtedly be received quite differently by group members. (p. 451)

Still another characteristic of effective short-term group therapists is their ability to quickly form positive relationships with group members so that such members will understand that the directiveness we have referred to comes from a position of an appropriate degree of caring. This will also further the ability of the therapists to offer themselves as behavioral models when this will be helpful to members.

Strategies in Structured Groups

In addition to the previously mentioned strategies that are used in most short-term groups, there are additional ones that are employed in structured groups. In these groups, the therapist creates an agenda for each session in order to help the members attain psychoeducational goals. The agenda is likely to include discussion topics, short lectures, exercises, and simulations. Depending on the therapist's approach, the plan for the session may be more or less rigidly followed. It is also possible for groups to have some structured and some unstructured sessions.

The social skills groups described in detail in the next chapter are one form of structured groups (Rose, Chapter 22 this volume). Other forms are task-centered groups (Garvin, 1985) and behavioral therapy groups (Rose, 1972, 1977). The purpose of such structured groups is to help the members acquire specific skills in order to attain specific goals. Although all short-term groups have goal specificity as a feature, in structured groups, the skills to attain the goals are usually predetermined.

In social skills groups the skills may be, for example, to act assertively, communicate effectively, or to cope with stress. In task-centered groups, the skills are those necessary to choose and carry out tasks that help the members to achieve their goals. And in behavioral therapy groups, the skills involve increasing or decreasing the performance of specified behaviors.

In a task-centered group whose purpose was to help seriously psychiatrically disabled patients involve themselves in productive activities, the therapist established the following agenda for the second session (Garvin, 1987b):

1. *Development of individual goals.* The idea of the "time line" that was presented at the previous meeting will be reviewed. Each member presents his or her previous day and, with the help of other group members, creates a time line on a sheet of paper. Members are asked whether that day was a typical one. If not, a more typical day may be substituted. The member is then asked what might be one way in which his or her use of leisure time on that day might have been enhanced (i.e., what is something she or her would have wished to do that would have been the way he or she wished to spend time). Members give feedback to each other (with the help of the therapists) in the form of suggestions. Members are asked whether this use of time is the one they wish to make their goal for the group experience. If not, with the help of time lines, other goals are considered. The object, however, is to create the goal in terms of a time line.

How the member wishes to spend her or his time may not necessarily be within his or her competency at the time. The purpose is to identify some way that the member will wish to use time at the end of the process. There may be several intermediate steps in the form of tasks; these can be placed on a time line also.

It is estimated that the previously described process may take 10 to 15 minutes per member so that the group will have to be subdivided into two subgroups of about four members. With this approach, the process will take about an hour. The therapists should try to create two subgroups with about equal distribution of members who are slow at the activity so that the two groups will finish at about the same time.

2. *Leisure time experience.* Because members will have been working hard, the last 15 to 30 minutes should be spent in some way that is reinforcing. This should be in the form of refreshments and a game. The game that we recommend is "Leisure Time Trivia." For this game, the group is divided into two subgroups. A series of questions have been devised such as the following: name three objects that are necessary for a baseball game; name one movie now playing in a local theatre.

3. *Evaluation of session.* The meeting should conclude with a discussion of feelings about the group and how things are going. The plan for the next meeting is described that will include a reaffirmation that the members wish to pursue the goals selected at this meeting and initial work on constructing tasks to attain these goals.

This agenda was constructed by the therapist based on her assessment of what the members were capable of, what the purposes of the group were, and how much time each activity was likely to take. The therapist must be competent in this kind of planning in order to work effectively with a structured group.

Strategies in Unstructured Groups

Unstructured groups are those in which the therapist helps the members to achieve their goals by guiding the process of the group as it unfolds. There is less effort than in structured groups on limiting what the process will be through the creation of an agenda. (We note, nevertheless, that "groups have lives of their own," and the therapist can never fully control processes as they emerge.) A particular focus is to help members to perceive how they affect and are affected by group processes so that they may experiment with new ways of behaving in social situations.

We know of no research that has established conclusively when and for whom structured and unstructured group therapy approaches work better. In unstructured groups, there is more emphasis on members discovering the meaning of social processes for themselves and on "fine tuning" their social responses. This allows for a great deal of variation in the issues on which members work. Consequently an unstructured approach may be required when members have dissimilar goals.

The emphasis in unstructured groups on cognition may make them more appropriate for people who function at good intelligence levels and whose problem-solving abilities are intact. Their motivation to work on interpersonal issues should also be strong.

We have used Yalom's (1985) process illumination procedures successfully in short-term group psychotherapy. He indicates that the therapist who uses this approach must be very sensitive to the relationship implications of both the verbal and nonverbal behaviors of members. Among the behaviors, therefore, that should be noted are seating patterns, eye contacts, contradictions between verbal and nonverbal responses, and so on. The therapist will make comments on this to any one or all of the members involved in the process or even to others to secure their perceptions. A progression that Yalom uses in deciding on such comments is the following:

> The comments for a progression from sense data commentary—observations of single acts—to a description of feelings evoked by an act, to observations about several acts over a period of time, to the juxtaposition of different acts, to speculations about the patient's intentions and motivations, to comments about the unfortunate repercussions of this behavior to the inclusion of more inferential data (dreams, subtle gestures), to calling attention to the similarity between his behavioral patterns in the here-and-now and in his outside social world. (p. 173)

Poey (1985) defines the therapist's role in unstructured short-term groups in analytic structural terms:

> The predominant focus of brief group work would be on the ego level—strengthening members' adaptive ego functioning and uncovering the "repressed positive ego." Some superego material is also appropriate, particularly when severe superego functioning is inhibiting healthy ego processes. Much less attention, however, should be directed toward primitive id material except in several specific instances. One instance in which the leaders might choose to attend to id expressions would be in an attempt to "normalize" such material or to help the members erect healthier defenses to cope with it. (p. 346)

Termination

Because the time limits for the group are stated in the beginning, termination issues are dealt with throughout the group. Therapists will frequently remind the members about the amount of time remaining and the tasks that the group must accomplish in view of this. In addition, they will focus specifically on termination during the last few sessions.

During this termination process, the therapist will seek to accomplish the following tasks:

1. The members will evaluate their degree of goal attainment. This can be accomplished through qualitative discussion or through the use of appropriate instruments (Garvin, 1987a). At times, members may also ask significant others outside the group to rate their progress, and these ratings will be discussed in the group.

2. The members will evaluate the group experience itself and will describe those aspects that were helpful and not helpful to them. This can also be done on a session-by-session basis either orally or in writing. This information helps the members to understand what has contributed to their progress so they can continue to make use of similar conditions. It also helps the therapist to plan better for future groups. We also recommend that the therapist ask for an evaluation of himself or herself.

3. Members will discuss "next steps." This will include both how they plan

on using what they have gained from the group as well as plans for future experiences to build upon these gains.

4. Members will cope with feelings they have about termination. Some of these will be pleasurable as members reflect on good experiences and how they have been helpful. Other feelings will include sadness as members say goodbye to each other and to the therapist. We believe that this expression of feelings helps members to deal fully with other aspects of the group experience as well as with other terminations they face.

STUDIES OF EFFECTIVENESS

In a review of evaluation studies of short-term group psychotherapy, Klein (1985, p. 311) found that "comparative studies of brief versus unlimited therapies administered on either an individual or a group level show essentially no differences in results." He cites studies by Lieberman (1976), Imber, Lewis, and Loiselle (1979), and Budman, Randall, and Denby (1981) that focused specifically on short-term groups. Poey (1985, p. 332) concludes that "there is clear indication that therapeutic change can and does occur in those specified areas on which the brief group focuses," and he cites studies by Budman, Randell, and Denby (1981) and from the University of Massachusetts Mental Health Service in support of this conclusion.

Garvin (1985) reports on a series of evaluations of task-centered groups with such populations as the chronically mentally ill, delinquents, and the elderly. The reports invariably were positive, although Garvin noted major weaknesses in the research designs. Rose (1972, 1977, 1980) demonstrates high effectiveness of behaviorally oriented short-term groups for a wide array of clients including children, the elderly, marital couples, and people deficient in social skills.

Despite these positive signs, many research gaps remain. We know little about the effects of different group lengths and group procedures on members with different characteristics when conducted by therapist with different attributes. Many complex issues still remain to be solved regarding any type of group therapy having to do with creating comparable groups, determining appropriate controls, and taking group conditions (group structures and processes) into consideration.

FUTURE ISSUES

Many of the principles we have presented in this chapter are informed opinions of short-term group therapists. Even though much of the research on group psychotherapy is performed on time-limited groups, the outcomes that can be expected from these as compared to long- and indefinite-term groups have not been examined through rigorous research. This type of research must be done if we are to see this modality, in which we have so much confidence, firmly established among the array of services.

Even though we have been speaking of short-term groups, there is considerable variation in the number of sessions held. This variation must be examined so that the time frame, the central feature of this modality, is not left to the therapist's idiosyncratic decision making.

Short-term group psychotherapy also must be analyzed along with all other therapeutic approaches in terms of the particular combination of client characteristics and problems, group compositions, and therapist interventions that produce desired outcomes. This type of work will necessitate that we further develop our typologies of therapist interventions and how they combine into overall group approaches so that one set can be compared to another in relationship to outcomes.

REFERENCES

Benne, K. D. (1964). History of the T group in the laboratory setting. In L. P. Bradford, J. R. Gibb, & K. D. Benne (Eds.), *T-group therapy and laboratory method* (pp. 80–135). New York: Wiley.

Bertcher, H., & Maple, F. (1985). Elements and issues in group composition. In M. Sundel, P. Glasser, R. Sarri, & R. Vinter (Eds.), *Individual change through small groups* (2nd ed.; pp. 180–202). New York: Free Press.

Budman, S. H., & Bennett, M. J. (1983). Short-term group psychotherapy. In H. I. Kaplan & B. J. Sadock (Eds.), *Comprehensive group psychotherapy* (2nd ed., pp. 138–143). Baltimore: Williams & Wilkins.

Budman, S. H., Clifford, M., Bader, L., & Bader, B. (1981). Experiential pre-group preparation and screening. *Group, 5*, 19–26.

Budman, S. H., Randall, M., & Denby, A. (1981). Outcome in short-term group psychotherapy. *Group, 5*, 37–51.

Butcher, J. N., & Koss, M. P. (1978). Research on brief and crisis-oriented therapies. In A. E. Bergin & S. L. Garfield (Eds.), *Handbook of psychotherapy and behavior change* (2nd ed., pp. 725–767). New York: Wiley.

Chu, J., & Sue, S. (1984). Asian/Pacific Americans and group practice. *Social Work with Groups, 7*, 23–36.

Davis, L. (1984). Essential components of group work with Black Americans. *Social Work with Groups, 7*, 97–109.

Dies, R. R. (1985). Leadership in short-term group therapy: Manipulation or facilitation. *International Journal of Group Psychotherapy, 35*, 435–455.

Edwards, E. D., Edwards, M. E., Daines, G. M., & Eddy, F. (1978). Enhancing self-concept and identification with "Indianness" of American Indian Girls. *Social Work with Groups, 1*, 309–318.

Garland, J. A., Jones, H. E., & Kolodny, R. (1965). A model for stages of development in social work groups. In S. Bernstein (Ed.), *Explorations in group work* (pp. 17–71). Boston: Boston University School of Social Work.

Garfield, S. L. (1978). Research on client variables in psychotherapy. in A. E. Bergin & S. L. Garfield (Eds.), *Handbook of psychotherapy and behavior change* (2nd ed., pp. 191–232). New York: Wiley.

Garvin, C. (1985). Practice with task-centered groups. In A. Fortune (Ed.), *Task centered practice with groups and families* (pp. 45–77). New York: Springer.

Garvin, C. (1987a). *Contemporary group work.* Englewood Cliffs, NJ: Prentice-Hall.

Garvin, C. (1987b). *A task-centered group approach to work with the chronically mentally ill.* Paper presented at the 9th Annual Symposium on Social Work with Groups, Boston, Mass., October 31, 1987.

Imber, S. D., Lewis, P. M. & Loiselle, R. H. (1979). Uses and abuses of the brief intervention group. *International Journal of Group Psychotherapy, 29*, 39–49.

Klein, R. H. (1985). Some principles of short-term group therapy. *International Journal of Group Psychotherapy, 35*, 309–329.

Lieberman, M. A. (1976). Change induction in small groups. In M. R. Rosenzweig & L. W. Porter (Eds.), *Annual review of psychology* (pp. 217–250). Palo Alto, CA: Annual Reviews, Inc.

Martin, P., & Shanahan, K. A. (1983). Transcending the effects of sex composition in small groups. *Social Work with Groups, 6,* 19–32.

Meadow, D. (n.d.) *Connecting theory and practice: The effect of pre-group preparation on individual and group behavior.* Mimeographed.

Navarre, E., Glasser, P. H., & Costabile, J. (1985). An evaluation of group work practice with AFDC mothers. In M. Sundel, P. Glasser, R. Sarri, & R. Vinter (Eds.), *Individual change through small groups* (2nd ed., pp. 391–407). New York: Free Press.

Poey, K. (1985). Guidelines for the practice of brief, dynamic group therapy. *International Journal of Group Psychotherapy, 35,* 331–354.

Rose, S. (1972). *Treating children in groups.* San Francisco: Jossey-Bass.

Rose, S. (1977). *Group therapy: A behavioral approach.* Englewood Cliffs, NJ: Prentice-Hall.

Rose, S. (1980). *A casebook in group therapy.* Englewood Cliffs, NJ: Prentice-Hall.

Rosenbaum, M. (Ed.). (1983). *Handbook of short-term therapy groups.* New York: McGraw-Hill.

Yalom, I. (1983). *Inpatient group psychotherapy.* New York: Basic Books.

Yalom, I. (1985). *The theory and practice of group psychotherapy* (3rd ed.). New York: Basic Books.

22

Social Skill Training in Short-Term Groups

Sheldon D. Rose

Social skill training is rapidly becoming one of the broadest applied therapeutic and educational approaches. Many people suffer the inconvenience or pain of not being able to deal with interpersonal relationships. Social skill training is designed to increase the client's competence in a wide variety of interactions with other people. The term *social skills* refers to the ability to perform a complex set of both verbal and nonverbal behaviors that compose a consistently effective response to a set of given social situations. It should be noted that social skills are situationally specific. That is, each type of situation has its unique requirements for an effective response. Persons may be skilled in responding to some situations but not to others. For example, some persons may be able to ask for help and express their feelings in situations that call for such behaviors but are not able to refuse others even when imposed upon. Others may be quite expert at all of the brief responses mentioned but falter in complex situations such as extended conversations, job interviews, or dating situations. Responses are considered effective if they help the client to move toward his or her own goals without imposing on the rights of others. Social skill training, therefore, focuses on both the learning of new behaviors appropriate to a given situation and the process involved in putting together a sequence of effective behaviors. Social skill training may be also used to eliminate or modify those behaviors that interfere with the attainment of personal goals. In training, the acquisition of specific social skills appropriate to given situations is often employed as a means of solving specific, imminent problems. It is an equally relevant means of helping clients develop a repertoire of appropriate nonverbal social skills (good eye contact, appropriate voice volume and modulation) that can be used in a wide variety of situations. Finally, it may serve to assist the client in improving long-term relationships as the client succeeds in meeting mutual goals for concrete situations with a partner.

The context of social skill training is the treatment dyad, the small group, or

---

Sheldon D. Rose • School of Social Work, University of Wisconsin–Madison, Madison, Wisconsin 53707.

the family. Most of the examples in this chapter will be drawn from the small-group context that is uniquely suited to social skill training for reasons that are described later. Social skill training may be a treatment in its own right or part of treatment with a more complex set of problems.

POPULATIONS SERVED AND PROBLEMS DEALT WITH

Although minor social deficiencies may be only a nuisance and source of brief personal stress, broad and persistent social skill deficits have been linked to a number of severe psychiatric disorders, such as schizophrenia, alcoholism, sexual dysfunction, marital discord, and depression. Although it is not clear what the role is of social skill deficits in the etiology and development of particular disorders, it is apparent that they contribute to the problems clients experience in coping with the effects of their disorders. Because of the link of social skill deficits to such disorders, social skill training procedures have been used with and shown to be effective in expanding the social skills of schizophrenics (Bellack, Hersen, & Turner, 1976); and in the treatment of unipolar depression (Hersen, Bellack, & Himmelhock, 1982); alcoholism (Miller & Eisler, 1977); social isolation and peer relationship problems in children (French & Tyne, 1982; Whitehill, Hersen, & Bellack, 1980); hyperactivity in children (Frederickson, Jenkins, Foy, & Eisler, 1976); communication problems of married couples (Buchler, 1979); and heterosocial failure and shyness (Galassi & Galassi, 1979). In addition, social skill training is often provided as a preventative mental health program in schools, industry, and other organizations as well as a remedial program in clinical settings. Specific social behaviors addressed by both practitioners and researchers are job interviewing, conversational skills, children's prosocial play behaviors, heterosexual date initiation behaviors, refusal assertion when imposed upon, giving praise and reinforcement to others, expressing feelings, and making requests. Clinicians report a far wider use, including helping people to approach authority persons, involving others in group discussions at work, setting limits on children, learning concrete parenting skills, asking for help from significant others, and disagreeing with others. However, almost any interactive behavior that occurs in an identifiable situation can be regarded as a legitimate target of social skill training.

THEORETICAL FOUNDATIONS OF SOCIAL SKILL TRAINING

Present-day social skill training seems to draw most heavily for its theoretical foundations on the social learning theory of Bandura (1977). According to social learning theory, except for some elementary reflex reactions, most behavior must be learned. Learning takes place either through direct experience or through observation of others as they behave in certain ways under certain circumstances. Social learning theory is primarily concerned with the mechanisms responsible for observational learning. These include attentional, retentional, motor reproduction, and motivational processes.

In social learning theory, the persons whose behavior and attitudes are being observed is referred to as a model. To learn a behavior performed by a model, clients must first attend to and perceive the modeled behavior accurately. Thus attentional processes, including characteristics of the observer and the person being observed, govern what is learned. For example, if a client is fatigued or is distracted by another event, he or she may not accurately attend to a particular behavior. If the potential model has extremely distasteful appearance or other characteristics as perceived by the observer, the behavior is unlikely to receive attention.

Retentional processes also govern how much is learned by observing a model. Clients are more likely to remember and, hence, reproduce a behavior if they have seen similar responses performed on several occasions by different models, or if they have used cues and other memory aids to help themselves remember what they have observed. Clients capacities also vary in this respect.

A third process that operates in observational learning is motor reproduction. To reproduce a modeled response, clients must have the physical capability and the skill needed to perform an observed behavior. No matter how much a person observes, he or she cannot reproduce a pole vault event without certain level of strength and prerequisite skills. Selection of initial targets for learning for which minimal motoric and technical skill prerequisite skills. Selection of initial targets for learning for which minimal motoric and technical skill prerequisites exist will facilitate reproduction of modeled behavior. In specialized or long-term treatment, shaping of more sophisticated skills may also be possible.

Motivation, a fourth process in observational learning, is affected both by observed consequences of the behavior and by the value system of the person making a given response. If the outcome of a given set of modeled behaviors is positive and the values of the model are compatible to that of the observer, the behaviors are more likely to be reproduced. The ability of the practitioner to establish a sound relationship certainly is an important consideration in establishing motivation. But the reverse is also true. An effective program seems to help build a relationship.

Social skill training is a program that incorporates all of the aforementioned principles into a set of strategies designed to increase the probability of learning social skills that are agreed upon by client and therapist.

ORGANIZATION FOR TREATMENT

When organizing a program, the practitioner must answer questions as to the number of sessions, length of sessions, number of session, and context of treatment. If the context is a group, the practitioner must also consider the number of therapists, the number of clients in the group, and the general composition of the group.

In general, social skill training has been considered a short-term treatment. Some research and practitioners report a 1-hour session per behavior treated, although eight sessions are more common. In the case of multiple deficiencies, long-term treatment is also more common. In individual treatment, the criteria for termination are whether the desired behaviors are being performed in the real world when they are called for.

Social skill training is often carried out in small groups. The research suggests that social skill training in groups is equivalent and in some cases superior to dyadic approaches (Kendall, 1982; Linehan, Walker, Bronheim, Haynes, & Yevzeroff, 1979). Group approaches provide various points of view in the form of social strategies and feedback to the client. Clients have an opportunity to help others as well as be the recipient of help. The group provides diverse role players for the roles of significant others in rehearsals and diverse models. In a group, however, it is somewhat more difficult to individualize the idiosyncratic needs of each client. The therapist must attempt to find common situations wherever possible. Care must also be taken that no one person dominate the discussion. Group problems such as low cohesion or intragroup conflict occasionally arise and should be brought to the attention of the members and dealt with.

There is usually one leader for groups (unless in a training situation). The groups vary in size, but a mean of seven to eight persons for adults and six or seven for children seems to be common. Groups tend to meet weekly for 2 hours for adults and 1 hour for children. The number of sessions varies a great deal, but eight sessions seem most common for members with shared goals. In respect to group composition, the greater the heterogeneity as to social skills required, the more time required. There appears to be no evidence that diversity in gender, race, socioeconomic background affects outcome.

Even if a group context is preferred, often no group is immediately available. In this case or in those situations in which greater individualization is required, the practitioner will work individually with the client. In individual treatment, the practitioner is required to be the model in all situations or to bring in others to the session as models. Drawing upon the same principles as in small groups, social skill training has also been carried out effectively in families and with couples (Buchler, 1979).

THE GENERAL TREATMENT PROCESS

The general strategical approach of social skill training consists of orientation, assessment, intervention, and generalization training. Although these four phases tend to overlap, they will be discussed in the following sections separately.

Orientation Strategies

Prior to and in the early sessions of treatment, the practitioner explains the assumptions of the approach and provides examples as to how treatment operates. In addition, he or she explains in brief how each of the procedures work and throughout treatment he or she continues to elaborate on the procedures just before they are used. Another strategy of treatment is the use of a treatment contract in which the expectations for both the practitioner and the client are explained in writing. This provides a basis for an honest and open working relationship.

Assessment Strategies

The primary purpose of assessment in the social skill training is to determine the specific client social skill attributes, deficiencies, and problematic situations in which he or she and significant others perceive his or her responses to be inappropriate or ineffective. Assessment also provides the practitioner with knowledge of potential personal and environmental resources available to the client in achieving his or her goals. Based on this preliminary information the therapist must also determine whether the social skill approach is appropriate to the presenting problem and whether the group or individual context is appropriate. In addition, motivation, environmental events, and specific physical conditions that impinge upon the present performance of the individual should be assessed. In order to achieve the first goal cited, a number of procedures can be used including individual and group interviews, naturalistic observations, observations of contrived or analog situations, self-reports, and standardized assessment instruments.

The Individual and Group Interview

Often prior to treatment a pretreatment interview is held in which the measures to be described are employed, and the client is interviewed in terms of situations he or she finds difficult or unsatisfying to cope with. The interviewer also enquires as to what the client thinks and feels during these situations, the relevance of these situations to the client's life, the societal and physical barriers to his or her performing more adequately in those situations, and the personal and societal resources for improving the client's performances. The same interview may be carried out in the first sessions of the group approach.

Interviews of Significant Others

With children, teacher and/or parents are usually interviewed prior to admission to the group to help ascertain the target of intervention or the specific skills that should be taught. The choice of interview depends on who referred the child or who is most concerned with his or her behavior. The content of the interview focuses on specific situations in which the child displays what the significant other perceives as problematic behavior.

Naturalistic Observations

In the case of institutionalized patients or children of school age, it may be possible for staff, family, or teachers to directly observe in the course of a few weeks the types of problematic social situations that occur and the nature of the responses of the client that follow. Obviously, the therapist cannot follow the noninstitutionalized adult client around in the course of the day to observe what are the problematic situations. However, on some occasions clients are sufficiently well motivated and skilled to observe themselves. In order to determine these situations and the client responses, a simulation or analog test may be used in which situations are presented to the client and he or she responds as if he or she were in that situation. A second approach would be to request the client to keep a diary of such events.

Analog Tests

There are two kinds of analog tests. The first is a brief role play in which a series of situations are presented one at a time to which the client is asked to respond as if in the given situation. For example, in a role-play test for children (see e.g., Edleson & Rose, 1978), each child is presented with eight situations, each calling for the demonstration of a particular social skill. The child is asked to respond as if he or she were in that situation. Because the responses of the child are taped, they can then be coded after the interview in terms of their effectiveness in dealing with the given situation. These tests, commonly used in social skill training, have been developed for various populations including psychiatric inpatients and outpatients, women (DeLange, 1976), children, adolescent delinquents (Freedman, 1974; Rosenthal, 1978), and the elderly (Berger, 1976). The second type of analog test is an extended role play and is used where the problem involves one extended or complex situation. For example, if the general problem is job interviewing, then a full-length simulated interview would provide the group worker and the group with a clear picture of what the client needs to work on (Kelley, 1982).

Diaries or Self-Report

In the diary, the clients are asked to describe recent difficult social situations in which they were either satisfied with their responses or dissatisfied. The diary points directly to the type of situations that the client will need to work on in subsequent sessions. The inclusion of successfully dealt with situations not only gives a picture of what the client views as success but also provides an opportunity for reinforcement from the practitioner and the group. Because self-monitoring is difficult even for the well-motivated client, clients are requested to describe in early sessions only one situation in which they were successful and one in which they were dissatisfied with their responses each week. In later sessions, clients are asked to describe several such situations.

Standardized Inventories

Instruments such as the Gambrill–Richey Assertive Inventory (1975) and the Rathus (1972) Assertiveness Inventory *are commonly used as a rapid means of* assessing the clients' social skills in various situations. Although there are a number of threats to internal validity, practitioners find these instruments easier to use than most of the other methods of collecting assessment data.

INTERVENTION PROCEDURES IN SOCIAL SKILL TRAINING PROGRAMS

Once social skill deficits, personal resources, and impediments to treatment have been identified, a social skill training program can be implemented. Although these programs (group, individual, or family) should be tailored to meet individual and group needs, the following common core of procedures and intervention strategies can be identified in most programs: orientation, situational analysis, modeling, behavioral rehearsal, feedback, coaching, reinforcement, and homework. It should be noted that orientation influences the effectiveness of treatment intervention but is not a direct intervention procedure in its own right. Furthermore, situational analysis is a kind of interphase between assessment and intervention.

Orientation

Social skill training is always initiated with a brief orientation of the clients to the theory behind it and the procedures to be used. At each session, the therapist provides a similar and more detailed rationale for any new procedures to be used at that session. Clients are given an opportunity to discuss these procedures or, if they so choose, to refuse to participate in them.

Situational Analysis

In many commonly occurring situations, the criteria for appropriate performance in those situations may be presented by the practitioner and discussed by the group. In situations unique to one or two persons, it may be first necessary to determine what the client's goal is in that situation through an evolution of this situation and the specific behavioral elements that might be required to achieve the goal. Often the client or therapist is aware of what these detailed steps might be. Occasionally, brainstorming among group or family members can be used to develop a number of potential responses that the client with the problem situation evaluates and then selects a set of behaviors to be performed. In the latter case, the client develops with the help of the practitioner and the group his or her own instructions through systematic problem solving. Let us look at a simplified example of situational analysis as it is used in social skill training:

Janet has difficulty in asserting herself in wide variety of service situations. Specifically, she presented a recent situation in which she has difficulty in returning a salad which was slightly spoiled. She didn't know what to say and noted that this was the kind of problem she often had difficulty with because of her passivity. When asked, the group suggested a number of strategies that included an angry response, exchanging the salad without talking to anyone, going over to the salad counter, calling the waitress and stating the problem, and then asking her to get another salad that was not spoiled. Janet chose the last situation because she felt it would achieve her goal of getting a new salad without excessively imposing on the waitress and because it was her right to have a good salad since she paid for it. The therapist suggested she would have to assertively get the attention of the waitress first by calling out to her in a loud clear voice as she passed. Janet agreed that that was a useful suggestion. Following another suggestion, Janet added she probably should sound as if she had every expectation that the exchange take place without a hassle.

Modeling

Central to social learning theory is the principle of frequent model presentation. In this program, it takes the form of a role-played demonstration by the practitioner and/or a group or family member. The responses demonstrated are based on the instruction or situational analysis already discussed. On occasion where no competent models are available who are similar to the clients, models are brought into the training sessions as special visitors. Let us continue with the preceding example and show how the therapist models the response for Janet:

Therapist: Let me show you how you might do that. Why don't you be the waitress, and let's role play the situation. I'll try to follow all the principles you thought were important in our earlier discussion.

Janet: OK, that would be helpful.

Therapist: (Looks at her imaginary plate, turns up her nose at it, and calls loudly to the waitress who happens to be passing.) Miss, Miss, (the waitress ignores her, then louder still, MISS, MISS (waitress looks), could you help me a minute?

Janet (as waitress):   Oh, sure what would you like?

Therapist: This salad, I'm afraid is spoiled. Could you get me another one, please, which is fresher? I would really appreciate that.

Therapist (as herself):   Is that something you might like to do?

Modeling does not always require role playing. Occasionally clients may observe someone in their real world with characteristics they would like to emulate. The therapist often can serve as assertive model across situations. Where role play is used, often repeated modeling is first required. Following whatever the form of modeling, if the client feels ready, she or he will rehearse the same situation in her or his own words.

Behavioral Rehearsal

This is a procedure in which the client practices or seeks to duplicate the behavior of the model or the instruction within a predefined situation. Usually, the role play is highly structured with the practitioner or another client playing the prescribed role of the significant other. In some situations, the behavior of the role players is only loosely prescribed or not prescribed at all. As treatment progresses, rehearsals tend to move from highly structured to relatively unstructured role plays. They also tend to become more complex and longer in later sessions. Initially the practitioner presents the situation to the client, and the role play partner narrates one or more comments to which the client is expected to respond as if he or she were in that situation. The actual rehearsal is often preceded by the client's review of what she or he is going to do as in the following example:

Therapist: Well, do you think you're ready to try it?

Janet: Yes, I'll give it a shot.

Therapist: Why don't you first review it for the group?

Janet: That's a good idea. First I have to get her attention, that's the hardest. Then using good eye contact and a loud voice I make my request in a way which implies I expect her to follow my request even if she is bored or busy. It's my right. And then I would thank her but without fawning as I usually do.

Therapist: Perfect, let's try it now. The rest of you should note what she does well, and anything she might consider doing differently. OK?

Janet (as herself): OK. Ah, er, (softly) waitress, (nothing happens then more loudly) Waitress. (She looks up.) Could you come here a minute please. (approaches Janet) This salad is spoiled. Would it be all right if you brought me another one, that is if you're not too busy? Would you?

In this example, there are some problems in Janet's performance. In order to make Janet aware of these problems the therapist and the group members provide her with corrective feedback.

Corrective Feedback

In order to reinforce the client, the therapist or group members first comment on what the client did well. This serves as support or reinforcement for her efforts. In order that the client be helped to improve her performance, the question is asked as to what the client might do differently. Feedback from the practitioner and the group is a powerful learning tool, but it can be counter productive as well if applied incorrectly. The group can devastate a client. In groups or families prior to giving feedback the first time, clients are trained through group exercises (see Rose, Hanusa, Tolman, & Hall, 1982, for examples of these exercises) in the giving and receiving of positive and corrective feedback. Not only are these skills necessary for facilitating the training procedures, they are important social skills in their own right. Let us look at the application of feedback procedures in the case of Janet:

Therapist: What did Janet do well in the role play in terms of meeting her own goals?

Clayton: Well, she got her attention, all right, that's for sure. And she spoke in a loud, clear voice.

Diann: She gave her good eye contact, that's something she has been working on.

Therapist: I have to agree with that, and I would add that she made the request she wanted. I wonder if there was anything she might consider doing differently in order to achieve her goals.

Marianne: I think she should be a little less apologetic. It tends to take away from the assertion of her belief that she has a right to make the request.

Others: (Nod agreement)

Janet: I agree, too, I was much too apologetic.

Therapist: Ok, then, when you do it this time, you'll continue to speak in a loud clear voice and give good eye contact. You'll make your request without any sense of apology. And you won't say, "Would that be all right." Does that seem to do it? (As she nods agreement), OK then let's give it another try.

After receiving feedback, the client usually repeats the rehearsal as he or she attempts to incorporate the suggestions received. Multiple trials are desirable in order to facilitate the retention of what the client has learned.

Coaching

This procedure involves the practitioner or a designated group member providing the client with suggestions as the client attempts to carry out his or her role in the behavioral rehearsal. For example, the coach might whisper to the client, "speak a little louder," "give eye contact," "be firmer," "you are doing great." Or more specifically, "tell him 'I won't do it, I'm sorry.'" The coach often sits directly behind the client to facilitate communication. Coaching is often used with relatively poorly functioning clients. Where coaching is used, it eventually is withdrawn. Because it requires more than two roles, it is usually used in small groups and families.

Reinforcement

Throughout training, clients receive reinforcement in the form of praise and recognition for a variety of small achievements such as a good suggestion, participation in the discussion, effective modeling, effective rehearsals, and the completion of homework assignments. The practitioner may praise the client directly, encourage others in treatment to be supportive of the client's efforts, or involve the client's family and friends in supporting and reinforcing an improved social skills repertoire. In children's groups, contingency contracts are used for satisfactory completion of homework assignments. In these contracts, clients receive points or direct rewards for their monitored achievement outside of the group on a contractual basis. One of the important principles of modeling is that if the client is reinforced for successful replication of the model's behavior, it is more likely that it will be replicated in the real world. Thus such reinforcement serves as one generalization strategy.

GENERALIZATION STRATEGIES

No intervention program is complete without extensive consideration of how the target behavior is to be transferred to the real world. A number of strategies have evolved for enhancing the maintenance and transfer of behaviors learned in the group. (See Rose & Edleson, 1987, for more examples and further explanation of these principles.) The foremost principle is that a plan is required to achieve transfer of change. It will not happen without external thought and effort. This plan consists of the following techniques, of which homework is one of the most important.

Homework

This involves designing with the client a number of tasks to be performed between training sessions. These assignments are usually prepared for during the session and include carrying out the assignment in a role play or, should the event occur, in real life. It might also include observing others who have the desired skills, reading about social skills, and/or keeping a diary of successful and unsuccessful interactions. Homework is one of the major procedures for facilitating the transfer of change learned in the group to the real world.

Multiple Trials

The reader may have noted that we have encouraged both multiple modeling demonstrations and multiple rehearsals. The more trials in the treatment context, the greater the likelihood that the target behavior will be performed outside the treatment context.

Variation in Treatment

If every session were exactly the same, it is likely that the clients would learn to perform only under those conditions. Variation in role play situations, in levels of difficulty, in types of homework assignments, in setting, and even in leaders appears to produce a greater likelihood of generalization (Goldstein, Heller, & Sechrest, 1966). One variation used with children, and sometimes with adults as well, is a social skill board game (see Rose & Edleson, 1987). Variation should also occur in such a way as to simulate as nearly as possible the real world.

Prepare for Uncertainty

Preparing clients solely for situations they expect to occur eliminates consideration of the vast majority of problematic situations that are likely to occur. For this, reason once clients are well prepared for predictable situations, practice through role play on situations for which no preparation is possible is included in the program. Sometimes former members are invited to talk about uncertain situations they experienced and how they handled them.

Prepare for Setbacks

The fact that new behavior is learned does not imply that it can always be applied. The client can expect both success and failure in dealing with the problematic situations. The goal is that the number of successes relative to setbacks gradually increase. In the last few sessions, a list of potential setbacks are developed with the members, and they discuss strategies on how to handle them.

Make Booster Sessions Available

Although no empirical support exists, where booster sessions exist for those attending such booster sessions, newly learned behaviors appear in practice to be more effectively maintained than where no such sessions exist.

All of these principles need to be investigated further to determine which set of these procedures seems to be most effective for which populations. Presently we try to implement all of them as much as possible.

FUTURE DIRECTIONS

Social skill training has become more sophisticated in recent years. The emphasis on rote acquisition of particular social skills through a highly structured and repetitive training agenda has decreased. A growing emphasis is presently being placed on learning to identify problematic events and to understand the processes that underlie the making of an effective social response to such events. There has been an increased concern with cognitions, emotions, and cultural values in social skill training and, as a result, practitioners are dealing with motivational issues and intentionality in the developing of responses. New procedures such as systematic problem solving, cognitive restructuring, and other cognitive procedures are being experimented with to supplement the intervention strategies described. Greater responsibility is being increasingly given to the client in and for the training process.

Still more attention needs to be placed on maintenance and the generalization of change because the results of research in this area are equivocal (Bellack & Morrison, 1982). Although some theory (Brown, 1982; Goldstein, Heller, & Sechrest, 1966) and principles have been proposed, it has not been adequately adhered to in practice. Greater attention to the social environment of the client may facilitate maintenance of skills learned in the training sessions. In the case of poorly functioning clients, programs need to be extended in duration and intensity from the usual 6- to 8-week program. Social skill training though important for the poorly functioning client is often necessary but seldom sufficient to obtain and maintain significant change. Incorporation of the training into other remedial programs may be required if major gains are to be achieved.

ACKNOWLEDGMENT. Partial support for the author in writing this chapter was provided by the Wisconsin Alumni Research Foundation of the University of Wisconsin.

REFERENCES

Bandura, A. (1977). *Social learning theory*. Englewood Cliffs, NJ: Prentice-Hall.

Bellack, A. S., Hersen, M., & Turner, S. M. (1976). Generalization effects of social skills training in chronic schizophrenics: An experimental analysis. *Behaviour research and therapy, 14*, 391–398.

Bellack, A. S., & Morrison, R. L. (1982). Interpersonal dysfunction. In A. S. Bellack, M. Hersen, & A. E. Kazdin, *International handbook of behavior modification and therapy* (pp. 717–747). New York: Plenum Press.

Berger, R. M. (1976). *Interpersonal skill training with institutionalized elderly patients*. Unpublished doctoral dissertation, University of Wisconsin, Madison.

Brown, M. (1982). Maintenance and generalization issues in skills training with chronic schizophrenics. In J. Curran & P. Monti (Eds.), *Social skills training* (pp. 90–116) New York: Guilford Press.

Buchler, G. R. (1979). Communication skills in married couples. In A. S. Bellack & M. Hersen (Eds.), *Research and practice in social skills training* (pp. 273–318). New York: Plenum Press.

DeLange, J. M. (1976). *Relative effectiveness of assertive skill training and desensitization for high and low anxiety women*. Unpublished doctoral dissertation, University of Wisconsin, Madison.

Edleson, J. L., & Rose, S. D. (1978). *A behavioral role-play test for measuring children's social skills*. Paper presented at the Twelfth Annual Convention of the Association for the Advancement of Behavior Therapy, Chicago.

Fredriksen, L., Jenkins, J., Foy, D., & Eisler, R. (1976). Social skills training in the modification of abusive verbal outbursts in adults. *Journal of applied behavior analysis, 9*, 117–125.

Freedman, B. J. (1974). *An analysis of social behavioral skill: Deficits in delinquent and non-delinquent adolescent boys*. Unpublished doctoral dissertation, University of Wisconsin, Madison.

French, D., & Tyne, T. (1982). The identification and treatment of children with peer-relationship difficulties. In J. Curran & P. Monti (Eds.), *Social skills training* (pp. 280–308). New York: Guilford Press.

Galassi, J., & Galassi, M. (1979). Modification of heterosocial skills deficits. In A. Bellack & M. Hersen (Eds.), *Research and practice in social skills training*. New York: Plenum Press.

Gambrill, E. D., & Richey, C. A. (1975). An Assertion Inventory for use in assessment and research. *Behavior Therapy, 6*(4), 550–561.

Goldstein, A. P., Heller, K., & Sechrest, L. B. (1966). *Psychotherapy and the psychology of behavior change*. New York: Wiley.

Hersen, M., Bellack, A., & Himmelhock, J. (1982). Skills training and unipolar depressed women. In J. Curran & P. Monti (Eds.), *Social skills training* (pp. 159–184). New York: Guilford Press.

Kelly, J. A. (1982). *Social skills training: A practical guide for interventions*. New York: Springer Publishing Company.

Kendall, P. (1982). Individual versus group control cognitive behavior self control training: one year Followup. *Behavior Therapy, 3*(2), 241–247.

Liberman, R., Nuechterlein, K., & Wallace, C. (1982). Social skills training and the nature of schizophrenia. In J. Curran & P. Monti (Eds.), *Social skills training* (pp. 5–56). New York: Guilford Press.

Linehan, M. M., Walker, R. O., Bronheim, S., Haynes, K. F., & Yevzeroff, Harriet. (1979). Group vs. individual assertion training. *Journal of Consulting Psychology, 47*(5), 1000–1002.

Miller, P. M., & Eisler, R. M. (1977). Assertive behavior of alcoholics: A descriptive analysis. *Behavior therapy, 8*, 146–149.

Mischel, W. (1973). Toward a cognitive social learning reconceptualization of personality. *Psychological Review, 80*(4), 252–283.

Monti, P., Corriveau, D., & Curan, J. (1982). Social skills training for psychiatric patients: Treatment and outcome. In J. Curran & P. Monti (Eds.), *Social skills training* (pp. 185–283). New York: Guilford Press.

Rathus, S. A. (1972). An experimental investigation of assertive training in a group setting. *Journal of Behavior Therapy and Experimental Psychiatry, 3*, 81–86.

Rose, S. D., & Edleson, J., (1987). *Working with children and adolescents in groups.* San Francisco: Jossey-Bass.

Rose, S. D., Hanusa, D., Tolman, Richard M. & Hall, J. A. (1982). *A group leader's guide to assertiveness training,* Crownsville, MD: Crownsville Hospital Center.

Rosenthal, L. (1978). *Behavioral Analysis of Social Skills in Adolescent Girls.* Unpublished doctoral dissertation. University of Wisconsin, Madison.

23

Short-Term Therapy Groups for Schizophrenics

NICK KANAS

Schizophrenia is a mental condition characterized by a disorder in thinking. Thought content frequently is disturbed and leads to psychotic symptoms such as hallucinations (hearing voices or seeing things that are not there) and delusions (beliefs that are not supported by reality). The thought process also is affected, leading to looseness in associating one idea to another. Because of the disturbances in thinking, schizophrenics often are unable to relate meaningfully with other people, resulting in a social isolation or inappropriate behavior. As a consequence of these problems, many schizophrenics have difficulties maintaining employment and generally are found at the lower ends of the socioeconomic spectrum, further compounding their difficulties. Although many of these patients have exacerbations of their symptoms that cause them to be hospitalized, the previously mentioned difficulties usually persist even between such acute episodes. For this reason, schizophrenia is seen as a chronic disorder, and it is very difficult for these patients to maintain a normal existence even when functioning optimally.

Antipsychotic medications have proven to be the single most effective treatment for schizophrenia, despite their sometimes serious side effects and the difficulties many patients have in taking the medications as prescribed. However, psychotherapy has been shown to be an important adjunct to medication in helping schizophrenics cope with their problems. In particular, group therapy has been shown to be an effective modality of treatment. In a review of 43 controlled studies, Kanas and Barr (1986) found that therapy groups were effective in 67% of the inpatient studies and 80% of the outpatient studies. In the inpatient setting, this treatment modality was especially useful in groups lasting more than 3 months. Of the nine inpatient studies evaluating short-term therapy groups lasting 16 or fewer sessions, five supported the conclusion that group therapy was more effective than no group therapy, three found no difference,

NICK KANAS • Department of Psychiatry, University of California, San Francisco, California 94143, and San Francisco Veteran's Administration Medical Center, 4150 Clement Street, San Francisco, California 94121.

and one found that more psychotic patients did worse in group therapy than in the no group therapy control condition. The review also found that in the inpatient setting, interaction-oriented approaches were significantly more successful than insight-oriented approaches, which were harmful for some schizophrenic patients. Of the 10 outpatient studies, two were considered to be short-term (defined as 16 or fewer sessions taking place in 4 months or less), and both of these were judged to be supportive of group therapy.

Given the fact that schizophrenia is a chronic disorder, as well as the evidence supporting the effectiveness of long-term schizophrenic groups, then why should one consider treating these patients in short-term therapy groups? The answer is essentially cost-effectiveness. Since the 1960s, the community mental health movement has led to the closure of long-term hospital beds and encouraged shorter term stays that are less expensive and less likely to produce the negative sequelae of institutionalization. This has meant that more patients are being treated in community outpatient facilities. More recently, economic pressures have encouraged treatment approaches that are effective but relatively inexpensive, thus allowing for more patients to be treated in briefer periods of time by fewer numbers of therapists. Provided that short-term therapy groups can be shown to be beneficial, then they would be an ideal treatment approach. As shown in this review, the effectiveness of short-term therapy groups for schizophrenics is respectable and warrants wider use in both inpatient and outpatient settings.

PATIENT SELECTION

Although schizophrenia is a chronic disorder, patients vary greatly in terms of proneness for acute exacerbations, diagnostic subtype, and various socioeconomic factors. In addition, some schizophrenics have a preponderance of positive symptoms, such as hallucinations and delusions, whereas others may have negative symptoms, such as social withdrawal and lack of initiative. Given this variability, which schizophrenic patients benefit the most from short-term group therapy? Although the answer to this question is not clear, some generalizations may be made. First, because group therapy is interpersonal in nature, those schizophrenics who are able to sit in a room and talk with others will benefit more than patients who are more withdrawn and isolated. Second, patients who are motivated to explore the nature of their problems using a discussion-oriented therapeutic approach would be more receptive to group therapy. Finally, one study found that short-term inpatient therapy groups were judged to be useful by significantly more schizophrenics who were below the median age than above and by significantly more nonparanoid than paranoid patients (Kanas & Barr, 1982). However, these demographic factors should be interpreted cautiously until they are replicated in other studies.

One issue that has stirred some controversy pertains to whether schizophrenics should be treated with patients of other diagnoses in heterogeneous groups, or whether they do better in homogeneous groups composed exclusively of schizophrenics. In reviewing the literature, there seems to be bias toward heterogeneous groups in inpatient settings and homogeneous groups in outpatient settings. However, it is my contention that schizophrenics do best in homogeneous groups in both settings, for several reasons. First, it is difficult to get a cohesive group where patients differ greatly from each other in terms of presenting problems, symptoms, and ego functioning. This is particularly true in short-term settings, where a major goal is to get patients interacting and relating with one another as soon as possible. Homogeneous groups allow cohesiveness to occur faster because patients have similar problems and perspectives. Second, the needs of psychotic schizophrenics are much different than those of nonpsychotic patients, and it is difficult to establish a group environment that can simultaneously address such conflicting needs. For example, patients who are trying to cope with loose associations and basic difficulties in relating with others would have no use for sophisticated confrontive techniques aimed at encouraging the expression of emotions and delineating causes of neurotic symptomatology. Homogeneous groups allow the use of techniques that are oriented toward specific needs in an efficient, relevant manner. Finally, some techniques that are helpful for nonpsychotic patients may be harmful for schizophrenics. For example, uncovering and self-disclosure, useful techniques for many neurotics, have been shown to be counterproductive for schizophrenic patients (Kanas, Rogers, Kreth, Patterson, & Campbell, 1980; Pattison, Brissenden, & Wohl, 1967; Strassberg, Roback, Anchor, & Abramowitz, 1975; Weiner, 1984). These techniques can be avoided in homogeneous groups of schizophrenics, and they can be replaced by more appropriate, safe interventions.

GOALS OF TREATMENT

As with other forms of brief therapies, it is important to have clear, relevant goals in conducting short-term therapy groups for schizophrenics. Given the nature of the problem faced by these patients, two specific goals are paramount. First, short-term groups should seek to help these patients improve their interpersonal relationships and contacts with others. Group therapy is ideal for this because it is a modality of treatment that is interpersonal in nature. Relationships may be improved in two ways. First, by discussing difficulties they have in relating with people, schizophrenic patients may learn strategies of interacting that they can practice outside of the group environment. For inpatients, this may include spending less time alone in their rooms, taking passes with other patients, and generally making an effort to be involved in the ward milieu. For outpatients, this may range from dealing better with family and friends to interacting better with salesclerks and bus drivers. Outside experiences may be brought back to the group session for feedback and support. A second way relationships can be improved is through the patient interactions themselves. By talking to one another, the group members are practicing social skills in the here and now, and they can give immediate feedback on each other's interpersonal skills as they are observed during the session. Sometimes relationship issues involving group members become the focus for the discussion. Examples include outside socializing and feelings patients have for each other. Thus, both extragroup and intragroup interpersonal contacts may be used in the service of improving relationships.

A second major goal of treatment for schizophrenics in short-term therapy groups consists of helping patients cope better with psychotic experiences. This generally involves two stages. First, patients must be made aware that hallucinations and delusions are not typical experiences of most people and that they represent breaks in reality. Once a patient is able to examine these experiences as being ego dystonic, then he or she is ready to proceed to the next stage, which consists of learning strategies of coping with these psychotic experiences. In supporting both reality testing and coping skills, other group members may provide important feedback. For example, a patient who believes that his food is poisoned may have this idea challenged by other patients who state that they once had the same belief but changed their minds as they got better with treatment. Although antipsychotic medications are important in helping patients deal with psychotic experiences, psychosocial strategies also may be helpful (Breier & Strauss, 1983; Cohen & Berk, 1985; Falloon & Talbot, 1981; Kanas & Barr, 1984). When psychotic symptoms are related to stressful external situations, then learning ways of avoiding stressors may help patients cope better with them. Some patients report that their voices are not so loud when they are less anxious. In a complimentary manner, boredom or isolation may make hallucinations or delusions more prominent. Finding things to occupy one's attention can be beneficial in this case. Sometimes patients offer unique strategies of coping. For example, in one inpatient group, a patient stated that his voices would go away when he would outyell them and tell them to depart in no uncertain terms! Many schizophrenic patients have learned successful ways of coping with psychosis, and their advice may be extremely beneficial to patients who are having difficulty in this area.

Structural Issues

Short-term inpatient schizophrenic groups usually are held from three to five times per week, with sessions typically lasting 45 to 60 minutes. On most acute care psychiatric units, new patients enter the group shortly after being admitted to the ward, provided that there is space due to the departure of other patients through discharge. This results in an open format, where during any given session a new patient may be entering or an old patient may be leaving. This creates some disruption in the group, and strategies need to be developed whereby these transitions may be addressed as quickly as possible so that the group can move on to other issues.

In the outpatient setting, short-term schizophrenic groups typically meet weekly in sessions lasting 60 to 90 minutes. Outpatient schizophrenics are able to tolerate being in a session for a longer period of time than their inpatient counterparts, and this helps to make up for the fewer number of sessions per week. Outpatient groups tend to be closed in that a group of patients will begin a group and continue to the end without adding new members. Closed groups have the advantage of allowing discussions to build on previous sessions in a stable environment where patients get to know one another as the group evolves.

In order to have enough patients to provide meaningful interactions, short-term therapy groups with schizophrenics should have at least four members. Inpatient groups usually can tolerate up to eight members. Numbers beyond this make it difficult for the therapists to keep track of interactions and maintain control of the group process. In the outpatient setting, up to 10 members can be accommodated because schizophrenic outpatients tend to be less disruptive and psychotic than their inpatient counterparts. However, in both settings, 6 to 8 patients represent an optimal range.

ROLE OF THE THERAPISTS

In dealing with schizophrenic groups, particularly in the short-term setting, therapists should be active, open, supportive, and consistent. At times, they need to direct the group process in order to help patients stay on a subject as well as to move discussions along in view of the limited number of sessions available. When in the service of assisting the discussion and modeling appropriate behavior, it is permissible for the therapists to reveal their own opinions and feelings about issues that arise. This may especially be useful in developing topics related to the primary goals of helping patient relate better with others and develop strategies of reality testing and coping with psychotic experiences. Therapists should not reveal their opinions for self-serving purposes or for reasons unrelated to the group members' needs.

Particularly in the inpatient setting, where patients may become quite disturbed and difficult to manage, co-therapy teams are useful. Having two therapists allows one to engage a given patient, whereas the other observes the reactions of this interaction on the other patients. Similarly, if one patient needs to leave the room accompanied by a therapist, the group can continue for a short time with the remaining therapist. Also, if one therapist becomes ill or is on vacation, then the group still can meet. Male–female teams offer an advantage in that some schizophrenic patients react better to members of one sex. Co-therapy teams are useful in the outpatient setting as well, although they are less critical from the management standpoint because outpatients tend to be less disruptive than inpatients. In settings where staff numbers are limited, then one therapist may be all that can be spared for the group. However, because schizophrenics are very needy and disorganized individuals, leading such groups can be psychologically taxing. For example, in one inpatient group, the patients began discussing the intricacies of a shared delusion involving a religious issue. The lone therapist was clearly odd man out, and he was left to ponder his own sense of reality. Having another nonpsychotic person in the group for support and reassurance is clearly desirable.

GROUP CONTENT

A number of discussion topics have been shown to be useful in short-term therapy groups with schizophrenics. In keeping with one of the primary goals of the group, topics involving relationships with others are fruitful and relevant to the needs of these patients. Many schizophrenics are involved in pathological relationships with family and friends where they are smothered and controlled on the one hand or rejected and abandoned on the other. Discussions over such issues may be emotionally loaded, and therapists should be prepared to deal with the sequelae. However, patients often given each other excellent advice on how to deal with significant others. In addition, they feel a sense of connectedness because problems with relationships are common among this patient population. Help also can be given in dealing better with more casual contacts, especially when distortions and fantasies are involved. For example, during one session of a short-term outpatient schizophrenic group, a patient described having a special relationship with a waitress who worked in a restaurant near his apartment. At the next session, he reported being somewhat shaken by her businesslike rebuff during the intervening week. The group members tried to give him some support while at the same time helping him see that this perceived amorous relationship was largely in his fantasies.

A second important topic area pertains to feelings of loneliness and despair. These emotions result from the sequelae of schizophrenia and the sense that one is isolated in the world with little to look forward to. By openly acknowledging such feelings, patients are able to see that they are not alone in having these emotions and that they at least can connect with other members of the group. At times, patients can learn to cope with these feelings, but usually this is not the case, and the major benefit of this discussion is for patients to see that others are in the same situation. However, sharing this sense of universality and cohesiveness has been found to be therapeutic in its own right (Maxmen, 1973; Yalom, 1975).

Learning ways to deal with hallucinations and delusions also are important group topics. As mentioned before, patients first need to perceive the experience as unreal before they can accept advice on coping strategies. Feedback from other patients usually is easier to accept than feedback from the therapists, especially around paranoid delusions. The here and now can be particularly useful in pointing out that no one else in the room is hearing a particular voice or sharing in a patient's belief system. For example, one patient had a delusion that people on the ward wanted to harm him, and he cited a poster on the dayroom wall that was particularly directed toward his demise. Because no one remembered the poster, the therapists asked all of the group members to leave the room and walk on to the ward to look at the sign. It was found to be an antinuclear power poster that pictured a nuclear reactor with a skull and cross-bones on it along with the words: "This could happen to you!" After returning to the group room, the members discussed the fact that this was a general reference to the dangers of nuclear power and did not relate specifically to any given person. The paranoid patient was forced to examine the reality of his belief system, and this led to a discussion of ways to cope with delusional thinking, such as checking out the belief with others.

A fourth topic area relates to the thinking processes of the patients. Acutely ill schizophrenics have trouble organizing their thinking, often leading to loose associations. For example, a patient in the group might begin discussing one issue but end up addressing something else or become lost in his own thinking. This phenomenon should be pointed out by the therapists, with some validation by other group members. Although patients cannot always control their thinking process, they can learn to be aware when they are getting lost or appreciate that others are not following them. This knowledge can be quite useful for patients, not only by helping them refocus on the topic but also by encouraging them to ask others to help them out with a comment such as: "I got lost here, what did you ask me again?"

Some discussion topics in the group have to do with practical issues, such as dealing with the side effects of medications, finding the right halfway houses, and exploring job opportunities. These discussions have a place in the group so long as patients give advice to each other based on their own experiences. Group time should not be used as question-and-answer sessions between the patients and the therapists. Professional advice more appropriately can be given after the session by the patient's doctor and other staff members.

Some topics have been shown to be unproductive or potentially harmful for patients. In particular, issues that lead to anger between group members may be toxic. Schizophrenics frequently have murderous fantasies and fears of being out of control, and anger-producing discussions stimulate both, sometimes leading to intolerable anxiety and a fear of acting out. For example, in one inpatient group, a new patient and an old patient began competing over a delusional issue. This quickly escalated into a confrontation, and the old patient suddenly clenched his fist and stood up in a threatening manner. One therapist quickly intervened, leading the patient out of the group room to cool off while the other therapist remained behind with the group. After 10 minutes, the patient came back in with the therapist, and the group finished with everyone discussing the importance of safety and remaining in control. Sexual material also may lead to difficult situations because some schizophrenic patients are delusionally conflicted over these issues. Discussions of sexual themes may make such patients anxious, with the possibility for regression and acting out. Finally, topics related to gaining developmental insight and exploring unconscious material have little value in a group of schizophrenics. These patients have difficulty enough coping with day-to-day existence. Dwelling on the past or risking anxiety through the use of uncovering techniques is not appropriate to their needs.

One way of facilitating the discussion of these topics is to proceed from the general to the specific. For example, schizophrenics frequently prefer to discuss an issue in nonpersonal terms first (e.g., hallucinations as symptoms), then relate it to their own situation (e.g., my hallucinations and problems I have in dealing with them). Another facilitating strategy is to point out that a given problem is held in common by many patients, then ask each patient to comment on how the problem specifically impacts on his or her life. This can be done in a go-around where each patient comments in turn. These techniques help the group members reveal and discuss personal issues by helping them see that they are not alone and that others are willing to share common problems with them.

GROUP PROCESS

The environment of the short-term schizophrenic group should be open and safe, with patients feeling free to discuss their problems with a minimum of pressure. Anxiety and severe confrontation may lead to turmoil and regression in a group of psychotic patients, and therapists should be careful to titrate the discussion in response to the degree of discomfort in the group. Sometimes this can be done by changing the subject, but at other times the therapists should acknowledge the potential dangers. For example, in one outpatient group where several patients were confronting another patient about his problems in a hostile, nonproductive manner, one of the therapists interrupted the discussion by stating that people seemed tense and that no one would benefit from a group where the members attacked each other. Another way of lowering anxiety is by discussing symptoms as manifestations of a mental disease and then asking patients to comment on how they cope with these symptoms. By abstracting the issue in medical terms, the therapists are able to depersonalize topics, thus making them safer for discussion.

Throughout the sessions, therapists should encourage patient-to-patient contact. At times, a directive approach is needed, whereby a therapist asks a patient to look at another person or directs him or her to ask for feedback from someone else. Particularly in inpatient therapy groups, there is a tendency for patients to make their comments to a therapist. In part, this is prompted by dependency issues and by the therapist's supportive, active style. It also may be due to patients' mistrust and isolation from each other. Therapists may discourage this behavior nonverbally by looking down or pointing at another patient. Sometimes they should be more explicit by stating that patients learn better from one another and should direct their conversations to each other wherever possible.

Yalom (1975) has stated that patients learn best when they can address an issue with each other during the group session rather than talking about past events involving people outside of the group. This here-and-now focus can be very powerful, and patients frequently learn a great deal from it. For example, one patient acknowledged that his voices were a problem for him. The therapist asked if he was hearing voices at the present time, and he said yes. The therapist then asked other members of the group to comment on whether they heard the voices, too. After several said no, the therapist redirected attention to the first patient, suggesting that perhaps his voices were real to him but did not represent reality to others. This then led to a discussion of ways to cope with voices. In discussing psychotic experiences in the hear and now, others may be asked to comment on the experience, and this consensual validation is a powerful reinforcer for the reality or unreality of a hallucination or delusion. At times, however, this can backfire. In one inpatient group, for example, a therapist asked the group members if they could relate to another patient's belief concerning the existence of multiple-dimension reality states. To the therapist's surprise, everyone became interested in this issue and began arguing as to how many dimensional states there really were. This became unproductive, and the therapist dealt with it by stating that such a decision could not be decided on in the group. He suggested that a more relevant topic should be considered, which was done.

At times, therapists will be asked questions about their personal life or their feelings concerning a topic being discussed. It is sometimes valuable for therapists to answer these questions directly, particularly when their responses serve as modeling behavior for the patients or enhance and further encourage work on the topic at hand. When to disclose is a difficult question, but a good rule of thumb is that when the answer is safe and seems to advance the discussion, then it probably is appropriate to respond to a patient's query. On the other hand, when the response does not serve such a purpose or when it is primarily therapeutic for the therapist, then changing the subject or turning the issue back to the patients would be more appropriate. Therapists sometimes offer opinions without being asked, and this can be very productive. For example, in a particularly confusing session, one of the therapists stated that he was having difficulty following the conversation and asked if others felt the same way. This led to a general discussion of disorganized thinking, with several patients admitting that they had been feeling particularly loose and that this was very difficult for them to tolerate. Issues involving coping then followed.

Ideally, schizophrenic patients in a short-term therapy group should learn to interact with one another freely and develop topics as fully as possible. However, this ideal is seldom realized, and at times it is important for the therapist to direct the process in order to accomplish these goals. When to intervene and when to remain silent depends upon the topic at hand and how patients are dealing with it. For example, in sessions where patients find it difficult to stay on track or where there is a great deal of anxiety present, therapists should structure the discussion by suggesting topics that are safe and relevant. On the other hand, when patients actively are discussing their problems with each other in an appropriate manner, then therapists should remain silent and intervene only to clarify and give support. Again, the rule of thumb is safety, and one way of assuring minimum anxiety is with structure. Unfortunately, too much intervention may choke off spontaneous discussion. One continually has to walk a fine line between too much and too little directiveness, according to what is currently going on in the group.

Sometimes a patient will be very quiet and will not respond to the topic being discussed. Such a patient should be invited to comment because it is desirable for every patient to participate in every session. The response may be limited to a statement that the quiet member does not want to talk today, but at least he or she learns what the expectation is and knows that others are concerned about the silence.

SPECIAL ISSUES

Prior to beginning the first session, each potential member should be oriented to the group. This is particularly important in short-term therapy groups for schizophrenics because the group goals and rules need to be made explicit to psychotic patients. They should be told that all of the patients have had difficulties in relating with others, hearing voices or seeing things that are not there, feeling suspicious, or having confused thoughts. They also should be told that they will be expected to participate in the sessions but that the group should be a safe place for everyone and that loud yelling or hitting the furniture or other patients is prohibited. Due to the short-term nature of the group, they should be on time and attend every session if they are to benefit.

During the first session, these orientation issues should be repeated in front of all the patients. In open groups, where new patients are admitted to ongoing groups as older patients depart, the new patient should be introduced to the other members and be asked what problems brought him or her into the group. An attempt should be made to find common symptoms between the new patient and members who have been there for some time. This beginning exercise serves to integrate a new member as soon as possible and can be completed within the first 5 to 10 minutes of the session. In closed groups, where all of the members start and end at the same time, the first session begins with the patients stating their names and describing their problems briefly in a go-around. Following this, the therapist tries to set an agenda based on the most common symptom or problem area, and the group is off.

Termination issues also are important. In an open group, a patient who is leaving should be given some time during his last session to say goodbye and describe his or her disposition. This gives closure to the patient's leaving, and it allows everyone to practice socially appropriate behavior around times of loss. In closed groups, where everyone terminates together, the go-around technique again is useful, with the members sharing their plans and stating what they have gained from the group experience. Discussions of termination may began two or three sessions before the last, allowing patients to separate from each other in a gradual manner.

Occasionally, a patient will need to leave a session to go to the bathroom or collect his or her thoughts in private. Therapists should always ask departing members why they are leaving and encourage them to stay if possible. However, if they need to leave, they should be allowed to do so with a clear statement that they should return when they feel ready. When this happens, the therapists should take immediate cognizance of the reentry and praise the patient for coming back. When more than one patient needs to leave, this may be an indication of general group tension, and this should be brought up as an issue.

The recent hospitalization or death of a member can create much anxiety in the group. When either of these events happens, patients frequently become concerned that the same fate will befall them and that the therapists may not have adequate control of the group. In a like manner, therapists often blame themselves and worry about the fate of the remaining patients. Dramatic events such as these need to be discussed at the next available session, with frequent reassurance that the group will continue and that the issues involved do not necessarily represent a danger to everyone else.

For some patients, a brief group therapy experience lasting 16 or fewer sessions will be adequate for them to accomplish a great deal of learning in service of the major group goals. Particularly for outpatients involved in closed groups, termination will represent a finality that will be sufficient, and they should give their new learning a try for a few weeks before considering another group. But on inpatient units, the departing members may desire another group therapy experience after leaving the ward. For these patients, it is probably a good idea to arrange this follow-up because they are less psychotic and may learn new things as outpatients. Furthermore, it has been found that longer term outpatient therapy groups are effective for schizophrenics and may lead to lower rehospitalization rates and decreased time spent in the hospital (Alden, Weddington, Jacobson, & Gianturco, 1979; Battegay & von Marschall, 1978; Shattan, D'Camp, Fujii, Fross, & Wolff, 1966). But short-term groups are useful for these patients, too, as is discussed next.

EFFECTIVENESS

Short-term therapy groups for schizophrenics based on this approach have been evaluated in both inpatient and outpatient settings. Three clinical studies were done on a 30-bed acute care psychiatric teaching unit at a Veterans Administration hospital, where the average length of stay was 21 days and where schizophrenic patients remained on the ward for an average of 35 days. In the first study (Kanas & Barr, 1982), 22 inpatient schizophrenics participated in an open, homogeneous group for an average of nine sessions each. At discharge, 95% of them rated their group experience as being "somewhat" or "very" helpful, with none of the patients stating that it had been harmful. Significantly more patients found the group to be very helpful who were below the median age and who were diagnosed as being nonparanoid schizophrenic. A rank ordering of 13 statements describing possible therapeutic factors revealed that the patients valued the group more as a place to express their feelings and learn ways of relating better with others rather than as a place to test reality or receive advice on medications, places to stay, or the nature of their illness. In the second study (Kanas, Barr, & Dossick, 1985), the Hill Interaction Matrix was used to evaluate group process from seven typical sessions. As compared with Hill's normative sample of 50 therapy group sessions, the inpatient schizophrenic group was characterized as allowing patients to confront one another related to general topics (at the 99th percentile) or related to personal problems (at the 96th percentile). Furthermore, the group environment supported mutual interactions and trust. There was little total group resistance, and emotions were able to be expressed. Reality testing was accomplished through the confrontation of distortions and delusional material. Typically, discussions would began with a general topic involving mental health but would then be applied to the patient's individual problems. There was a minimum of social amenities. The therapists were found to play an important role in shaping the process of the group. In the third study (Kanas & Barr, 1986), 22 patients were evaluated over 34 sessions of the group in a study using the short form of the Group Climate Questionnaire. Compared with a normative sample of 12 long-term, outpatient therapy groups composed primarily of neurotics, the inpatient schizophrenic gorup scored significantly lower in the Engaged and Conflict dimensions. The low Engaged score probably reflected the isolated nature of the patients and the rapid turnover of the members in the group. The low Conflict score probably resulted from the attempts made by the therapists to discourage interpersonal friction and anger in the here and now in order to facilitate a safe group environment. Also in this study, important discussion topics were written down after each session, and a content analysis revealed that they could be placed in four topic clusters. In order of decreasing frequency, these clusters were (1) encouraging contact with others, (2) expression of emotions, (3) reality testing, and (4) advice giving.

Two studies have evaluated the effectiveness of a short-term outpatient therapy group for schizophrenics using an approach lasting 12 sessions and predicated upon the techniques and goals described. The first of these (Kanas, Stewart, & Haney, 1988) was an uncontrolled study of a group conducted at a university outpatient clinic. In this study, it was found that the patients experienced a significant drop on the Social Anxiety and Distress Scale from beginning to end of the group. During the sessions, issues aimed at improving and encouraging contact with others were brought up most frequently, followed by topics related to reality testing, advice giving, general group therapy issues, and expression of emotions. A rank ordering of 13 therapeutic factor statements revealed that the top five statements concerned issues of helping patients relate better with others or cope more effectively with psychotic experiences. Both of these findings were consistent with the goals of the group. In a structured telephone interview conducted 4 months after the group ended, four of the five patients noted positive gains in their ability to relate with other people, and two believed they were better able to cope with psychotic experiences. The second study (Kanas, Deri, Ketter, & Fein, 1989) compared 12 schizophrenics who participated in two short-term therapy groups with nine similar waiting list control patients at a Veterans Administration outpatient clinic. The attendance rate was 88.9%. Again, the content analysis revealed that topics related to encouraging contact with others and coping with psychotic experiences were first and second in terms of frequency. On the SCL-90, the group patient scores dropped on all nine symptom dimensions pre- to postgroup, and two of these drops were statistically significant as compared to the controls (Anxiety and Somatization). In a 4-month follow-up, all of the group patients rated their experience as somewhat or very helpful, and significantly more group patients than controls reported improvement in ability to relate with others ($p < .01$) and cope with psychotic experiences ($p < .03$).

Although further empirical verification needs to be done in larger replicated studies, these findings support the value of a short-term group therapy format for schizophrenics in both inpatient and outpatient settings. The group environment appears to be safe and relevant to the needs of the patients. Attitudinal and symptomatic improvement has occurred, and some of the benefits persist for several months after the group ends. Should this approach continue to be shown effective in future studies, it offers a safe, cost-effective therapeutic method for treating schizophrenic patients in conjunction with antipsychotic medication and long-term follow-up.

REFERENCES

Alden, A. R., Weddington, W. W., Jr., Jacobson, C., & Gianturco, D. T. (1979). Group aftercare for chronic schizophrenia. *Journal of Clinical Psychiatry, 40,* 6–12.

Battegay, R., & von Marschall, R. (1978). Results of long-term group psychotherapy with schizophrenics. *Comprehensive Psychiatry, 19,* 349–353.

Breier, A., & Strauss, J. S. (1983). Self-control in psychotic disorders. *Archives of General Psychiatry, 40,* 1141–1145.

Cohen, C. I., & Berk, L. A. (1985). Personal coping styles of schizophrenic outpatients. *Hospital and Community Psychiatry, 36,* 407–410.

Falloon, I. R. H., & Talbot, R. E. (1981). Persistent auditory hallucinations: Coping mechanisms and implications for management. *Psychological Medicine, 11,* 329–339.

Kanas, N. (1986). Group therapy with schizophrenics: A review of controlled studies. *International Journal of Group Psychotherapy, 36,* 339–351.

Kanas, N., & Barr, M. A. (1982). Short-term homogeneous group therapy for schizophrenic inpatients. A questionnaire evaluation. *Group 6*(4), 32–38.

Kanas, N., & Barr, M. A. (1984). Self-control of psychotic productions in schizophrenics. *Archives of General Psychiatry, 41,* 919–920.

Kanas, N., & Barr, M. A. (1986). Process and content in a short-term inpatient schizophrenic group. *Small Group Behavior, 17,* 355–363.

Kanas, N., Rogers, M., Kreth, E., Patterson, L., & Campbell, R. (1980). The effectiveness of group psychotherapy during the first three weeks of hospitalization: A controlled study. *Journal of Nervous and Mental Disease, 168,* 487–492.

Kanas, N., Barr, M. A., & Dossick, S. (1985). The homogeneous schizophrenic inpatient group: An evaluation using the Hill Interaction Matrix. *Small Group Behavior, 16,* 397–409.

Kanas, N., Stewart, P., & Haney, K. (1988). Content and outcome in a short-term therapy group for schizophrenic outpatients. *Hospital and Community Psychiatry, 39,* 437–439.

Kanas, N., Deri, J., Ketter, T., & Fein, G. (1989). Short-term outpatient therapy groups for schizophrenics. *International Journal of Group Psychotherapy,*

Maxmen, J. S. (1973). Group therapy as viewed by hospitalized patients. *Archives of General Psychiatry, 28,* 404–408.

Pattison, E. M., Brissenden, E., & Wohl, T. (1967). Assessing special effects of inpatient group psychotherapy. *International Journal of Group Psychotherapy, 17,* 283–297.

Shattan, S. P., D'Camp, L., Fujii, E., Fross, G. G., & Wolff, R. J. (1966). Group treatment of conditionally discharged patients in a mental health clinic. *American Journal of Psychiatry, 122,* 798–805.

Strassberg, D. S., Roback, H. B., Anchor, K. N., & Abramowitz, S. I. (1975). Self-disclosure in group therapy with schizophrenics. *Archives of General Psychiatry, 32,* 1259–1261.

Weiner, M. F. (1984). Outcome of psychoanalytically oriented group psychotherapy. *Group, 8*(2), 3–12.

Yalom, I. D. (1975). *The theory and practice of group psychotherapy* (2nd ed.). New York: Basic Books.

24

Brief Crisis Therapy Groups

Stanley D. Imber and Karen J. Evanczuk

The special effort to provide rapid and effective relief to patients in acute crisis is a profoundly urgent, yet routinely familiar activity in every established program offering psychiatric services, whether that program is located in the intake-reception area of a large urban psychiatric hospital, a suicide prevention unit, a community mental health center, a counseling service, or a small social agency. The presentation of the crisis *per se* demands expeditious and sharply focused professional attention.

It is the rare clinic, however, that can furnish an appointment time within a day or two, even for the crisis patient, because of overwhelming case loads and long wait lists. The crisis patient may be given priority but quite likely that will still mean a wait of several weeks. In short, most often and for most crisis patients, there is an interim period of some considerable length before treatment ensues, and it is not uncommon during that crisis period for patients to experience mounting tension approaching the state that brought them to the hospital in the first instance. Paradoxically, it is in this very critical period when, as crisis theory dictates, the most efficacious work can be accomplished, that many, if not most patients do not have ready access, by way of appointment, to the professional help they require. For reasons of high costs and limitations in the use of precious staff time, psychiatric centers tend to consider it not feasible to maintain a cadre of highly skilled professionals whose primary or sole responsibility is to maintain a roster of crisis patients whom they are expected to see frequently over a period of 5 to 6 weeks, the most frequently observed and traditionally cited length of a crisis period (Caplan, 1961). This scenario of the fate of typical crisis patients has its location in the intake (or emergency) area of the large psychiatric institution, but the events and consequences outlined are in general not dissimilar from those found at other sites that provide psychiatric services, such as small local agencies and community mental health centers, except that these sites may attempt to absorb the emergency patient within their own systems that have even more limited resources for the continuing care of the patient.

Stanley D. Imber • School of Medicine, University of Pittsburgh, Pittsburgh, Pennsylvania 15213. Karen J. Evanczuk • Western Psychiatric Institute and Clinic, 3811 O'Hara Street, Pittsburgh, Pennsylvania 15213.

As the literature review indicates, a frequently noted motivation for the use of crisis groups has been cost-effectiveness, often described as efficiency in staff utilization because a far larger number of patients can be seen, over a stipulated time period, in a group than on an individual basis. Although we know of no objective efforts to document the presumed economic advantages of crisis groups, a more important but usually neglected consideration in the choice of a group approach lies in the theoretical and pragmatic advantages accruing to group techniques. A major objective of this chapter is to describe these special positive functions (and limitations) of the brief group modality in working with crisis patients.

The chapter will begin with a brief overview of crisis theory, pointing toward a working definition of the term *crisis* that will permit a consensual understanding of that concept as it is addressed in the chapter. This will be followed by a selective review of the literature in the use of crisis group methods, with an emphasis on relatively recent clinical and research papers and texts—those published since 1978. Drawing from our own clinical experience, we shall describe next two separate series of crisis groups conducted at different times in the same setting over the period of a decade. We will depict the organization and operation of these groups, including certain similarities and differences. In the two final sections, we will discuss the principal advantages as well as the limitations of brief crisis groups, basing our commentary on the relevant literature as well as our own clinical experience.

WHAT IS A CRISIS?

Perhaps the earliest scholarly formulation of the concept of crisis theory (and a recognition of its relevance for dealing with catastrophic events) can be found in the brilliant work of Erich Lindemann (1944). A more current highly influential student of crisis work is Gerald Caplan, who has been a central figure in the ongoing development of crisis theory over the past 30 years. The definition Caplan offers for crisis is that it exists "when a person faces an obstacle to important life-long goals that is, for a time, insurmountable through the utilization of customary methods of problem solving. A period of disorganization ensues, a period of upset, during which many abortive attempts at solution are made" (Caplan, 1961). This general definition has been narrowed in more current applications to clinical settings by crisis workers, such as Donovan, Bennett, and McElroy (1979), who describe a crisis group candidate as one "who has experienced the acute onset of significant symptoms—i.e., sleeplessness, inability to work—in connection with a definable precipitating event or stress." This specification of the terms *acuteness*, *symptomatology*, and *stressors* is critical for the clinician in that these terms suggest concrete approaches to intervention. Subsequently this definition of crisis has been expanded by Budman and Bennett (1983) to incorporate the notion of felt or actual loss, which they identify as the most common problem or event that serves to stimulate the acute onset of crisis. These writers make one further significant addition to the defined conditions of crisis when they note than an individual's adaptive style may fail due to repeated or cumulative stress rather than merely a single stressful event.

There are a number of additional factors that some authors consider to be central to a full understanding of the nature of psychiatric crisis. For example, Bancroft (1986) suggests that change problems (which other writers may interpret as loss or separation issues) and interpersonal and conflict problems frequently tend to be present in the acute crisis situation. Although it will be noted in the literature review that, among different writers, there are certain minor variations and emphases in what is regarded as a crisis, for the most part there is common agreement with the following statement, which represents a kind of distillate of the descriptions cited. As a referential guideline for our purposes in this chapter, *crisis* refers to a highly distressed state of the individual, characterized by an acute onset; the individual experiences symptoms that disrupt the usual equilibrium and coping adequacy, and there is an identifiable stressor, or series of stressors, that precipitated the state.

THE CRISIS GROUP AND RELATED LITERATURE: A SELECTED REVIEW

Although reports of techniques used to help people in emotional crisis can be traced to the earliest writings on psychopathology, the deliberate and systematic use of group methods is a relatively recent phenomenon, and much of the literature has appeared in the past decade or so. In this section, our review of published material covers mainly theoretical papers, clinical reports, and research findings that have appeared since 1978, although several earlier articles and texts that have had important influence on recent work will receive attention. The review falls into two categories: (1) publications dealing directly with brief crisis therapy groups, the focal topic of the chapter; and (2) publications having to do with other subject matter or activities that have had significant impact on the theory and practice of crisis groups, such as currently promulgated techniques for the conduct of short-term group psychotherapy, individual approaches to crisis work, and developmental crisis models.

Among earlier references to the planned use of groups for patients in crisis are articles by Sadock, Normand, and their associates (Norman, Fensterheim, Tannenbaum, & Sager, 1963; Sadock, Newman, & Normand, 1968). The setting for their work was a walk-in clinic, patients were seen for 6 to 10 visits and cotherapists were used. They described the approach as "ameliorative rather than curative" and indicated the emphasis was on understanding the presenting problem and providing as much relief as possible in the limited time available. The tactics mainly involved what they termed *environmental modification*, although they carefully note they also attended to "interpersonal and intrapsychic events." Sessions were held on a weekly basis, and it is noted that no diagnostic class was excluded except for the "extremely paranoid patient."

A few years later, an article by Allgeyer (1970) emphasized what she considered to be the unique advantage of crisis groups for the economically impoverished and the minority poor in our society, people, she writes, who do not

ordinarily seek assistance until crisis has overwhelmed them. She also advocated that these people be treated in peer groups within their own geographical
areas, where they would be most likely to seek out and accept treatment. In
Allgeyer's (1970) program, patients rotated in and out of the meetings (that is,
there was "open" membership) and were expected to remain a maximum of 6
weeks, a period explicitly selected to be in accord with Caplan's (1961) model
postulating crisis resolution within that time frame. Every patient underwent a
pregroup assessment during which the crisis and the precipitating event was
identified. It is noteworthy that the clientele in the Sadock groups described also
were drawn from an economically deprived area, suggesting the possibility that
patients may have been seen in groups, rather than individually, largely because
they could not pay fees, whatever theoretical or clinical advantages might also
have been considered (Sadock *et al.*, 1968).

Trakas and Lloyd (1971) present an early outcome study of a short-term
group experience with the emergency management of patients in a walk-in
clinic. Their stated intention was to provide care "for as many people as possible, by a small number of staff and in a limited number of sessions." The group
met weekly with a limit of 10 patients and a maximum of six sessions per patient.
The therapeutic approach was somewhat unusual in that a multiplicity of interventions were applied, including directive and supportive techniques as well as
individual and group (process) interpretations, family casework, vocational re-
habilitation, and medication. Treatment goals, as in most other brief crisis group
efforts, were to quickly restore patients to their previous functioning levels,
provide rapid symptom relief, and make appropriate disposition for patients in
need of further care. In addition, the authors developed a research design to
evaluate treatment outcome of their patients. Their findings indicated twice as
many group-treated patients reported improvement as control patients (treated
with several other methods). In the results of a follow-up of patients discharged
from the group as improved, not one patient indicated any worsening of his or
her condition over a 6-month period, a remarkably stable and positive finding in
the psychotherapy outcome research literature. Although the effort to assess
systematically the consequences of their work was laudable, unfortunately the
findings reported must be viewed as somewhat questionable because the research design itself was seriously flawed (e.g., nonrandomization of treatment
assignment, unreliable rating criteria, absence of independent evaluations,
probable bias of the follow-up samples, etc.). Nonetheless, this article had the
merit of a rare early effort to evaluate outcome, and the treatment represented
an unusual multimodal effort with crisis patients in a brief group format.

In a second paper that followed the one cited, Allgeyer (1973) elaborated
further on her crisis group work, noting particularly that in outpatient settings it
is important to exclude patients who present as suicidal or homicidal risks and
individuals likely to disrupt the group proceedings. She also indicated the sali-
ence of a pregroup interview with each patient for the purpose of exploring
actual or anticipated loss of "life roles" or significant others and advocated
encouraging group members to actively engage fellow patients in the sessions
and assist them in developing alternative coping mechanisms.

In 1979, the senior author of this chapter described the uses and abuses of the brief intervention group (Imber, Lewis, & Loiselle, 1979), about which we will have more to say. Although the group experience outlined in that paper served psychiatric patients with a variety of disorders, a considerable portion were essentially in crisis, and a central focus of the group process dealt directly with that emergent condition. The major purpose of the article was to provide a succinct guideline for the practicing therapist in meeting the challenges and demands of that kind of group. In our discussion, we shall reappraise that guideline from the perspective of almost a decade later, revising some of our thoughts and recommendations and expanding on others. We take quick note of the earlier work here because it fits at this point in the sequence of the literature review.

In the early 1970s the Harvard Community Health Plan in Boston initiated an outpatient crisis program and over the next several years provided a series of reports on the organization, development, and functioning of the activity that included the establishment of a crisis group (Donovan et al., 1979; Donovan, Bennett, & McElroy, 1981; Budman & Bennett, 1983). The group met twice each week, just prior to and following the weekend, for a total of eight sessions over a 4-week period. Candidates were all individuals who presented acute symptoms that seriously and adversely affected their usual functioning, except that homicidal, suicidal, and psychotic patients were not accepted. All sessions were led by co-therapists, one of whom routinely interviewed each patient before admission. The preparation done in the intake interview apparently was a critical step in the process of determining patient eligibility and was designed to facilitate the patient's subsequent participation in group activities. During intake, the therapist ascertained that basic qualifying criteria were met but principally spent time exploring the nature of the patient's crisis, defining it with the patient and providing a meaningful explanation for its occurrence, connecting it to current stressful events and attempting to give it a psychodynamic basis. The therapist provided a description of the way the group functioned, preparing the patient for expected role activities of both patient and therapist, and finally they discussed and came to agreement on workable goals to be accomplished during the upcoming 4-week period. The therapist's objective during this fairly extensive intake interview was to establish a working alliance and a common viewpoint with the patient prior to the first meeting in the group. It was a crucial feature of the program plan that co-therapist roles be shared among all professional staff members, and therefore there was regular rotation of assignment among staff, and the schedule was arranged so that one of the two therapists terminated every four sessions. Therapist techniques were described as active, directive, supportive, and task-oriented, and group process received only secondary attention. Also according to the authors, "there was little reliance on medication" (Donovan et al., 1979). With respect to adherence to time limits for patient stay in the group, the writers make special note that the group was not insight oriented and the patient was expected to present the crisis problem promptly, get support and advice, "take steps to resolve [it], improve and leave" (Donovan et al., 1979, p. 909).

The Harvard plan staff examined the results of their extensive treatment program for a subsample of patients seen over a 26-month period (Donovan *et al.*, 1981). Although this apparently was an "in-house" study, lacking certain key aspects of adequate research design (e.g., a control group), the findings at treatment termination and at 1-year follow-up demonstrated impressive benefits, as reported by the patients. The writers observed that, despite the active and often directive roles assumed by therapists, patients themselves seemed to attribute benefits to the "group culture" rather than to the therapists. Moreover, in spite of the brevity of the crisis group experience, they posit cohesiveness as a curative factor in the group, in addition to universality, that is, patient awareness that other people have difficulties similar to their own. It is of particular interest that the authors explicitly remark that the group model may not be especially economical and specifically when co-therapists are used. Nonetheless, they continue to recommend the co-therapy arrangement for the crisis situation because of the "fast-paced and acute nature of the difficulties and the large number of patients" (Donovan *et al.*, 1981).

The most recent retrospective account of the Harvard plan crisis group (Budman *et al.*, 1984) places emphasis on the special relevance of Mann's theoretical position (Mann, 1973) regarding time limits and the utility of that concept in group as well as individual forms of therapy. In the crisis group, it is seen as a powerful motivating force toward rapid resolution of the crisis problem. Because, as we have already noted, loss and separation, accompanied by feelings of low self-esteem, are probably the most common presenting problems among crisis patients, it has special usefulness in promoting the progress of group work because it is one issue very likely to be shared by nearly every patient.

A short-term group for suicidal patients represents a specialized crisis group format. Faberow and Marmor (1983) report a successful daily "drop-in" group at a suicide prevention center. In this life-threatening situation, there were no limits on the number of sessions a patient could attend, but in fact more than half the patients came for only one session. As one might expect, the major objective was to help the patient survive the immediate emergency, and the focus inevitably was on the here and now. Problem themes had to do with rejection, separation, and loss, including the depletion of concrete resources (e.g., money, jobs, housing). Therapists adopted an active position in which the provision of information, specific suggestions, and encouragement were deemed of central import. A cadre of therapists was available for assignment to the group leadership, and generally any one therapist did not lead the group more than once per week. According to the authors, the constant turnover of participating patients and the rotation of therapists paradoxically proved not to be disadvantageous because the routine movement of people in and out from session to session stimulated patients to focus on themselves, to make full use of the meeting for their own immediate purposes, and to feel an obligation to no one but themselves.

Another variant of the crisis group has been described by Lonergan (1985). This group was set up for patients already placed on a wait list for individual therapy but who were undergoing some particular crisis that indicated imminent need for professional assistance while awaiting the individual treatment appointment. There was minimal preparation of patients for the group, frequent turnover of members, and little attention given to group composition. What was quite unusual in this crisis group was the in-depth group interaction reported to have occurred in the sessions and the deliberate use of negative and positive interpretations. However, it should be noted that this group experience was rather atypical in a number of ways. First, the membership had previously been screened and found acceptable for individual psychotherapy; the urgency of the crisis that brought most of them to the group may well have been qualitatively different and less severe than the conventional crisis patient; the average patient stay was 10 sessions, longer than that for most patients in crisis groups, and some patients remained for as many as 42 sessions. These differences may account for the somewhat uncommon dynamics that transpired. One important attribute for the successful therapist of a crisis group, highlighted by this writer, is versatility in the form of a repertoire of differential techniques that may be applied, depending on the composition and stage of the group.

The significance of this versatility is also stressed by Prazoff, Joyce, and Azim (1986) who advocate that therapists have at their disposal a variety of therapeutic modes to manage the different diagnostic categories of patients who present in crisis and their dissimilar levels of psychological crisis. However, the writers point up the limits of insight techniques in the short-term context and indicate a preference for cognitive and behavioral interventions, such as reframing and redefining the presented crisis problem. The setting in which this work was done was a psychiatric walk-in clinic, but some patients had to wait as long as 3 weeks for entry into the group that usually comprised 12 members. Both the size of the group and the 3-week wait, even if only an occasional occurrence, are not typical of most short-term crisis groups. As is increasingly the case with recent crisis group reports, Prazoff and colleagues (1986) make note of the prominence of loss and separation among patient problems and the special relevance of the time-limited approach.

This then represents the résumé of the literature specifically on the brief crisis group, and we turn for the remainder of this section to a review of several publications on related topics having important implications for, and influence on, the contemporary theory and practice of crisis groups. Over a decade ago Ewing (1978) published a splendid, concise text on crisis intervention that has not received the attention it merits. The author furnishes a lucid account of the history and principles of crisis theory and the more commonly used current intervention methods as well as a critique of evaluative research. He explicates several features shared by just about all intervention methods but not always recognized by practitioners, among them the principle that intervention must be readily available and that, by its very nature, it is bound to be brief. Ewing (1978) notes that intervention addresses a wide range of human problems, and this has led to a sometimes controversial effort by some practitioners to broaden the definition of the "in-crisis" individual to include anyone seeking mental health services. He further indicates that all intervention strategies have the ultimate objective of preventing future crises and that effective crisis work requires therapists to feel comfortable in taking nontraditional roles, such as educator, advisor, partner, and model. As relevant as most of his commentary is for the operation of crisis groups, it is noteworthy that Ewing (1978) made no reference in his text to the use of group methods, except perhaps in terms of family work. This may be because group approaches were perceived as relatively rare activities among crisis workers, a condition that probably still obtains today. Current crisis theory continues to put emphasis on the unique quality of the crisis problem as it is presented and on the import of individual coping mechanisms, all of which may lead some clinicians to assume that only individual-centered methods may be appropriate.

Zimet (1979) has outlined an attractive theoretical model derived from the seminal work of Erikson (1959), advocating the use of short-term groups in part to test the utility of that model for the prevention of psychopathology. He proposed a set of developmental task and crisis groups for people in "everyday life," with a focus on the transition between the critical stages in development from childhood to old age. He saw the groups as permitting participants to grasp and overcome the special (crisis) issues at each stage and considered the approach to be essentially preventive in its effects, reducing the probability of later psychiatric disorders. The term *crisis*, of course, had a somewhat different meaning for Zimet (1979) and for Erikson (1959) than our usage in this chapter, although there is the common notion of the distressed state of the individual whose coping skills are inadequate in the face of significant stressors. Budman and his associates (Budman, Bennett, & Wisneski, 1980) took this conceptual model one step further by applying it directly to a clinical population, forming four types of short-term groups: young adults, midlife, postmidlife, and couples groups. Again here group members were not necessarily in clinical crisis, but the objective was to help patients recognize the serious problematic issues that are faced at different life stages and to assist them in working out their own solutions to the issues sufficiently well so that possibilities of psychological disturbance would be reduced and future episodes of acute crisis might be prevented.

In a comprehensive review of the literature in short-term group therapy, Klein (1985) lays out a set of recommended principles for the conduct of brief groups and specifies the goals of treatments. Although he gives only passing attention to the particular conditions of the crisis group, it is apparent that the principles and goals enunciated correspond to those of that type of group. Thus Klein (1985) indicates the goals of the short-term group include amelioration of distress, reestablishment of previous emotional equilibrium, and promotion of the use of patient resources and coping skills. In terms of particular technique recommendations, Klein (1985) points to the basic requirement, now adopted almost without exception in short-term work, that the therapist be active, directive, and flexible and hold the group to a here-and-now atmosphere. In addition, he signals the importance of assisting patients in the shaping of improved coping strategies, cautions the therapist to be sensitive to the more disturbed patient who will need a more supportive orientation, and advises against the use of the group process approach in a brief group setting.

In a companion piece published in the same journal issue as the work of

Klein, there is a set of quite practical guidelines offered by Poey (1985) that are specific to the conduct of brief groups with a psychodynamic orientation. This article also makes only cursory reference to crisis theory and strategy, but many of the suggestions are appropriate to the nondynamic crisis group. In particular, there is extended discussion of two topics that have not usually received adequate attention—therapist burnout and conditions of effective co-therapist arrangements. With respect to the burnout phenomenon, Poey (1985) notes this condition can be recognized when the therapists "see each new group as a burden . . . and experience members' neediness as intolerable . . . [and feel] increasingly ineffective and guilty that they are only doing 'band aid' work and begin to withdraw from involvement" (Poey, p. 348). He emphasizes that the complexities of brief therapy and the intensive techniques required are considerably greater than in long-term approaches. Partly for these reasons, he urges the use of co-therapists. However, Poey (1985) makes it clear that the choice of co-leaders should be deliberate and made in accord with certain criteria. Thus he recommends co-therapists be equal in professional status, rather than, for example, a staff member–trainee pairing. Equally important, they should have similar theoretical orientations but contrasting interpersonal style (in terms of interaction within the group). He stresses the importance of therapists establishing a working relationship prior to initiation of the group and that they meet for 15 to 30 minutes before and after each session to review, take notes, and "diffuse their feelings and to plan" (Poey, p. 349). He also suggests weekly supervision/consultation because that would provide still another skilled individual to consider the complex aspects of treatment sessions.

Finally, we note the current and succinct writing of Bancroft (1986) on crisis intervention. He sees the occurrence of a crisis as prime evidence of individual failure in coping and advocates a cognitive framework as offering the most promising possibilities for a remedy. He describes problem-solving techniques in some detail and adds a touch of what professionals sometimes too easily overlook when he explicitly notes the high significance of practical common sense in crisis work. Like Ewing (1978), however, Bancroft's understanding of crisis resolution seems to encompass only individual methods. He, too, makes no mention of the group as an available technique.

Perhaps the most important conclusion that may be drawn from this summary overview of the literature is that in the history of crisis work individual methods always have been the predominant form of treatment and that group techniques have received sparse attention. In the past two decades, however, there has been some increase in published works that deal explicitly with crisis groups, and these have provided useful theoretical underpinning to that approach. In addition, the literature demonstrates a gathering consensus on the most effective strategies and techniques for group crisis workers. Unfortunately, there is no convincing empirical evidence for the efficacy of crisis groups, a situation not considerably different from findings on crisis techniques in general. Estimates of efficacy continue to be based mainly on anecdotal reports and uncontrolled clinical studies. The few systematic efforts at outcome research have been plagued with serious methodological deficiencies.

EXPERIENCE WITH TWO CRISIS GROUPS IN A DECADE

Separated by almost exactly 10 years, two series of crisis groups were formed and conducted at the Western Psychiatric Institute and Clinic in the Department of Psychiatry, University of Pittsburgh, the first in 1975–1977 with the senior author as organizer and initial therapist (there were others subsequently) and the second with the chapter co-author as one of two co-therapists and with the senior author as supervisor/consultant. We will present brief accounts of each group series because, although there are basic similarities, there also are interesting differences in approach and management that took place over the 10-year period.

In the first group, all patients over the age of 18 who, after initial evaluation, required immediate treatment (but not hospitalization) and other clinical services were not then available, received a referral to the brief group program. Overtly psychotic, addicted, or retarded patients were excluded, as were individuals viewed as imminent suicidal and homicidal risks. Other operational exclusion criteria were inability to communicate clearly and/or likelihood of behavior disruptive to the group. Patients were placed in the group usually within 1 to 4 days of referral. All patients received a prior individual screening and preparatory interview, in which emphasis was placed on a description of the group activities, the expected group role of patient and of therapist, and the understanding that the group commitment was for six weekly sessions of 1½ hours each. The group was an open one, with new patients usually joining each session and some departing. The same single group therapist remained as group leader over long periods of time. Ordinarily there were between four to six patients in each session, some leaving before the contracted six sessions and a few remaining, with therapist approval, beyond that point. Although the group was not conceptualized originally as a specialized service for patients in a crisis state, in fact it became very rapidly a clinic resource that dealt almost exclusively with the crisis patient. The therapist used multiple procedures in working with the changing group membership and the variety of problematic issues, but he tended to focus on inducing patients to examine their current skills and social support systems, with the objective of moving the patient to use these in developing a plan for resolving the present tense situation. The therapist was active, goal oriented, and ahistorical, with a focus on here-and-now behavior within the group and an insistence on each patient's responsibility for progress of the group as a whole and for the provision of assistance to others as well as receiving it.

In addition to its primary objective of providing immediate patient care, the group did serve other functions within the clinic, which at some level influenced the manner in which it proceeded. For example, although for the vast majority of patients, this group experience constituted their full treatment experience at least for this episode, there were a number of patients whose emotional status and intricate problems were such that it became obvious that further treatment would be necessary following the six-session experience. Some of these people remained with the group until their referral was completed. Also, although the group was not designed for wait purposes, it did serve that function for a few patients whose condition was considered sufficiently critical (in crisis) that it was considered in their best clinical interest that they participate in a brief group experience until the appointment date in their assigned clinic. Further, observation of the group was open, with permission of the patients for therapists conducting long-term groups as an opportunity for them to recruit appropriate new patients. The opportunity to observe present group behavior, a good predictor of subsequent group behavior, allowed therapists to make more sound patient selections for their ongoing groups than the usual written intake evaluation reports.

The second and more recent group was conducted in the same setting as the one just described. Patients were drawn from the emergency walk-in clinic formally established in the past few years and from other clinic services in the institute. Unlike the first group, this one was set up specifically for patients in crisis, defined as patients requiring immediate treatment and who presented in a highly disturbed state, with serious difficulty in managing an ongoing or recent stressful event. In patient recruitment announcements to other clinic services, a stressful event was described in terms of actual or anticipated loss (e.g., death of a significant other, job dismissal, etc.) or a transitional development problem (e.g., retirement or midlife crisis, etc.). All patients 18 or older who were in crisis, therefore, qualified, with the exception of imminent suicidal and homicidal risks and those likely to disrupt group process because of behavior difficult to control. A pregroup screening and orientation interview by two co-therapists was arranged for every patient and took place on the first workday after the referral was made. The interview served to assess the precipitating stress event, formulate the nature of the crisis and provide some understanding of it with the patient, explore available coping mechanisms, and finally to prepare the patient for the experience in the group. The group met three times per week for 90 minutes and was open-ended with one or more new patients admitted nearly every session. Patients understood they could remain in the group for 10 sessions, although only a few stayed that long. The therapists were two experienced nurse–clinicians. One continued in the role of co-therapist for the nearly year and one-half that this series of group sessions ran. Her co-therapists rotated approximately every 3 months. It is important to note here that over time the co-therapists began to experience fatigue and the stress of burnout with the demands of the three weekly group sessions, the screening-preparatory sessions for new candidates and weekly supervisory-consulting sessions, all this in addition to their other major professional responsibilities.

The work of the therapists in this second group centered on efforts to work directly with patients on their crisis problems. Patients were encouraged to explicate the details of the crisis, the events surrounding it, and especially to begin to develop alternate methods for resolving the situation. Advice and guidance were routinely provided by therapists and by peer group members. Different problem-solving strategies were considered for each patient, and a concrete step-by-step tactic was encouraged, with patients expected to report outside applications at the next succeeding group session. Although there was a certain degree of patient-to-patient interaction, the predominant form of interaction was between individual therapist and patient, reflecting a general patient preference. The senior author of this chapter served as supervisor-consultant to the co-therapists throughout this group series, meeting with them on a weekly basis.

The description of the two brief crisis groups indicates that, despite their formation and operation some 10 years apart, they were essentially similar in objectives and in clinical techniques. Both dealt mainly with the crisis patient, although only the more recent group was explicitly organized to deal with crisis, especially in terms of loss and separation issues. Also, the second series was more structured than the first, particularly in the directed effort to assist patients to develop and test new skills in problem solving. The earlier group, on the other hand, tended to focus more attention on group process and to stimulate patient interaction, that is, it was more group centered. Yet that first series, even with a more group-centered framework, quite directly dealt with crisis problems and means for their resolution. In addition, there were certain technique differences between the groups, for the most part minor ones, such as a single versus a co-therapist arrangement, a 3-session as opposed to a 1-session-per-week schedule, and a 6 versus a 10-session limit for patient attendance. Although there were no systematic outcome evaluations done for either group series, the clinical impression of the therapists and the results of an informal follow-up patient survey indicate that most patients profited from the group treatment, and there were no outstanding differences in outcome between the two series.

SIGNIFICANT ADVANTAGES OF THE BRIEF CRISIS GROUP

The treatment of patients in crisis tends still to be done principally on an individual basis, but there are important reasons why crisis workers will find a group approach at least equally advantageous. Drawing from the previously cited literature as well as from our own direct experience with crisis groups, we outline in seven categories the special advantages of the group for crisis patients.

Relief of Acute Distress

Patients in crisis present themselves to an intake service at a particularly high point of distress and demoralization. Their objective is to find assistance in combating this state, and the provision of quick and expert attention in the screening interview and especially the rapid placement in treatment are actions that generally have the effect of diminishing the discomfort of patients quite promptly. Upon first entering the group, most patients find the concern and ministrations of the group reassuring, and their morale is further boosted as they quickly become aware that some fellow patients have begun to emerge from their high crisis state as a consequence of work accomplished in the group. For the newly admitted patient, this commonly experienced reduction in discomfort provides a sound basis for reevaluation of their own problems and the consideration of alternative solutions.

The Function of Universality

Within the group setting and in the presence of other individuals undergoing similar states of tension and despair, the crisis patient quickly becomes aware that profound loss and separation are shared, universal, even lifelong issues, and that there are effective means of managing them and surviving. New patients also recognize there are certain symptoms and even some stressful events present in their experience that others in the group are also undergoing. A consequence of the phenomenon of universality discovered in the group is the reduction of feelings of isolation and victimization that so frequently torment the person in crisis.

The Function of Cohesiveness

For the crisis patient, the feeling of belonging, which is the essence of cohesiveness, is a direct function of a successful group and helps considerably in counteracting the pervasive feelings of loss and separation almost routinely found in the crisis patient. By virtue of joining a new group of people, the patient in fact is adding new people to those few who are accessible for support and assistance in the period of emergency, even if they do not immediately replace the loss of significant others. In the group, as other patients offer encouragement and begin to give advice, new patients in turn tend to offer their own suggestions to others. The fact that this advice usually is taken quite seriously and even acted on tends to provide an enormous boost of confidence and self-esteem as the patient becomes aware that he or she retains the ability to develop practical plans and solutions. The involvement in the problems of other people, even if only very briefly, also provides the patient with a kind of release from envelopment in the tension of self-preoccupation.

Interaction with Other People

Interpersonal disputes and conflicts very often lie at the roots of crisis problems that confront the patient. The group setting provides a safe place for crisis patients to begin to examine their ongoing interpersonal relationships not only by describing their outside contacts with people but also by beginning to observe the characteristics of their interactions with others in the group itself. The safe group setting also allows patients to begin to alter maladaptive styles by practicing alternatives, under the guidance of the therapist.

Learning from Others in Crisis

We have already alluded to the advantage for patients in having the opportunity to observe other patients address the specifics of their problems and work out alternative solutions. We make special note of this activity here because it is the very setting of the group that can stimulate a patient to capitalize on the opportunity. Patients are only too well familiar with professionals offering suggestions and even laying out detailed plans for them and, far more often than appreciated, the patient rejects this advice because the professional is perceived as an individual who has never experienced the deep anxieties and the events encountered by the patient. In the crisis group setting, however, the patient recognizes the presence of others much like themselves undergoing a similar severe crisis. The solutions worked out by these peers and the suggestions and advice they offer each other often will be more easily considered and even acted on than identical proffers from the therapist. This is indeed a considerable by-product of the group arrangement.

Time Limits, an Incentive and Learning Tool

Time limits in the crisis group have the singular importance of pressing all patients to work actively and efficiently toward dispelling the crisis problem and avoiding delays because the period when aid is available has a set termination date. Equally important, however, under the guidance of the therapist, patients begin to appreciate they can learn to deal more effectively with loss and separation by confronting and working out those issues as they occur in the group, where different members depart nearly every session and especially as they must prepare for their own separation in the impending future.

Some Potential Indirect Advantages

Depending on how the group is organized, there are additional uses to which it can be put, three of which we will mention here: student instruction, diagnostic observation, and patient preparation for long-term treatment. With respect to instruction, students in training for group work rarely have the opportunity to observe directly the complete therapy experience of a set of patients or the life of a group. The brief group allows students to examine the complete development of the group experience within a time period consistent with the needs of most students. Concerning diagnostic observation, the intake procedures at many outpatient clinics often provide insufficient information to draw up adequate treatment plans or to reliably make some other disposition. The observation of patients interacting with others over a limited period of time provides a good opportunity for the clinician to formulate a diagnosis and treatment plan, making use of interpersonal data not usually forthcoming in individual interviews. Finally, during the course of the brief group experience, patients acquire familiarity with many of the phenomena that take place during longer term groups, including interactions with other patients, therapist in group behaviors, and the group process itself. These can be expected to allow patients to engage more efficiently in further therapy experience, including longer term groups, to which they may be assigned.

LIMITS AND ADMONITIONS IN THE USE OF BRIEF CRISIS GROUPS

In our view, the principal limits to the brief crisis group remain much as we described them in an earlier article (Imber *et al.*, 1979). With some elaboration and one or two added concerns, we recapitulate those prior cautionary qualifications.

Maintenance of Therapeutic Commitment

The constant flow of patients in and out of the group produces not only discontinuity in the group process but makes it all but impossible for the therapist to work intensively with the patients as individuals. Moreover, therapists only rarely have any follow-up information on the fate of people deeply troubled when they were seen in treatment, and at times these patients may begin to seem like metaphorical ships that pass in the night. In addition, should the therapist conduct sessions two or three times in a week, the sense of constant change in the people present and in the discussion content most surely poses a continuing challenge to therapists seeking to maintain high levels of therapeutic commitment.

Pressures on the Therapist and "Burnout"

The burden on the therapist responsible for the monitoring and care of a large number of patients all of whom are in crisis simultaneously can only be described as intense. Beyond that is the fact that it is not unusual for therapists to conduct an overlapping series of such groups for very long periods of time (and, as noted, sometimes conducting them two or three times weekly). The obvious need for periodic relief for the crisis group therapist often is overlooked in emergency settings where most staff feel harassed and overworked. Nonetheless, the danger of early "burnout" for the crisis group therapist is real, and group work probably can be done best by having available a cadre of competent therapists to share and rotate leadership.

Restraint on Group Process Development

We made mention of the advantages to the patient that are generated by group cohesiveness and universality, phenomena that emerge in the course of the development of process in a successful group. These phenomena are sufficiently important to be called *therapeutic factors* by Yalom (1985). Yet it must be acknowledged that the promotion of process within the strict time limits of a brief group is an achievement that probably only highly experienced therapists can manage with facility. For many therapists who may be process centered in their orientation, the restricted time sequence and circumscribed patient interaction in this format may be seen as permitting only tentative and difficult-to-preserve group process.

Dangerous Territory for the Novice Therapist

As several of the remarks indicate, we are of the strong opinion that only the most skilled and experienced group therapists can do the job adequately. The telescoped time period, the need for prompt diagnostic decisions, the constant change in group membership, the multiple patient problems attendant to the crisis, and the uncertainties of process and direction within the sessions all call for a repertoire of techniques and flexibility of style that only the more talented and seasoned therapists possess.

Ruleouts for the Brief Group

In terms of exclusion from short-term groups, patients who are imminent suicidal risks and those who are homicidal, as well as patients too disorganized to communicate clearly, represent the more obvious ruleouts. There are still other kinds of patients, however, who present in crisis and in the past were quite likely to be included in the brief group but now tend to be excluded, although most probably are responsive to other forms of crisis treatments. We refer here to patients with frequently recurring crises, patients diagnosed as primary personality (character) disorders, and patients who have serious difficulty in controlling behavior disruptive to group progress, such as substance abusers. The crises of these people are every bit as real as others deemed qualified for the brief group, but probably the best disposition for them is one of the alternative forms of longer term treatment.

A Continuing Need for Treatment

Despite the impression of positive outcome we previously noted in our own recent crisis group work and positive reports by other clinicians summarized in prior sections, in sober retrospect and in the absence of adequate controlled studies, we are constrained to take a more conservative position. It is our judgment that a very large portion of patients seen in crisis groups require further treatment at a later time. To some observers, this conclusion is not surprising and may be consistent with their own expectations. After all, many patients who come for help in crisis are likely to have critical and complex problems that have long gone unattended. These will not be resolved in any form of brief crisis treatment, whether that involves group or individual procedures or medication. And for those crisis group workers who may be discouraged at this conclusion and question their own wisdom in expending so much energy and emotion in this work, we would note that the crisis group does remain an expeditious means of problem resolution at least for *some* patients and yields a marked reduction in symptoms and distress for most of the others.

SUMMARY

The short-term group is an increasingly common intervention method for the treatment of patients in crisis. In this chapter we first provided a résumé of crisis theory in general and then defined the crisis state, a critical condition that often is misunderstood. Following this, we presented a selective review of the literature of brief crisis groups, centering on materials published since 1978. In drawing conclusions from the review, we observed that individual treatment methods for crisis patients have always been favored over group approaches, but the latter are becoming more prominent. We also noted the absence of convincing empirical evidence for the efficacy of crisis groups, an unfortunate deficiency that seems also to hold for other crisis treatment methods as well. Among the major advantages of crisis groups we described the following: the prompt relief of acute patient distress, the functions of universality and of cohesiveness, the importance of opportunity for interaction with other people and learning from others in crisis, and the special incentive of time limits in the group. Finally, we pointed out a number of significant limitations in the use of brief crisis groups, including difficulties in maintaining therapist commitment, the danger of therapist burnout, restraint on group process development, the requirement for experienced therapists, the inappropriateness of the group for some people in crisis, and the probability that most patients still need further treatment even after crisis management.

REFERENCES

Allgeyer, J. M. (1970). The crisis group—its unique usefulness to the disadvantaged. *International Journal of Group Psychotherapy, 20,* 235–239.

Allgeyer, J. M. (1973). Brief communications: Using groups in a crisis-oriented outpatient setting. *International Journal of Group Psychotherapy, 23,* 217–222.

Bancroft, J. (1986). Crisis intervention. In S. Bloch (Ed.), *An introduction to the psychotherapys* (2nd ed., pp. 113–132). New York: Oxford University Press.

Budman, S. H., & Bennett, M. J. (1983). Short-term group psychotherapy. In H. I. Kaplan & B. J. Sadock (Eds.), *Comprehensive group psychotherapy* (2nd ed., pp. 138–144). Baltimore: Williams & Wilkins.

Budman, S. H., Bennett, M. J., & Wisneski, J. J. (1980). Short-term group psychotherapy: An adult developmental model. *International Journal of Group Psychotherapy, 30*(1), 63–76.

Budman, S. H., Demby, A., Feldstein, M., & Gold, M. (1984). The effects of time-limited group psychotherapy: A controlled study. *International Journal of Group Psychotherapy, 34*(4), 587–603.

Caplan, G. (1961). *An approach to community mental health.* New York: Grune & Stratton.

Donovan, J. M., Bennett, M. J., & McElroy, C. M. (1979). The crisis group: An outcome study. *American Journal of Psychiatry, 136*(7), 906–910.

Donovan, J. M., Bennett, M. J., & McElroy, C. M. (1981). The crisis group: Its rationale, format, and outcome. In S. H. Budman (Ed.), *Forms of brief therapy* (pp. 283–303). New York: The Guilford Press.

Erikson, E. H. (1959). *Identity and the life cycle.* New York: International Universities Press.

Ewing, C. P. (1978). *Crisis intervention as psychotherapy.* New York: Oxford University Press.

Faberow, N. L., & Marmor, K. (1983). Short-term group psychotherapy with suicidal patients. In M. Rosenbaum (Ed.), *Handbook of short-term therapy groups* (pp. 337–355). New York: McGraw-Hill.

Imber, S. D., Lewis, P. M., and Loiselle, R. H. (1979). Uses and abuses of the brief intervention group. *International Journal of Group Psychotherapy, 29*(1), 39–49.

Klein, R. H. (1985). Some principles of short-term group therapy. *International Journal of Group Psychotherapy, 35*(3), 309–330.

Lindemann, E. (1944). Symptomatology and management of acute grief. *American Journal of Psychiatry, 101,* 141–148.

Lonergan, E. C. (1985). Utilizing group process in crisis-waiting-list groups. *International Journal of Group Psychotherapy, 35*(3), 355–372.

Mann, J. (1973). *Time-limited psychotherapy.* Cambridge, MA: Harvard University Press.

Normand, W., Fensterheim, H., Tannenbaum, G., & Sager, C. J. (1963). The acceptance of the psychiatric walk-in clinic in a highly deprived community. *American Journal of Psychiatry, 120*(6), 533–539.

Poey, K. (1985). Guidelines for the practice of brief, dynamic group therapy. *International Journal of Group Psychotherapy, 35*(3), 331–354.

Prazoff, M., Joyce, A. S., & Azim, H. F. A. (1986). Brief crisis group psychotherapy: One therapist's model. *Group, 10*(1), 34–40.

Sadock, B., Newman, L., & Normand, W. C. (1968). Short-term group psychotherapy in a psychiatric walk-in clinic. *American Journalof Orthopsychiatry, 38*, 724–732.

Trakas, D. A., & Lloyd G. (1971). Emergency management in a short-term open group. *Comprehensive Psychiatry, 12*(2), 170–175.

Yalom, I. D. (1985). *The theory and practice of group psychotherapy* (3rd. ed.). New York: Basic Books.

Zimet, C. N. (1979). Developmental task and crisis groups: The application of group psychotherapy to maturational processes. *Psychotherapy: Theory, Research and Practice, 16*(1), 2–8.

25

Psychodrama in Short-Term Psychotherapy

Ray Naar

Like most psychiatric concepts *time-limited* or *short*-term psychotherapy may be understood in many different ways. The simplest is to define short-term psychotherapy as a psychotherapeutic intervention of brief duration. While meeting operational requirements, this definition is vague and wanting in terms of applicability and outcome. Indeed, it says nothing of the goals to be achieved.

In order to make a case for the use of psychodrama in short-term psychotherapy, I shall enlarge upon the preceding definition and render it more specific. I shall, then, attempt to show how psychodramatic interventions may achieve the goals explicitly stated in my definition.

I shall define "time-limited psychotherapy" as a brief psychotherapeutic intervention that strives to achieve one or more of the objectives listed next. The intervention consists of one single session during which the goal is achieved, followed by a few more sessions to integrate and consolidate the patient's gains. The objectives are:

1. To change a circumscribed area of behavior, that is, a recurring dream, a phobia, a specific unassertive behavior, and the like.
2. To enable an individual to start making decisions again instead of remaining fixated into a rigid, emotional position.
3. To resolve an unexpected crisis in one's life.
4. To enable an individual to go through a therapeutic, dynamic cycle, that is, gain insight into the motivation for nonconstructive behaviors, achieve a needed emotional catharsis, and adopt new, more spontaneous, more constructive behavior patterns.

This conceptualization of time-limited psychotherapy offers the additional advantage of bypassing the controversy of long-term versus short-term therapy. Indeed, when one of the aforementioned goals has been achieved, the patient may choose to terminate therapy or to set a different set of goals with the same

RAY NAAR • Medical Center East, 211 Whitfield Street, Suite 635, Pittsburgh, Pennsylvania 15206.

or different therapists. In this chapter, I propose to dispel some widely held misconceptions regarding the use of psychodrama, describe with appropriate examples some of the key psychodramatic techniques, and illustrate the preceding definition with case histories from my practice.

While retaining a loyal group of adherents, psychodrama was never as widely disseminated as other psychotherapeutic modalities. Moreno's charismatic, sometimes overwhelming personality, his rift with Slavson, may have been contributing factors. It is more likely, however that the zeitgeist was not right. Therapists of the 1920s through the 1950s were wary of an approach that promoted action instead of talk and were more interested in interpreting dreams than—as Moreno once told Freud—"giving people the courage to dream again."[1]

Even today, psychodrama is only partially understood. Yalom (1983, p. 29) cautions against its application with an inpatient population because it encourages catharsis and regression. Yet, in a subsequent chapter of the same book (Yalom, 1983), he advocates the use of psychodramatic techniques (i.e., a variation of *doubling* on p. 154 and *role reversal* on p. 158) without labeling them as such and without giving Moreno proper credit (Moreno, 1944, 1959b).

It is true that psychodrama is a powerful tool that can release the floodgates of emotion. To promote affect, however, is but only one of the objectives that an effective use of psychodrama can achieve. Psychodrama, as developed by Moreno, has sound theoretical underpinnings and, as a psychotherapeutic modality, aims at helping the individual break old, rigid cognitive patterns, develop new patterns, and, as a result, engage in new, creative behaviors (Fox, 1987). Psychodrama may also be viewed as a set of techniques but of such elegance and flexibility that they can be used within many different theoretical frameworks (Naar, 1981). The dangers in using psychodrama with a fragile population are not inherent in the method but in the manner in which it is used and its appropriateness to the contract established with the patient. In an excellent discussion of the precautions necessary in utilizing action methods, Passariello (1987) points out that in a psychotherapy group geared toward personality changes, catharsis and regression may be totally appropriate. In a group of hospitalized patients, on the other hand, geared toward shoring existing defenses, psychodrama can be used as an instrument to refine social skills, identify existing strengths, and investigate available options. It is this marvelous flexibility that makes psychodrama appropriate for all ages, all cultures, all kinds of people in all diagnostic categories.

The founder of psychodrama was J. L. Moreno, and the highlights of his life and career have so often been covered in both factual and anecdotal fashions (Fox, 1987; Leutz, 1985) that I only wish, here, to acknowledge a debt of gratitude to the man who, for almost half a century, dominated the field of group psychotherapy. As stated earlier, however, I shall describe some of the key concepts and techniques in psychodrama, then illustrate their use in brief psychotherapy with appropriate case histories.

---

[1]Zerka Moreno, personal communication.

ELEMENTS OF PSYCHODRAMA[2]

A classical psychodrama consists generally of three stages: the warmup, the drama, and the sharing phase.

The warmup is a group of exercise that primes the group for action, puts members in touch with their feelings, quickly builds group cohesiveness, and leads to the choice of a protagonist. A very moving warmup demonstrated in my presence by James Sacks is described:

Director to group: We often talk about "unfinished business" in people's lives. For me, "unfinished businesses" refer to all the times in my life when I could have said something but did not, I could have done something but did not. It means the unexpressed feelings, the missed opportunities and most always, it is in relation to another person. We all have "unfinished businesses" in our lives. I would like each of you to remember one unfinished business, and in your fantasy, place the person to whom the unfinished business relates on this empty chair. Then we'll go around the circle and share with each other whatever we feel comfortable in sharing and no more.

These instructions usually evoke a considerable amount of poignant memories, and some typical responses are listed next:

I wish I could have told my grandparent how much I loved him/her before he/she died. I'll never forget my third grade teacher. She gave me more self-confidence than any other person in my life. I wish I knew where she is so I could tell her that I've done well.

The Protagonist

As stated before, the warmup leads to the choice of a protagonist. The protagonist is the center figure of the drama, the person around whom the action unfolds.

It must be remembered that, although psychodrama is usually associated with group psychotherapy, psychodramatic techniques can also be used in individual therapy. In such case, the protagonist is simply the patient.

The Soliloquy

The soliloquy is, exactly, what the term implies. The protagonist (or any other member of the drama) is asked to soliloquize, i.e., talk to him- or herself, to verbalize thoughts and feelings. Usually the protagonist is asked to imagine himself or herself in the place where, as a child (or even as an adolescent or an adult), he or she would feel safe and use as a retreat. At other times, the protagonist may be asked to stop an ongoing interaction and go into a soliloquy as illustrated in the following example:

[2]For an expanded discussion of this section, see R. Naar (1981). *A Primer of Group Psychotherapy.* New York: Human Sciences Press.

Protagonist: (to older brother) You never paid any attention to me. I was nonexistent for you. "Shithead," that's what you would call me, and you never let me play with any of your friends.

Older brother: My friends were all I had, shithead, and I wasn't about to let you take them away from me as you did Mom and Dad. Did it ever occur to you that, from the day you were born, I no longer mattered. It was Jason here, Jason there. Take care of Jason. Well, piss on Jason. At least he wasn't about to take my friends.

Director: (to protagonist) Jason, I want you to go into a soliloquy about what just happened.

Protagonist: (soliloquizing) Well, he may have a point there; come to think of it, I would always run to Mom when I wanted to get at him. I never knew he felt as strongly about it. Really, I think he should work it out with Dad and Mom. But, it bothers me . . . it really does . . . he hates me.

Protagonist: (to brother) You know I care for you . . . I really . . . well, it was partly my fault. . . .

Auxiliary Egos

All participants in the drama, with the exception, of course, of the protagonist are called auxiliary egos. Their function is to help expand the protagonist's intellectual and affective awareness. It is also to help the protagonist develop new behavioral ways of coping with old and new situations.

The Double

One auxiliary ego serves a very special function and is called the double. The most important function of the double is to expand the protagonist's awareness. The double "becomes" the protagonist and talks "as if" he or she were the protagonist whenever the double feels that the protagonist is not completely in touch with or not quite able to verbalize feelings and ideas. There are many different ways to double, and some fairly elementary doubling techniques are described below.

DOUBLING AS A CLIENT-CENTERED REFLECTION OF FEELINGS

Protagonist: I went to pick her up and, well . . . she told me to kiss off. Well, that's the way it goes. I didn't know what to do . . . and . . .

Double: It felt awkward . . . felt more than awkward . . . it hurt

Protagonist: Yes, it did . . . right then and there I felt like bursting into tears.

DOUBLING AS A MATCHING OF WORDS, FEELINGS, AND TONE OF VOICE

Protagonist (in a matter-of-fact tone of voice): So, my little girl is not so little anymore. She got married and left home.

Double (in a very soft tone of voice):   She left home.
Protagonist: (Nods with tears in her eyes.)

Doubling as Incomplete Sentences

Protagonist: What I told him was that I was sorry, and that I would be more careful next time.
Double: What I wanted to tell him was . . .
Protagonist: What I really wanted to tell him was "Fuck off, you big tub of lard."

Role Reversal

The role reversal is a procedure in which two people in the drama (usually the protagonist and an auxiliary ego) reverse roles and assume each other's identity. The role reversal may be very brief or may last for several minutes and may serve many purposes, some of which are described next.

Role reversal helps the auxiliary ego become acquainted with his or her role. The protagonist is asked to play the part of the person to be depicted by the auxiliary ego.

A role reversal helps an individual reincorporate one's projections.

Protagonist: In our fifteen years of married life, you never once trusted me.
Director: Please, reverse roles.
Protagonist (as wife):   You never trusted me either. You are a jealous husband.
Director: Reverse roles.
Protagonist: That is kinda true. . . .

A role reversal especially helps an individual understand and feel what it is like to be someone else, to see the world from someone else's point of view. This is poignantly illustrated in the following lines from Moreno:

> A meeting of two; eye to eye, face to face
> And when you are near I will tear your eyes out
> and place them instead of mine.
> and you will tear my eyes out
> and will place them instead of yours,
> then I will look at you with your eyes
> and you will look at me with mine
> —*Motto* (Moreno, 1964)

The Drama

There is, of course, no formula for the drama. It unfolds and may go into any direction according to the needs of the protagonist, the spontaneity of the participants, and the knowledge and imagination of the director. Some psychodramatic scenes are moving and poignant; others may be plodding and boring. The movement and affect displayed by the participants are not always a measure of the benefit derived by the protagonist. A psychodrama may appear slow and uninteresting and still be a journey in exploration of one's feelings, thoughts, and attitudes.

The Sharing Phase

When a protagonist goes through the drama of his/her life, no one in the audience has gone through precisely the same experiences. Almost everyone, however, can resonate to the protagonist's hurt, sadness, anger, and joy. The feelings thus stimulated have to be worked through. At the conclusion of the drama, the members of the groups are asked to share and discuss their feelings with each other and with the protagonist.

These are some of the very basic concepts and techniques in psychodrama. There are many more, of course (Moreno, 1959a, 1965b; Naar, 1977; Sacks, 1965, 1974), and they are limited only by the skills and ingenuity of psychodramatists. The simplicity of the techniques described may be deceiving. The use of a single technique may be effective occasionally, but a psychodramatist must know how to use all of these in combination with each other and, always, within a coherent theoretical framework.

Before illustrating the use of these techniques in the psychotherapeutic process, it may be appropriate to discuss some of the contexts within which they can be used.

Psychodrama and Moreno have been traditionally associated with group psychotherapy and, indeed, it is within the context of psychotherapy in groups that psychodrama is most often used. It has, however, several additional applications, including its employment in individual therapy as well as in marital and family therapy. Psychodrama can also be used as a surgical intervention when a therapist, having reached an impasse with a patient in individual therapy, refers that patient to a psychodrama group for a few sessions in order to break the logjam in ways that will be described later in this chapter. It would be irrelevant and too time consuming to illustrate the use of psychodrama within each of the previously mentioned contexts. An example of how one psychodramatic technique (i.e., doubling) can be used in individual therapy, however, is provided next[3]:

Therapist: You are very silent, Ginger.

Ginger: I was just thinking—(silence of 3 minutes)

Therapist: Sometimes, it feels better to just think by oneself rather than talk.

Ginger: Yea, it is—(silence of 2 minutes)

Therapist: Could you think out loud? I'll just move next to you, out of your field of vision so I won't disturb you. Occasionally, if I feel that there is something you want to say but cannot put it into words, I might say it for you, just as if I were you. But remember, if you don't agree with something I say you must tell me.

[3]The interaction described is reproduced from R. Naar (1981). Psychotherapeutic intervention: A nonschool approach. In C. J. Golden, S. S. Alcaparras, F. D. Strider, & B. Graber (Eds.), *Applied techniques in behavioral medicine* (pp. 19–47). New York: Grune & Stratton.

Ginger: OK, I was thinking of my father—why did he have to do that?—(sighs) (brief silence)

Therapist: It saddens me to think of it.

Ginger: Yes, it does—because I loved him and he loved me very much. But it always puzzled him that I could be good in math (silence).

Therapist: It even made him feel uncomfortable.

Ginger: It did, indeed. He could not understand that. For him a good woman should cook, stay at home, and all that crap. Until he died, I was 22, I was still his "baby doll." (silence)

Ginger: He couldn't see me as a woman.

Therapist: Sometimes, I have trouble seeing myself as a woman, I am afraid to follow through.

Ginger: Twice, I signed up for a course in math and twice I withdrew. Yet, I knew I could do the work—in fact, I could do better than half the jerks in the class.

Therapist: It was as if . . .

Ginger: As if I was afraid to displease my father—as if I let him down (Ginger hits the chair with her fist).

Therapist: Damn—that pisses me off.

Ginger: It really does—what I want—(silence)

Therapist: What I want is to show the whole goddamn world that I am as good as any man, as good as anybody.

Ginger: (turns around to face the therapist and smiles) You know I was thinking exactly that but I was afraid to put it into words.

One of the interventions that I shall now describe occurred within the context of individual therapy; the other three occurred in a group.

Case I—Changing a Specific Behavior

Linda, a 35-year-old physician had been sexually molested by her father when she was 7 or 8. Her father would come into her bedroom at night, insert his hand under her nightgown and caress her without saying a word. The child was petrified, too frightened to protest and had never shared that experience with anyone until she entered therapy. The incidents of molestation occurred only a few times, stopped, and never occurred again. In all other respects, Linda's father's behavior was appropriate: He provided well for his children, never abused them, and always displayed appropriate care and concern for their welfare. Linda's relationship with her father, while civil, had remained tense and stilted through the years. She had never been able to confront him with her anger and hurt and never been able to show any affection toward him. The psychodrama described next occurred shortly before Thanksgiving. Linda had, wistfully, expressed her desire to feel comfortable in her father's presence, at least once in her life. At my suggestion she agreed to become the protagonist in a psychodrama dealing with that period of her life. It was my belief that Linda's unexpressed anger stood in the way of a more relaxed interaction between her father and herself. An attempt to encourage a confrontation and a release of anger proved futile. Linda's affect, usually quite appropriate, would become flat and, whenever requested to talk to her father, she would sound distant and detached. I decided to experiment with a variation of the Playback Theater, an approach that basically consists of the spontaneous enactment by members of the group, of a protagonist's personal drama (Fox, 1987; Salas, 1982). The following interaction took place:

Director: Linda, would you please pick two people who could play your father and you at the age of 7.

Linda: (She points to Eva and Joe.)

Director: And now, Linda, all I want you to do is sit on the chair, be the "raconteuse." Describe what happened and watch, enacted in front of you, a slice of your life. Feel free, however, to come in whenever you like. When did this take place?

Linda: In my bedroom.

Director: Could you describe it?

Linda: My bed is against the window. There is a dresser there and on the other side a chest of toys.

Director: Could you describe the walls?

Linda: They are pink; there is a picture there, but I can't remember it.

Director: What time is it?

Linda: It is late; it is dark and I am in bed.

(Director dims the lights and Eva lays down on three pillows arranged as a bed.)

Director: How do you sleep? On your stomach, your back?

Linda: On my side. (silence)

Director: What happens then, Linda?

Linda: The door opens; I am really scared. He comes close to me. (Joe gets on the floor and comes close to Eva.)

Linda: (screaming) Get away, get away from her.

Director: (insisting) What happens, then, Linda?

Linda: He puts my hand under my nightgown. (Joe pretends to insert his hand under Eva's shirt.)

Linda: (screaming) Leave her alone, you hear, you bastard, leave her alone.

Director: Help her, Linda, help her.

Linda: (screaming) Damn you, damn you . . . (She flies off her chair, grabs Joe who offers no resistance, beats him with her fists, propels him to the door, and throws him out of the room. She comes back into the room, gets on the floor, bursts into tears, cradles Eva's head against her breast, and moans.) Oh, my baby, my baby, what have they done to you, what have they done to you. . . .

After Linda's tears subsided, her father was brought back into the room, tied to a chair, gagged, and Linda talked to him for a long time, in a calmer but assertive and not detached tone of voice. She told him how angry she had been at him, how much she had been damaged by what he had done, how hurt and sad she still was at not ever being able to have a true father–daughter relationship.

When Linda returned to the group 2 weeks later, she was bubbling with excitement. For the first time in her life, she had felt at ease in the presence of her father. She stated that she did not feel "closer to but more comfortable with him." It was as if having shed the weight of unexpressed anger, she could move more freely. It was my belief, later corroborated in an individual session, that two more important events also occurred. Witnessing, rather than just experiencing, the harm that had been done to her, enabled her to overcome the unconscious and irrational guilt that so often plagues the victims of rape and incest. Finally, she was able to give to herself, through the medium of Eva, the love and understanding which she had hitherto denied herself.

As a result of these three factors, that is, the overt expression of anger, the overcoming of guilt, and the expression of self-love, a circumscribed area of behavior (Linda's feelings toward her father and her behavior in his presence) had dramatically been altered. Although Linda was a member of an ongoing group, her case is typical of the surgical intervention mentioned earlier when a therapist having reached an impasse with a patient in individual therapy refers that patient to a psychodrama group to get the therapeutic process moving again.

Case II—Enabling an Individual to Start Making Decisions Again Instead of Remaining Fixated into a Rigid, Emotional Position

I saw Judith for the first time in 1969.[4] At that time she was in religious life. Approximately 30 years old, neatly dressed, rather attractive albeit quite heavy, she sat on the edge of her chair and seemed to make great and successful efforts at controlling her tension. She conveyed an almost painful impression of muscular rigidity. She had difficulty verbalizing problems and/or goals. She spoke of herself as being "encased in ice," "extremely lonely," and "unable to relate to anyone." She then added, "I can't go on like this, I've got to do something about this."

Rejection and loneliness were the overriding themes in her reminiscences. According to Judith, her parents never held her and never touched her except to administer physical punishment. Her father would never talk to her, and her mother addressed her only to scold and threaten. She remembers as a child, spending entire evenings, and sometimes part of the night, wandering alone and daydreaming through the neighborhood cemetery.

I began meeting with Judith on an individual basis in 1969 and our interaction was client-centered in nature. At the end of her first year in therapy, Judith and I agreed that it would be greatly rewarding if she could establish with other people the kind of relationship which she enjoyed with me. She agreed to join a group that was being formed. The group, composed of Judith and seven other sisters, became an intensive and powerful experience. The group was always supportive, never critical, and offered her the first opportunity to express and receive love verbally as well as nonverbally. She learned to relate and became very close to all the group members.

Several weeks before the group terminated, a tragic incident occurred. Judith talked about her father, and for the first time was able to ventilate anger at him. This very unusual behavior on her part was reinforced by the other members of the group. Approximately an hour after the group had left, there was a knock at my office door. Judith, trembling and white as a sheet, was standing at the threshold. I helped her in, and she explained that while she was expressing anger at her father with the group in my office,

---

[4]For a full description of Judith's story, see R. Naar (1979). What, when and for what: A successful multi model approach to therapy. *Psychology: Theory, Research and Practice, 16,* 1.

he was dying (in fact, had died) of a sudden heart attack in the emergency room located in another part of the building.

In an understandable illustration of paratoxic thinking, Judith held herself responsible for her father's death. It did not help to find, on her way back from the funeral, an old letter which her father had written and hidden in a bible, and in which he stated that he loved her but never knew how to express that love.

Judith became obsessed with the memory of her father. She dreamed of him every night and thought of him constantly during the day. During our sessions, however, she refused to talk about her experiences with him except to point out that he was a good man and that she had been a terrible daughter for having accused him and being angry at him. This went on for several months, and it seemed as if therapy during that time remained at a standstill. I made no effort to point out to her the incongruity of her attitude, feeling very strongly that any such attempt on my part would alienate her. Eventually, approximately 8 months later, she came to the session and brusquely stated that she could stand this no longer, that she realized that her father was not what she pretended, and that she wanted to do something to cure herself of that unbearable obsession.

It was my feeling that the way in which this could be accomplished was for Judith to come to grips honestly with her anger at her father, that is, to accept, experience, and express it freely but also to become accessible to whatever positive feelings existed toward her father and experience them, not to alleviate her guilt, but because she truly felt them. I was hoping that my goal could be achieved in a psychodramatic fashion using the theoretical concept of "surplus reality" coined by Moreno (1965b) and the technique of the reformed auxiliary ego described by Sacks (1970). According to the concept of "surplus reality," there is in psychodrama a note of experience which goes beyond reality and provides the subject with a new and more extensive experience of reality. (Moreno, 1965). As for the reformed auxiliary ego technique, it is specially conceived to bring into awareness both a repressed love and repressed needs for love (Sacks, 1970). What the technique entails will become clear as the psychodrama which unfolded is described.

Believing very strongly that the planned intervention should occur within the context of extreme emotional support, I contacted the members of the group which had disbanded several months earlier (Judith had remained in individual therapy), and they all agreed to return for one more session. A colleague, Dr. Paul Levy, trained in psychodrama, was willing to assist me and play the part of Judith's father. The group met in a new office into which I had moved and which had no windows. I turned no lights on and, in the almost total darkness, only shadows could be seen. (The absence of lights can be rationalized on many grounds: In this case, I insisted on darkness because of Judith's still great difficulty in expressing personal feelings in front of a stranger, that is, Dr. Levy. In the darkness, he maintained anonymity, and his identification with Judith's father was easier.)

The drama began with a dialogue between Judith and her father. At the beginning of the interaction, Judith was subdued and talked in a very soft voice, sounding apologetic and fearful. As the exchange continued, however, Judith's anger began to mount. Using the "shut-up" technique developed by Sacks (1976), which essentially consists of initially thwarting the patient's efforts at expressing his/her feelings and reinforcing increments of anger, Dr. Levy was successful in helping Judith become extremely angry. Suddenly, she literally exploded and, screaming at the top of her lungs, spewed forth a torrent of accusations and abuse, at last telling her father all the things which she had wanted to but had been afraid to tell him throughout her life, all the anger, all the hate, all the rejections, the hurts for which he had been, in part, responsible.

When she was finally exhausted, Dr. Levy, as her father, became a reformed parent

(Sacks, 1970), changed his attitude and softly, gently stated that "maybe she was right and truly he wanted to hear her at last." Then, somewhat wistfully and sadly, she spent many minutes sharing with him, this time without anger, the hurt which he had caused her, the pain, the fear, the loneliness, the walks through the cemetery, the times which she would do anything to get his attention and would never get it, and, when she was finished, she was sobbing, again an emotional manifestation extremely rare in her. In the darkness, she embraced her father and, to my question replied that it was now alright for him to die and leave. Dr. Levy walked out of the door, and it is somewhat unsettling to think that, after this powerful, intense experience, they could run into and never recognize each other.

As Dr. Levy left, the other sisters gathered around Judith, put their arms around her and literally rocked her like a child, for more than an hour, sharing their feelings with her, until she felt comfortable and ready to leave. We spent the next few sessions reliving that experience and discussing it from a cognitive point of view. Since that time, Judith has no longer been obsessed with the memory of her father. She can think of him with a good feeling, knowing that there is still some love in her for him, but she is fully aware of the damage which he had caused her. Several weeks later, Judith sent me a note, excerpts of which are quoted next:

"He [the father] was with me all the time, like haunting me. I couldn't get away from him. In the psychodrama, for the first time in my life, what I was feeling and what I was saying were together. For the first time I was feeling anger and expressing it verbally. This may not seem like much, but to me it was one of the greatest experiences of my life. Before that day, the only feeling I had for my father was strong hatred. Only after expressing my anger did I not only realize that I loved him but I also felt that love."

Although the cases of Linda and Judith offer many similarities, one major difference sets them apart. In the case of Linda, a specific, circumscribed area of behavior needed to be corrected. Judith's life, on the other hand, however, had been on hold since her father's death. The psychodramatic intervention enabled Linda to improve her relationship with her father. Judith's psychodrama enabled her to start living again.

CASE III—RESOLUTION OF AN UNEXPECTED CRISIS IN A PERSON'S LIFE

Jane was a 25-year-old psychiatric nurse who had come to therapy approximately 5 years ago while in nurse's training.[5] At that time she was complaining of a general dissatisfaction with life and particularly her schoolwork, poor family relationships, loneliness, depression and "alienation." She remained in therapy for approximately 2 years and did quite well in the sense that her zest for life was reawakened, she successfully completed her training and was able to wean herself away from her family while maintaining friendly relations with family members. Approximately 2 years later she married a young physician, shortly before his being drafted into the service and assigned to an Army post near a thriving midwest metropolis. Eventually, Jane and her husband, aware of many incompatibilities, decided to divorce. The divorce was amicable, and the two parties remained on friendly terms. In the meantime, however, Jane had become the administrator of a small psychiatric hospital, a well-paid and responsible position which she thoroughly enjoyed. She wanted very much to keep her job but was very frightened

[5]For a full theoretical discussion of Jane's case, see R. Naar, Psychodramatic Intervention (footnote 2).

at the thought of being alone, without the emotional and psychological support provided by her husband. She returned to Pittsburgh for a brief vacation, and we met once. We spent part of the hour discussing the pros and cons of remaining in the midwest in her present position versus returning to Pittsburgh where she had many friends and acquaintances. Twenty minutes before ending the session, she was asked to have a fantasy. The following interaction took place:

T: I would like you to close your eyes and imagine yourself back in time, as far as you can go. It's like climbing on a time machine and seeing your life like a motion picture projected in reverse. Experience yourself becoming younger, younger yet, much much younger, a very little girl. Can you see yourself?

J: (Nods)

T: How old are you?

J: About 5.

T: Get acquainted with yourself, look at the way you are dressed. Feel your face, your hair. Imagine yourself in a large empty room with a large size mirror. Can you see the mirror?

J: Yes.

T: You know that anything can happen in a fantasy. After all, it's only a fantasy. As you look into the mirror, you see that it is a very unusual mirror. You don't see your reflection in it. Instead, you see a vague, indistinct silhouette. As you keep staring at it, it becomes clearer, and . . . clearer. It is now quite distinguishable. It is you, but you today, you as an adult. The adult You steps out of the mirror, into the room and stands right next to the child You. Be the adult first and talk to the child.

J: (as the Adult) Hi! What are you doing there?

T: Now be the child.

J: (as the Child) I don't know.

T: I want you to look at the child's face. Can you tell me what you see?

J: I see loneliness and fear.

T: Tell her.

J: (as the Adult) Why are you so afraid? Things can't be so bad.

T: Now be the child and look at the grownup. What do you want from her?

J: (as Child) I want to stay here. Don't go away. Don't leave me.

T: What do you feel now, Jane?

J: I'd like to tell her . . .

T: (interrupting) Tell her.

J: (as Adult) I won't leave you. Don't be afraid. I'll stay with you as long as you want me to.

T: Look at the child's face. What do you see now?

J: More peaceful but still a little afraid.

T: What do you want to tell her?

J: I want to tell her . . . (voice trails off) . . . everything will be OK. Don't cry. I'll help you. I . . .

T: How do you feel about the child?

J: I like her very much. I want to help her.

T: Tell her.

J: (as Adult) I love you very much . . . very much.

T: What do you want to do, Jane?

J: I'd like to put my arm around her and hold her.

T: Kind of difficult, isn't it? She is so small, and you are so big.

J: I could kneel.

T: Go ahead. . .

J: (Puts her arms around herself and cries silently, rocking gently right and left)

T: It feels good, doesn't it? Stay together for as long as you want to. Then blend together into one and open your eyes.

(After a while, Jane's tears subside. She opens her eyes, looks very peaceful, smiles.)

J: You know, I found out something.

T: What's that?

J: I found out that I don't need someone to be with me and love me all the time. I am perfectly capable of loving myself. I mean . . . I can hack it.

Jane was indeed quite capable of "hacking it." She returned to her post and did quite well.

It was stated earlier that psychodramatic techniques are of such flexibility and elegance that they can be used within any theoretical framework. The intervention, described was, of course, based on transactional analysis concepts (Berne, 1964). One of the implications of the transactional analysis conception of personality is that "every individual was once younger than he is now and that he carries within him *fixated relics from earlier years which can be activated under certain circumstances* (Berne, 1964, p. 24).

In the case of Jane the "fixated relics from earlier years" included fear, weakness, and vulnerability as she had experienced them as a child. Under the stress caused by her divorce, these Child ego states were reactivated. The fantasy helped Jane realize that she was neither as vulnerable nor as weak as she had felt as a child and that such feelings (at least at that level of intensity), while legitimate in a child, were less appropriate for an adult. To use her own words, "I don't need someone to be with me and love me all the time. I am perfectly capable of loving myself. I mean . . . I can hack it."

Unlike the psychodramas involving Linda and Judith, this intervention was conducted within the context of individual therapy. Since Jane had to return to her home base no follow-up sessions were possible. I saw Jane a few years later, however, when she told me again that her session had been a milestone in her life.

CASE IV—ENABLING AN INDIVIDUAL TO GO THROUGH A THERAPEUTIC DYNAMIC CYCLE, THAT IS, INSIGHT, CATHARSIS, AND ADOPTION OF NEW BEHAVIORS

Unlike the three previous cases involving patients, this fourth illustration involved mental health professionals engaged in a group psychotherapy and psychodrama course. Also, unlike the previous cases in which copious notes were taken and transcripts made immediately after the sessions, this fourth psychodrama was reconstituted from very sketchy notes.

Anna, a talented social worker, discussed with the group her relationship with a close friend. Her friend had a crippled leg and would constantly ask Anna to do things for her such as her shopping, chores, house cleaning, and so forth. Anna liked her friend very much yet felt very often put upon and taken advantage of. At the same time, she felt unable to confront her friend with these feelings and asked to explore the relationship in a psychodrama.

Director: Anna, let us have a feel for how it would be like were you to try a confrontation, and pick someone to be Barbara (Anna's friend).

(Anna picks a group member called Mimi.)

Director: Anna, where would this confrontation take place?

Anna: In Barbara's living room.

Director: OK. Anna, make that living room come to life. (With the director's help, Anna describes the living room in great detail.)

Director: Of course, Mimi has never seen Barbara, so would you reverse roles a few times and give Mimi an idea of what Barbara would say, how she would stand, talk, etc. (Anna and Barbara reverse roles a few times.)

Director: (to Mimi) Do you have a feel for Barbara?

Mimi: I think so.

Director: Let us have some action.

Anna: Barbara, there is something I want to tell you.

Mimi: (as Barbara, henceforth referred to as Barbara) What is it?

Anna: You know, when you ask me to do your shopping and all those other things. . . .

Barbara: Well . . .

Anna: Well . . . I . . . (silence)

Anna: (to Director) I just can't . . . I can't tell her.

Director: OK, let Barbara go for a while and tell me what you are experiencing now.

Anna: It's like a feeling of heaviness . . . futility.

Director: Where in your body do you experience that feelings?

Anna: Right in the middle of my chest.

Director: Stay with that feeling . . . don't let go of it. You know situations change in people's lives, but feelings always remain the same. I would like you to hang on to your feeling and go as far back as you can in your memory, way, way back and see if you can remember the first time ever, you experienced that same feeling in your chest.

Anna: (after a long silence) I remember being a little girl and feeling that way when mother would ask me to go to the store. She had a heart condition and was supposed to avoid exertion.

Director: Is your mother still alive?

Anna: Yes, she is 82 now and her heart still bothers her. She'll probably live to be 102, and her heart still will bother her.

Director: OK Anna, how about picking someone to play the part of your mother.

(Anna picks Sue, describes the place where she would conceivably talk to her mother, and reverses roles with Sue a few times.)

Director: OK Anna. Your task will be to confront your mother and tell her that, even though you love her, you feel that she has manipulated you and taken advantage of you all these years.

Anna: OK. I'll try but I can't promise anything.

Anna: (to Mother) Mom, you have had a heart condition for as far as I can remember.

Sue: (henceforth referred to as Mother) I have done my best to take care of it. I was so afraid to leave you and Dad alone.

Anna: But Mom . . .

Mother: I always followed the doctor's orders, deprived myself of so many opportunities so that I wouldn't exert myself. It wasn't easy you know.

Anna: Yeah, I know. Mom . . . I know. . . . (silence)

Director: Anna, I would like you to select a double (This being a training group, the psychodramatic concepts of *double, soliloquy, role reversal,* etc. did not need to be explained.) I also would like you to imagine that I pull down a curtain between you and mother so that she can neither see nor hear you. Get in touch with what you are feeling and thinking and go into a soliloquy.

Anna: She does it to me every time. I know it has been tough for her, and I don't want to hurt her feelings. (silence)

Double: I don't want to hurt her feelings, yet there are times when I want to say . . .

Anna: Enough, already, mother . . . enough. . . .

Double: I get so godamned angry sometimes. . . .

Anna: That is true . . . but how can I . . . (silence)

Double: How can I get angry at an 82-year-old woman. . . . I am afraid that if I raise my voice or contradict her, her heart will stop and I will have killed her. . . .

Anna: Nonsense, her heart is stronger than mine. . . .

Double: Of course it is, of course it is. . . . So all these years . . .

Anna: All these years, I've been an idiot.

Director: Anna, I am now going to pull the blind back up. She can see you and hear you now.

Anna: (to mother—in an assertive tone of voice) Mother, I must tell you that I did not appreciate using your heart as an excuse all these years to make me

Mother: (interrupting) Anna, how can you?

Anna: (interrupting) Quiet, mother, let me talk. You made me wait on you hands and feet, always feeling guilty that if I didn't you would keel over and die.

Mother: (in a loud tone of voice) But, Anna, I am sick.

Double: Bullshit.

Anna: Bullshit, you are healthier than I am, and you will live for many years.

Director: Reverse roles, but Anna, as your mother, state your fantasy of what your mother is thinking, feeling but not willing to say.

Anna: (as her mother) She really does not love me.

Director: Reverse roles and, Anna, pretend that you heard what she said.

Anna: Oh, mother, I love you so much. But I love you for who you are, for all the love you have given me, all the care you have shown me. I don't need to love you out of guilt. That only made me resent you and made me feel so sad.

Mother: Do you, do you really love me?

Anna: Of course, Mom.

Director: Reverse roles.

Anna: (as mother) I feel like I want to cry, but not from sadness. It's like a huge weight lifted off my shoulders.

Director: Reverse roles.

Anna: (as herself) Oh! Mom. (She cries, puts her arms around her mother and hugs her for several seconds.)

Director: Now, let us bring Barbara back in and try that confrontation again.

Anna: Barbara, there is something I want to tell you.

Barbara: What is it?

Anna: You ask me to do too many things for you. I like you a lot, but sometimes, I feel put upon, and I resent it.

Barbara: I guess you are right. Sometimes my leg really hurts, but sometimes, I am real lazy, and you never seemed to mind.

Anna: I don't mind doing for you when it's necessary, but at other times, it really pisses me off.

Barbara: Let us make a deal. I'll try not to ask when I don't have to but you will level with me and tell me honestly when it is an imposition.

Anna: It's a deal. You mean . . . we're still friends?

(At that moment, the group bursts into laughter at the expression on Anna's face.)

Barbara: Of course, you dummy.

It would, of course, be naive to pretend that this brief psychodrama explored in depth the dynamics of Anna's relationship with her mother. It did, however, accomplish what it set out to achieve, that is, a minidynamic cycle. Indeed, Anna became aware of the transferential aspect of her relationship with Barbara; she overcame that transference through the intervening confrontation with her mother and learned to relate to Barbara in a more constructive way.

Although these four vignettes[6] describe the manner in which psycho-dramatic techniques may be used as brief interventions to achieve specific goals in therapy, psychodrama is far from being a panacea. Although diagnostic categories, age, cultural background, and the like, are not contraindications for its applicability, other factors may stand in the way of successful interventions, such as the therapist's training or the patient's willingness to be the protagonist. Psychodrama can be a very seductive modality, and the group pressure may also have subtle but powerful effects. It is incumbent upon the director to determine whether the reluctant protagonist is simply asking for some encouragement or really unwilling to become involved. Pressure, subtle or direct, will not only inhibit spontaneity thereby achieving the opposite results but may also strip protagonists of their dignity. An utmost respect for each protagonist, a care and sensitivity for and to their feelings are a *sine qua non* for a psychodrama (in fact for any kind of therapy) to be effective.

[6]I wish to express my gratitude to Linda and Anna for having allowed me to submit their psycho-dramas for publication.

It is also realized that many of the assumptions upon which the use of psychodrama, as described in this chapter, is based have not been proved experimentally and, although logically consistent, must for the time being, be taken on faith. There is a paucity of research and the possible reasons are extensively discussed by Kipper (1978). In addition to problems of methodology, definitions, contaminations of the dependent, and independent variables, there is also the psychodramatists' tendency to rely on case histories and descriptions of therapeutic strategies rather than research studies to substantiate their claims. Kipper, however, concludes his review by stating that (1) although more evidence is needed, past research shows encouraging signs, and (2) the effectiveness of psychodrama is amenable to experimental investigation. At this time, Kipper is engaged in an update of his review of research trends in psychodrama covering the years 1978 to 1987.

There is, too often, a tendency among mental health professionals to think of themselves as omniscient and to experiment with new techniques after only perfunctory exposure to them. Although a solid, generic training in a mental health field is an indispensable foundation for the use of psychodrama, it is, by no means, sufficient. Psychodrama is such a powerful modality that, not unlike some modern drugs, it can help or harm according to how it is used. Within the past few years, uniform guidelines for the training of psychodramatists were established and are administered by the American Board of Examiners in Psychodrama, Sociometry and Group Psychotherapy. In addition to certification of individuals, the board of examiners also certifies training institutions by reviewing the credentials of the teaching staff and the quality of training offered.

In retrospect, this chapter leaves me with a sense of incompleteness. Indeed, any attempt at incapsulating psychodrama can only be incomplete. Whether it is viewed as a philosophy of life, a theory of personality and behavior, or a therapeutic modality, its ramifications, implications, and potential are so rich and vast that no one book, let alone a single chapter can cover them adequately. Like the phoenix born of its ashes, the more exhaustive a discussion of psychodrama, the more one becomes aware of new possibilities and new usages. Perhaps, the best one can do is to make some concrete, specific points; the points which I tried to make can be summarized as follows:

1. Psychodrama as a therapeutic modality is of such flexibility that it can be used with all kinds of populations and diagnoses.
2. Psychodrama can be used to achieve specific therapeutic goals very quickly. In this respect, it is admirably suited for the practice of short-term psychotherapy.
3. Although empirical evidence has been accumulating over the years, experimental data is lagging behind. The little research data available, however, is promising and tends to support the claims of psychodramatists.
4. Psychodrama is a powerful modality which can be used for better or worse. Uniform and intensive training for psychodramatists is available at accredited training institutions.

REFERENCES

Berne, E. (1964). *Games people play*. New York: Grove Press.

Fox, J. (1982). Playback theater: The community sees itself. In R. Courtney & G. Schattner (Eds.), *Drama for therapy* (Vol. II, pp. 295–306). New York: Drama Books Specialists.

Fox, J. (1987). (Ed.). *The essential Moreno*. New York: Springer.

Kipper, D. A. (1978). Trends in the research on the effectiveness of psychodrama: Retrospect and prospect. *Group Psychotherapy, Psychodrama and Sociometry, 31*, 5–18.

Leutz, G. A. (1985). *Mettre sa vie en scene: Le Psychodrame*. Paris: Epi.

Moreno, J. L. (1944). "A Case of Paranoia," *Sociometry, 7*, 325.

Moreno, J. L. (1959a). *Psychodrama* in *American Handbook of Psychiatry* (Vol. 1, pp. 1375–1396). New York: Basic Books.

Moreno, J. L. (1959b). A survey of psychodramatic techniques. *Group Psychotherapy, 12*, 5–14.

Moreno, J. L. (1964). *Psychodrama* (Vol. I, rev. ed.). New York: Beacon House.

Moreno, J. L. (1965a). Psychodramatic rules, techniques and adjunctive methods. *Group Psychotherapy, 18*, 73–86.

Moreno, J. L. (1965b). Therapeutic vehicles and the concept of surplus reality. *Group Therapy, 18*, 211–216.

Moreno, J. L. (1970). *Psychodrama*, (Vol. 1, 3rd ed.). New York: Beacon House.

Naar, R. (1977). A psychodramatic intervention within a T. A. framework in individual and group psychotherapy. *Group Psychology, Psychodrama and Sociometry, 30*, 127–134.

Naar, R. (1981). *A primer of group psychotherapy*. New York: Human Sciences Press.

Passariello, N. M. (1987). *Psychodrama on the short-term inpatient unit*. Unpublished paper.

Sacks, J. M. (1965). The judgment technique in psychodrama. *Group Psychotherapy, 18*, 69–72.

Sacks, J. M. (1970). The reformed auxiliary ego technique: A psychodramatic rekindling of hope. *Group Psychotherapy, 23*, 118–126.

Sacks, J. M. (1974). The letter. *Group Psychotherapy and Psychodrama, 27*(1–4), 184, 190.

Sacks, J. M. (1976). The "shut-up" technique for releasing inhibited anger. *Group Psychotherapy, Psychodrama and Sociometry, 29*, 52–62.

Salas, J. (1982). Culture and community: Playback theater. *The Drama Review, 27*(2), 15–25.

Yalom, I. D. (1983). *Inpatient group psychotherapy*. New York: Basic Books.

Index

ISBN 0-306-43270-6

90000

9 780306 432705